MW01042082

Electroconvulsive and Neuromodulation Therapies

This ground-breaking new text is the definitive reference on electroconvulsive and neuromodulation therapies. It comprehensively covers the scientific basis and clinical practice of ECT as well as comparisons between ECT and medication therapies, including the new generation of antipsychotic drugs. It also provides readers with administrative perspectives and specific details for the management of this modality in clinical practice. The new forms of nonconvulsive electrical and magnetic brain stimulation therapy are also covered in detail, in a separate section. The chapter authors are leading scholars and clinicians.

DR. CONRAD M. SWARTZ is a board-certified psychiatrist, elected Fellow and past president of the Association for Convulsive Therapy, and two-time recipient of the Clinical Research Award from the American Academy of Clinical Psychiatrists for studies involving ECT. His extensive scholarly publications about electroconvulsive therapy and clinical pharmacology reflect his combining doctoral skills in engineering with medical psychiatry to find new practical solutions to clinical problems. He has directed ECT programs at several medical schools as well as research, education, and clinical programs. He is a co-author of the recently published title *Psychotic Depression* (Cambridge University Press, 2007).

Electroconvulsive and Neuromodulation Therapies

Edited by

CONRAD M. SWARTZ
Oregon Health and Science University
and
Southern Illinois University

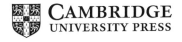

CAMBRIDGE
UNIVERSITY PRESS

CAMBRIDGE UNIVERSITY PRESS
Cambridge, New York, Melbourne, Madrid, Cape Town, Singapore, São Paulo, Delhi

Cambridge University Press
32 Avenue of the Americas, New York, NY 10013-2473, USA

www.cambridge.org
Information on this title: www.cambridge.org/9780521883887

© Cambridge University Press 2009

This publication is in copyright. Subject to statutory exception
and to the provisions of relevant collective licensing agreements,
no reproduction of any part may take place without the written
permission of Cambridge University Press.

First published 2009

Printed in the United States of America

A catalog record for this publication is available from the British Library.

Library of Congress Cataloging in Publication data

Electroconvulsive and neuromodulation therapies / edited by Conrad M. Swartz.
    p. ; cm.
Includes bibliographical references and index.
ISBN 978-0-521-88388-7 (hardback)
1. Electroconvulsive therapy.   2. Electric stimulation.   3. Magnetic brain stimulation.
I. Swartz, Conrad M.   II. Title.
[DNLM: 1. Electroconvulsive Therapy.   2. Mental Disorders – therapy.   3. Electric Stimulation
Therapy.   4. Transcranial Magnetic Stimulation. WM 412 E377 2009]
RC485.E38   2009
616.89′122–dc22   2008034119

ISBN 978-0-521-88388-7 hardback

Cambridge University Press has no responsibility for the persistence or
accuracy of URLs for external or third-party Internet Web sites referred to in
this publication and does not guarantee that any content on such Web sites is,
or will remain, accurate or appropriate. Information regarding prices, travel
timetables, and other factual information given in this work are correct at
the time of first printing, but Cambridge University Press does not guarantee
the accuracy of such information thereafter.

Every effort has been made in preparing this book to provide accurate and
up-to-date information that is in accord with accepted standards and practice at the time
of publication. Nevertheless, the authors, editors, and publisher can make no warranties
that the information contained herein is totally free from error, not least because clinical
standards are constantly changing through research and regulation. The authors, editors,
and publisher therefore disclaim all liability for direct or consequential damages
resulting from the use of material contained in this book. Readers are strongly advised to
pay careful attention to information provided by the manufacturer of any drugs or
equipment that they plan to use.

Contents

Contributors		*page* ix
Color Plates		xv
Preface		xvii

Part I   **Scientific and experimental bases of electroconvulsive therapy**

1   Electricity and electroconvulsive therapy   3
Conrad M. Swartz

2   Nonelectrical convulsive therapies   17
Niall McCrae

3   Neurochemical effects of electrically induced seizures: Relevance to the antidepressant mechanism of electroconvulsive therapy   45
Renana Eitan, Galit Landshut, and Bernard Lerer

4   Hypothesized mechanisms and sites of action of electroconvulsive therapy   75
Nikolaus Michael

5   Brain imaging and electroconvulsive therapy   94
Kathy Peng and Hal Blumenfeld

6   Evidence for electroconvulsive therapy efficacy in mood disorders   109
Keith G. Rasmussen

7   Clinical evidence for the efficacy of electroconvulsive therapy in the treatment of catatonia and psychoses   124
Gabor Gazdag, Stephan C. Mann, Gabor S. Ungvari, and Stanley N. Caroff

8   Hormonal effects of electroconvulsive therapy   149
Conrad M. Swartz

Part II   **Historical, societal, and geographic perspectives**

9   History of electroconvulsive therapy   167
Edward Shorter

v

10   Electroconvulsive therapy in biographical books and movies   180
      Andrew McDonald and Garry Walter

11   Professional barriers to providing electroconvulsive therapy   197
      William H. Reid

12   Legislation that regulates, limits, or bans electroconvulsive therapy   207
      Alan R. Felthous

Part III   International perspectives

13   Electroconvulsive therapy availability in the United States   227
      Michelle Magid and Barbara M. Rohland

14   Electroconvulsive therapy in Scandinavia and the United Kingdom   236
      Susan Mary Benbow and Tom G. Bolwig

15   Electroconvulsive therapy in continental Western Europe:
      A literature review   246
      Pascal Sienaert and Walter W. van den Broek

16   Electroconvulsive therapy in Asia   256
      Sidney S. Chang

17   History of electroconvulsive therapy in the Russian Federation   266
      Alexander I. Nelson and Nataliya Giagou

18   Electroconvulsive therapy in Latin America   276
      Moacyr Alexandro Rosa and Marina Odebrecht Rosa

Part IV   Administrative perspectives

19   Electroconvulsive therapy hospital policy and quality assurance   287
      Barry Alan Kramer

20   Staff management and physical layout for electroconvulsive therapy   314
      Jerry Lewis

21   Electroconvulsive therapy forms   326
      Jerry Lewis

Part V   The clinical manual

22   Patient selection and electroconvulsive therapy indications   341
      Conrad M. Swartz

23 Electroconvulsive therapy or antipsychotic drugs (or benzodiazepines for catatonia)   362
Conrad M. Swartz

24 Informed consent   384
Peter B. Rosenquist

25 Electroconvulsive therapy in the medically ill   401
Keith G. Rasmussen and Paul S. Mueller

26 Anesthesia for electroconvulsive therapy   412
Charles H. Kellner, Dongchen Li, and Limore Maron

27 Stimulus electrode placement   430
Conrad M. Swartz

28 Stimulus dosing   447
W. Vaughn McCall

29 Electroencephalogram monitoring and implications   468
Hideki Azuma

30 Heart rate and electroconvulsive therapy   477
Conrad M. Swartz

31 Cognitive side effects and psychological testing   485
James Stuart Lawson

32 Electroconvulsive therapy in children and adolescents   498
Garry Walter, Colleen Loo, and Joseph M. Rey

33 Postelectroconvulsive therapy evaluation and prophylaxis   505
T. K. Birkenhäger and Walter W. van den Broek

34 Ambulatory and maintenance electroconvulsive therapy   515
Charles H. Kellner and Unnati D. Patel

Part VI   Neuromodulation treatment

35 Transcranial magnetic stimulation   527
Oded Rosenberg and Pinhas N. Dannon

36 Vagus nerve stimulation: Indications, efficacy, and methods   543
Shawn M. McClintock, Kenneth Trevino, and Mustafa M. Husain

37   Deep brain stimulation: Methods, indications, locations, and efficacy   556
      Thomas E. Schläpfer and Bettina Heike Bewernick

38   Transcranial direct current stimulation   573
      Julie A. Williams and Felipe Fregni

      Index   583

Contributors

Hideki Azuma, MD, PhD
Lecturer, Department of Psychiatry
  and Cognitive-Behavioral Medicine
Nagoya City University Graduate
  School of Medical Sciences
Nagoya, Japan
Nagoya City University Hospital
Nagoya, Japan

Susan Mary Benbow, FRCPsych
Professor of Mental Health and Ageing
Centre for Ageing and Mental Health
Staffordshire University
Stafford, United Kingdom
Consultant Psychiatrist (Old Age
  Psychiatry), Penn Hospital
Wolverhampton, United Kingdom

Bettina Heike Bewernick, Dr. rer. nat.
Research Assistant, Department of
  Psychiatry and Psychotherapy
University Hospital Bonn
Bonn, Germany

T. K. Birkenhäger, MD, PhD
Associate Professor, Department of
  Psychiatry
Erasmus Medical Centre
Rotterdam, The Netherlands

Hal Blumenfeld, MD, PhD
Director of Medical Studies
Clinical Neurosciences
Associate Professor, Departments of
  Neurology, Neurobiology, and
  Neurosurgery
Yale University School of Medicine
New Haven, Connecticut

Tom G. Bolwig, MD, DMSc
Professor, University of Copenhagen
Copenhagen, Denmark
Professor, Department of Psychiatry
Copenhagen University Hospital
Copenhagen, Denmark

Stanley N. Caroff, MD
Professor, Department of Psychiatry
University of Pennsylvania
Philadelphia, Pennsylvania
Chief, Inpatient Section, Behavioral
  Health Service
Veterans Affairs Medical Center
Philadelphia, Pennsylvania

Sidney S. Chang, MD
Staff Psychiatrist, Department of
  Psychiatry
Shin Kong Memorial Hospital
Taipei, Taiwan

Pinhas N. Dannon, MD
Associate Professor (Clinical),
  Department of Psychiatry
Tel Aviv University
Tel Aviv, Israel

Director, Research Department and
  Brain Stimulation Unit
Beer Yaakov Mental Health Center
Beer Yaakov, Israel

Renana Eitan, MD
Instructor, Department of
  Psychiatry
Hebrew University – Hadassah
  Medical School
Jerusalem, Israel
Biological Psychiatry Laboratory,
  Department of Psychiatry
Hadassah – Hebrew University
  Medical Center
Jerusalem, Israel

Alan R. Felthous, MD
Professor and Director, Forensic
  Psychiatry Division, Department of
  Neurology and Psychiatry
Saint Louis University School of
  Medicine
St. Louis, Missouri
Professor Emeritus, Department of
  Psychiatry
Southern Illinois University
Springfield, Illinois

Felipe Fregni, MD, PhD
Berenson–Allen Center for
  Noninvasive Brain Stimulation
Department of Neurology
Beth Israel Deaconess Medical Center
Harvard Medical School
Boston, Massachusetts

Gabor Gazdag, MD, PhD
Chief, Inpatient Section, Department
  of Psychiatry
Jahn Ferenc Hospital
Budapest, Hungary

Nataliya Giagou, MD
Resident Physician
Department of Psychiatry
Southern Illinois University School of
  Medicine
Springfield, Illinois

Mustafa M. Husain, MD
Professor, Department of Psychiatry
  and Internal Medicine
University of Texas Southwestern
  Medical Center
Dallas, Texas

Charles H. Kellner, MD
Professor, Department of Psychiatry
UMDNJ–New Jersey Medical School
Director, Electroconvulsive Therapy
  Service
Department of Psychiatry
University Hospital
Newark, New Jersey

Barry Alan Kramer, MD
Medical Director of Electroconvulsive
  Therapy
Department of Psychiatry and
  Behavioral Neurosciences
Cedars-Sinai Medical Center
Los Angeles, California
Adjunct Assistant Professor of
  Pharmacy Practice
University of Southern California
  School of Pharmacy
Los Angeles, California

Galit Landshut, MSc
PhD Student, Department of
  Psychiatry
Hebrew University – Hadassah
  Medical School
Jerusalem, Israel

James Stuart Lawson, PhD
Professor Emeritus and Adjunct I,
  Department of Psychiatry
Queen's University
Kingston, Ontario, Canada
Honorary Researcher, Department of
  Psychiatry
Providencecare Mental Health
  Services
Kingston, Ontario, Canada

Bernard Lerer, MD
Professor, Department of Psychiatry
Hebrew University – Hadassah
  Medical School
Jerusalem, Israel
Director, Biological Psychiatry
  Laboratory
Department of Psychiatry, Hadassah –
  Hebrew University Medical Center
Jerusalem, Israel

Jerry Lewis, MD
Clinical Associate Professor
Director of Electroconvulsive Therapy
  Services
Department of Psychiatry
University of Iowa Hospitals and
  Clinics
Iowa City, Iowa

Dongchen Li, MD
Assistant Professor, Department of
  Anesthesiology and Perioperative
  Medicine
UMDNJ–New Jersey Medical School
Newark, New Jersey

Colleen Loo, MB BS, MD, FRANZCP
Associate Professor, School of
  Psychiatry
University of New South Wales

The St. George Hospital
Kogarah, New South Wales, Australia

Michelle Magid, MD
Assistant Professor, Department of
  Psychiatry
Austin Medical Education Program,
  University of Texas Medical Branch,
  Austin
Director of Electroconvulsive Therapy,
  Department of Psychiatry
Seton Hospital – Shoal Creek
Austin, Texas

Stephan C. Mann, MD
Clinical Professor, Department of
  Psychiatry and Behavioral Sciences
University of Louisville School of
  Medicine
Louisville, Kentucky
Medical Director
Central Montgomery Mental Health
  and Mental Retardation Center
Norristown, Pennsylvania

Limore Maron, MD
Physician Resident, Department of
  Psychiatry
UMDNJ–New Jersey Medical School
Newark, New Jersey

W. Vaughn McCall, MD, MS
Professor and Chair, Department of
  Psychiatry and Behavioral
  Medicine
Wake Forest University Health
  Sciences
Winston-Salem, North Carolina
Chief of Psychiatry
North Carolina Baptist Hospital
Winston-Salem, North Carolina

Shawn M. McClintock, PhD
Postdoctoral Fellow, Department of
   Psychiatry
University of Texas Southwestern
   Medical Center
Dallas, Texas
New York State Psychiatric
   Institute
Columbia University
New York, New York

Niall McCrae, MSc, RMN
Clinical Trial Manager, Health Services
   Research Department
Institute of Psychiatry, King's College
   London
London, United Kingdom

**Andrew McDonald, BMed,
   FRANZCP**
Consultant Psychiatrist, Westminster
   Adult Services
Central and North West London, NHS
   Foundation Trust
London, United Kingdom

Nikolaus Michael, MD
Associate Professor, Department of
   Psychiatry
Westfälische Wilhelms-Universität
Münster, Germany
Chief, Department of Psychiatry III,
   Evangelische Stiftung
   Tannenhof
Remscheid, Germany

Paul S. Mueller, MD
Associate Professor, Department of
   Medicine
Mayo Clinic
Rochester, Minnesota

Alexander I. Nelson, MD, PhD
Chief, Regional Center of
   Psycho-Reanimatology
Moscow Regional Psychiatric Hospital
   No. 23
Moscow, Russia

Unnati D. Patel, MD
Physician Resident, Department of
   Psychiatry
UMDNJ–New Jersey Medical School
Newark, New Jersey

Kathy Peng, BA
Department of Neurology
Yale University School of
   Medicine
New Haven, Connecticut

Keith G. Rasmussen, MD
Associate Professor, Department of
   Psychiatry
Mayo Clinic
Rochester, Minnesota

William H. Reid, MD, MPH
Clinical Professor of Psychiatry
University of Texas Health Science
   Center
San Antonio, Texas
Adjunct Professor of Psychiatry
Texas A&M College of Medicine
Temple, Texas
Texas Tech School of Medicine
Lubbock, Texas

**Joseph M. Rey, MB BS, PhD,
   FRANZCP**
Honorary Professor, Discipline of
   Psychological Medicine
University of Sydney
New South Wales, Australia

Barbara M. Rohland, MD
Associate Professor, Department of
  Psychology and Psychiatry
Mayo Clinic College of Medicine
Staff Consultant
Department of Psychiatry and
  Psychology
Saint Mary's Hospital
Rochester, Minnesota

Marina Odebrecht Rosa, MD, MS
Chief, Department of
  Electroconvulsive Therapy
Hospital Saint Paul
São Paulo, Brazil

Moacyr Alexandre Rosa, MD, PhD
Instructor Professor, Department of
  Medical Psychology and
  Psychiatry
Faculdade de Ciências Médicas da
  Santa Casa de São Paulo
São Paulo, Brazil
Assistant Doctor, Centro de Atenção
  Integrada à Saúde Mental
  (CAISM)
Irmandade da Santa Casa de
  Misericórdia de São Paulo
São Paulo, Brazil

Oded Rosenberg, MD
Research Department
Doctor in Research Unit
Beer Yaakov, Israel

Peter B. Rosenquist, MD
Associate Professor, Department of
  Psychiatry and Behavioral
  Medicine
Wake Forest University School of
  Medicine
Winston-Salem, North Carolina

Thomas E. Schläpfer, MD
Vice Chair and Professor of Psychiatry
  and Psychotherapy
Department of Psychiatry and
  Psychotherapy
University Hospital, Bonn
Bonn, Germany
Departments of Psychiatry and Mental
  Health
The Johns Hopkins University
Baltimore, Maryland

Edward Shorter, PhD
Hannah Chair in the History of
  Medicine/Professor of Psychiatry
History of Medicine Program, Faculty
  of Medicine
University of Toronto
Toronto, Ontario, Canada

Pascal Sienaert, MD
ECT Department and Department of
  Mood Disorders
University Psychiatric
  Center–Catholic University Leuven
  (campus Kortenberg)
Kortenberg, Belgium

Conrad M. Swartz, PhD, MD
Affiliate Associate Professor,
  Department of Psychiatry
Oregon Health and Science University
Portland, Oregon
Professor Emeritus, Department of
  Psychiatry
Southern Illinois University
Springfield, Illinois
Staff Physician Honorary
Department of Psychiatry
St. John's Hospital
Springfield, Illinois

Kenneth Trevino, BA
Clinical Psychology Doctoral
    Candidate
Department of Psychiatry
University of Texas Southwestern
    Medical Center
Dallas, Texas

Gabor S. Ungvari, MD, PhD
Professor, Department of Psychiatry
Chinese University of Hong Kong
Hong Kong, SAR, China
Honorary Consultant, Department of
    Psychiatry, Shatin Hospital, Ma On
    Shan
Shatin, NT, China

Walter W. van den Broek, MD, PhD
Associate Professor, Department of
    Psychiatry

Erasmus Medical College
Rotterdam, The Netherlands

**Garry Walter, MB BS, BMedSc, PhD,
    FRANZCP**
Professor and Chair of Child and
    Adolescent Psychiatry
Discipline of Psychological Medicine,
    University of Sydney
Area Clinical Director, Child and
    Adolescent Mental Health Services
Northern Sydney Central Coast Health
New South Wales, Australia

Julie A. Williams, MA
Research Associate, Department of
    Neurology
Beth Israel Deaconess Medical Center
Boston, Massachusetts

Color Plates

I.   Hierarchical levels of brain function (Chapter 4)

II.   Seizure induction and ensuing effects (Chapter 4)

III.   Induced seizures disrupt neuronal activity (Chapter 4)

IV.   Sketch (hypothetical) of imbalanced activity (Chapter 4)

V.   Ictal cerebral blood flow changes (Chapter 5)

VI.   Focal ictal subcortical cerebral blood flow increases (Chapter 5)

VII.   Evidence for ictal propagation (Chapter 5)

VIII.   Interictal (postictal) cerebral blood flow (Chapter 5)

IX.   Subject receiving tDCS over the occipital cortex (Chapter 38)

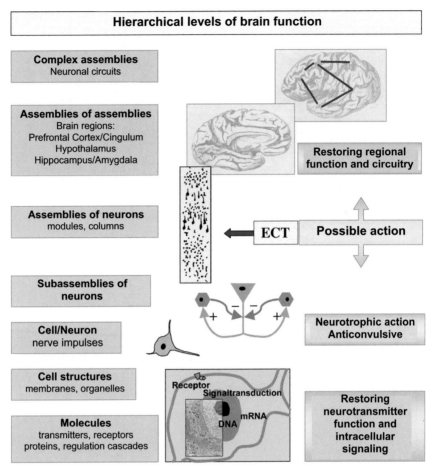

Hierarchical levels of brain function

Complex assemblies
Neuronal circuits

Assemblies of assemblies
Brain regions:
Prefrontal Cortex/Cingulum
Hypothalamus
Hippocampus/Amygdala

Restoring regional function and circuitry

Assemblies of neurons
modules, columns

ECT **Possible action**

Subassemblies of neurons

Cell/Neuron
nerve impulses

Neurotrophic action Anticonvulsive

Cell structures
membranes, organelles

Receptor
Signaltransduction
mRNA
DNA

Restoring neurotransmitter function and intracellular signaling

Molecules
transmitters, receptors
proteins, regulation cascades

Plate I   The brain is organized in different hierarchical levels, and electroconvulsive therapy (ECT) is likely to affect functions on every level. mRNA, messenger RNA. (See Chapter 4.)

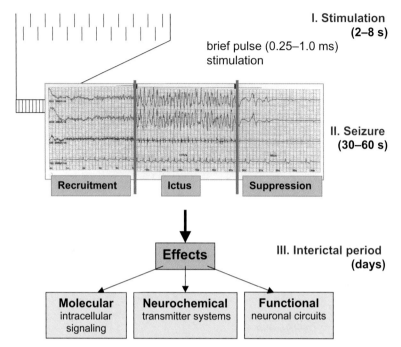

I. Stimulation
(2–8 s)

brief pulse (0.25–1.0 ms)
stimulation

II. Seizure
(30–60 s)

Recruitment   Ictus   Suppression

Effects

III. Interictal period
(days)

Molecular
intracellular
signaling

Neurochemical
transmitter systems

Functional
neuronal circuits

Plate II   Seizure induction and ensuing effects. The actual treatment consists of the stimulation,
which takes a few seconds (I). The seizure (II), its limitation, and the resulting effects (III)
are the brain's work. (See Chapter 4.)

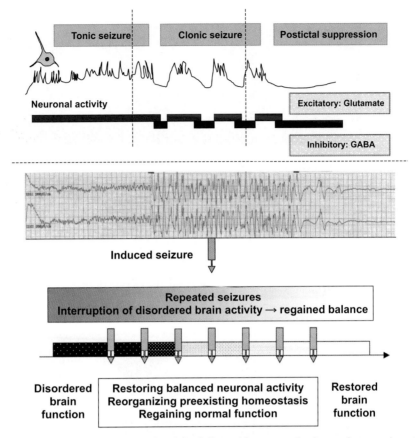

Plate III   Induced seizures disrupt neuronal activity, followed by reorganization and restoration of normal function. It is perhaps the repeated disruption of disordered activity and the rebuilding of ordinary balanced neuronal activity from postictal suppression that are essential for efficacy. GABA, gamma-aminobutyric acid. (See Chapter 4.)

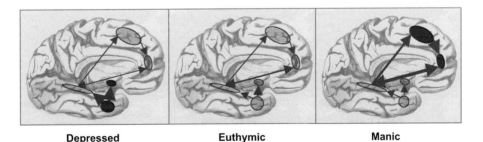

Depressed   **Euthymic**   **Manic**

Plate IV   Sketch (hypothetical) of imbalanced activity within a neuronal circuit. Clinical syndromes may result from distinct patterns of dysregulated (= imbalanced) neuronal circuitry, in other words, overactivated as well as underactivated regions contribute to a complex constellation of symptoms (e.g., manic, depressive, catatonic, and psychotic symptoms). Color intensity and thickness of arrows indicate disordered activity. (See Chapter 4.)

A. Bitemporal ECT

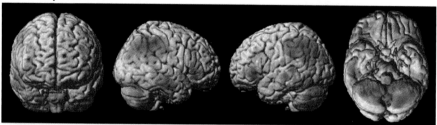

B. Right Unilateral ECT

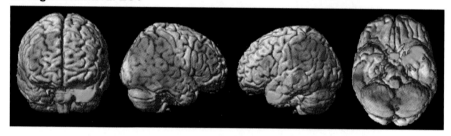

C. Bifrontal ECT

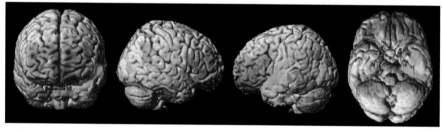

Plate V   Ictal cerebral blood flow changes during bitemporal, right unilateral, and bifrontal electroconvulsive therapy (ECT-)induced seizures. (A) Bitemporal ECT-induced seizures ($n = 10$). (B) Right unilateral ECT-induced seizures ($n = 8$). (C) Bifrontal ECT-induced seizures ($n = 4$). For (A) – (C), ictal images were compared with interictal images using SPM99. Focal single photon emission computed tomography increases (**red**) and decreases (**green**) were seen during ECT-induced seizures compared with baseline scans done under the same conditions. SPM extent threshold, $k = 125$ voxels and height threshold, $p = .02$ (equivalent to a z score > 2.05), using a two-sample t-test model. For further details of methods, see Blumenfeld et al. (2003a, 2003b). (A) and (B) modified with permission from Blumenfeld et al. (2003b); (C) modified with permission from Blumenfeld et al. (2003a). (See Chapter 5.)

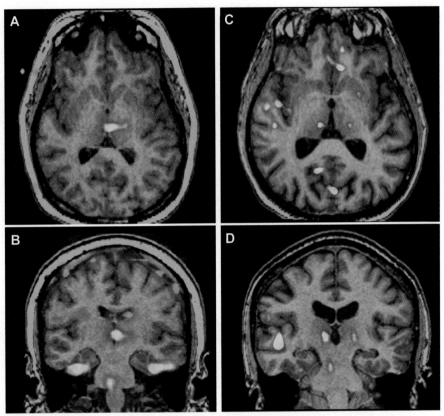

Plate VI   Focal ictal subcortical cerebral blood flow (CBF) increases in bitemporal and right
unilateral electroconvulsive therapy (ECT-)induced seizures. (A) and (B) single photon
emission computed tomography (SPECT) ictal–interictal difference imaging in a bilateral
ECT-induced seizure, axial and coronal images, showing bilateral medial, thalamic, CBF
increases. (C) and (D) SPECT ictal–interictal difference imaging in a right unilateral
ECT-induced seizure, axial and coronal images, showing asymmetric involvement of the
medial thalamus. CBF increases are displayed on each patient's high-resolution
T1-weighted magnetic resonance imaging scan. **Orange:** Increases of 55%; **purple:**
increases of 35% relative to interictal scan. The right side of each image corresponds to
the left side of the brain. Reproduced with permission from Blumenfeld et al. (2003a).
(See Chapter 5.)

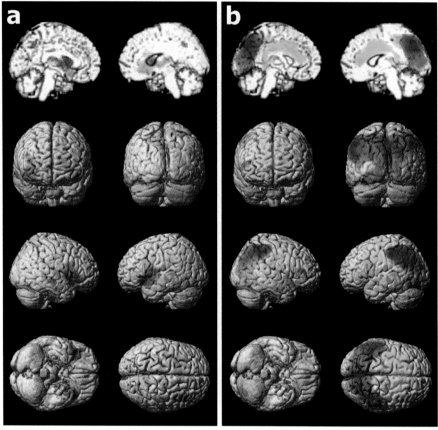

Plate VII   Evidence for ictal propagation: Early cerebral blood flow (CBF) increases in frontal cortex
and late CBF increases in parietal cortex with bitemporal electroconvulsive therapy (ECT).
Single photon emission computed tomography (SPECT) images of significant CBF changes
during bitemporal ECT-induced seizures. Statistical parametric maps depict CBF increases
(hyperperfusion) in **red** and decreases (hypoperfusion) in **green**. (a) CBF changes in
patients with ictal injections at onset (0 s after ECT stimulus). Increases occur in the
bilateral inferior frontal gyrus, anterior insula, putamen, and thalamus. No significant
decreases were found ($n = 4$). (b) Changes in patients with ictal injections 30 s after ECT
stimulus. Increases occur in bilateral parietal and occipital cortex, whereas decreases occur
in the bilateral cingulate gyrus and left dorsolateral frontal cortex ($n = 7$). For (a) and (b),
extent threshold, $k = 125$ voxels (voxel size $= 2 \times 2 \times 2$ mm). Height threshold, $p = .01$.
Equivalently, only voxel clusters > 1 cm^3 in volume and with z scores > 2.33 are
displayed. Reproduced with permission from Enev et al. (2007). (See Chapter 5.)

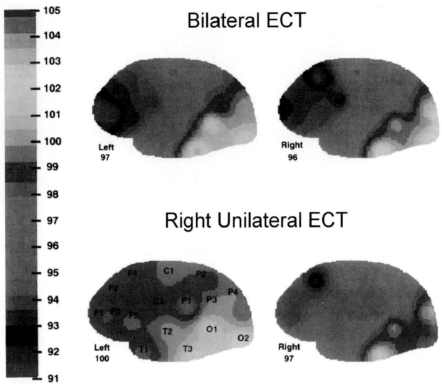

Plate VIII   Interictal (postictal) cerebral blood flow (CBF) patterns following bitemporal and right unilateral electroconvulsive therapy (ECT). Xenon-133 regional CBF (rCBF) 50 minutes after ECT compared with 30 minutes before ECT. Values of 100 indicate no change. The ratio scores were color coded so that **purple** and **blue** correspond to postictal CBF reductions, whereas **orange** and **red** correspond to postictal CBF increases (scale on left). Mean CBF percent changes are indicated next to each hemisphere. Positions of the rCBF detectors are labeled at bottom left. Reproduced with permission from Nobler et al. (1994). (See Chapter 5.)

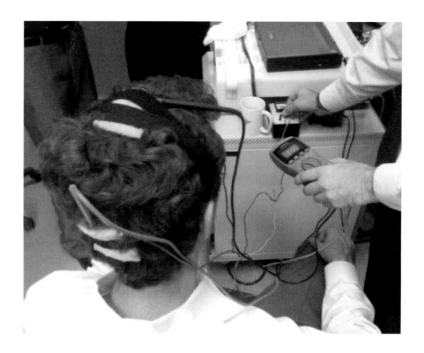

Plate IX   Subject receiving tDCS over the occipital cortex – the reference electrode is placed on Cz. (See Chapter 38.)

Preface

This book is dedicated to describing how electroconvulsive therapy (ECT) treats mental illness. Besides treating mental illness, ECT can prevent mental illness in several ways. First, ECT interrupts psychosis and catatonia and thereby prevents episodes of these from persisting and becoming chronic. Genetic data have identified similarities rather than distinctions between psychotic mood disorders and schizophrenia (e.g., Kishimoto et al., 2008; Taylor, 1992). These data complement epidemiologic–phenomenological studies that find continuous variation between psychotic mood disorders and schizophrenia, without a point of rarity to demarcate them. In other words, there is no known difference between schizophrenia and a psychotic (or catatonic) episode that has persisted. We should make every effort to interrupt these episodes before they become entrenched. In this way, ECT should prevent chronic schizophrenia.

Second, but just as important, ECT circumvents using antipsychotic drugs in patients who would otherwise receive them. As detailed in Chapter 23, "Electroconvulsive therapy or antipsychotic drugs (or benzodiazepines for catatonia)," these medications can cause a variety of serious psychiatric, neurological, and medical impairments. It takes a powerful lot of faith to believe that patients with psychosis who receive antipsychotic medications will indeed achieve remission and then maintain it after these medications are stopped. In reality, the data show the opposite. Virtually 100% of patients started on antipsychotic medications for psychosis eventually receive the diagnosis of schizophrenia on follow-up. Psychiatric diagnosis is simply not this reliable. It should not be this reliable for a diagnosis of exclusion such as schizophrenia, especially when the exclusion is not made rigorously. These data point to schizophrenia as often (but not always) the result of an "antipsychotic trap." After all, what psychiatrist can boldly face the liabilities of discontinuing antipsychotic drugs on an outpatient? These issues are reviewed in detail in Chapter 23.

Third, if ECT is used early in a serious psychiatric episode, it prevents or abbreviates further threatening experiences associated with the illness, including stigmatization, loss of control over life course and job performance, self-injurious behavior, loss of control of thoughts, separation from home and family, and exposure to psychiatric wards. Decreasing these threats prevents or diminishes the development of anxiety disorders such as post-traumatic stress disorder (PTSD). Accordingly, ECT is a treatment that should be used early; it is not merely a last resort. Several chapters in this volume elaborate on this message.

Causation of anxiety disorder by serious psychiatric illness is a pervasive, serious, and underrecognized problem in psychiatric patients. It can fall under several different diagnoses and guises besides anxiety disorders. It is called resistant depression, residual depression, chronic depression, and institutional dependency. It has been called "bipolar depression," a chronic depression that gradually develops and worsens among patients with bipolar disorder. This is not the rapid-onset episode with melancholic or psychotic features that was once known as the type of depressive episode that bipolar type I patients suffered. In my clinical experience, this PTSD from bipolar disorder often underlies the deteriorating course of bipolar disorder. I urge readers to evaluate for comorbid anxiety disorders in patients who have serious Axis-I diagnoses, including patients who receive ECT. Often, comorbid anxiety disorders are missed, and their symptoms are attributed to resistant depression or allegedly genetic panic disorder.

The course of treatment with ECT is analogous to that with antibiotics in patients with acute infections. Treatment typically brings the patient to remission and is then stopped. Any side effects then disappear over days to weeks. The patient receives a persistent benefit, the removal of active disease. The illness can recur, but steps can be taken to prevent it.

ECT is also analogous to surgery. Surgery can be controversial, some surgeries have been overused, surgical procedures become more effective and safer with technological progress, and patients who undergo surgery wish there were an easier way. Throughout, there is no doubt of its frequent necessity, its effectiveness in professional hands, and the right of the patient and doctor to choose it. Indeed, I recommend a surgeon's lecture, a recording of surgeon Sherwin Nuland, MD, eloquently describing his personal experience receiving ECT. This program clearly illustrates the value of ECT to our patients; it is on the Internet at: http://www.ted.com/index.php/talks/sherwin_nuland_on_electroshock_therapy.html (accessed January 17, 2009).

Several chapters here contend with obstacles to ECT, their development, and the influences of politics. In my professional lifetime, the strongest negative influence about ECT on the public is Milos Forman's movie, *One Flew over the Cuckoo's Nest*. Despite the completely fictional nature of this film, through dramatic suggestion it imparts a negative impression of ECT. Yet, even in the movie, ECT itself was not alleged to have caused injury or persisting brain changes. The issues were the crude appearance of unanesthetized ECT, forced nonconsenting administration, the absence of observable psychiatric illness, and a punitive environment. ECT was presented as a whiplashing in medical guise. This has nothing whatsoever to do with modern ECT as medical treatment for a psychiatric condition that has seriously impaired the patient and caused him to appear sickly, disorganized, and emotionally drained.

Psychiatry is notorious for wide variations in concepts and practice, particularly concerning diagnostic formulations and its explanations. No one person's views encompass what is thought best or even what is proper in psychiatry. My own perspectives are influenced by extensive training in physical science before entering medicine and psychiatry. So it seemed that a wide variety of other authors should be included in this book, and they are. This book is divided into several major sections, and each section has several chapters. Ethics considerations are integrated into the book chapters, rather than collected from them into a separate or redundant chapter, just as ethics are integrated into our clinical and scientific work.

The section on "Scientific and experimental bases of electroconvulsive therapy" begins with my essay on ECT and electricity. Much of this material is new and perhaps surprising. Choosing efficient stimulus pulse width and frequency is included, with an evaluation of ultrabrief stimuli.

In describing historical events in Chapter 2, Niall McCrae reveals the details of how "Nonelectrical convulsive therapies" are experimental bases for ECT and specifically how electrical induction is preferable. Along the way this chapter reflects on many pearls about medical practice, for example, "diagnostic practice is determined by available treatment," and it is much more than a history.

Writing on the neurochemical effects of seizure and implications for ECT mechanism in Chapter 3, Drs. Renana Eitan and Bernard Lerer and Ms. Galit Landshut will bring you up to date in this wide-ranging and fast-moving area. The numerous alterations in the hippocampus with ECT suggest its involvement in ECT mechanism, but this part of the brain is particularly given to change. This tendency to change together with its involvement in memory suggest that the hippocampus may be involved in ECT cognitive side effects as well as efficacy.

In Chapter 4, Dr. Nikolaus Michael explains and integrates the latest concepts in how seizure generalization, anatomical sites, and neuronal changes are implicated in ECT mechanism.

The photos and descriptions of Dr. Hal Blumenfeld and Ms. Kathy Peng correspond to localized brain effects of ECT stimulus placement and how anatomy is an important consideration in ECT. Their Chapter 5 evaluates the various technologies used in imaging the brain after ECT.

We know ECT works for depression, but the state of clinical evidence establishing that ECT is effective in mood disorders is a scientific matter. It is critically reviewed by Dr. Keith Rasmussen in Chapter 6.

Although there are no double-blind randomized ECT studies of catatonia or schizophrenia, "catatonic features" is the only psychiatric syndrome in DSM that requires verifiable observable evidence – and nothing but – in making the diagnosis.

So studies of ECT efficacy in catatonia have an aspect of objectivity missing from other treatment studies in psychiatry, including those of major depression, and this objectivity provides clear evidence of ECT efficacy. The state of knowledge about ECT efficacy in catatonia (with or without schizophrenia) and schizophrenia is reviewed in Chapter 7 by Drs. Gabor Gazdag, Stephan Mann, Gabor Ungvari, and Stanley Caroff.

Bypassing speculations without evidence, I reviewed only the known effects and patterns of ECT-induced hormone changes in Chapter 8, "Hormonal effects of electroconvulsive therapy."

Beginning the section on "Historical, societal, and geographic perspectives," in Chapter 9 historian Edward Shorter summarizes both the fascinating history of ECT and variations in modern professional opinions about aspects of ECT practice. This is a living history of ECT, not merely a past. For more details, please see his book on the topic.

Movies mentioning ECT comprise most peoples' entire awareness of it, which is one reason to read Chapter 10 by Drs. Andrew McDonald and Garry Walter on popular books and movies about ECT. They explain how such portrayals are impressionistic rather than factual.

Strong barriers to ECT stand within the professional world as well as outside it, as Dr. William Reid elucidates in Chapter 11. To confront them or even operate next to them, it is important to understand their nature. Moreover, Dr. Reid identifies several likely surprises, including the requirements for residency training in the United States.

Legislation in some countries and U.S. states deprives many patients of access to ECT, regardless of their medical needs. Notably, some of this legislation was motivated by followers of L. Ron Hubbard ("Scientology") or was in reaction to ECT use that is now understood as not appropriate. In Chapter 12, Dr. Alan Felthous reviews these issues and explains how it remains useful to understand them.

The "International perspectives" section begins in the United States with a review of availability by Drs. Michelle Magid and Barbara Rohland in Chapter 13. Dr. Susan Benbow begins Chapter 14 by describing recent conflicts and misleading acronyms in the UK that represent an apparent assault on psychiatry by nonpsychiatric physicians. Famous for its tolerance, Scandinavia seems to have a more stable medical environment for ECT, as reviewed by Dr. Tom Bolwig in the conclusion of Chapter 14. Drs. Pascal Sienaert and Walter van den Broek similarly describe the generally receptive environment for ECT in Western Europe in Chapter 15. Ironically, the environment for ECT is difficult in Italy, where ECT originated.

In contrast, ECT availability and quality are widely variable in Asia, as noted by Dr. Sidney Chang in Chapter 16. In Russia ECT has been strongly influenced by national politics, according to details provided by Drs. Alexander Nelson and

Nataliya Giagou in Chapter 17. In South America, the ECT environment reflects variability in sociocultural and economic conditions, as reviewed by Drs. Moacyr and Marina Rosa in Chapter 18.

Although it is relatively brief, the "Administrative perspectives" section should provide valuable assistance in facing the bureaucratic expectations of administrating an ECT service. In Chapter 19, Dr. Barry Kramer offers detailed archetype documentation for "Electroconvulsive therapy hospital policy and quality assurance." In Chapters 20 and 21, Dr. Jerry Lewis describes a salt-of-the-earth perspective on everyday concerns in "Staff management and physical layout for electroconvulsive therapy" and prototype forms for ECT service operation. These concerns include making privacy, efficiency, and completeness routine for both inpatient and ambulatory ECT.

The next section is a practical guide to the clinical aspects of ECT practice, in effect an ECT practice manual. As the first step is patient selection and ECT indications, this appears next as Chapter 22. In describing who is suitable for ECT and who is not, selectively, it differs fundamentally from the American Psychiatric Association (APA) Task Force Report, which aimed to allow rather than select.

Antipsychotic drugs are the medications most used in patients who should receive ECT but do not. I review how this differs from using these drugs in chronic schizophrenia in Chapter 23, "Electroconvulsive therapy or antipsychotic drugs (or benzodiazepines for catatonia)." This chapter elucidates how and why long-term antipsychotic drugs should be reserved as the last resort in psychiatric management.

Informed consent is required in the United States. Obtaining understanding by patients and families can involve psychological insight as well as knowledge about the procedures, and in Chapter 24, Dr. Peter Rosenquist aims to help achieve it. This chapter systematically presents ECT consent within the general considerations of informed consent.

Drs. Keith Rasmussen and Paul Mueller consider how to identify and reduce the wide variety of risks associated with concurrent medical conditions as part of the pre-ECT evaluation, in Chapter 25.

Anesthesia for ECT has basic differences from surgical anesthesia and cannot merely be delegated to an anesthesiologist because many details potently influence the psychiatric outcome. In Chapter 26, Drs. Charles Kellner, Dongchen Li, and Limore Maron present what the psychiatrist needs to know about anesthesia in ECT.

Regarding the electrical stimulus, two main considerations are where to place it and how to dose it. I present placement in Chapter 27, and Dr. Vaughn McCall reviews dosing in Chapter 28, but these chapters cannot be entirely separate from each other or from Chapters 1 and 31. These chapters describe variations in opinion that correspond to common variations in clinical practice. Perhaps the reader should scrutinize my views most strongly because I have influenced this book as the editor.

Moving on to monitoring, the intricacies of the ECT seizure as displayed on the electroencephalogram (EEG) are demystified and systematically described by Dr. Hideki Azuma. Chapter 29 elucidates both the structure of the seizure and EEG terminology, which should assist communications about EEGs among ECT practitioners. In Chapter 30 on heart rate, I analogously discuss the pattern of heart rate acceleration and deceleration that accompanies the ECT seizure along with its clinical meanings and uses.

The cognitive effects and concerns associated with ECT are explained by Dr. James Stuart Lawson in Chapter 31, along with cognitive testing that can be performed to monitor it and identify when the patient has completed convalescence. Dr. Lawson discusses how cognitive effects from symptomatic psychiatric illness and medications can affect cognitive testing and how intellectual testing results can improve with ECT.

Lately, antipsychotic medications have been widely promoted for use in children and adolescents, even in those who do not have schizophrenia. These medications have never been established as safer than ECT in children and – as outlined in the chapter on antipsychotics earlier in this section – seem far more dangerous. So we include a timely review by Drs. Garry Walter, Colleen Loo, and Joseph Rey on ECT methods particular to adolescents and children in Chapter 32.

Post-ECT evaluation and medication prophylaxis and its consequences are elucidated by Drs. T. K. Birkenhäger and Walter van den Broek in Chapter 33. Drs. Charles Kellner and Unnati Patel note that ambulatory ECT usage is growing rapidly and might now be as common as inpatient ECT, especially in urban settings. Accordingly, their review of its efficacy and clinical specifics in Chapter 34 should be of interest to most readers. Some additional details that concern ambulatory ECT appear in Chapters 20 and 33.

The final section focuses on the newest somatic treatments in psychiatry. Transcranial magnetic stimulation (TMS) is explained and reviewed by Drs. Oded Rosenberg and Pinhas Dannon in Chapter 35. Vagus nerve stimulation is presented in Chapter 36 by Drs. Shawn McClintock and Mustafa Husain and Mr. Kenneth Trevino. Deep brain electrical stimulation through implanted electrodes is described by Drs. Thomas Schläpfer and Bettina Bewernick in Chapter 37. Perhaps less well-known than these other treatments, but also promising, transcranial direct current stimulation (tDCS) is presented by Ms. Julie Williams and Dr. Felipe Fregni in Chapter 38. Several studies comparing different methods of tDCS have reported varying efficacy and efficacy greater than sham treatment, and this suggests that tDCS may be useful clinically. The details here imply that tDCS differs from alternating (bidirectional) low-level currents, such as delivered by devices for transcutaneous electrical nerve stimulation (TENS).

I will take an editor's prerogative to state a few medical concepts in this preface. First is my rationalization of how and why ECT works, the "Reboot Theory." This is followed by my preferences in ECT clinical practice.

The reboot theory of ECT mechanism and its implications

How electrical current induces seizure is presented in Chapter 1. The clinical question is how the seizure produces psychotropic benefits. I will first summarize the "reboot theory"and then explain it; I believe its initial mention was by Swartz (1984). This mechanism of ECT effect is inherently tied to the phenomenon of seizure, and it has two phases: seizure and recovery from seizure. In the first phase, ECT grand mal seizure depletes brain neurotransmitters by causing neuronal depolarization and neurotransmitter release. In the second phase, this depletion is corrected by replenishment of neurotransmitters according to gene transcription. The induction of replenishment is stimulated by homeostatic mechanisms operating in response to the depletion. This mechanism meshes closely with the details of Chapter 4 and is compatible with the other scientific chapters.

By definition, there is no ECT therapeutic effect without preexisting psychiatric illness. In this mechanism, the psychiatric illness is mediated by a pathological pattern of neurotransmitters in the brain. This pattern resulted from interactions between the patient's genes and the environment. These interactions are life experiences that affect body physiology, such as activation of the sympathetic nervous system. The patterns of illness that result from this interaction can result from combining severely pathological genes with mild life stresses. Such defective genes represent a fragile patient and a highly heritable illness. Illness can also result from combining mildly pathological genes with severe life stresses; this combination represents severe or repeatedly severe adverse life experiences. Alternatively, illness can result from moderate gene predisposition and moderate life stresses.

Eventually, if not interrupted, this pathological pattern of neurotransmitters can begin conversion into a structural pattern, and in time this structural pattern can become established more deeply, essentially worn in. The stronger the structural pattern, the more resistant it is to change, including the changes that ECT can make. When the pathological pattern is primarily in neurotransmitters, the illness has a good prognosis if treated. When the pattern is strongly established in cell structure, it is, for example, chronic schizophrenia. Even when a psychiatric illness is established structurally it should have some neurotransmitter components that can be mitigated by depletion and replacement.

The basic characteristic of grand mal seizure, as in ECT, is the widespread depletion of central nervous system (CNS) neurotransmitters until a change occurs to stop the seizure. Seizure termination is apparently related to neurotransmitter depletion or to the extensive release of neurotransmitters, itself concomitant with neurotransmitter depletion. As the ECT seizure depletes neurotransmitters, their pathological patterns and networks are disrupted and so is the expression of illness they mediate. With repeated ECT seizures, the pathological patterns are progressively depleted and disrupted. Eventually the pathological pattern fades, and so does the illness.

This therapeutic effect is buttressed by replenishment of neurotransmitters according to gene transcription that is activated by neurotransmitter depletion, neurotransmitter release, or both. With repeated ECT seizures, this replacement and its patterns become stronger and more extensive, and they gradually displace the pretreatment pathological pattern of neurotransmitters and eventually become dominant. This pattern of replenishment and replacement reflects only the genes, not effects of the environment or any interaction with the environment, and thereby differs from the pretreatment pathological pattern.

The benefit of neurotransmitter depletion and replacement should persist as long as the gene–environment interaction effects do not accumulate sufficiently to overcome it. Maintenance ECT should work by depleting accumulations of gene–environment interaction effects on neurotransmitters. Perhaps lithium works by diminishing the effect of the environment on neurotransmitter patterns; such a mechanism for lithium is consistent with its effect of decreasing second messenger activity.

The gradual and progressive processes of neurotransmitter depletion and replacement correspond to the gradual improvement and eventual achievement of remission along a course of several ECT sessions. It is somewhat analogous to rebooting (restarting) a computer, suggesting a name for this mechanism. In this analogy, psychiatric illness resembles errors accumulating in random access memory during computer operation. These errors eventually produce malfunctions. ECT is analogous to clearing the computer memory by restarting it from the bootstrap memory (read-only memory [ROM]), in other words, rebooting. This is a nondestructive process.

In this mechanism, ECT restores brain neurotransmitter patterns and function to a normal preillness state. This mechanism differs from the mechanisms of medical interventions that obstruct aspects of brain function, for example, psychosurgery, deep brain electrical stimulation, antipsychotic drugs, and slow TMS. It also differs from treatments that stimulate aspects of brain operation, such as vagal nerve stimulation, stimulant drugs, and rapid TMS (rTMS).

According to this mechanism of ECT, the seizure and its therapeutic effects are inseparable. It is hard to imagine how a medication could accomplish similar neurotransmitter depletion and replacement actions without inducing seizure, and there is no conceivable equivalent treatment or substitute for convulsive therapy (or ECT). Aspects of the convulsive therapy procedure might change in how it is induced, its intensity, and its location, but seizure – neurotransmitter depletion and replacement – is the essence of ECT therapeutic effect and not just its means.

This mechanism accounts for a broad range of ECT phenomena, including providing therapeutic benefits in several different neuropsychiatric disorders. Presumably each disorder has its own pathological pattern of neurotransmitters. The nonspecific nature of neurotransmitter depletion should disrupt any neurotransmitter-mediated illness. It corresponds to the gradual and cumulative clinical effect of giving several ECT treatments and the possible involvement of multiple neural networks, anatomic locations, and neurotransmitters. It is consistent with the stronger therapeutic effect generally seen with greater seizure generalization, including bilateral ECT and higher stimulus doses. The mechanism accounts for ECT cognitive side effects, as recent memory resides in labile neurotransmitters whereas remote memory is structural. It meshes with the genetic–environmental interaction theories of mood disorders and the greater resistance to treatment of longer-lasting illnesses. It explains the corrective therapeutic action of ECT, in which remission typically continues despite discontinuation of the treatment, analogous to antibiotic treatment of infection. Finally, this mechanism and its aspects can be tested and developed further, and its elements can be explained briefly and simply to patients and their families.

ECT surely causes neurochemical changes besides depleting neurotransmitters, such as generating anticonvulsant activity and briefly releasing hormones from the pituitary and other glands. The anticonvulsant activity might help to relieve psychopathology caused by seizure disorders or focal brain irritability. Because several anticonvulsant medications treat mania or diminish somatic tension anxiety, so might the anticonvulsant effects of ECT. However, anticonvulsant activity from ECT persists for only several weeks and so does not explain the persistent remission that typically continues after ECT is stopped.

My ECT clinical preferences

Approach to informed consent

I aim to harness the ECT strength so that it specifically helps patients whose illness is visible. Even seriously ill patients are concerned about personal appearance and privacy. Together, these observable features provide concrete, accurate, and persuasive information about the benefits of ECT.

First, I examine for noticeable signs of illness. These include poverty of speech, motor retardation, masked facies, exhaustion, pained expression, difficulty in solving problems, withdrawal, and malnutrition. Then I describe what I see back to the patient. I typically describe deficits in initiating conversation, physical movement, and emotional expression. A patient only rarely disputes my saying that other people easily see that he or she is ill, and that his or her illness is not private.

I mention that we have a treatment that should help him or her look normal, feel healthier and stronger, and manage his or her own life as before the illness. This is usually persuasive.

I believe that my obtaining informed consent is helped by my maintaining good outcomes with only rare side effects. These good outcomes require strict patient selection and avoidance of bitemporal ECT as a routine. On the ward, patients watch each other. When obviously ill patients improve, other patients notice the difference. When ECT patients show confusion, they also notice – and can feel threatened. When I started using left anterior right temporal (LART) placement, my ECT patients improved without showing confused behavior, and other patients began requesting ECT.

Sedation for sleep on the night before ECT

Promethazine (Phenergan) 25 to 50 mg at bedtime. It is a highly sedating antihistamine and a mild antiadrenergic and antidopaminergic. Yet, it does not inhibit seizure. At 50 mg (25 mg in elderly patients), mild drowsiness can continue in the morning. This drowsiness helps to blunt pre-ECT anxiety. I avoid benzodiazepines because they are anticonvulsant. Zaleplon (Sonata) is too weak for inpatients but should be useful for ambulatory ECT patients.

Pre-ECT intramuscular medication

Glycopyrrolate 0.0044 mg/kg, 1 to 3 hours prior to ECT. When I omit it, saliva secretion usually interferes with treatment and seemingly risks aspiration. I prefer intramuscular (IM) to intravenous (IV) because patients seem drier and some anesthesiologists object to IV.

Pre-ECT oral medication (two to four hours prior to ECT with water sip)

Many patients develop sore muscle headache after ECT. For them, I first try either ibuprofen (400 mg) or acetaminophen (500 to 1,000 mg). Headache patients usually assert their preference, and I order accordingly. Heat and massage can help.

Atropinic agent IV

If glycopyrrolate was not given IM, I give it IV.

Routine narcosis agent, dose range

My preference is methohexital (0.4 to 0.7 mg/kg). My aim is only to obtund the patient from awareness of succinylcholine paralysis. Higher doses can inhibit seizure, but patients with past heavy drinking often require them. If methohexital is not available, I prefer etomidate. For patients younger than 30 years, for the first few ECT sessions I don't mind propofol, about 1 mg/kg. I avoid propofol in elderly patients because of anticonvulsant effects and aspiration risk if the patient takes an antipsychotic or has parkinsonism.

Routine muscle relaxant, dose

In the succinylcholine routine, I prefer 1 mg/kg in muscular or lean patients, 0.7 mg/kg for average patients, and 0.4 mg/kg in the morbidly obese. If the patient has past postictal excitement, I use 1.1 mg/kg (more if the anesthesiologist is willing).

Other common pre-ECT IV agents

When pre-ECT acetaminophen or ibuprofen does not control post-ECT headache, I use ketoprofen (Toradol; 15 to 30 mg). I rarely give other drugs pre-ECT. For patients who show hypertension or tachycardia after ECT seizure, esmolol or labetalol given 30 seconds poststimulus does not inhibit the seizure. Given before the stimulus they can shorten seizure.

Extra steps (if any) for patients taking benzodiazepines

I have not seen flumazenil help obtain a seizure in patients taking benzodiazepines, so I avoid it. I prefer gradually discontinuing benzodiazepines (to avoid withdrawal) but not delaying ECT for this. As the first ECT treatments show the most vigorous seizures, it is still timely to stop benzodiazepines by the third or fourth ECT treatment. In older patients, I additionally compensate for recent benzodiazepines by increasing stimulus dose.

Oxygenation

I prefer maximum hyperventilation from the time of obtundation until the stimulus, regardless of oximeter readings. Higher oxygen and lower carbon dioxide levels promote seizure. Ventilation according to oxygen saturation alone unfortunately allows carbon dioxide levels to accumulate and inhibit seizure. After the stimulus, I aim for a pink patient and an oxygen saturation of at least 97%.

Other anesthetic considerations

Minimizing antipsychotic use in elderly patients cuts aspiration from parkinsonian dysphagia. I avoid propofol in patients on an antipsychotic, those with Parkinson's disease, those receiving no atropinic agent, and elderly patients in general. In patients with postictal excitement despite a succinylcholine dose of 1.1 mg/kg, I administer an additional methohexital (30–50 mg) or propofol bolus immediately after the motor seizure.

Electrode placement

LART placement is my routine. If I avoid excessive electrical dosage, cognitive side effects are usually impalpable. Lower side effects should result from both its asymmetry and its physical separation from the working memory functions of the left dorsolateral prefrontal cortex.

However, if the patient is actively suicidal or violent, I use bitemporal ECT. When the patient has a history of severe ECT confusion, I use right unilateral placement unless it produced this problem. If the patient shows no improvement after four good-quality ECT treatments, I usually switch to bitemporal ECT.

Stimulus dose method

I use the Benchmark Method to adjust the stimulus dose along the course of treatment, with peak heart rate and tonic motor seizure as the physiological indicators. The stimulus dose at the first ECT is "half age %Energy" at 900 mA and 0.5-ms pulse width with LART or bitemporal placement. This dose has a charge of 2.5 mC/year of age at a 900-mA current. I increase this dose if seizure-inhibiting influences are present, for example, anticonvulsants and benzodiazepines. For unilateral ECT, I start with "full age %Energy" (5 mC/year). At 800 mA the equivalent charge is 4 mC/year for any bilateral ECT and 8 mC/year for unilateral ECT.

I monitor heart rate during seizure and motor seizure. If no tonic motor activity occurs, it is not a good benchmark seizure and I increase stimulus dose. I also increase the electrical dose if peak heart rate is less than 140 bpm, unless the patient is older than 80 years or has a specific medical reason for low heart rate (e.g., propofol anesthesia, atherosclerotic cardiovascular disease). Otherwise, the peak heart rate becomes the initial benchmark. If peak heart rate at later ECT treatments is within 6 bpm of that benchmark and at least 140 bpm, the stimulus dose is high enough. If peak heart rate is lower, I increase stimulus dose. Likewise, if there is no tonic motor activity, I increase the electrical dose. I follow EEG signs of seizure intensity (such as postictal suppression), but it only rarely adds guidance.

Stimulus potentiation (after maximum stimulus dose is reached)

My first approach is basic: medication discontinuation, clear airways, maximal hyperventilation, minimizing methohexital dosage, and considering promethazine at bedtime before ECT. Next, I switch to etomidate anesthesia. If this is not enough, I usually give two stimulus doses, one right after the other. Traditional ECT devices do not prevent this. Even a gap of 5 seconds between the two stimuli should not prevent their effects from combining. In this double stimulus method, each stimulus should not exceed a four-second duration, so the total does not exceed eight seconds. If this is inadequate, I switch to ketamine anesthesia and use a single maximum stimulus dose. The next step after this is a double stimulus. My final step, in addition to everything else, is IV caffeine pre-ECT, 500 mg for an elderly patient or 1,000 mg for other patients.

Caffeine is last because of adverse histological CNS neural effects (Enns et al., 1996). This toxicity occurred with high caffeine doses alone, so it is probably the same effect caused by any exposure to amphetamine or methylphenidate and should not prevent IV caffeine when truly needed.

Physiological monitoring (and specific signs)

I monitor tonic motor activity and peak heart rate during the seizure. If there is no tonic motor activity, total motor duration is less than 18 seconds, or peak heart rate decreases as described in "Stimulus dose method," I strongly consider increasing stimulus dose. If peak heart rate is within 10 bpm of baseline heart rate and motor duration is less than 10 seconds or equivocal, I restimulate under the same anesthesia. I do not restimulate for weak EEG morphology alone, but if it weakens I increase the dose at the next session.

If motor seizure exceeds 60 seconds or EEG seizure exceeds 120 seconds, I administer IV methohexital, propofol, or midazolam to terminate the seizure.

Recovery from ECT

Unpleasant feelings of agitation from postictal excitement dispose patients to withdraw consent, so I treat this vigorously, but with drugs eliminated from the body by the next ECT. I use midazolam (1 mg IV), monitoring carefully for apnea. After the patient can swallow, I give oral oxazepam, with another dose four to five hours later. For the next ECT, I plan to prevent postictal excitement with higher doses of succinylcholine and sometimes a second dose of methohexital at the end of the seizure, as noted earlier.

Ward management

With any catatonic or moderately or severely depressed inpatient, I weigh him or her daily; monitor orientation, initiation of speech, psychomotor activity, and emotional expression; and describe changes since ECT was started.

Discharge considerations

I try to enforce a minimum ECT course of six sessions. My median is seven. I treat to plateau, with one to two extra sessions for patients who are risky, resistant, or long ill. Then I evaluate for anxiety disorder. This evaluation is routine because patients can develop PTSD from the experience of having a severe psychiatric illness. I investigate discrepancies between improvements I see and patient self-assessments. If psychomotor activity normalized but the patient complains of continuing "depression," low mood, dissatisfaction, apprehension, or persistent unpleasant thoughts, then anxiety disorder is likely. ECT probably temporarily decreases somatic tension anxiety, but in patients with anxiety disorder, somatic tension still needs treatment and selective serotonin reuptake inhibitors do not reliably mitigate it.

I advise that patients avoid making major life or financial changes within two months of the end of an ECT course because ECT can temporarily induce an orbital–frontal syndrome or dysexecutive syndrome and it can be subtle, but it should fade within five to six weeks.

Acknowledgments

My deep and unending gratitude goes to my wife Cynthia for inspiration and encouragement; to Barbara Walthall for forgiving patience; to Marc Strauss for keen insight in initiating this project and producing it; to Ned Shorter for starting me on the path; and to each and every chapter author for truly admirable fortitude, flexibility, and scholarship.

Conrad M. Swartz

References

Enns, M., Peeling, J., and Sutherland, G.R. 1996. Hippocampal neurons are damaged by caffeine-augmented electroshock seizures. Biol Psychiatry 40: 642–47.

Kishimoto, M., Ujike, H., Motohashi, Y., et al. 2008. The dysbindin gene (DTNBP1) is associated with methamphetamine psychosis. Biol Psychiatry 63: 191–96.

Swartz, C.M. The justification for ECT. 1984. Behavioral Brain Sci 7: 37.

Taylor, M. A. 1992. Are schizophrenia and affective disorder related? A selective literature review. Am J Psychiatry 149: 22–32.

Part I

Scientific and experimental bases of electroconvulsive therapy

Electricity and electroconvulsive therapy

Conrad M. Swartz

Information about electricity helps ensure electroconvulsive therapy (ECT) safety and efficacy and limit side effects. It bears on seizure generation, stimulus dose, and stimulus efficiency. Efficiency refers to how stimuli of the same dose differ in generating seizures or side effects. Although electricity specific to ECT is our focus, regular safety practices should be used. Do not use frayed cables or electrical equipment that is or was wet, do not pull on wires, and avoid becoming part of an electrical circuit by contacting the patient at more than one place during the stimulus.

Basic electrical facts and safety

Electricity, the flow of electrons, is basically specified by its current and voltage, and how they vary with time. "Current" is the number of electrons flowing per second. Amperes ("amps") are electrons per second multiplied by a conversion factor. "Voltage" is the electrical force that pushes these electrons to flow. "Charge" is the number of electrons passing during the period of interest; if current is constant, charge equals current multiplied by time. In an analogy between electron flow (electricity) and water flow, current is analogous to water volume flowing per second, voltage is analogous to water pressure, and charge is analogous to total water volume passing during the period of interest. Greater pressure or voltage produces proportionately greater current. For electricity, the proportionality constant between voltage and current is impedance, that is, voltage equals current times impedance. The famous "Ohm's law" is the special case in which all impedance is resistance.

Just as it takes energy to pump water, energy is carried in electric current. All energy in the ECT stimulus is eventually converted into heat, and the amount of energy is described in the same units used for heat. Risk from electricity comes from temperature increases that correspond to the rate of heat liberation. A separate safety issue is that electricity applied near the heart can cause arrhythmias, but we avoid this problem at ECT by applying electricity only on the head.

Electrical energy is the product of voltage, current, impedance, and time; the electric company charges us for this product. Just as with a tank of gasoline, energy has no built-in time rate; you can use a particular amount quickly or slowly. In contrast, power has a time factor, power is the rate of energy use, and power corresponds to temperature changes. For an ECT stimulus that we plan to apply, we can know in advance only the current or the voltage (but not both) because we do not know the patient's impedance to the stimulus before it is delivered. After the stimulus, when we know the current we can use the relationship that energy equals the product of current squared, impedance, and time. When we know the voltage we can use energy equals voltage squared multiplied by time and divided by impedance.

These basic facts apply to ECT in several ways. There are three types of ECT stimulus generators ("ECT machines"): constant current, constant voltage, and fixed charge. All commercially available modern stimulus generators supply a constant (and therefore limited) current. This means that voltage increases with impedance because current remains fixed. This is generally safer than constant voltage because of the possibility of a short circuit between the electrodes (as from sweat, gel, water, or if electrodes are too near each other). With constant current, a short circuit produces impedance near zero and thereby a voltage near zero. No burn can occur because the rate of energy release is low, as it equals impedance times current squared. In this circumstance impedance is low and current does not change, so their multiplication product is low.

In contrast, with a constant-voltage stimulus the rate of energy release equals voltage squared divided by impedance. This means that low impedance increases the rate of energy release and thereby the risk of skin burn. Indeed, a study that placed electrodes only 5 cm apart with constant-voltage stimuli produced unacceptable skin burns (Abrams and Taylor, 1973). This is one reason why constant-voltage ECT devices are obsolete.

Fixed-charge devices gradually build up ("fully charge") a large capacitor; the stimulus is then delivered from the capacitor. Cardiac defibrillators are fixed-charge devices. Before they can deliver a shock, a "charge-up" button must be pressed, and there is a wait for the capacitor to fill with electrons. Defibrillators are notorious for skin burns that result because their current is not limited. Fixed-charge ECT stimulus generators are not currently commercially available.

Skin burns can occur with constant-current ECT. This can happen in the circumstance that is the opposite of a short circuit: extremely high impedance between the two electrodes. In practice, this occurs only when there is poor contact between the electrode and the skin or between the electrode and the ECT instrument itself. Poor contact means high impedance. There is a one-to-one relationship between high impedance and high heat release. If higher impedance is present where the stimulus electrode meets the skin, a higher temperature will surely develop there. Conversely, a skin burn occurring during an ECT stimulus specifically indicates that high impedance was present where the burn occurred. In one situation in which I used a rubber head strap with steel plate electrodes, after the stimulus I noticed that one of the electrodes had slipped onto its edge. Under the electrode edge I saw a thin straight red line – a mild burn. It healed quickly but left me a mental picture of the need to keep impedance down.

The energy in constant-current ECT stimuli is far too small to produce a burn anywhere but where the electrode meets the skin. Even if all the electrical current were to enter the brain and liberate 100 joules in its path, brain tissue temperature would increase by less than 0.1°C (Swartz, 1989). However, only about 1% of the electrical current crosses the bony skull into the brain because skull impedance is about 100 times higher than skin impedance (Weaver et al., 1976). That is, about 99% is shunted through the scalp and the skin and never enters the brain, and 99% of the stimulus energy is dissipated as heat in the skin and scalp. Accordingly, brain temperature increases by less than 0.001°C. Still, a skin burn can occur, but only if the connection between the electrode and the skin is not good, that is, the impedance of the connection is high. The clinician can act to lower the impedance of the skin, the electrode, and the connection between them by removing sources of high impedance. These include oils, rust, dirt, cosmetics, skin lotions, crust, and hair. Removing natural skin oils with organic solvents such as alcohol or acetone increases impedance. Salt-containing gels and fluids decrease impedance.

In medication therapy, we are concerned about how close our therapeutic dosage approaches the toxic range. Analogously, how high would an ECT stimulus have to be to cause injury? Electrical injury derives from the heat of electrical energy dissipation. Because 99% of the current is shunted through skin (including scalp), it is the vulnerable site in the electrical path. Troublesome skin injury would occur at far lower stimulus energy than could cause thermal injury inside the skull, as long as the skull is intact. For brief-pulse stimuli, if liquid electrode gel were applied between the electrode and the skin, the heat liberated by each pulse would be conducted into the gel and dispersed through it before the next pulse arrived (Swartz, 1989). If a metal electrode were involved, it would be included in this heat dispersal. This means that no skin burn could occur until the entire gel and metal electrode mass reached scalding temperature, approximately 60°C, about 35°C higher than room temperature. A typical metal electrode weighs 20 g. Assuming a gram of gel, the total weighs 42 grams for two electrodes. Supposing the worst case – all energy dissipation at the skin to electrode junction – each 100-joule stimulus would raise electrode temperature by 0.57°C. Raising the heat of the electrodes to scalding temperature would require 6,100 joules, or 61 maximal brief-pulse ECT stimuli. A very conservative safe upper limit for ECT stimulus energy regarding the most vulnerable site, the skin, is 10% of this, 610 joules. There are 4.187 joules per calorie; 100 joules = 24 calories.

For the small amount of electric current that passes through the skull and the brain, virtually all energy dissipation occurs within the skull because impedance is far higher through skull than through brain. Brain tissue would not be electrically heated until skull impedance breaks down from heat damage. Before brain tissue would be subject to electrical heating it would be exposed to heat that diffuses from the electrically heated skull. This analysis leads to a useful result: Before brain tissue could be injured by electrical heating, the skull would become painfully hot. Of course in ECT practice skull heating does not occur. Accordingly, no electrical brain injury occurs. If you have wondered why execution by electrocution sometimes does not occur despite massive amounts of electrical energy, now you know. There is more lethality in cardiac arrhythmia.

Before the ECT stimulus dose is applied, some stimulus generators can apply a tiny and impalpable electrical current to examine the electrical connection. The resulting number is the "static impedance." A high impedance risks skin burn. The "dynamic impedance" printed after the treatment results from measuring both the current and voltage of the ECT stimulus. A typical dynamic impedance is 220 ohms, and an ordinary range is 100 to 320 ohms. A higher dynamic impedance indicates poor connection to the patient, for example, an electrode slipped out of place after the static impedance test.

Seizure generation

ECT efficacy derives from the generalized seizure (Ottosson, 1960). Seizure includes both neurotransmitter release and electrical currents, and, because they are inseparable in the seizure, therapeutic benefit corresponds to both. Still, there is a basic difference between the electricity of the seizure and the electrical stimulus. In modern ECT, the electrical stimulus only induces seizure and by itself is not substantially therapeutic.

The process that connects the seizure to the electrical stimulus is the mechanism of seizure induction. The mechanism described here may seem surprising. The purpose of this mechanism is to identify what it is about electricity that represents the ECT stimulus dose. It also provides the opportunity to understand how the ECT seizure develops from the stimulus, but the following dose formula can be clinically used without understanding.

The modern ECT stimulus consists of a series of electron pulses flowing between two electrodes (see Figure 1.1). The pulses strictly alternate in direction. This electron flow is called "bidirectional" or "alternating" current. Each pulse is typically 0.5 to 1 ms in duration. Electrical silence between pulses typically lasts for 6 to 16 ms,

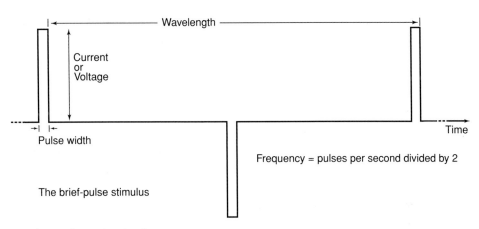

Figure 1.1   The modern ECT stimulus.

about 10 times longer than the pulse. A typical ECT stimulus has 100 to 1,000 pulses and is one to three times as long as the minimum that would generate a seizure, so a single pulse is not strong enough to induce a seizure by itself.

The time that passes between pulses is long enough for any polarization, depolarization, or other directional charge effect induced by a pulse to dissipate before the next pulse. Moreover, this next pulse is in the opposite direction and thereby neutralizes any possible remaining polarization, and any other effect associated with electron flow in a particular direction. Taken together, these basic facts indicate that the modern bidirectional ECT stimulus cannot induce seizure primarily through electrical depolarization.

Traditionally, electrical depolarization has been the stated mechanism for ECT seizure generation. It was rationalized only by analogy to direct-current depolarization of a single neuron (Sackeim et al., 1994). With a single neuron at rest, the inner surface of the cell membrane has a negative voltage relative to the outer surface, by 70 mV. When this polarization is reversed by the current from a small negative electrode applied to the outside of the cell body, the single neuron immediately fires, that is, it immediately transmits a wave of depolarization along its axon that extrudes neurotransmitters onto an adjacent neuron. Analogous firing of many neurons by depolarization has never been proven as the mechanism for seizure with a bidirectionally pulsed stimulus. The analogy is not reasonable because a human brain is 11 orders of magnitude larger than a single neuron. Extrapolating from a mouse to an elephant is much closer, yet lethal (e.g., West et al., 1962).

As an ECT seizure cannot be induced primarily by electrical depolarization, the simplest known remaining possible mechanism is rapid kindling. Kindling means that the seizure threshold progressively decreases with each stimulus pulse. Eventually, it becomes low enough for enough neurons to depolarize to initiate a seizure.

This process is similar to how a seizure is generated by increasing levels of proconvulsant pharmaceuticals, such as stimulant drugs, pentylenetetrazol, and flurothyl. The ECT stimulus pulse evidently disrupts the neuronal cell membrane and the operation of the sodium–potassium exchange pump across it. Normally sodium is actively pumped from the cell; the cell membrane is only slightly permeable to sodium inflow, and the intracellular sodium level remains very low. Presumably, with each ECT stimulus pulse intracellular sodium levels would increase, whether from greater sodium permeability or decreased sodium–potassium pump effectiveness. In turn, this decreases the negative voltage on the inner membrane surface. This is rapid kindling. Eventually, the effects of pulses aggregate into producing neuronal depolarization. The depolarized neurons depolarize adjacent neurons, and a wave of depolarization sweeps through the brain.

If there were no kindling, that is, no decrease in seizure threshold in the brain, and the seizure were generated solely by electrical depolarization, there would be no more than one wave of neuronal depolarization after the end of the ECT stimulus. However, a seizure is much more than a single wave of neuronal depolarization, and it is much more than the depolarization of a single neuron by – and solely during – an applied voltage. Rather, the ECT seizure consists of 2 to 5 waves per second lasting 20 to 60 seconds. In a manner separate from previous discussion, this reasoning also indicates that electrical depolarization of neurons is not the principal means of ECT seizure induction. Rather, the ECT seizure must be built upon rapid kindling. The kindled neurons from which waves of depolarization spread are the seizure foci.

The rapid kindling mechanism applies as well to unidirectional pulse stimuli for the same reasons. It applies because the interval between pulses is long enough to dissipate polarization (or depolarization) effects from any pulse before the next pulse. It applies also because the waves of seizure continue long after the electrical stimulus ceases. If rapid kindling develops only at the anode (the positive electrode), an ECT seizure induced by unidirectional stimuli would begin at one electrode, rather than from both electrodes, as with bidirectional stimuli.

The rapid kindling mechanism implies that the stimulus titration method for measuring seizure threshold embodies a systematic error if two or more stimuli are administered in succession. In this method, progressively higher electrical stimuli are administered until a convulsion develops. If a stimulus is not followed by a convulsion within 20 seconds, another stimulus is administered. However, subconvulsive ECT stimuli contribute to kindling for at least 1 minute (Swartz, 1990). So the "method of limits" measurement of seizure threshold underestimates it more with each additional stimulus administered. Additional internal inconsistencies in using seizure threshold to help set the stimulus dose are discussed elsewhere (Swartz, 2001).

Brief-pulse stimulus dose

This section updates a previous report (Swartz, 2006). Even several times the amount of electrical charge and energy in an ECT stimulus applied to the skin would be impalpable if given over several hours. If it were applied to the head that slowly it would not affect consciousness and certainly it would not generate a seizure because the electrical voltage and current are too small. That is, a certain minimum voltage is needed to induce disruption of the neuronal cell membrane and kindling and eventually produce neuronal depolarization. Using the charge as the stimulus dose ignores the effect of voltage. Expressing stimulus dose as energy (e.g., joules) is similarly inadequate because it represents only the total heat liberated by the electrical stimulus, not even the rate of heat liberation that affects the temperature.

To reflect seizure-inducing capability, the unit of stimulus dose must be related to the desired result, the induction of a generalized brain seizure. That is, the stimulus dose is reflected by the (three-dimensional) volume of seizure foci it produces. The minimum volume of seizure foci that induces a generalized brain seizure is the "seizure threshold." To reach this threshold, the voltage across the electrodes must be high enough to induce kindling and a sufficient number of electrons (that is, charge) must pass between the electrodes.

Modeling real-world phenomena with equations ordinarily begins with identifying reasonable approximations that can be represented by physically meaningful mathematical terms. One such approximation is that the two stimulus electrode sites are far enough apart that the neuronal effects around each are separate from the other site. Another is that each electrode site is small compared with the distance between the electrodes and so can be represented by a point. A third approximation is that the electrical impedance of the brain is uniform. This implies that the voltage drops linearly between the two electrodes. Conversely, a particular voltage drop corresponds to a particular physical distance. A final approximation is that the volume of seizure foci is much smaller than the entire brain, so that the geometry of the skull bordering each electrode can be approximated as a plane.

The approximation of separation is compatible with all three versions of bilateral ECT: bitemporal, bifrontal, and left anterior right temporal (LART). In these placements, the two electrodes are in two widely separated planes. Each electrode site can be considered very small because small differences in electrode placement produce clinically observable changes. In specific, relocating each of the electrodes of bitemporal ECT forward by merely 2.5 cm significantly increased post-ECT cognitive function scores and significantly decreased the variability of these scores. The lower variability indicates that fewer patients had marked cognitive dysfunction.

Consider a voltage E as the minimum sufficient to kindle neurons. As noted earlier, a particular voltage corresponds to a particular physical distance. The brain *volume* within a hemisphere of *radius E* around the electrode site is $(2/3)\pi E^3$. The *volume* of kindled brain equals the *volume* within this voltage hemisphere multiplied by the number of voltage carriers, that is, the *charge*. The kindled brain *volume* – which represents the stimulus dose – increases with the cube of the *voltage* multiplied by the *charge*. As voltage increases, this *volume* increases in proportion to *voltage* cubed.

The stimulus dose can be expressed in terms of current instead of voltage by using Ohm's law, *voltage E* equals *current I* times *impedance Z*. Replacing E with I (current) times Z (impedance) indicates that the kindled brain *volume* – that is, the stimulus dose – increases in proportion to the cube of the *current* multiplied by the *charge*.

With bilateral ECT, at the same charge a stimulus of *current I3* has $(I3/I2)^3$ times the seizure-inducing dose as a stimulus of *current I2*. To illustrate, a 900-mA stimulus has 1.42 times the seizure-inducing dose of an 800-mA stimulus at the same charge. This calculation indicates a strong difference between a 900-mA ECT instrument and an 800-mA instrument. Consistent with this 142% calculation, direct randomized comparisons involving 88 patients receiving bitemporal ECT found that 900-mA stimuli had 1.61 times the seizure-inducing effects of stimuli of 800 mA or less at the same charge and a pulse width of 1 ms (Chanpattana, 2001).

Unlike the bilateral placements (bitemporal, bifrontal, LART), the Lancaster right unilateral placement locates the electrodes in the same plane and near each other. In this circumstance the volume of seizure foci increases in two dimensions – rather than three – as the current increases. The stimulus *dose* is then proportional to *charge* times the *current* squared, rather than cubed. In the modern right unilateral placement, with electrodes at the right temple and vertex, there is more separation than in the Lancaster placement but less than in bilateral ECT. Accordingly, the *volume* of seizure foci should increase proportionally to an exponential power of *current* larger than 2 (as for Lancaster) and less than 3 (as for bilateral). As a first approximation, this exponential power is 2.5. Corresponding to this, a 900-mA current would have 1.34 times the dose of an 800-mA current at the same charge.

For bilateral ECT, the result of multiplying *charge* in millicoulombs (mC) by *current* cubed produces an unfamiliar number. For example, a 504-mC charge at 0.9-A current gives 367.4 raw dose units. To have a familiar number as the result, simply use a constant coefficient of 1.372 on the raw dose units to produce foci units, that is, 376.7 times 1.372 equals 504. As another example, a 574-mC charge at 0.8 A is 405 foci units. In other words, by definition, the *charge* and the foci units are the same at 0.9 A; however, they will differ for other at other currents. *Bilateral Dose* (foci units) $= 1.372 \times$ *charge* in mC $\times$ (*current* in A)^3 and *Unilateral Dose* (foci units) $= 1.372 \times charge$ in mC $\times (current$ in A$)^{2.5}$. Unlike charge alone, these doses are relative, not absolute. In other words, a bilateral dose can be compared only with other bilateral doses, not with a unilateral dose.

Sine wave stimulus dose

The dose of a sine wave stimulus is more complex to express, because its current and voltage constantly vary. *Current* to the third power multiplied by *charge* for the brief-pulse stimulus is basically integration over *time* of *current* to the fourth power. Expressing the sine wave current as $A \, sin(t)$, where A is the peak current and t is the time, and integrating the fourth power of current over one wavelength yields the stimulus dose for one wave as $(3/8)LA^4$, where L is the wavelength. Replacing L with the stimulus duration T gives the dose for an entire sine wave stimulus.

Stating the stimulus dose as the charge alone vastly and incorrectly understates the dose of sine wave stimuli, especially in elderly patients. This understatement is best understood by comparing typical doses of brief-pulse and sine wave stimuli. For a brief-pulse stimulus, the stimulus duration T is calculated as the total time of all pulses. For typical stimuli of 100 to 250 mC at 900 mA, current total time is 0.11 to 0.28 seconds. This range is equivalent to sine wave stimuli of 0.29- to 0.75-seconds duration with the same peak current as the brief-pulse stimuli. Sine wave stimuli of 170 root-mean-square (RMS) volts reach 240 volts at peak. At the average human dynamic impedance of 200 ohms, the peak current is 1200 mA. Corresponding to this peak current, the dose of a 1-second 170-volt sine wave stimulus is 0.78 raw units [that is, $(1.2)^4 \times (3/8) \times 1$]. The current and dose are far higher for patients with lower impedance, specifically elderly patients (Sackeim et al., 1987). At 150 ohms impedance – typical for elderly patients – peak current is 1.6 A and corresponding dose is 2.46 raw units. At 120 ohms – still within normal range – peak current is 2 A and dose is 6 raw units. These much higher doses at low impedance apparently explain why sine wave devices effectively induced seizures in elderly patients. Excessive dose might explain why some patients experienced severe cognitive side effects.

In comparison, maximum doses are 0.37 raw units for a 504-mC brief-pulse device at 900 mA and 0.29 raw units for a 576-mC brief-pulse device at 800 mA. These lower raw unit doses show that sine wave devices delivered far higher maximum stimulus doses than present brief-pulse devices do. Per the previous paragraph illustration, this is 2.1 and 2.7 times the maximum dose at average impedance and 6.6 and 8.5 times the maximum dose for typical elderly patients (150 ohms). The problem with sine wave stimuli was inefficiency. Inefficiency is why sine wave stimuli need high doses to succeed, and it is presumably why they also produce substantially greater cognitive side effects than do brief-pulse stimuli.

Stimulus efficiency

The ECT electrical stimulus has two separate attributes that influence seizure intensity: dose and waveform efficiency. Returning to the gasoline analogy, stimulus dose corresponds to gallons of gasoline, stimulus efficiency to miles per gallon, and seizure induction to a particular trip. With low efficiency, a higher dose (more gasoline) is needed to reach the goal. By definition, the characteristics of a waveform that is more clinically effective at the same stimulus dose are more efficient.

Before we consider these characteristics, there is a basic question about the virtues of stimulus efficiency. Compare two stimuli that are equally effective in producing ECT seizures but the efficiencies of which differ. For equal effectiveness, the less efficient stimulus is administered at a higher dose. The question is: Does the less efficient higher dose stimulus have more side effects? A related question is: For the higher dose stimulus, does the extra electricity cause adverse effects? The lower efficiency stimulus is analogous to driving with the parking brake on. In view of this analogy (and because of the higher dose), some of the less efficient stimuli presumably interfere with seizure generation, so we should expect that less efficient stimuli have more side effects, and the most efficient stimuli are the most clinically desirable. This expectation is clearly true in the comparison between brief-pulse and sine wave stimuli, and it is presumably true in general.

Basic waveform characteristics include wave shape (e.g., rectangular or sine), continuous or pulsed train, phase width, wave frequency, and charge rate. The phase width is the width of the stimulus wave. For rectangular waves, it is pulse width. For sine waves it is half the wavelength. Mathematically, wavelength equals the number 1 divided by wave frequency, and charge rate is the average absolute value of the current. Charge rate is the amount of stimulus charge delivered per second counting intervals when the current is off. In contrast, stimulus current refers only to periods when the current is on. Specifying any two of charge rate, pulse width, and frequency at a specific current determines the third, by the following mathematical relationship: *charge rate* (mC/s) $= 2 \times$ *frequency* (Hz) $\times$ *pulse width* (ms) $\times$ *current* (A).

Sine wave versus brief-pulse stimuli

The report that brief-pulse stimuli have milder side effects and use less charge than sine wave stimuli do is well known (Weiner et al., 1986). However, the result was never proven as just stated. Although the comparison found milder side effects and less charge with brief-pulse stimuli, there were large electrical differences between stimuli outside of wave shape. There are several reasons why the clinical differences are more logically attributable to differences in phase width and charge rate, that is, to efficiency.

It is understood that brief-pulse stimuli are rectangular in shape, commonly called square waves. The brief-pulse stimulus had a 0.75- to 2-ms phase width and a 72- to 168-mC/s charge rate. The sine wave stimulus had an 8.3-ms phase width and an expected average of 700-mC/s charge rate. These phase widths and charge rates differ by an order of magnitude and so are not similar. Other studies published since have shown that – within the range of 0.5 to 1.5 ms – shorter pulse widths are more efficient and have greater physiological impact at the same charge (Swartz, 2000; Swartz and Larson, 1989; Swartz and Manly, 2000). Likewise, within the range of 0.75- to 1.5-ms pulse width, lower charge rate is more efficient.

Moreover, within the brain, sine wave and square wave stimuli differ little in shape because of the effects of skull capacitance. This capacitance smooths out abrupt changes in the current, so that the current increase at the start of a pulse is not vertical but sloped positively, and likewise at the end of a pulse the current decrease is sloped negatively. Furthermore, skull capacitance rounds off the sharply angular upper shoulders and lower bases of a square wave pulse. Combined, skull capacitance and short pulse width smooth a square wave stimulus to resemble a sine wave stimulus. With little difference in wave shape between sine wave and square wave stimuli but large differences in phase width and charge rate, the clinical differences are more attributable to phase width and charge rate. Finally, a direct comparison of sine wave and square wave stimuli at the same phase width and charge rate has never been conducted, so there is no evidence that square wave stimuli differ in effects from brief-pulse stimuli of the same phase width, current, and charge.

Efficiency of brief-pulse stimuli

Efficiency varies substantially within brief-pulse stimuli, not just between brief pulse and sine wave. Two studies compared several different stimuli of identical dose on the same group of patients in randomized order. This "repeated measures" method compensates for variations from one patient to the next. Repeated measures analysis of variance found that a 0.5-ms pulse width was significantly more effective than 1 ms at the same charge and current. When using fixed "half-age" stimulus dosing (2.5 mC/year at 900-mA current), abortive or failed motor seizures occurred in 8% of treatments at a 0.5-ms pulse width, but in 23% of treatments at 1 ms of the same stimulus charge and current (Swartz and Manly, 2000). There was no difference in effect between a 30- and 60-Hz frequency at either 0.5- or 1-ms pulse width. These data point to preferring stimuli of 0.5-ms pulse width.

An earlier study similarly compared a different range of stimuli at a fixed 1,440-mC charge and 800-mA current. These were 0.75-ms pulse width 60 Hz for 2 seconds, 1.5-ms pulse width 30 Hz for 2 seconds, and 1.5-ms pulse width 60 Hz for 1 second. Failed motor seizures occurred in 4.8%, 14.3%, and 47.6% of stimuli, respectively (Swartz and Larson, 1989). Here, using the wider1.5-ms pulse width frequency had a strong effect, whereas the later study showed no observable difference between 0.5- and 1-ms pulse widths. Over both studies, narrower pulse width was more efficient (ranging from 0.5 to 1.5 ms), lower charge rate was at least as efficient and usually more efficient (ranging from 27 to 144 mC/s), and lower frequency was at least as efficient and sometimes more efficient (ranging from 30 to 60 Hz).

Ultrabrief pulse

By definition, brief-pulse stimuli are of pulse width 0.5 ms to 2.0 ms, and ultrabrief-pulse stimuli are less than 0.5 ms. Because skull capacitance puts a slope on square waves and rounds off their tops, in effect it decreases both pulse width and pulse amplitude. Decreasing pulse width decreases charge, and lowering amplitude decreases current and charge. As previously noted, any decrease in current is magnified to the fourth power, an extreme influence on stimulus dose. This strong effect of current on stimulus dose implies that there is a minimum pulse width (in milliseconds) below which the ECT stimulus becomes clinically ineffectual. This minimum surely varies among patients and probably differs between bilateral and unilateral electrode placements, analogous to how seizure threshold varies. The higher the current, the narrower this minimum effective pulse width will be, because higher current compensates for current attenuation by skull capacitance. Consistent with this, greater current was required for ultrabrief stimuli to induce seizure in the (larger) brain of the pig than in that of the rabbit (Hyrman et al., 1985).

By analogy to the ineffectuality of right unilateral ECT at a minimal dose (near seizure threshold), ultrabrief stimuli may be clinically ineffectual despite inducing a grand mal seizure. The induced seizure should be weak and poorly generalized through the brain. In a direct comparison of bilateral ECT among low-energy ultrabrief stimuli, mid-energy brief pulse, and high-energy chopped sine wave (a variation of brief pulse), ultrabrief stimuli averaged less improvement per ECT than did the other two, which had equal efficacy (Robin and De Tissera, 1982). Although the waveforms of this study differ from modern instruments, a recent study reported similar results with right unilateral ECT. Specifically, 0.3-ms ultrabrief ECT produced significantly less improvement per ECT than at 1-ms pulse width and needed an average of 12 rather than 8 ECT sessions (Loo et al., 2007). This number of ECT sessions is undesirably large. Remission was achieved in only 4/30 = 13% of the ultrabrief group, far below what is expected for ECT and usually reported in ECT studies. The response rate to unilateral ECT was only about 50% for both groups, which is also less than expected for ECT. This method of ultrabrief ECT is not sufficiently effective for regular clinical use.

Peculiarly, one report claimed that, with ultrabrief stimuli, right unilateral ECT is more effective than bilateral ECT (Sackeim et al., 2008). This result is not consistent with the overwhelming preponderance of data – and understanding – that unilateral ECT aspires to equal bilateral ECT in efficacy but does not surpass it. This inconsistency suggests that 0.3-ms stimuli are well below the typical minimum effective pulse width for bilateral but not unilateral ECT. This situation is analogous to unilateral ECT having a lower seizure threshold than bilateral ECT. Alternatively, there might have been an unidentified method error.

This study (Sackeim et al., 2008) is not relevant to clinical practice for several other reasons. The bitemporal brief-pulse stimulus dose it used, 2.5 times seizure threshold, is excessively high and causes unnecessary cognitive side effects. Likewise the comparison pulse width used, 1.5 ms, is inefficient and generates unnecessary cognitive side effects. Both bitemporal ECT at 2.5 times threshold and stimuli of 1.5 ms pulse width are clinically undesirable. Accordingly, comparisons of ultrabrief stimuli with them cannot demonstrate any justification of ultrabrief stimuli for clinical use. No justification has ever been presented for using 0.3-ms pulse width in place of the desirable 0.5-ms pulse width, so that 0.3-ms pulse width remains entirely speculative and experimental.

The average and range of the minimum effective pulse width in human patients have not been specifically identified. In view of the clear superiority of 0.5-ms pulse width to 1.0-ms pulse width in seizure induction as well as peak heart rate elevation over baseline (Swartz and Manly, 2000), this minimum pulse width is at or below 0.5 ms. The basic question is: What is the narrowest pulse width that is reliably at least as effective as 0.5 ms? Clear evidence should be obtained from studying patients whose severity of illness is verifiably observable, for example, retarded melancholia, catatonia, or acute mania. Until studies are done with such patients, the efficacy of ultrabrief stimuli will not be clearly established. There is no point in taking the gamble of using an ultrabrief pulse width until it is tested against 0.5-ms pulse width, and it is hard to imagine there could be a sizable advantage over 0.5 ms.

References

Abrams, R. and Taylor, M. A. 1973. Anterior bifrontal ECT: A clinical trial. Br J Psychiatry 122: 587–90.

Chanpattana, W. 2001. Seizure threshold in electroconvulsive therapy: Effect of instrument titration schedule. German J Psychiatry 4(3): 51–6.

Hyrman, V., Palmer, L. H., Cernik, J., and Jetelina, J. 1985. ECT: The search for the perfect stimulus. Biol Psychiatry 20: 634–5.

Loo, C., Sheehan, P., Pigot, M., and Lyndon, W. 2007. A report on mood and cognitive outcomes with right unilateral ultrabrief pulsewidth (0.3 ms) ECT and retrospective comparison with standard pulsewidth right unilateral ECT. J Affect Disord 103: 277–81.

Ottosson, J. O. 1960. Experimental studies of the mode of action of convulsive therapy. Copenhagen: Munksgaard.

Robin, A. and De Tissera, S. 1982. A double-blind controlled comparison of the therapeutic effects of low and high energy electroconvulsive therapies. Br J Psychiatr 141: 357–66.

Sackeim, H. A., Decina, P., Kanzler, M., et al. 1987. Effects of electrode placement on the efficacy of titrated, low dosage ECT. Am J Psychiatry 144: 1449–55.

Sackeim, H. A., Long, J., Luber, B., et al. 1994. Physical properties and quantification of the ECT stimulus: I. Basic principles. Convuls Ther 10: 93–123.

Sackeim, H. A., Prudic, J., Nobler, M., et al. 2008. Effects of pulse width and electrode placement on the efficacy and cognitive effects of electroconvulsive therapy. Brain Stimulation 1: 71–83.

Swartz, C. M. 1989. Safety and ECT stimulus electrodes: I. Heat liberation at the electrode-to-skin interface. Convuls Ther 5: 171–5.

Swartz, C. M. 1990. Repeated ECT stimuli and the seizure threshold. Convuls Ther 6: 181–2.

Swartz, C. M. 2000. Physiological response to ECT stimulus dose. Psychiatry Res 97: 229–35.

Swartz, C. M. 2001. Stimulus dosing in electroconvulsive therapy and the threshold multiple method. J ECT 17: 87–90.

Swartz, C. M. 2006. ECT stimulus dose expressed as volume of seizure foci. J ECT 22: 54–8.

Swartz, C. M. and Larson, G. 1989. ECT stimulus duration and its efficacy. Ann Clin Psychiatry 1: 147–52.

Swartz, C. M. and Manly, D. T. 2000. Efficiency of the stimulus characteristics of ECT. Am J Psychiatry 157: 1504–6.

Weaver, L., Williams, R., and Rush, S. 1976. Current density in bilateral and unilateral ECT. Biol Psychiatry 11: 303–12.

Weiner, R. D., Rogers, H. J., Davidson, J. R. T., and Squire, L. R. 1986. Effects of stimulus parameters on cognitive side effects. Ann NY Acad Sci 462: 315–25.

West, L. J., Pierce, C. M., and Thomas W. D. 1962. Lysergic acid diethylamide: Its effects on a male Asiatic elephant. Science 138: 1100–2.

2

Nonelectrical convulsive therapies

Niall McCrae

Introduction

This chapter reviews nonelectrical convulsive therapy (non-ECT) procedures, including pentylenetetrazol (PTZ) and cyclohexylethyltriazol, flurothyl inhalation, and insulin coma therapy, which also had epileptoid effects. Evidence from the period of application is presented, followed by a contemporary analysis of therapeutic mechanisms. Factors are considered that might explain the observed superiority of PTZ and insulin, in some conditions, over ECT. Lessons may yet be drawn from treatments condemned to the historical annals of psychiatry.

Historical background

The advent of shock treatment must be placed in the context of psychiatry in the 1930s. In 1918 Julius von Wagner-Jauregg had boosted morale with his malarial treatment for neurosyphilis, a condition affecting approximately one quarter of patients in mental hospitals, but this was an oasis in a therapeutic desert. Admission to public mental institutions was not necessarily a life sentence, but a paucity of effective treatments meant that the best hope was self-remission. Recurring psychosis inevitably led to prolonged incarceration in the neglected "back wards." Asylum stalwarts, paraldehyde and bromides, maintained a semblance of order, but the drab institutional regimen was regularly colored by wild psychotic behavior. Life on the wards featured force-feeding of stuporous patients, constant surveillance of suicidal cases, and regular use of padded seclusion rooms (Rollin, 1990). Schizophrenia was regarded as an untreatable hereditary disorder, and many leading psychiatrists were affirmed eugenicists, emphasizing the role of the mental institution in preventing procreation of tainted stock. The growth of psychoanalysis, with speculative theories arguably closer to art than medicine, had limited practical relevance in hopelessly understaffed hospitals. The holy grail of orthodox psychiatry was identified by Bumke in his textbook of 1929, in which he stated, "I am convinced that every attempt to reduce dementia praecox to psychological

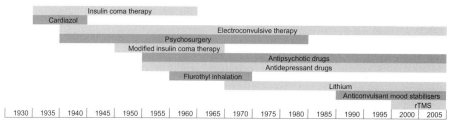

Figure 2.1   Periods of application of somatic treatments (approximate).

terms will become superfluous as soon as we discover the organic basis for these disorders."

Faith in the disease model, hostility toward psychoanalytic incursions, and desperation to stem the relentless tide of chronicity made psychiatry particularly receptive to the revolutionary somatic treatments for schizophrenia. Manfred Sakel announced insulin shock treatment in Vienna in 1933; a year later, in Budapest, Ladislas Meduna launched convulsive therapy. The widespread interest in these coinciding developments was driven not by their dubious theoretical rationale, but by results. Such treatments increased the prospects of bringing psychiatry closer to general medicine, but also met scepticism. A leading figure in American psychiatry, Adolph Meyer, warned against a lurch toward a somatic model, and practitioners of psychoanalytic leanings reacted with dismay, but their tortuous pursuit of the underlying roots of mental disorder appeared impotent against the dramatic new physical treatments. Max Müller made his clinic in Münsingen, Switzerland, a world center for evaluation of shock therapies; his clinic hosted the First International Meeting on Modern Treatment of Schizophrenia in 1937. Literature on the new methods mushroomed. A timely manual devoted to shock therapy by Jessner and Ryan appeared in 1941, followed by lengthier texts by Sargant and Slater in 1944 and by Kalinowsky, Hoch, and Lewis in 1946, both of these running to several editions, appending psychosurgery and drugs to their contents (Figure 2.1). At last psychiatry had a technology of its own.

Chemical convulsants

Meduna's line of enquiry followed interesting observations on the relationship between psychosis and epilepsy (Kennedy, 1937). In 1929, Müller observed improvement in two patients with schizophrenia after spontaneous epileptic fits. Nyirö and Jablonszky observed that epileptic patients with schizophrenic features had remission of psychosis during periods of frequent seizures, and in 1931 Glaus remarked on the near absence of epilepsy in 6,000 patients with schizophrenia. The idea that the conditions might be mutually exclusive suggested the possibility of curing one disease with the other. In 1932 Nyirö transfused blood from epileptic patients into patients with schizophrenia, but without success. Meduna (1934) believed that artificially induced seizures would produce biochemical changes that might arrest the progress of schizophrenia. In animal experiments he identified a candidate analeptic to test his theory. Camphor had already been used in mental disease, by Weickhardt, whose *Medizinisches Praktisches Handbuch* of 1798 recommended its use in lunatics to the point at which seizures occurred, and by French and English physicians of the same era (Kennedy, 1937). Meduna's first recipient had been immersed in catatonic stupor for four years. After an anxious wait of 45 minutes following injection, a full epileptic seizure ensued, and after four further treatments, the patient was transformed. Meduna (1934) published his first series of results later that year. However, camphorated oil, administered intramuscularly, presented significant technical difficulties, with seizure sometimes delayed for up to three hours. A synthetic camphor, PTZ, was already in use as a cardiac stimulant, manufactured by Knoll under the trade name Cardiazol (Metrazol in the United States). Being soluble in water, this compound was suitable for intravenous use, producing a seizure soon after injection.

Procedure

To facilitate a seizure, PTZ was injected rapidly through a wide-bore needle. As a 20% concentration caused local pain and coagulation; the standard delivery was diluted to 10%. Excessive haste risked rupture or thrombosis. The optimum dose for each patient (usually around 5 mL) was found by trial and error. The needle was usually left in situ so that a further dose could be administered if no fit occurred within 20 seconds. Attendants stood on each side, applying pressure to restrain limbs and prevent flexion of the neck. First signs of seizure appeared within 10 seconds as the patient turned pale and rigid and emitted a cough or cry. On loss of consciousness, invariably the mouth opened wide for several seconds, a characteristic feature of PTZ treatment. This allowed insertion of a mouth gag to avert the common casualty of jaw dislocation. The ensuing grand mal seizure began with major tonic spasms lasting about 10 seconds, followed by a clonic stage of about 40 seconds, ending with brief apnea and livid cyanosis. On waking from a few minutes of comatose sleep, the patient was monitored by attendants until any confusion subsided.

As patients were subjected to a frightening sensation between injection and seizure, apprehension toward further treatments was alleviated by paraldehyde or hyoscine, but these drugs increased the likelihood of an unsuccessful injection. Some practitioners administered PTZ during insulin sopor to avoid the unpleasantness (Sands, 1939); Neustatter et al. (1939) used general anesthesia. However, such techniques complicated the treatment, and most clinicians relied on coercion to continue courses. PTZ was given intramuscularly in resistive patients or where veins were obliterated, but absorption rate was unpredictable. Unsuccessful additional doses left patients in a confusional twilight state for several hours, often causing marked anxiety. The unpleasantness of PTZ encouraged trials of alternative compounds, of which the best known was cyclohexylethyltriazol, brand named Triazol. Of lesser bulk, it could be injected with less haste, and despite a longer wait between injection and fit, patients found the treatment less distressing (Mayer-Gross and Walk, 1938). Similar advantages were reported with ammonium chloride and picrotoxin (Bleckwinn et al., 1940), but substitute products were hampered by technical shortcomings.

Indications and results

Remission figures of more than 70% were claimed at the Münsingen conference in 1937. However, results diverged between treatment centers, and meaningful evaluation was hindered by differences in application and recording. Whereas some practitioners targeted the most amenable cases, others showed indiscriminate faith in PTZ as a specific treatment for schizophrenia. Loosely defined outcome categories made results prone to exaggeration; recovery might mean anything from cessation of symptoms to modest improvement, and "social remissions" was a particularly nebulous entity. Notwithstanding these anomalies, consistent themes emerged. Duration of illness became a major determinant of treatment success, as did the presentations of schizophrenia; consequently, writers subdivided treatment groups by using Bleuler's (1924) classification based on symptoms and prognosis (simple, hebephrenic, catatonic, and paranoid). PTZ produced the best results during catatonic stupor, but proved less effective during catatonic excitement and in paranoid patients.

Initially, overall results appeared to match those of insulin therapy, leading to the suggestion that PTZ would supersede insulin because of its simplicity and safety (Wyllie, 1938). Pullar-Strecker's (1938) review of European data found 37% complete or incomplete remissions for schizophrenia after PTZ treatment, compared with 40% after insulin. Reitmann (1939), restricting his analysis of European and American results to 840 cases of fewer than 18-months duration, found an average complete remission rate of 52%, considerably better than that achieved with insulin. In 3,000 cases of similar duration from 75 American and European hospitals, Meduna and Friedman (1939) also reported 52% remissions, plus another 20% improved, although in cases of more than 18 months only 10% recovered. As data accumulated, judgments became more sober. From a large survey of New York state hospitals, Ross and Malzberg (1939) found that PTZ produced outcomes starkly inferior to those of insulin, and no better than in an untreated control group. These figures were extremely disappointing, but the sample was

Table 2.1 Outcomes of somatic treatments and controls (Ross and Malzberg, 1939)

Treatment	Cases	Recovered	Much improved	Improved	Unimproved	Died
Insulin	1757	11.1%	26.5%	26.0%	35.2%	1.1%
PTZ	1140	1.6%	9.9%	24.5%	63.5%	0.5%
Control	1039	3.5%	11.2%	7.4%	73.3%	4.6%

Note: PTZ, pentylenetetrazol.

imbalanced: Only 15% of the PTZ group had been ill for less than one year (Table 2.1).

Meduna accepted that his treatment was symptomatic rather than curative, but believed that results reinforced its role in the battle against schizophrenia (Meduna and Rohny, 1939). The limitations of PTZ were underlined by the tendency for relapse. In their haste to publish their successes, early writers had given insufficient time to assess sustainability of remissions. Notkin et al. (1940) found that only 18% of 100 patients with schizophrenia were well six months after PTZ treatment, compared with 8% of controls. Psychotherapeutic opportunities were presented as patients became accessible, but the reality of understaffed institutions left doctors little time for formal adjunctive psychotherapy, and Kalinowsky et al. (1946) found psychological work precluded by postictal confusion. Many practitioners persevered with the treatment in chronic schizophrenia, particularly in hospitals yet to introduce insulin. Although full recovery was unlikely in cases of advanced deterioration, PTZ temporarily increased social performance and made wards more manageable (Wyllie, 1940). However, Bain (1940) warned against judging patients to have benefited when they had merely improved in conduct. He described one man who, prior to PTZ treatment, had continually pestered doctors for his release. Although marked as "greatly improved," on closer examination he had lost all interest in his future, his will crushed by the mental trauma of repeated convulsive treatments. Observing several cases of deterioration following treatment, Bain explained that, for the patient with schizophrenia, fantasy was preferable to reality, and that such a disturbing stimulus did more harm than good.

Although PTZ was valued as an early intervention for schizophrenia, its full potential was revealed by practitioners straying beyond the initial indication. The first report of PTZ to treat affective disorders was by Verstraeten (1937). Finding dramatic results in cases of depression, Cook (1938a) concluded that convulsive therapy removed morbid reaction states, whether occurring in schizophrenia or other disorders. Low and colleagues (1938) successfully treated manic-depressive psychosis at either pole, noting that duration of illness had little influence, unlike with schizophrenia. Bennett (1940a), after terminating two thirds of manic states and achieving cures in nearly all cases of psychotic depression, claimed that the true indication for convulsive therapy was affective disorders. In depression, just five seizures were sufficient for full recovery (Kalinowsky et al., 1946), and the debilitating condition of involutional melancholia was particularly amenable to convulsive therapy. Indeed, convulsive therapy proved so reliable in arresting a depressive episode that it became a diagnostic aid: Positive outcome within six shocks confirmed affective disorder, whereas tardy response suggested deeper psychopathology.

How had convulsive therapy initially appeared so effective in schizophrenia? Targeted against acute catatonic reactions, it attacked cases with the best prospects of spontaneous recovery. According to Dynes (1939), affective sequelae such as elation in some patients following PTZ treatment raised doubts about diagnostic accuracy. Good (1940) attributed earlier results to erroneous classification of patients with mania and depression as those with schizophrenia. Aubrey Lewis (1938/2003) observed that Meduna and followers painted schizophrenia with a broad brush. At that time schizophrenia was diagnosed more frequently in Europe than in the United States (Jessner and Ryan, 1941) and in Britain, where the older pessimistic label "dementia praecox" was applied, usually only after confirmation by repeat episodes. By urging treatment as soon as symptoms appeared, rather than wasting time in confirming a diagnosis, Meduna probably encouraged a schizophrenic salient into affective disorders (McCrae, 2006), illustrating a phenomenon noted by Braslow (1997), whereby diagnostic practice is determined by available treatment. Although PTZ undoubtedly brought remissions in true cases of acute schizophrenia, unwittingly mixed groups of patients would at least partly explain the inconsistency in results.

Complications

Fatalities during PTZ treatment were uncommon. Müller (1937) reported one death in 495 patients; a larger survey found a mortality of 0.1% (Kolb and Vogel, 1942). Risks were minimized by excluding patients with cardiovascular disease. Convulsive treatment sometimes reactivated pulmonary tuberculosis, a leading cause of mortality in squalid mental institutions. The immediate hazard of status epilepticus was exacerbated when practitioners supplemented unsuccessful doses, potentially increasing the convulsant to dangerous levels. This was a particular problem with cyclohexylethyltriazol, which took longer to produce seizure, and after several deaths many practitioners reverted to PTZ (Kalinowsky et al., 1946). Toxic sequelae included vomiting, delirium, and psychomotor excitement. Euphoria was common on the following day, and florid symptoms sometimes appeared (Kennedy, 1937). Neuropathological effects were initially reported as negligible and limited to transient functional disturbance and memory loss. However, reflecting the ongoing debate on ECT, concerns were raised about lasting impairment, especially in patients receiving lengthy courses (Dynes, 1939). Animal tests showed cortical damage from prolonged application. Amnesia appeared similar to that found in organic psychoses (Jessner and Ryan, 1941). Although intellectual deficits were scarcely discernible in most patients, Tooth and Blackburn (1939) warned of them in highly educated persons. Others argued that the benefits of shock treatment outweighed any permanent damage to nervous tissue (Wyllie, 1940).

The worst complications were related to the severity of the seizure, which Wyllie (1938, p. 271) described as "to the novice greatly alarming." Unlike those in idiopathic epilepsy, the tonic spasms had a lightning onset. Incidence of skeletal injuries was high, including fractures to the neck of femur, humerus, and thoracic vertebrae (Pollock, 1939). Preventative measures included various manual restraint techniques and ensuring hyperextension of the spine before injection. Morphine or hyoscine made posture less rigid prior to seizure (Cook, 1938b), but necessitated a higher analeptic dose, risking status epilepticus. Bellinger (1939) issued calcium supplements, attributing fractures to deficiencies in the hospital diet. The treatment came under fire at the American Psychiatric Association conference in 1939, after x-rays revealed hairline vertebral fractures in an alarming 43% of patients (Polatin et al., 1939). Most radiologically identified fractures were symptomless and caused no permanent disability (Read, 1940), but despite these assurances the damage was done. With the treatment facing abolition in America, clearly the only resolution was to reduce the severity of seizure. A pioneer of fracture prevention was Abram Bennett (1940b) in Nebraska. He had used insulin to administer PTZ during a state of drowsiness and muscular dystonia, and also tried spinal anesthesia. Bennett was using curare to relieve spastic paralyses in children, when Walter Freeman, of later eminence in psychosurgery, encouraged him to try it in greater strength as a muscle relaxant in PTZ therapy (Sneader, 1985). Curare reduced motor severity without apparent dilution of treatment effects. However, originally used by South American Indians for arrow poison, curare was a dangerous substance, its clinical and fatal dose very close, with respiratory failure a serious risk. Increased mortality in convulsive therapy was blamed on curare, its dangers evidently worse than the fractures it was meant to prevent (Charlton et al., 1942). Other substances with curarelike action were found equally hazardous, until the short-acting succinylcholine was introduced in 1951 (Holmberg and Thesleff, 1952). The psychological aspects of convulsive therapy are considered later in this chapter.

Replacement by ECT

Ugo Cerletti and his assistant Bini (1937) announced electroshock therapy at Münsingen in 1937, demonstrating it in Rome in the following year. Although it seemed drastic, the electrical method offered clear advantages over PTZ. Perhaps most persuasively, as patients lost consciousness on activation of electrodes, the dreadful aura was avoided, thus improving cooperation. By the end of the decade, ECT was beginning to replace chemical convulsants, its introduction delayed only by lack of available apparatus. Lacking toxicity, ECT could be safely administered in outpatient clinics. Moreover, seizures appeared less violent, bringing a timely reduction in musculoskeletal injuries: Hemphill and Walter (1941) reported just one fracture in more than 200 patients, and on x-ray Lingley and Robbins (1947) found a 23% incidence of vertebral fractures with "straight" ECT, half that reported with PTZ. No new theory of action was offered; the principal indication remained schizophrenia, for which Cerletti promoted lengthy courses, generally avoided with PTZ. By the time ECT was introduced, the application of convulsive therapy had shifted toward affective disorders. After their first year of using ECT on a mixed group, Hemphill and Walter confirmed that patients with depression and mania fared best and stated, "*The original conception that convulsion therapy had its principal use in the treatment of schizophrenia is now abandoned and early hypotheses on its mode of action cannot be upheld*" (1941, p. 270). However, they suggested that convulsive therapy retain a place in psychosis, adding that "*the possibility of improving the large numbers of old schizophrenics that fill the chronic wards of every large hospital is of special interest*" (p. 273). Kalinowsky et al. (1946) stated that ECT had an assured role in schizophrenia, matching the remission rates initially found with PTZ in acute cases.

Just as PTZ was being abandoned, Bianchi and Chiarello (1945) reported outcomes superior to those of ECT, a finding supported in a large-scale study by Fasanaro (1947). PTZ was believed to produce seizures of deeper impact, and some practitioners valued its potency in cases of stupor and food refusal (Dax, 1951). In addition, there was initial apprehension among patients toward ECT, perhaps because of connotations with the "electric chair." However, by the late 1940s ECT was established as the standard convulsive method. Some years later, Berg and Robbins (1959) introduced a new chemical compound. Tetramethyl-succinamide (PM-1090) was administered orally or intravenously, but despite promising results it was discontinued because of unpredictable delay before seizure, precluding use of muscle relaxants (Kalinowsky and Hoch, 1961). As a last remnant, in the final edition of their somatic treatment manual, Sargant and Slater (1972) retained PTZ for severely agitated depressive or stuporous states.

Insulin coma treatment

Soon after its isolation in 1922, insulin began to be used for symptomatic purposes in psychiatry, initially to increase weight in anorectic patients, but it was also found to alleviate agitation (Wortis, 1959). Sakel, who had been using insulin to treat morphine addiction, beginning in 1928 began deliberately inducing hypoglycemic states. Observing that an inadvertent coma had a beneficial impact on psychotic symptoms, Sakel hypothesized a hypoglycemic cure for schizophrenia. The eminent Professor Otto Pöetzl allowed him to develop his work at the university psychiatric clinic in Vienna, where the first cases were treated in 1933 (Wortis, 1959). A preliminary report in 1934 met a barrage of scepticism, but Müller began a major evaluation of the treatment at Münsingen, supervised by Dussik, a previous colleague of Sakel. Impressive results from several centers were presented at the international conference in 1937. However, the complexity and hazards of Sakel's treatment contrasted sharply with PTZ therapy. Whereas PTZ injections took a few minutes, insulin coma therapy required constant medical attendance for several hours. Special units were established, with skilled nurses deployed. Although insulin showed greater promise in treating schizophrenia, its introduction was constrained by its demand for resources (e.g., Colomb and Wadsworth, 1941). Because of wartime shortages, many British hospitals did not initiate insulin coma therapy until 1945 or later (McCrae, 2006).

Procedure

Insulin was administered intramuscularly, and the patient became increasingly drowsy, falling into a deep coma in the fifth hour. Courses began with gradual titration aimed at finding the minimum coma dose before a lengthy series of deep comas was induced. Typical courses entailed 50 to 60 treatments, but sometimes more than 100. Coma was not consistently defined. As physical signs varied enormously, Küppers (1937) demarcated the precoma phase by conscious reaction. One hour of deep coma was preferred, extended to 90 minutes by some practitioners. Coma was interrupted with glucose by nasogastric or intravenous tube. As it brought sudden arousal, intravenous glucose was reserved for emergencies. In later years coma was terminated with glucagon, a pancreatic hormone, which had a gradual action and could be given intramuscularly, thereby avoiding risk of thrombosis (Kalinowsky and Hippius, 1969). Pursuit of improved efficacy and efficiency led to modifications to Sakel's procedure. W. Kraulis in Latvia prolonged the coma for up to 12 hours by administering small amounts of glucose throughout, and Joseph Wortis for up to 24 hours, but protracted coma risked permanent brain damage (Kalinowsky and Hoch, 1961). Ambulatory insulin treatment, whereby the patient remained alert and mobile except during the peak of hypoglycemia, was applied by Polatin et al. (1940a), and many of these courses stretched to several years.

Indications and results

Insulin evaluation suffered from shortcomings similar to those of its contemporary developments of the 1930s, with inconsistencies in diagnosis; targeting of the treatment, intensity, and duration of courses; and outcome measurement. From the

Table 2.2 Full and partial remissions from insulin therapy

Duration of illness	Müller	Ross and Malzberg
0 to 6 months	59%	59%
7 to 12 months	52%	51%
13 to 24 months	27%	38%

outset, Sakel (1935) acknowledged that the treatment had a considerably reduced impact on chronic schizophrenia, as confirmed by Müller (1937), whose survey found full recovery in 73% of early cases, 50% in cases of duration between 6 and 18 months, but only 0.5% in longer-term cases. Results of a larger series by Müller (1939) showed remarkable concordance with those of an extensive survey by Ross and Malzberg (1939) at New York state hospitals (Table 2.2). Ross and Malzberg concluded, "*it is quite evident that we have obtained a potent agent to deal with dementia praecox.*"

Although insulin and PTZ showed overall equivalence in reversing acute schizophrenia, in subacute cases insulin was demonstrably superior. Its value was greatest in catatonic excitement and paranoid cases, the latter subtype being resistant to PTZ and least amenable to naturalistic recovery. Simple and hebephrenic types were less responsive, but despite such limitations, insulin was believed to intervene with the disease process. However, results varied widely between treatment centers. Frostig (1940) associated poorer outcomes with deviations from Sakel's technique, noting that some practitioners tended to interrupt coma prematurely. Bond and Rivers (1944) found a stark contrast between their results of 1936 to 1938 and those of later years, when deeper and longer comas were produced; remission rates increased from 46% to 79%. Shorter courses may have contributed to the less favorable outcomes reported by Rennie and Fowler (1943) and Gottlieb and Huston (1951), who gave an average of 36 and 30 treatments, respectively. Evidence suggested that remissions outlasted those effected by PTZ therapy. Examining data on more than 1,000 cases per year after treatment, Ross and colleagues (1941) found that patients who had made full recoveries mostly remained stable. Bond and Rivers (1944) obtained 55% remissions at the end of treatment, decreasing to 42% one year later and to 31% after three years. Reviewing 10 years of data, Freudenberg (1947) reported 56% full and social remissions compared with 34% in untreated patients. Not only did insulin produce roughly double the rate of spontaneous recoveries, but several writers described a higher quality of emotional, social, and intellectual improvement than in self-remissions.

Yet, as the relatively convenient ECT was increasingly applied as frontline treatment in schizophrenia, practitioners began to reserve insulin for resistant cases, thus limiting its potential effectiveness. Sakel's optimistic report to the International

Congress of Psychiatry in Paris in 1950 met criticism; Mayer-Gross (1951) stated that insulin was ineffective in half of the treated cases. Comparing three treatment groups receiving brief psychotherapy, insulin, and ECT, Gottlieb and Huston (1951) reported no difference in outcomes after four years, rejecting the claim that insulin had a lasting impact on schizophrenia. An influential article, *The Insulin Myth* (Bourn, 1953), attributed positive results to flaws in evaluation. David (1954) argued that 20 years of insulin coma therapy had not produced conclusive evidence of its merits. Use of insulin coma was already in gradual decline by the early 1950s, and its death knell was sounded by Ackner et al. (1957), whose randomized, blinded study of insulin- versus barbiturate-induced coma found no difference in outcomes. Clearly insulin was not the specific agent. The demise of insulin was hastened by the pharmacological revolution. Fink and colleagues (1958) compared chlorpromazine with insulin for four months and found no difference, but the convenience of the "wonder drugs" made insulin treatment an unnecessary hazard and expense.

As insulin treatment was reappraised, many advocates were swayed by the notion that a therapeutic vibe, rather than any physiological action, explained its effects. Just as early appraisal had been skewed by excessive optimism, insulin therapy came to be rashly dismissed. Contrasting with the acceptance of neuroleptics as maintenance regimens, insulin was unfairly measured as a curative procedure. Realistically, insulin was an effective symptomatic therapy: A single series often produced lasting remission, and although relapses often necessitated repeat courses, lengthy periods free from biological intervention were possible. Kalinowsky and Hoch (1961) continued their endorsement, and some centers persevered with insulin through the 1960s. In the last revision of the manual on physical treatment in 1969, Kalinowsky and Hippius appealed, "*Since the technical difficulties and dangers of insulin coma have been diminished, this method should be retained as an important tool in the treatment of schizophrenia*" (p. 299). Markowe et al. (1967) issued fresh evidence that the results of insulin matched those of chlorpromazine. However, even in the largest hospitals, demand fell below the critical mass to justify special treatment units. In the Soviet Union, orthodox insulin therapy remained the treatment of choice, but elsewhere, as coma was contraindicated during neuroleptic therapy, the ambulatory method became favored. Sargant and Slater had initially restricted this procedure to neuroses, believing that schizophrenia required full coma and that positive results in this condition may have been skewed by unanticipated comas. However, in their 1972 text, Sargant and Slater deemed sopor sufficient, stating, "*we now believe it wise to give every early schizophrenic the benefit of a full course of ECT while he is under one or other of the phenothiazines, and to make sure the patient's weight is restored to normal or above normal by modified insulin therapy.*" This use of insulin to produce general physical improvement revived the original work of the 1920s.

Complications

Unquestionably, insulin therapy was a perilous procedure. In a Canadian survey, Kinsey (1941) reported 90 deaths in 12,234 patients, compared with 43 in 18,543 PTZ patients. In the spirit of the times, writers assured that relieving morbidity of the multitude trumped mortality of a few. As physicians gained experience with the procedure, the fatality rate fell, from 1.29%, reported by Ross and Malzberg (1939) in New York hospitals, to 0.85% in 305 hospitals surveyed by Kolb and Vogel (1942), and to around 0.5% by the late 1940s (e.g., Müller, 1949). The catastrophe of irreversible coma emphasized the need for careful titration of insulin units, but insulin coma therapy remained a hazard even with experienced application. Emergencies were caused by vasomotor collapse or respiratory distress, and sometimes large doses of glucose failed to arouse the patient. The use of glucagon, according to Kalinowsky and Hippius (1969), virtually eliminated fatalities. In 1972, Sargant and Slater boasted of only one death since 1937. The possibility of neurological damage was discussed, but there was consensus that intellectual impairment was of lesser severity and duration than in convulsive therapy. According to Polatin et al. (1940b), clinical symptoms, electroencephalographic (EEG) imaging, and psychological performance tests showed only temporary cerebral disturbance. The convulsive aspect of insulin therapy will be discussed in depth later in this chapter.

Combined insulin and chemical convulsants

Sharing the same indication, but with different impact, insulin and convulsive treatments were sometimes synergized. In cases failing to respond to the initial intervention, Erb (1936) crossed treatments. Hebephrenic schizophrenia cases were given insulin followed by a series of PTZ shocks before a further course of insulin; in catatonic cases, the sequence was reversed. James et al. (1937), after noting better outcomes in patients having seizures during hypoglycemia, administered PTZ on insulin rest days. Georgi and Strauss (1937) maximized therapeutic potential by administering PTZ during insulin coma treatment and presented their "summation treatment" at Münsingen in 1937, reporting good results in patients responding insufficiently to insulin alone. Their method removed the unpleasant experience of PTZ therapy, and as fits were less severe, fewer injuries resulted. Furthermore, the seizure threshold was lowered by insulin, enabling Georgi and Strauss to obtain a 72% occurrence of seizures compared with 66% with PTZ alone. A favored model was von Braunmühl's block method, entailing a course of 20 to 30 insulin comas, then a brief series of PTZ injections during hypoglycemia, followed by a further 10 insulin treatments.

Procedure

Georgi and Strauss administered PTZ during the second hour of hypoglycemia, when motor irritability appeared as blood sugar dipped to its lowest level. Unless a spontaneous fit had occurred first, Tillim (1940) induced seizures as consciousness clouded in the third hour. As seizure threshold was lowered by hypoglycemia, half the normal PTZ dose sufficed, and even less for patients exhibiting myoclonic activity. It was generally agreed that coma should be interrupted after seizure to prevent dangerous strain on the cardiovascular system, but Tillim allowed patients to return to coma, which he terminated in the fifth hour as usual. Some practitioners induced seizures during deep coma, but high doses of PTZ or electrical current were required, and fits were atypical (Kalinowsky and Hoch, 1961). Although otherwise supplanted by ECT, chemical convulsants were often preferred in combined treatment (Polonio and Slater, 1954).

Indications and results

Induced seizures appeared to significantly boost the effectiveness of insulin, particularly in resistant cases. Von Braunmühl (1942) produced 56% remissions in acute schizophrenia, 51% in cases of six months to one year, and 26% in cases of one to two years duration. The best results were in catatonic excitement (66%), although the condition showing most benefit compared with insulin alone was stupor. Chapuis (1942) reported lower rates of relapse at Georgi's hospital, where patients received around 10 to 20 shock treatments within a course of 70 to 80 insulin comas. Full remissions were obtained in 71% of cases, and after five years most of these patients remained stable. Russell (1938) recommended routine use of PTZ to shorten courses of insulin therapy, but Jessner and Ryan (1941) reserved summation treatment for cases responding inadequately to insulin alone. Kalinowsky et al. (1946) were not convinced of any improvement on single methods, but as the combined method tended to be reserved for patients failing to respond to ECT or insulin alone, a preponderance of treatment-resistant cases would have significantly detracted from its effectiveness. Sakel generally opposed combined treatment, accepting its use only in catatonic stupor (Wortis, 1959). As results in other disorders were disappointing, the combined method, like insulin alone, was restricted to schizophrenia. Mayer-Gross (1951) endorsed the method in schizophrenia with an affective component.

Complications

By all accounts the combined method was relatively safe. Von Braunmühl recorded only 0.37% fatalities, far lower than even centers of excellence achieved with insulin alone. The main reason was the reduced risk of irreversible coma, despite the larger amount of insulin required in combined courses, as hypoglycemia was usually terminated after seizure. The fear and fractures of conventional PTZ therapy were also avoided.

Flurothyl inhalation

Through serendipity, a new method of convulsive therapy emerged in the late 1950s. During research on anesthesia, Krantz and colleagues (1957) observed convulsive properties in a light concentration of fluorinated ether. In 1956, Krantz began work with Esquibel and Kurland at Spring Grove State Hospital in Maryland to test the compound flurothyl as convulsive therapy, where it was found as effective as ECT (Esquibil et al., 1958), well tolerated, and indeed preferred by some patients, particularly those with apprehension about electric shock (Kurland et al., 1960). Marketed as Indoklon, it became generally available in 1961 (Arce, 1970). Flurothyl was also administered intravenously, but following reports of venous sclerosis and risk of thrombus, the inhalational method was favored. Around 0.5 to 1 mL was administered through a vaporizer, connected to an oxygen bag and a tightly fitted face mask. The bag was squeezed repeatedly until seizure occurred, usually within 40 seconds (Arce, 1970). The anesthetic action of flurothyl meant that the patient lost consciousness before the seizure. Initially the treatment was administered in unmodified form, as the need for respiratory effort precluded use of muscle relaxants, but incidence of fractures was high. Karliner and Padula (1959) resolved this problem by simultaneous administration of succinylcholine. Onset of seizure was slower than in ECT. A period of myoclonic activity was followed by a tonic–clonic convulsion, with a prolonged clonic phase. EEG investigations by Small and Small (1972) showed that ECT and flurothyl seizures were basically similar, but the latter produced fits lasting an average of 104 seconds, compared with 45 seconds in ECT.

Unlike its precursors in the 1930s, flurothyl was subjected to robust scientific evaluation, with use of sensitive neuropsychological instruments. Several studies supported its effectiveness in clinical practice. Dolenz (1965) obtained positive outcomes with a sample of mostly patients who were schizoaffective or depressed who had failed to respond to ECT, whereas Lapolla and colleagues (1965) reported improvement without complications in all 40 cases of severe mental disorder, with an average of only six treatments. Collating data from six studies using the inhalational method between 1958 and 1970, Arce (1970) found 78 excellent recoveries, 144 good results, and only 10 failures. A review by Small and Small (1972) confirmed that the results of flurothyl use matched those of ECT. Some writers recommended Indoklon on the basis of reduced postictal confusion and memory impairment, possibly because of oxygen in the gas mixture.

Yet the treatment failed to replace ECT, mainly because of technical difficulties. Leakage from ill-fitting masks caused incomplete seizures. Restricted by thiopental and barbiturates, fits were not always obvious (Gander et al., 1967). The dissolved gas lingered in the bloodstream, and secondary seizures occurred in around one quarter of treatments (Kalinowsky and Hoch, 1961). From their experience, Kalinowsky and Hippius (1969) disagreed that flurothyl, compared with ECT, produced less marked confusion and memory deficits. Dolenz (1967) observed delayed confusional states. Headaches were worse after flurothyl, with severe cases reported by Gander and colleagues (1967). Nausea frequently required injection of an antiemetic (Kalinowsky and Hippius, 1969). In their manual of 1961, Kalinowsky and Hoch suggested that "Indoklon might easily replace ECT" (p. 128), but in the 1969 edition its application was restricted to patients hostile to ECT. Arce (1970) regarded flurothyl as a useful alternative to ECT for severe depression, schizoaffective states with depressive symptoms, and acute schizophrenia with excitement or catatonic stupor. Sebag-Montefiore (1974) reported excellent results in depression, but the procedure remained on the sidelines. Sargant and Slater omitted any mention in their 1972 manual. With limited commercial prospects, Indoklon was soon discontinued by its manufacturer.

Theoretical implications

As the modus operandi of insulin and convulsive therapy was never identified, both treatments remained empirical. Sakel produced an unwieldy working hypothesis for insulin (1935), relating to suppression of excitation in the nervous system, and Meduna (1935) based convulsive therapy on biological antagonism, but several alternative theories were postulated. Cobb (1938) suggested that both treatments worked by destroying swathes of the cerebral cortex. Other physiological theories related to anoxia, sugar metabolism, and cardiovascular effects, but none reached general acceptance. The advent of shock treatments coincided with the psychoanalytic zenith, and some practitioners suggested that therapeutic effects resulted not from biochemical action but as a psychological response to severe bodily assault.

The fear factor in convulsive therapy

Insulin and PTZ therapies presented quite different experiences for the patient. The tender atmosphere of the insulin ward, where even seemingly impenetrable patients with schizophrenia responded to intense medical and nursing attention in an otherwise impersonal institution, contrasted sharply with the brief violence of PTZ. Writers candidly told of terror and hostility from patients. Bewilderment immediately after injection was followed by a steadily building apprehension as the drug reached the central nervous system (CNS), causing sensations of flashing lights and heat circulating in the body (Good, 1940). Intense dread was terminated by loss of consciousness and seizure, unless a subconvulsive dose had been administered. Despite remarks to the contrary by Meduna, Gillespie (1939) found that most patients feared the treatment, typified by the quote: *"the very thought of it makes me shrink with horror."* Many patients were unwilling to discuss their trauma afterward. Good (1940) witnessed extreme efforts to escape: Patients struggled with attendants, jumped through windows, climbed on to the hospital roof, and even attempted suicide.

The relationship between fear and outcome was a matter of much interest. Several writers were convinced that psychological trauma was the therapeutic mechanism (Abse, 1944; Good, 1940). Meduna himself believed that fear contributed to treatment success, but others disagreed. Jessner and Ryan (1941) observed that apprehensive patients tended to show least improvement. Blaurock et al. (1939) investigated the extent to which results of PTZ therapy were influenced by the seizure, pharmacological effects, or fear. Comparing groups treated with convulsive doses, nonconvulsive doses, or sodium chloride, they found no evidence that fear was associated with therapeutic benefit. Cohen (1939) administered PTZ slowly to 20 patients with schizophrenia, increasing the preparoxysmal period to several minutes or even hours, then administered a conventional course one month later with significantly better outcomes. However, both of these studies had flaws. The comparator courses in the first study would not have generated the same level of fear, whereas the second study inflicted such cruelty that patients were surely relieved to receive an immediately convulsant dose!

Contrasting with the mild impact of insulin coma, Silbermann described PTZ therapy as "a violent thunderstorm," giving "a far more vehement shock" (1940, p. 179). He noted that insulin therapy produced better results when seizures occurred, and believed that the psychotic ego required a strong force for its disruption. He quoted one patient's experience of death and resurrection: *"I have never in all my life felt such a terrible thing as after the injection . . . now I feel I am a new person, entirely changed, as though I had been born again"* (p. 187). Euphoria following treatment was attributed to the overwhelming relief of having survived helpless submission to mortal danger, but there was a deeper psychological impact. Schilder (1939) believed that PTZ overcame libido fixations, leading to reconstruction of emotions. Freed from superego suppression, patients who were previously psychotic came to rationally reappraise reality. Abse (1944) explained that seizures disrupted the process of introversion in schizophrenia, the defensive reaction against trauma stimulating repression of primal anxiety; he believed that cases of fixed delusions or extreme apathy were least amenable to this mechanism. Another psychoanalytic theme was the fulfillment of punishment desire, although cleansing of sins would have little lasting impact on ingrained masochistic attitudes (Silbermann, 1940).

A problem in explaining the psychogenic impact of treatment is that responses vary widely: For one patient fear may be absent or inconsequential; for another it might significantly influence the outcome. Reactions changed during courses. Perhaps as patients were lifted from stupor, they became more alert to the full terror of the treatment. PTZ may have operated, unwittingly, as a form of behavior modification; it would then make sense that remission rates were highest in early cases, whereas more established patients with schizophrenia might have been less able to adapt their behavior to avoid further trauma. Jessner and Ryan (1941) found that continuing courses beyond a satisfactory level of improvement was counterproductive.

Since the 1950s, several trials have shown superiority of ECT over sham treatment (Sartorius et al., 1993), suggesting that ECT has little psychological impact. Anxiety was minimized by refinement in premedication, and apprehensive patients are soon reassured by the painless experience of ECT (Freeman and Cheshire, 1986). As evidence suggests that chemical convulsants were more effective than ECT for catatonic stupor, was fear the difference? The terror associated with PTZ may have stimulated positive change, but lasting benefits were unlikely. By today's ethical standards, subjecting patients to a treatment that British psychiatrist Henry Rollin reflected on as "mediaeval torture" (Valentine, 1996, p. 80) would be unthinkable.

The convulsive factor in insulin coma therapy

Epileptiform phenomena frequently arose during insulin coma therapy. Frostig (1940) reported an incidence of only 2.8%, but Fink (2003) stated that grand mal seizures happened during around 10% of insulin treatments. Gross-May (1938) reported that 37 of his 105 patients experienced at least one seizure. As with other neurological responses to insulin treatment, seizures were unpredictable, occurring at any time during hypoglycemia and arising in patients without known epileptic susceptibility. Some patients had multiple convulsions (Sargant and Slater, 1954). All individuals have epileptic potential, and insulin coma therapy presented two conditions physiologically associated with seizures: hypoglycemia and deep sleep. In hypoglycemia, the brain is starved of its main energy source, stimulating electrical and biochemical reactions. Seizures stimulate a sudden increase in blood sugar, of around 15%. Almost half of epileptic patients have fits only while sleeping, and prior to refined anticonvulsant medication, daytime naps were discouraged in sleep-sensitive epileptic patients. Insulin coma therapy lowered the seizure threshold, but the therapeutic value of epileptic events remains inadequately understood.

Sakel (1935) described two types of response to insulin treatment: a "moist shock," with profuse perspiration; and a "dry shock," marked by epileptiform activity. Initially, Sakel regarded spontaneous seizures as a hazard, despite having witnessed their therapeutic potential; he later recalled a case in 1933 of a psychotic man who, on escaping from hospital, had jumped off a wall on to live electricity wires, causing violent convulsions, but for the next two weeks his schizophrenic symptoms vanished. Perhaps swayed by other practitioners such as Georgi and von Braunmühl, Sakel began administering PTZ during insulin treatments, but he soon abandoned chemical convulsants, reinforcing hypoglycemia as the sole mechanism. Followers of Sakel often witnessed his resentment toward convulsive therapy, a coinciding development that had diverted attention from insulin coma and a potential Nobel prize (Wortis, 1959). Yet having incidentally induced seizures in patients with schizophrenia before Meduna's work, Sakel (1938) felt justified in claiming convulsive therapy as his own discovery.

Müller minimized the therapeutic value of spontaneous seizures, a stance supported by data from Ross and Malzberg (1939). Plattner and Fröhlicher (1938) reported seizures in 4.3% of unimproved cases but only in 1.6% of recovered cases. However, a careful study over a five-year period by Hoenig and Leibermann (1953) produced strong evidence that spontaneous seizures were advantageous in cases with good prognosis and that recoveries from insulin treatment correlated with epileptic activity. Epileptic phenomena including twitching, myoclonus, or seizures occurred in one third of insulin comas, but in patients who recovered the rate was 41%, compared with 23% in unimproved cases. For seizures, the figures were 38% and 15%, respectively, suggesting that epileptic activity played an important therapeutic role in insulin coma therapy. Reappraising the treatment, Fink (2003, p. 288) attributed recoveries to the regular occurrence of grand mal seizures, stating that insulin "is best appreciated today as an inefficient form of convulsion therapy."

Antagonism revisited

The efficacy of seizures in insulin coma therapy should be considered in relation to the perceived relationship between epilepsy and schizophrenia, which evolved in 20th-century psychiatric literature. Affinity was the prevailing notion in Kraepelin's time. Not only did a large number of patients in mental hospitals have epilepsy, but symptoms of his trinity of psychotic disorders, comprising dementia praecox, manic-depressive psychosis, and epileptic insanity, frequently overlapped. Kraepelin (1919) observed epileptic features in 18% of patients with schizophrenia. Meduna attracted few adherents for his incompatibility thesis, the conditions apparently placed as discrete natural disease entities at opposite poles of a psychoneurological continuum. However, as Wolf and Trimble (1985) illuminated, Meduna's theory has tended to be misrepresented, partly because his writings often lacked precision. Well aware of the coexistence of psychosis and epilepsy from research at his same institution in Budapest by Nyirö and Jablonszky (1929), Meduna saw therapeutic implications in that epileptic patients with psychotic features tended to have a favorable prognosis. His treatment did not induce epilepsy but its major manifestation, and in his idea of mutual exclusivity he probably meant symptomatic antagonism operating within syndromic affinity.

By the 1940s, epilepsy and schizophrenia were regarded as coincidental (Hoch, 1943). The proportion of epileptic patients in mental hospitals diminished after the introduction of phenytoin (Merritt and Putman, 1938), and as psychiatry discarded the concept of epileptic insanity, epilepsy was ceded to neurology. However, a higher propensity to mental disorder among epileptic patients is generally recognized, although the relationship remains inadequately understood. Shortly after the birth of convulsive therapy, EEG imaging enabled Gibbs et al. (1938) to show that epileptoid changes were common in patients with schizophrenia. On finding that subcortical discharges correlated with the recovery process in schizophrenia, Hill (1945) proposed a "homeostatic theory" in which psychosis was corrected by seizures, and vice versa. In 1953, Hans Landolt discovered that the emergence of behavioral disturbance in epileptic patients during seizure-free periods was associated with normality in EEG readings, a phenomenon that he called "forced normalisation" (Schmitz, 1998). Slater et al. (1963) identified an excess prevalence of schizophrenic illness in epileptic patients. Noting that in all 69 of Slater's cases schizophrenia had followed epilepsy, by an average of 14 years, Reynolds (1968) suggested a delayed inhibitory mechanism. Several writers have argued that biochemical disturbances in either condition have a protective effect; Stevens (1998) presents a "yin and yang" relationship, whereby seizures and schizophrenia are an excessive response to imbalance in excitatory and inhibitory networks. Such theories remain controversial; Fenwick (1998) saw insufficient evidence for antagonism, being observable in only a few patients. A major confounding factor is the routine use of maintenance medication in both conditions. Neuroleptic drugs can trigger seizures, whereas highly retardant anticonvulsants such as phenobarbitone and phenytoin can seem to be psychotogenic. Pharmacological control of grand mal seizures sometimes leads to complex partial seizures associated with psychotic symptoms. However, an inhibitory mechanism cannot be dismissed. Inhibition was first demonstrated as an active biological process by Russian physiologist Sechenov in the 19th century, and neurological studies have shown that manipulation of the CNS can produce excessive response, possibly resulting from disruption of inhibitory circuits (Valenstein, 1973). A putative inborn antagonism might be complemented or counteracted by medicinal and shock treatments.

Convulsive therapy has proved an effective remedy for severe depressive illness, but although positive outcomes have been achieved in schizoaffective states, its value in schizophrenia appears limited (Ottoson, 1981), and it is not recommended for lengthy courses because of neurological sequelae. Repeated applications of PTZ or ECT, although producing transient improvement, might have blunted an innate inhibitory response. Instead of a sudden generalized tonic–clonic seizure, insulin treatment exposed patients to a mild but prolonged epileptogenic situation. Frostig (1940) recorded clonic twitchings in the third hour in 79% of cases, and in the fourth hour 83% had tonic spasms, but the implications of subconvulsive seizure activity may have been underestimated by practitioners. An antagonistic mechanism may have been stimulated, but left intact, by insulin coma therapy. Hoenig and Leibermann (1953) observed that seizure threshold fluctuated with progress of symptoms, being highest in stupor, and lowest at point of recovery. Catatonic patients with schizophrenia might therefore benefit from an initial course of convulsive therapy followed by a gentler analeptic over a longer duration. Studies in the 1950s refuted the idea that full motor effects were necessary for the therapeutic process in convulsive therapy. Recently, transcranial magnetic stimulation (TMS) has emerged as a possible therapy. Entering neurology in the 1980s as a diagnostic tool, TMS can trigger seizures in persons with a low threshold and was found to elevate mood in healthy subjects (Bickford et al., 1987). Repetitive low-frequency TMS entails a prolonged stimulation of around 20 minutes, generating submotor activity. As well as its possible antidepressant performance (Kolbinger et al., 1995), it has shown promise in schizophrenia. Lee et al. (2005) reported a reduction in psychotic symptoms in treatment-resistant patients with schizophrenia after 10 daily treatments. Side effects are confined to fleeting headache and amnesia, disappearing within minutes. Further research on TMS is warranted (Goodwin and Jamison, 2007), but results suggest that mild stimulation may be a more effective means of therapy in schizophrenia than are the generalized seizures induced by ECT, and may explain the possible superiority of insulin over ECT in treating this condition.

In his monograph, Meduna (1937) described schizophrenia as a heterogenous condition. Unlike the reactive endogenous type, the inherited symptomatic type responded well to convulsive therapy, often requiring lower doses for seizure. Meduna's observations were possibly skewed by patients misdiagnosed with depression, but his antagonistic theory could yet be revived by further investigation of epileptic potential in psychotic patients. The value of convulsive therapy in the affective component of schizophrenia may have been underestimated. In recent years, the extent of overlap in the functional psychoses has raised tentative challenge to Kraepelin's dichotomy (Craddock and Owen, 2005), and although such debate lies beyond the scope of this chapter, of relevance is the presence of epileptic patterns in bipolar as well as in schizophrenic illness. A hypothesized affinity between manic-depressive disorder and epilepsy dates from the Hippocratic corpus, and a common etiology and periodicity has interested psychiatrists and neurologists since epileptoid equivalents were described in the mid-19th century (Berrios, 1979). Interictal conditions have been described (Himmelhoch, 1984), but a wider subepileptic population may exist among psychotic patients. Anticonvulsants are increasingly used to augment or replace lithium therapy in bipolar disorder (Post and Speer,

2002); indeed carbamazepine, initially developed as an antidepressant, has been described as "a drug in search of a disorder" (Himmelhoch, 1984, p. 44). Such stabilizing treatment may have implications for a dynamic relationship between functional psychosis and epileptiform symptoms. Furthermore, fresh inferences might be drawn from insulin coma therapy.

A deeper understanding of the role of seizures in mental disorder requires a closer relationship between psychiatry and neurology. Yet these specialties have developed in parallel, polarized by a Cartesian dichotomy of mind and brain, reinforced by advances in diagnostic technology in neuroscience and the influence of psychodynamics (Price et al., 2000). Biological psychiatrists since the 1960s, encouraged by neuroanatomical advances, have pursued collaboration beyond a few conditions in "no man's land." Generally, psychiatry has shown limited interest in a rapprochement with neurology, perhaps fearing encroachment of naïve physical science on its esoteric cognizance of mental disorder, and a threat to its status was psyche to be marginalized in etiology, assessment, and treatment. Focusing on behavioral constructs without visible pathology, psychiatry has eschewed verifiable evidence; for example, in its classification of mental disorders. The danger of its value-laden approach is demonstrated by an uncritical acceptance and rejection of treatments such as insulin coma therapy and reactions to the ethical crusades on ECT. Consequently, the status of psychiatry has been hindered within a wider profession founded on scientific rigor (Cunningham et al., 2006). As knowledge accumulates on interaction between psychiatric symptoms and neurological processes, whatever the nature and direction of the relationship, much may be gained from a coalescence of psychiatric and neurological expertise. ECT may be fertile ground.

Conclusions

Unlike insulin, ECT survived modern scientific scrutiny to establish its place as a mainstream treatment in psychiatry. Chemical convulsants produced a basically similar seizure but may have had additional effects through psychological distress inflicted in preparoxysmal aura. Of greater relevance today is the convulsive aspect of hypoglycemic coma, inadequately understood in the heyday of insulin treatment units. If Fink was correct, and if prolonged epileptic activity as in TMS transpires as an effective therapeutic mechanism in functional psychosis, modern psychiatry may be as indebted to Sakel as to Meduna.

Acknowledgment

The author appreciates helpful comments by Mike Philpot and Michaela Poppe at the Institute of Psychiatry, King's College London.

References

Abse, W. 1944. Theory of the rationale of convulsion therapy. Br J Med Psychol 20: 33–50.

Ackner, B., Harris, A., and Oldham, A. J. 1957. Insulin treatment of schizophrenia. Lancet i: 607–11.

Arce, L. 1970. Indoklon: convulsive therapy: Experimental-clinical studies. Psychosomatics 11: 358–60.

Bain, A. J. 1940. The influence of Cardiazol on chronic schizophrenia. J Ment Sci 86: 502–13.

Bellinger, C. H. 1939. Discussion. Psychiatr Q 13: 569–73.

Bennett, A. E. 1940a. Metrazol convulsive shock therapy in affective psychoses: A follow up report of results obtained in 61 depressive and 9 manic cases. Am J Med Sci 198: 695–701.

Bennett, A. E. 1940b. Preventing traumatic complications in convulsive shock therapy by curare. JAMA 114: 322–4.

Berrios, G. E. 1979. Insanity and epilepsy in the nineteenth century. In Psychiatry, genetics and pathography: A tribute to Eliot Slater (eds. Roth, M. and Cowie, V.). London: Gaskell.

Berg, S. and Robbins, E. S. 1959. A pharmacological report on PM-1090. J Neuropsychiatr, 1: 32–4.

Bianchi, J. A. and Chiarello, C. J. 1945. Shock therapy in the involutional and manic-depressive psychoses. Psychiatr Q 18: 118–27.

Bickford, R. G., Guidie, N., Fertesque, P., and Svenson, M. 1987. Magnetic stimulation of human peripheral nerve and brain: Response and enhancement by combined magneto electrical technique. Neurosurgery 20: 110–16.

Bini, L. 1937. Richerche sperimentali nell'accesso epilettico da corrente elettrica. Schweizer Arch Neurol Psychiatr 39(supplement): 121–2.

Blaurock, M. F., Low, A. A., and Sachs, M. 1939. Influence of fear, pharmacological action and convulsion in metrazol therapy. Arch Neurol Psychiatry 42: 233–6.

Bleckwinn, W. J., Hodgson, E. R., and Herwick, R. P. 1940. Clinical comparison of picotroxin, metrazol and coriamyrtin used as analytics and as convulsants. J Pharmacol Exp Ther 69: 81–8.

Bleuler, E. 1924. Textbook of psychiatry. New York: Macmillan.

Bond, E. D. and Rivers, T. D. 1944. Insulin shock therapy after seven years. Am J Psychiatry 101: 62–3.

Bourn, H. 1953. The insulin myth. Lancet ii: 964–8.

Braslow, J. 1997. Mental ills and bodily cures: Psychiatric treatment in the first half of the twentieth century. Berkeley: University of California Press.

Bumke, O. 1929. Lehrbuch des Geisteskrankheiten. München: Bergmann.

Chapuis, R. 1942. Cinq ans d'insulino et de convulsivo-therapie chez 210 malades mentaux. Schweiz Arch Neurol Psychiatr 52: 1–12.

Charlton, G. E., Brinegar, W. C., and Holloway, O. R. 1942. Curare and metrazol therapy of psychoses. Arch Neurol Psychiatry 48: 267–70.

Cobb, S. 1938. Review of neuropsychiatry for 1938. Arch Intern Med 62: 883–99.

Cohen, L. H. 1939. The therapeutic significance of fear in the Metrazol treatment of schizophrenia. Am J Psychiatry 95: 1349–57.

Colomb, H. O. and Wadsworth, G. L. 1941. An analysis of results in the Metrazol shock therapy of schizophrenia. J Nerv Ment Dis 93: 53–62.

Cook, L. C. 1938a. The range of mental reaction states influenced by Cardiazol convulsions. J Ment Sci 84: 664–7.

Cook, L. C. 1938b. Cardiazol convulsion therapy in schizophrenia. Proc R Soc Med 31: 567–84.

Craddock, N. and Owen, M. J. 2005. The beginning of the end for the Kraepelinian dichotomy. Br J Psychiatry 186: 364–6.

Cunningham, M. G., Goldstein, M., Katz, D., et al. 2006. Coalescence of psychiatry, neurology and neuropsychology: From theory to practice. Harv Rev Psychiatry 14: 127–40.

David, H. P. 1954. A critique of psychiatric and psychological research on insulin treatment in schizophrenia. Am J Psychiatry 110(10): 774–6.

Dax, C. E. 1951. Indications for shock therapy. J Ment Sci 97: 142–4.

Dolenz, B. J. 1965. Indoklon: A clinical review. Psychosomatics 4: 200–5.

Dolenz, B. J. 1967. Flurothyl (Indoklon) side effects. Am J Psychiatry 123: 1453–5.

Dynes, J. B. 1939. Undesirable mental sequelae to convulsant drug therapy. J Ment Sci 85: 493–7.

Erb, A. 1936. Über die Möglichkeiten der kombinierten Insulin-Cardiazolbehandlung der Schizophrenie. Arch Psychiatr 16: 1762–3.

Esquibil, A. J., Krantz, J. C., Truitt, E. B., et al. 1958. Hexafluorodiethyl ether (Indoklon): Its use as a convulsant in psychiatric treatment. J Nerv Ment Dis 126: 530–4.

Fasanaro, G. 1947. La prognosi nella schizophrenia con le moderne terapie. Acta Neurol 2: 813–20.

Fenwick, P. 1998. Does forced normalization exist and how relevant is it to the psychiatrist? In Forced normalization and alternative psychoses of epilepsy (eds. Trimble, M. R. and Scmitz, B.). Petersfield, UK: Wrightson Biomedical. 209–20.

Fink, M. 2003. 'A Beautiful Mind' and insulin coma: Social constraints on psychiatric diagnosis and treatment. Harv Rev Psychiatry 11: 284–90.

Fink, M., Shaw, R., Gross, C. E., and Coleman, F. S. 1958. Comparative study of chlorpromazine and insulin coma therapy of psychosis. JAMA 166: 1846–50.

Freeman, C. P. L. and Cheshire, K. E. 1986. Attitude studies on electroconvulsive therapy. Convuls Ther 2: 31–42.

Freudenberg, R. 1947. Ten years' experience of insulin therapy in schizophrenia. J Ment Sci 93: 9–22.

Frostig, J. P. 1940. Clinical observations in insulin treatment of schizophrenia: The symptomology and therapeutic factors of the insulin effect. Am J Psychiatry 96: 1167–90.

Gander, D. R., Bennett, P. J., and Kelly, D. H. W. 1967. Hexafluorodiethyl ether (Indoklon) convulsive therapy: A pilot study. Br J Psychiatry 117: 1413–18.

Georgi, F. and Strauss, R. 1937. Krampfproblem und Insulintherapie: Berücksichtigung klinischer und humoralpathologischer Gesichtspunkte. Schweizer Arch Neurol Psychiatr 39 (supplement): 49–55.

Gibbs, F. A., Gibbs, E. L., and Lennox, W. G. 1938. The likeness of the cortical dysrhythmias of schizophrenia and psychomotor epilepsy. Am J Psychiatry 95: 255–69.

Gillespie, J. E. O. N. 1939. Cardiazol convulsions: The subjective aspect. Lancet i: 391–2.

Glaus, A. 1931. Über Kombinationen von Schizophrenie und Epilepsie. Zeitschrift für die gesamte Neurologie und Psychiatrie 135: 450–500.

Good, R. 1940. Some observations on psychological aspects of Cardiazol therapy. J Ment Sci 86: 491–501.

Goodwin, F. K. and Jamison, K. R. 2007. Manic-depressive illness: Bipolar disorders and recurrent depression. New York: Oxford University Press.

Gottlieb, J. S. and Huston, P. E. 1951. Treatment of schizophrenia; a comparison of three methods: Brief psychotherapy, insulin coma and electric shock. J Nerv Ment Dis 113: 237–46.

Gross-May, G. 1938. Über epileptiforme Anfälle bei der Insulintherapie der Schizophrenie. Nervenarzt 11: 400–13.

Hemphill, R. E. and Walter, W. G. 1941. The treatment of mental disorders by electrically induced convulsions. J Ment Sci 87: 256–75.

Hill, D. 1945. The relationship of electroencephalography to psychiatry. J Ment Sci 91: 281–9.

Himmelhoch, J. M. 1984. Major mood disorders and epileptic changes. In Psychiatric aspects of epilepsy (ed. Blumer, D.). Washington: American Psychiatric Press, pp. 271–91.

Hoch, P. H. 1943. Clinical and biological interrelations between schizophrenia and epilepsy. Am J Psychiatry 99: 507–12.

Hoenig, J. and Leibermann, D. M. 1953. The epileptic threshold in schizophrenia. J Neurol Neurosurg Psychiatr 16: 29–34.

Holmberg, G. and Thesleff, S. 1952. Succinyl-choline-iodide as a muscular relaxant in electroshock therapy. Am J Psychiatry 108: 842–6.

James, G. W. B., Freudenberg, R., and Cannon, A. T. 1937. Insulin shock treatment of schizophrenia. Lancet i: 1101–4.

Jessner, L. and Ryan, V. G. 1941. Shock treatment in psychiatry: A manual. New York: Grune & Stratton.

Kalinowsky, L. B. and Hippius, H. 1969. Pharmacological, convulsive and other somatic treatments in psychiatry. New York: Grune & Stratton.

Kalinowsky, L. B. and Hoch, P. H. 1961. Somatic treatments in psychiatry. New York: Grune & Stratton.

Kalinowsky, L. B., Hoch, P. H., and Lewis, N. D. C. 1946. Shock treatments and other somatic procedures in psychiatry. New York: Grune & Stratton.

Karliner, W. and Padula, L. J. 1959. Indoklon combined with pentothal and anectine. Am J Psychiatry 116: 358.

Kennedy, A. 1937. Convulsion therapy in schizophrenia. J Ment Sci 83: 1–20.

Kinsey, J. L. 1941. Incidence and cause of death in shock therapy. Arch Neurol Psychiatry 46: 55–8.

Kolb, L. and Vogel, V. H. 1942. The use of shock therapy in 305 mental hospitals. Am J Psychiatry 99: 90–100.

Kolbinger, H. M., Höflich, G., Hufnagel, A., et al. 1995. Transcranial magnetic stimulation (TMS) in the treatment of major depression: A pilot study. Hum Psychopharmacol 10: 305–10.

Kraepelin, E. 1919. Zur Epilepsiefrage. Zeitschrift ges Neurologie 52: 107–16.

Krantz, J. C., Traitt J. R., Speers L., and Ling A. S. C. 1957. New pharmacoconvulsive agent. Science 126: 353–4.

Küppers, E. 1937. Die Insulinbehandlung der Schizophrenie. Dtsch Med Wochenschr 63: 377–84.

Kurland, A. A., Krantz, J. C., and Traitt, E. B. 1960. The treatment of schizophrenia with sustained exposure to hexafluorodiethyl ether. J Nerv Ment Dis 130: 155–9.

Lapolla, A., McBurney, R. D., Sutton, C. E., and Nash, L. R. 1965. A clinical report on Indoklon. Dis Nerv Syst 26: 735–8.

Lee, S.-H., Kim, W., Chung, Y.-C., et al. 2005. A double blind study showing that two weeks of daily repetitive TMS over the left or right temporoparietal cortex reduces symptoms in patients with schizophrenia who are having treatment-refractory auditory hallucinations. Neurosci Lett 376: 177–81.

Lewis, A. 1938/2003. Aubrey Lewis's report on visits to psychiatric centres in Europe in 1937. In European psychiatry on the eve of war: Aubrey Lewis, the Maudsley Hospital and the Rockefeller Foundation in the 1930s (eds. Angel, K., Jones, E., and Neve, M.). Supplement 22 to Medical History. London: Wellcome Trust Centre for the History of Medicine, pp. 64–147.

Lingley, J. R. and Robbins, L. L. 1947. Fractures following electroshock therapy. Radiology 48: 124–8.

Low, A. A., Sonenthal, I., Blaurock, M., et al. 1938. Metrazol shock treatment of the functional psychoses. Arch Neurol Psychiatry 39: 717–36.

Markowe, M., Steinert, J., and Heyworth-Davis, F. 1967. Insulin and chlorpromazine in schizophrenia: A ten year comparative survey. Br J Psychiatry 113: 1101–6.

Mayer-Gross, W. 1951. Insulin coma therapy of schizophrenia: Some critical remarks on Dr Sakel's report. J Ment Sci 97: 132–5.

Mayer-Gross, W. and Walk, A. 1938. Cyclohexyl-ethyl-triazol in the convulsion treatment of schizophrenia. Lancet i: 1324–5.

McCrae, N. 2006. 'A violent thunderstorm': Cardiazol therapy in British mental hospitals. Hist Psychiatry 17: 67–90.

Meduna, L. 1934. Über experimentalle Kampherepilepsie. Arch Psychiatr 102: 333–9.

Meduna, L. 1935. Versuche über die biologische Beeinflussung des Ablaufes der Schizophrenie. Zeitschrift für die gesamte Neurologie und Psychiatrie 152: 235–62.

Meduna, L. 1937. Die Konvulsionstherapie der Schizophrenie. Halle: Carl Marhold.

Meduna, L. and Friedman, E. 1939. Convulsive-irritative therapy of psychoses: Survey of more than 3000 cases. JAMA 112: 502–9.

Meduna, L. and Rohny, B. 1939. Insulin and Cardiazol treatment of schizophrenia. Lancet i: 1139–42.

Merritt, H. H. and Putman, T. J. 1938. New series of anti-convulsant drugs tested by experiments on animals. Arch Neurol Psychiatry 39: 1003–15.

Müller, M. 1937. Le traitement de la schizophrénie par l'insuline (Société Médico-Psychologique séance du 23 Novembre). Ann Med Psychol (Paris) 94: 34–8.

Müller, M. 1939. Die Insulin- und Cardiazolbehandlung in der Psychiatrie. Fortschr Neurol Psychiatr Grenzgeb 11: 361–76.

Müller, M. 1949. Prognose und Therapie der Geisteskrankheiten. Stuttgart: George Thieme.

Neustatter, W. L., Lond, M. B., and Freeman, H. 1939. The prevention of fear in Cardiazol therapy by preliminary anaesthesia with cyclopropane or with nitrous oxide. Lancet ii: 1071–2.

Notkin, J., DeNatale, F. J., Niles, C. E., and Wittman, G. 1940. Comparative study of Metrazol treatment and control observations of schizophrenia. Arch Neurol Psychiatry 44: 568–77.

Nyirö, G. and Jablonszky, A. 1929. Einige Daten zur Prognose der Epilepsie: Mit besonderer Rücksicht auf die Konstitution. Psychiatrisch-Neurologische Wochenschrift 31: 547–9.

Ottoson, J. O. 1981. Convulsive therapy. In Handbook of biological psychiatry, Part VI (eds. Van Praag, H. M., Lader, M. H., Rafaelsen, O. J., and Sachar, E.J.). New York: Marcel Dekker, pp. 419–54.

Plattner, P. and Fröhlicher, E. 1938. Zur Insulinschockbehandlung der Schizophrenie. Arch Psychiatr Nervenkr Z Gesamte Neurol Psychiatr 160: 735–41.

Polatin, P., Friedman, M. M., Harris, M. M., and Horwitz, W. A. 1939. Vertebral fractures produced by Metrazol-induced convulsions in treatment of psychiatric disorders. JAMA 112: 1684–7.

Polatin, P., Spotnitz, H., and Wiesel, B. 1940a. Ambulatory insulin treatment of mental disorders. N Y State J Med 40: 843–8.

Polatin, P., Strauss, H., and Altman, L. L. 1940b. Transient organic mental reactions during shock therapy of the psychoses: a clinical study with electroencephalographic and psychological performance correlates. Psychiatr Q 14: 925–31.

Pollock, H. M. 1939. A statistical survey of 1140 dementia praecox patients treated with Metrazol. Psychiatr Q 13: 558–73.

Polonio, P. and Slater, E. 1954. A prognostic study of insulin treatment in schizophrenia. J Ment Sci 100: 442–50.

Post, R. M. and Speer, A. 2002. A brief history of anticonvulsant use in affective disorders. In Seizures, affective disorders and anticonvulsant drugs (eds. Trimble, M. and Schmitz, B.). Guildford, UK: Clarius, pp. 54–81.

Price, B. H., Adams, R. D., and Coyle, J. T. 2000. Neurology and psychiatry: Closing the great divide. Neurology 54: 8–14.

Pullar-Strecker, H. 1938. A comparison of insulin and cardiazol convulsion therapies in the treatment of schizophrenia. Lancet i: 371–3.

Read, C. F. 1940. Consequences of metrazol shock therapy. Am J Psychiatry 97: 667–76.

Reitmann, F. 1939. Cardiazol therapy of schizophrenia: Some statistical data. Lancet i: 439–40.

Rennie, T. A. C. and Fowler, J. B. 1943. Prognosis in manic-depressive and schizophrenic conditions following shock treatment. Psychiatr Q 17: 654–61.

Reynolds, E. H. 1968. Epilepsy and schizophrenia: Relationship and biochemistry. Lancet i: 398–401.

Rollin, H. R. 1990. Festina lente: A psychiatric odyssey. London: Br Med J Publications.

Ross, J. R. and Malzberg, B. 1939. A review of the results of the pharmacological shock therapy and the Metrazol therapy in New York State. Am J Psychiatry 96: 297–316.

Ross, J. R., Rossman, J. M., Cline, W. B., et al. 1941. A two year follow-up study from the New York state hospitals with some recommendations for the future. Am J Psychiatry 97: 1007–23.

Russell, L. W. 1938. Insulin and Cardiazol: Experiences of the combined method. J Ment Sci 84: 672–6.

Sakel, M. 1935. Neue Behandslungmethode der Schizophrenie. Vienna: Verlag Moritz Perles.

Sakel, M. 1938. The pharmacological shock treatment of schizophrenia (Nervous & Mental Disease Monograph Series 62). New York: Nervous & Mental Disease Publishing.

Sands, D. E. 1939. Insulin premedication in convulsion therapy. Lancet ii: 250–1.

Sargant, W. and Slater, E. 1944. An introduction to somatic methods of treatment in psychiatry. Baltimore: Williams & Wilkins.

Sargant, W. and Slater, E. 1954. An introduction to somatic methods of treatment in psychiatry (3rd edn). Baltimore: Williams & Wilkins.

Sargant, W. and Slater, E. 1972. An introduction to physical methods of treatment in psychiatry, 5th edn. Edinburgh: Churchill Livingstone.

Sartorius, N., de Girolamo, G., Andrews, G., et al. 1993. Treatment of mental disorders: A review of effectiveness. Washington, DC: World Health Organization.

Schilder, P. 1939. Notes on psychology of metrazol treatment of schizophrenia. J Nerv Ment Dis 89: 133–44.

Schmitz, B. 1998. Forced normalization: History of a concept. In Forced normalization and alternative psychoses of epilepsy (eds. Trimble, M. R. and Schmitz, B.). Petersfield, UK: Wrightson Biomedical, pp. 7–24.

Sebag-Montefiore, S. E. 1974. Flurothyl (Indoklon) in depression. Br J Psychiatry 124: 616–17.

Silbermann, I. 1940. The psychical experiences during the shocks in shock therapy. Int J Psychoanal 21: 179–200.

Slater, E., Beard, A. W., and Glithero, E. 1963. The schizophrenia-like psychoses of epilepsy. Br J Psychiatry 109: 95–150.

Small, J. G. and Small, I. F. 1972. Clinical results: Indoklon versus ECT. Semin Psychiatry 4: 13–26.

Sneader, W. 1985. Drug discovery: The evolution of modern medicines. Chichester, UK: Wiley.

Stevens, J. R. 1998. Seizure or psychosis: Alternative brain responses to the physiological events of puberty, the reproductive period, brain injury or malformation. In Forced normalization and alternative psychoses of epilepsy (eds. Trimble, M. R. and Scmitz, B.). Petersfield, UK: Wrightson Biomedical, pp. 121–41.

Tillim, S. J. 1940. Combined insulin and metrazol in treatment of psychoses. Psychiatr Q 14: 81–102.

Tooth, G. and Blackburn, J. M. 1939. Disturbance of memory after convulsion treatment. Lancet ii: 17–20.

Valenstein, E. S. 1973. Brain control: A critical examination of brain stimulation and psychosurgery. New York: Wiley-Interscience.

Valentine, R. 1996. Asylum, hospital, haven: A history of Horton Hospital. London: Riverside Mental Health Trust.

Verstraeten, P. 1937. La thérapeutique convulsivante de la psychose maniaco-depressive (Société de Médecine Mentale de Belgique: séance du 23 octobre 1937). Ann Med Psychol (Paris) 95: 700.

von Braunmühl, A. 1942. Fünf Jahre Schock - und Krampfbehandlung in Eglfing-haar. Archiv Psychiatr 114: 410.

Wolf, P. and Trimble, M. R. 1985. Biological antagonism and epileptic psychosis. Br J Psychiatry 146: 272–6.

Wortis, J. 1959. The history of insulin shock treatment. In Insulin treatment in psychiatry (eds. Rinkel, M. and Himwich, H. E.). New York: Philadelphia Library.

Wyllie, A. M. 1938. Treatment of mental disorders by Cardiazol. Glasgow Med J 129: 269–79.

Wyllie, A. M. 1940. Convulsion therapy of the psychoses. J Ment Sci 86: 248–59.

3

Neurochemical effects of electrically induced seizures: Relevance to the antidepressant mechanism of electroconvulsive therapy

Renana Eitan, Galit Landshut, and Bernard Lerer

Introduction

The mechanism of action of electroconvulsive therapy (ECT) has intrigued psychiatrists and neuroscientists since the treatment was first introduced. Ladislas Meduna, the inventor of convulsive therapy, suggested that chemically induced seizures were effective in the treatment of schizophrenia by "changing the chemical composition of the brain" (Meduna, 1936). In the course of ECT, an electrical current traverses brain tissue and a grand mal seizure ensues; it is inevitable that events such as these will have major physiological consequences.

Research into the mechanism of action of ECT should take into account clinical aspects of the treatment that have a potentially important impact in the research context. The first consideration is that long-standing changes induced by repeated administration of electroconvulsive shock (ECS) are more likely to be relevant to the therapeutic mechanism of ECT than are transient effects of a single ECS. The therapeutic spectrum of ECT is another highly relevant consideration. In addition to its antidepressant properties, ECT has antimanic, antipsychotic, anticatatonic, antiepileptic, and anticonvulsant effects and is used clinically for all these indications. It is highly implausible that a single mechanism of action will explain all these varied and (in some cases) opposite clinical effects. In considering the antidepressant mechanism of ECT, it is also important to note that ECT is substantially more effective than antidepressants; more than 50% of patients who have not responded to at least two adequate trials of antidepressant medication will respond to ECT. Furthermore, ECT is effective in patients with psychotic depression whereas antidepressant drugs are not, unless administered in conjunction with an antipsychotic.

Modern neuroscience focuses on four brain regions in the regulation of normal emotions, in the pathologic processes of depression, and in the antidepressant effect of ECT or other antidepressants. These areas are the prefrontal cortex, the anterior cingulate cortex, the hippocampus, and the amygdala. Thus, it is important to note that ECT has specific effects on specific processes in different brain areas. All these observations provide some explanation of why a definitive understanding of the mechanism of action of ECT has proved so elusive despite the enormous efforts that have been invested.

This chapter addresses the neurochemical effects of ECT and their possible role in the antidepressant effect of ECT, specific neurochemical theories of ECT, and the evidence that has been gathered in support of them. One important research direction has been the effect of ECT on neurotransmitters, receptors, and postreceptor signaling mechanisms in the brain. The emphasis has been primarily on serotonergic, noradrenergic, and dopaminergic systems with some consideration of gamma-aminobutyric acid (GABA)-ergic and glutamatergic mechanisms. A second research direction has been the effect of ECT on neuropeptides. Recent intriguing findings regarding the effect of ECT on gene transcription, neurotrophic factors, synaptic plasticity, and neurogenesis will also be discussed.

The effect of ECT on neurotransmitters and receptors in the brain

Neurotransmitters, receptors, depression, and ECT

Over several decades and using a variety of technologies, there has been extensive research on the effect of ECT on neurotransmitters, receptors, and postreceptor signaling mechanisms in the brain, particularly mechanisms that are also implicated in the action of antidepressant drugs. The emphasis has been primarily on monoamines (serotonergic, noradrenergic, and dopaminergic systems), because monoamine depletion is one of the most common theories of depression (Mongeau et al., 1997). Monoamine systems regulate many aspects of behavior such as mood, cognition, anxiety, aggression, arousal, sleep, appetite, and libido. Other neurotransmitter mechanisms that have been studied in relation to ECT include GABA-ergic and, more recently, glutamatergic mechanisms (Donati and Rasenick, 2003). Although many studies provide evidence that implicates specific neurotransmitters or receptors in the pathogenesis of depression or the mechanism of action of antidepressant treatments, more recent theories emphasize the complexity of the different systems and the extensive interactions between them (Mongeau et al., 1997). For a more comprehensive presentation of many of the older studies referred to in the next sections, and for references to specific studies, the reader is referred to previous reviews on the neurochemical mechanisms of ECT (Lerer, 1987; Mann, 1998; Newman et al., 1998; Sackeim et al., 1995).

The serotonergic pathway

Serotonin, depression, and the effects of ECT

Dysregulation of the serotonergic system is one of the most widely studied patho-physiological theories of depression. Serotonin (5-HT) is produced in cells of the raphe nuclei and regulates many brain regions that might be related to depression, such as prefrontal and cingulate cortex, hypothalamus, thalamus, hippocampus, amygdala, and basal ganglia. The effects of serotonin on depression are mediated by presynaptic and postsynaptic receptors, mainly 5-HT1a, 5-HT1b, 5-HT2a, 5-HT2c, 5-HT3, and 5-HT7. After release from the presynaptic nerve terminal, serotonin binds to presynaptic or postsynaptic receptors or is taken up into the presynaptic terminal by the serotonin transporter and either repackaged into a new terminal vesicle or degraded by monoamine oxidase (MAO).

Serotonin metabolites in the peripheral blood and in the cerebrospinal fluid (CSF) were found to be lower in depressed patients than in nondepressed subjects and in postmortem brain samples from depressed patients who committed suicide compared with controls. Further evidence connects the serotonergic system with depression, such as lower platelet serotonin uptake and serotonin uptake sites and higher receptor levels in the brains of suicide victims. Many antidepressant drugs block the serotonin transporter or regulate serotonergic receptors or serotonin degradation enzymes, and the effects of antidepressants can be reversed by tryptophan depletion.

Interstitial serotonin level was found to be increased by ECS in the hippocampus of freely moving rats by use of in vivo microdialysis (Zis et al., 1992). However, no statistically significant effect of ECT on serotonin metabolites in the CSF of patients has been reported. Serotonin transporter (5-HTT) number was found to be increased by acute and chronic ECS in the frontal cortex of rats and also in the platelets of patients after a course of ECT. However, 5-HTT messenger RNA (mRNA) expression was decreased after acute and chronic ECS in rat raphe nucleus (Shen et al., 2001). An association between depression and a functional polymorphism in the promoter region for the serotonin transporter gene (Collier et al., 1996), and an association between this polymorphism and response to antidepressant drug treatment, have been reported (Serretti et al., 2007). Association with response to ECT has not been tested.

Effects of ECS on serotonin receptors

There is great variability in the effect of ECS on serotonin receptors as well as regional differences (Dremencov et al., 2002, 2003). Repeated ECS did not affect the sensitivity of 5-HT1a or 5-HT1b autoreceptors, which regulate 5-HT release;

the firing activity of 5-HT neurons; or the sensitivity of somatodendritic 5-HT1a autoreceptors in the dorsal raphe and terminal 5-HT1a receptors in the hypothalamus (Blier and Bouchard, 1992). Similarly, chronic ECS did not change basal 5-HT levels or alter sensitivity to the 5-HT1a receptor agonist, 8-hydroxy-2-(di-n-propylamino) tetralin (8-OH-DPAT), in rat frontal cortex and hippocampus, measured by in vivo microdialysis. The effect of administration of the mixed 5-HT1a and 5-HT1b antagonist, pindolol, to increase 5-HT levels in hippocampus, was also not affected by chronic ECS (Newman et al., 1998). In contrast, repeated ECS attenuated 8-OH-DPAT–induced hypothermia in mice (in which the effect is presynaptic) and also in rats (in which the effect is postsynaptic) (Blier and Bouchard, 1992). Hippocampal 5-HT1a receptor mRNA was found to be decreased in CA4 and increased in dentate gyrus by single or chronic ECS, with parallel alterations in [3H]8-OH-DPAT binding site densities.

The most studied effect of ECS on brain serotonergic systems in rodent brain is sensitization of postsynaptic 5-HT1a receptors and a consequent increase in serotonergic transmission. Long-term ECS increased the responsiveness of postsynaptic neurons to the microiontophoretic application of 5-HT or the selective 5-HT1a receptor ligand 8-OH-DPAT. The increased sensitivity of postsynaptic 5-HT1a receptors may be caused by an increase in postsynaptic 5-HT1a receptor number; quantitative, autoradiographic analysis showed that repeated ECS significantly increased [3H]8-OH-DPAT binding sites in the dentate gyrus of the hippocampus and in the cerebral cortex, although other studies did not confirm these reports. In contrast, biochemical studies that measured the second messenger, adenylate cyclase, in the postsynaptic neuron, demonstrated that postsynaptic 5-HT1a receptor activity is decreased after ECS. However, these measurements of adenylate cyclase could be influenced by the activity of other postsynaptic receptors, such as 5-HT4, 5-HT6, and 5-HT7 (Mongeau et al., 1997).

Receptors of the 5-HT2a type are located postsynaptically in the neocortex. Post-mortem studies of brains of suicide victims as well as long-term ECS in animals have shown an increase in 5-HT2a receptor number in cortex, whereas antidepressant treatment reduced 5-HT2a receptor number. The ECS-induced increase in 5-HT2a receptor number was correlated with increased levels of 5-HT2a receptor mRNA. In another report, ECS-induced increase in 5-HT2a receptor number was found only in male rats but not in female rats. ECT has also been reported to increase 5-HT2a receptor number in the platelets of depressed patients. ECS was found to reduce rather than increase 5-HT2 receptor binding in nonhuman primates (5-HT2a and 5-HT2c subtypes). In this study, adult male rhesus monkeys treated with chronic ECS were examined with positron emission tomography (PET) and the radiotracer [18F]-setoperone. 5-HT2 receptor binding was significantly decreased 24 hours and

1 week post-ECS, but returned to baseline four to six weeks posttreatment (Strome et al., 2005).

In a neuroendocrine challenge study of depressed patients, fenfluramine (a serotonin-releasing agent) induced a twofold increase in plasma prolactin levels, and this response was significantly enhanced after an ECT series (Shapira et al., 1992). The release of prolactin is thought to be via postsynaptic 5-HT2a and 5-HT2c receptors in the hypothalamus. In rats, 1-(2,5-dimethoxy-4-iodophenyl)-2-aminopropane (DOI; a 5-HT2a agonist) produced dose-dependent increases in plasma adrenocorticotropin (ACTH); this response was enhanced after ECT (Gartside et al., 1992).

ECS was found to increase 5-HT3 receptor activity in rats (Ishihara and Sasa, 2001). The selective 5-HT3 receptor antagonist, ondansetron, was found to inhibit the effect of ECS on behavioral tests (open field test) in rats. In one study, ECS did not modify 5-HT4 receptor functions (Ishihara and Sasa, 2004), but in another study ECS attenuated the effects of 5-HT4 receptor activation by zacopride (a 5-HT4 receptor agonist) in hippocampal slices (Bijak et al., 2001). Another serotonin receptor, 5-HT7, has been implicated in such processes as phase shifting of circadian rhythms and induction of sleep, disturbances of which often accompany affective disorders. Down-regulation of 5-HT7 receptors occurs in rat suprachiasmatic nucleus after chronic treatment with a number of antidepressants (Neumaier et al., 2001). Most recently, it has been demonstrated that chronic but not acute ECS enhances the excitatory effect of the activation of 5-HT7 receptors (Pitra et al., 2007). 5-HT7 mRNA was not found to be changed after acute or chronic ECS in the hippocampus (Burnet et al., 1999).

The noradrenergic (norepinephrine) pathway

Norepinephrine, depression, and the effects of ECT

A role for norepinephrine (NE) dysregulation in the pathophysiology of depression was suggested in parallel with the serotonergic theory. NE is primarily produced in cells of the locus ceruleus that project to subcortical and cortical brain areas. The effects of NE are mediated by presynaptic and postsynaptic α- and β-adrenergic receptors. Similarly to serotonin, after release from the presynaptic nerve terminal, NE binds to presynaptic or postsynaptic receptors or is taken up into the presynaptic terminal by the norepinephrine transporter (NET) and either repackaged into a new terminal vesicle or degraded by MAO.

The role of NE in the mechanism of ECT has been afforded less prominence than that of serotonin. Most studies have not found any significant effect of ECT on NE metabolism. Chronic ECS has been found to decrease the level and mRNA expression of tyrosine hydroxylase, the rate-limiting enzyme of NE and dopamine formation, in the locus ceruleus. Thus, ECS might down-regulate NE transmission at the presynaptic level. Peripheral effects of ECS include reports of decreased number of platelet NE α2 receptors and normalization of lymphocyte NE β receptor responsivity.

Effects of ECT on NE receptors

There was intense interest in the effects of ECT on NE neurotransmission during the 1980s and early 1990s. A number of studies were performed that examined the effect of ECS on α2-adrenoceptors in the locus ceruleus that control the release of NE from presynaptic neurons and on β-adrenoceptor and α1-adrenoceptors post-synaptic receptors. These studies included receptor-binding studies to examine the density and affinity of these receptors and functional studies such as cyclic adenosine monophosphate (cAMP) accumulation following stimulation of β-adrenoceptor by NE or adrenergic agonists and the release of NE from presynaptic terminals following stimulation of α2-adrenoceptors. Effects of ECS were examined in different brain areas with different effects being observed according to the different brain areas examined. There are differences between brain areas in terms of the effect of ECS on NE receptors, and within brain areas reported effects are not always consistent. All these considerations preclude a simple conclusion as to whether ECS enhances or reduces NE neurotransmission in the brain after chronic administration to rats.

Some pivotal findings regarding the effects of ECS on NE receptors merit specific mention. Initially, ECS was hypothesized to reduce NE neurotransmission. This hypothesis was based on findings that ECS induced β-adrenoceptor down-regulation, reduced the sensitivity of β-adrenoceptors, and reduced the generation of cAMP in response to NE or β-adrenoceptor agonists. However, subsequent studies, reviewed by Newman et al. (1998), demonstrated that the postsynaptic effect of ECS is to increase NE neurotransmission. ECS was found to functionally increase NE neurotransmission by increasing postreceptor-mediated adenylate cyclase activity, by increasing cAMP levels and by increasing the formation of the second messenger inositol phosphate in response to α1-adrenoceptor stimulation. In addition, ECS was found to reduce presynaptic α2-adrenoceptor sensitivity and thus to increase NE neurotransmission because these receptors have an inhibitory role in NE release from the presynaptic terminal. These effects could indicate that ECS increases NE neurotransmission, but they are limited to the cortex and do not necessarily reflect NE neurotransmission in the hippocampus or in other brain areas.

In recent years, the focus of interest has shifted from direct effects of ECS on neurotransmission and postreceptor signaling and more distal effects on gene transcription. As a consequence, the intriguing body of results regarding effects of

ECS on NE neurotransmission and the theories derived from them has not matured into a definitive conceptualization.

The dopaminergic pathway

Although long-term ECT was not generally found to elevate the dopamine metabolite homovanillic acid (HVA), a few studies reported elevated HVA level after chronic ECT. It has been shown that there is a significant increase of dopamine in the rat striatum after ECS but not after chemically (fluorothyl-) induced seizures. As mentioned earlier, chronic ECS decreases the level and mRNA levels of the rate-limiting enzyme of NE and dopamine formation, tyrosine hydroxylase, in the locus ceruleus; thus, ECS might regulate dopamine transmission at the presynaptic level. ECS increases activity in the dopaminergic systems of the rat brain, as measured by behavioral tests that are specific for the dopaminergic systems (such as locomotion, rearing, grooming, and yawning). Increased dopaminergic function by ECT is a finding that is consistent with the anti-parkinsonian effects of the treatment but difficult to reconcile with its antipsychotic action.

Dopamine receptor D1 binding has not been found to be changed by ECS. Chronic ECS as well as antidepressants increased D3 receptor mRNA and binding in the shell of nucleus accumbens, a major projection area of the mesolimbic dopaminergic system, whereas D1 receptor and D2 receptor mRNA were increased by some other antidepressants, but not by ECS (Lammers et al., 2000). In another recent study, ECS has been found to enhance striatal dopamine D1 and D3 receptor binding and to improve motor performance in parkinsonian rats (Strome et al., 2007).

The GABA pathway

It has been suggested that ECT-induced increase in brain GABA levels may underlie the antidepressant as well as the anticonvulsive effect of ECT. Chronic ECS has been shown in most studies to increase GABA concentration in the striatum, hypothalamus, hippocampus, and cortex (Bowdler et al., 1983), whereas other studies suggest that repeated ECS leads to a substantial inhibition of release in the striatum and hippocampus and a long-term inhibition of GABA synthesis in these regions (Wielosz et al., 1985). Pretreatment with antagonists of GABA (such as bicuculline or pentylenetetrazol) stopped the increase in the concentration of GABA in the corpus striatum, usually seen after repeated ECS. CSF and plasma GABA levels are low in depressed patients. Moreover, plasma GABA levels decreased acutely after ECT, and this could reflect decreased levels of GABA in brain extracellular space or decreased brain turnover. Most interesting, compared with ECT nonresponders, ECT responders had higher GABA levels at both baseline and after a course of ECT (Devanand et al., 1995).

Repeated ECS increases the function and the number of the GABA-B receptors in the frontal cortex modulating 5-HT release (Lloyd et al., 1985) and nonspecifically alters the function of the GABA-A receptor (Cupello et al., 1993). ECS was found to reversibly increase the GABA-A receptor subunit mRNAs in several brain regions (Kang et al., 1991).

Glutamatergic systems

Excitatory amino acid carrier 1 (EAAC1) is a transporter of glutamate, which is the major excitatory neurotransmitter in the central nervous system (CNS). EAAC1 is located on neurons and is known to down-regulate the concentration of glutamate and thus avoid associated neurotoxicity in the hippocampus. EAAC1 mRNA was found to be up-regulated by ECS in the dentate gyrus granule cell layer but not in the CA1, CA2, or CA3 pyramidal cell layers of the hippocampus (Ploski et al., 2006). Glutamate transporter 1 (GLT-1) is another glutamate transporter that is predominantly located on glial cells. GLT-1 mRNA was found to be up-regulated by ECS in the molecular layer of the hippocampus (Ploski et al., 2006).

The effect of ECT on neuropeptides

Background

Neuropeptides such as neuropeptide Y (NPY), neural calcium sensor-1 (NCS-1), neuroserpin, neurotensin, corticotrophin releasing factor (CRF), somatostatin, calcitonin gene-related peptide (CGRP), and tachykinins (neurokinin A and substance P) have multiple CNS functions and are involved in many mental disorders. ECT was found to affect neuropeptide levels in human CSF. For example, chronic ECT was found to elevate NPY-, somatostatin-, CRF-, and endothelin-like immunoreactivity (Mathé, 1999). In animal models, ECS was found to elevate NPY-, neurokinin A-, and somatostatin-like immunoreactivity, but did not change neurotensin-, substance P-, or CGRP-like immunoreactivity in the hippocampus, frontal cortex, and occipital cortex. These effects on neuropeptides were found only in the hippocampus, frontal cortex, and occipital lobe, but not in other brain areas, such as the striatum (Mathé, 1999). In this section, the effects of ECT on neuropeptides are discussed; related hormonal changes are summarized briefly because they are discussed in another chapter in this book.

NPY

NPY is a 36-amino-acid peptide that belongs to the pancreatic polypeptide family named after a peptide found during the process of isolating insulin from pancreatic islets. NPY is differentially distributed in brain regions and, compared with other neuropeptides, its concentrations in the CNS are high (Bolwig et al., 1999).

NPY has antidepressant effects, anticonvulsant effects, and also angiogenic- and neurogenesis-promoting effects (Mathé et al., 2007). Decreased NPY concentrations have been associated with depression and anxiety. In animal models, antidepressants, lithium, and ECS were found to elevate NPY level in many brain areas. Chronic ECS was found to increase NPY-like immunoreactivity in the hippocampus and frontal cortex. The antidepressant-like effects of NPY are thought to be mediated by activation of NPY-Y1 receptors and inactivation of NPY-Y2 receptors. The angiogenic pattern induced by NPY is similar to that of fibroblast growth factor-2 (FGF-2) rather than that of vascular endothelial growth factor (VEGF): NPY induces a distinct vascular treelike structure showing vasodilation. NPY was also found to be important to hippocampal neurogenesis. The angiogenesis and neurogenesis effects of NPY are related to structural, functional, and behavioral effects of chronic antidepressant and ECS treatments (Bolwig et al., 1999; Mathé et al., 2007).

The NPY gene was found to be up-regulated after chronic ECS in the frontal cortex, dentate gyrus, and CA3 of the hippocampus (Altar et al., 2004; Mikkelsen and Woldbye, 2006; Newton et al., 2003; Ploski et al., 2006). Both peptide and mRNA NPY were found to increase, whereas NPY-Y1 receptor binding was found to decrease (Jiménez-Vasquez et al., 2007). The increased synthesis of NPY after repeated ECS results in a net increase in NPY signaling despite reduced levels of NPY-sensitive binding (Christensen et al., 2006).

NCS-1

NCS-1 is a neuropeptide that detects and transmits calcium signals across several cellular responses. NCS-1 was demonstrated to mediate desensitization of D2 dopamine receptors, and the NCS-1-D2 receptor interaction may serve to couple dopamine and calcium signaling pathways, thereby providing a critical component in the regulation of dopaminergic signaling (Kabbani et al., 2002). NCS-1 expression was found to be up-regulated after chronic ECS in the cerebellum but not in the frontal cortex or hippocampus (Rosa et al., 2007).

Neuroserpin

Neuroserpin is a serine protease inhibitor that is implicated in the regulation of synaptic plasticity, neuronal migration, and axonogenesis in the CNS. Tissue distribution analysis reveals a predominantly neuronal expression during the late stages of neurogenesis and, in the adult brain, in areas where synaptic changes are associated with learning and memory (synaptic plasticity). The role of neuroserpin in mood regulation was deduced from overexpression and underexpression of the neuropeptide in genetically modified mice, which showed increased anxiety and novelty-induced hypolocomotion. Neuroserpin mRNA expression was found to be up-regulated by chronic ECS (Tanaka et al., 2006).

Neurotensin

Neurotensin is a neuropeptide that, via activation of neurotensin receptor subtype 1 (NTS1), promotes and reinforces endogenous glutamate signaling in discrete brain regions. Neurotensin is involved in the amplification of glutamate-induced neurotoxicity in mesencephalic dopamine and cortical neurons. Whereas dopamine agonists and antagonists affect neurotensin synthesis and metabolism, ECS was not found to affect neurotensin level (Mathé, 1999).

Tachykinins

The tachykinins – substance P, neurokinin A, and neurokinin B – are found in the nervous system where they act as neurotransmitters and neuromodulators. Their respective receptors are NK1, NK2, and NK3 receptors. The NK1 receptor antagonist (MK869, aprepitant) was demonstrated to have antidepressant and antiemetic activities, and the NK3 receptor antagonist was demonstrated to have antipsychotic activity. Chronic ECS was shown to up-regulate neurokinin A-like immunoreactivity, but this effect was not found regarding substance P (Mathé, 1999).

The effect of ECT on gene transcription and neurotrophic factors

Overall effects

ECS has been found to alter gene transcription in many brain areas including the hippocampus and frontal cortex. ECS-regulated genes are related to many cellular functions such as growth factor signaling and neurogenesis, transcription factors and kinases, neurotransmitter signaling, angiogenesis, and vasodilation. Some are immediate early genes, and others are of unknown function.

Altar et al. (2004) studied the effects of single versus repeated ECS on gene transcription and concluded that acute and chronic ECS influence the expression of different genes and that genes in the hippocampus and the frontal cortex respond differently to ECS. A large set of gene expression changes in the hippocampus and frontal cortex were identified with gene microarrays and confirmed with real-time, reverse transcriptase–polymerase chain reaction (RT–PCR). The following are principal findings of this fundamental work:

- A total of 120 different genes were differentially expressed in ECS-treated rats compared with controls.
- Nineteen of these genes were regulated similarly by acute and chronic ECS in the hippocampus and frontal cortex.
- Seventy-nine genes were differentially regulated in the hippocampus after a single acute ECS and thirty-three in the frontal cortex.

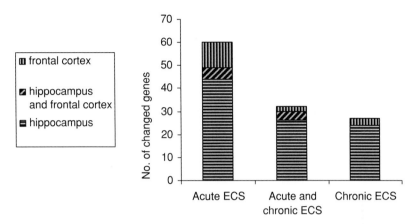

Figure 3.1   Number of changed genes in the hippocampus and the frontal cortex after acute and chronic electroconvulsive shock (ECS). Some genes change only in the hippocampus or the frontal cortex, but other genes change both in the hippocampus and in the frontal cortex. Some genes change only after acute or chronic ECS, whereas other genes change after both acute and chronic ECS.

- Fifty-seven genes were differentially regulated in the hippocampus after chronic ECS; half of these were different from the seventy-nine genes that were regulated after a single ECS.
- Only nine genes were differentially regulated in the frontal cortex after a chronic ECS.

Figure 3.1 illustrates the distribution of changes in the 120 unique genes in the frontal cortex and hippocampus after acute or chronic ECS. Thus, at the genomic level, it seems that the hippocampus rather than the frontal cortex mediates the chronic effects of ECS.

In the context of these findings it is noteworthy that, according to recent reports, several genes that were not found to be regulated by ECS in the hippocampus as a whole are regulated in the dentate gyrus (which is thought be the main site of effect of ECS in the hippocampus) (Ploski et al., 2006). Also noteworthy is that the four genes that were codirectionally changed after chronic and acute ECS in the hippocampus and frontal cortex were *BDNF, COX-2, Narp (neuronal activity-regulated pentraxin)*, and *TIEG (transforming growth factor beta [TGF-β]–inducible early growth response)*, all of which are pivotally implicated in neuroplastic processes that have been linked to the mechanism of action of ECT. Some of the major genes that have been found to be regulated by ECS (and their hypothetical function that might be relevant to the mechanism of ECT) are subsequently discussed. Selected gene pathways and genes that are regulated by ECT are summarized in Table 3.1.

Table 3.1 Selected genes and gene pathway that are regulated by chronic electroconvulsive shock (ECS)

Gene name	Gene function	Change by ECS	Brain region
Brain-derived neurotrophic factor/cAMP response element binding (BDNF/CREB) pathway			
BDNF	Cellular signal transduction, involved in neuronal survival and protection	Up-regulated	Frontal cortex
CREB	A transcription factor, involved in long-term memory and in cognitive and affective disorders	Up-regulated (in most studies) Phosphorylation or occupancy are changed acutely	Hippocampus Frontal cortex, hippocampus, striatum
c-jun	Immediate early gene in CREB pathway	Down-regulated or unchanged	Cortex and hippocampus
b-jun	Immediate early gene in CREB pathway	Up-regulated	Cortex and hippocampus
FosB	Transcription factors, involved in neuronal plasticity	Unchanged	Frontal cortex, hippocampus
c-fos	Transcription factors involved in neuronal plasticity	Up-regulated	Frontal cortex, hippocampus
Vesl/homer	Involved in synaptic activity during cortical development	Up-regulated	Frontal cortex, hippocampus
Neuritin	Involved in enhanced neurite outgrowth	Up-regulated	Hippocampus
Growth arrest and DNA damage inducible gene 45-beta (Gadd45-beta)	Involved in blood cell development and response to stress	Up-regulated	Hippocampus
Grb-2	Involved in cell growth and differentiation	Up-regulated	Hippocampus, cortex
Arachidonic acid cascade			
cPLA2	Releases arachidonate from phospholipids	Up-regulated	Hippocampus
Cox-2	Catalyzes the conversion of arachidonic acid to prostaglandins; involved in cell proliferation and plasticity, angiogenesis, vasodilation, and inflammation	Up-regulated	Hippocampus, cortex, amygdala
Prostaglandin D synthase	Involved in neurotoxicity	Down-regulated	Frontal cortex, hippocampus

Angiogenesis-, metabolism-, and homeostasis-regulating genes

Gene	Function	Regulation	Brain region
VGF	Involved in energy balance and homeostasis	Up-regulated	Hippocampus
vascular endothelial growth factor (VEGF)	Involved in angiogenesis stimulation, neurogenesis, and neuroprotection	Up-regulated	Hippocampus

Other genes

Gene	Function	Regulation	Brain region
Fibroblast growth factor-2 (FGF-2)	Involved in angiogenesis and neurogenesis	Up-regulated	Hippocampus, frontal cortex
Nerve growth factor (NGF)	Involved in neurogenesis and neuroprotection	Up-regulated	Hippocampus, striatum
		Down-regulated	Frontal cortex
Activity-regulated cytoskeleton (Arc)	Related to decline in memory consolidation after electroconvulsive therapy	Down-regulated	Hippocampus
ERK5-MEF2C	Involved in neuronal survival and neuroprotection	Unchanged	Frontal cortex, hippocampus
Thyrotropin-releasing hormone (TRH)	Regulates thyroid hormone function; involved in neuroprotection	Up-regulated	Hippocampus
Tissue inhibitors of metalloproteinases-1 (TIMP-1)	Involved in inflammation, neuroprotection; related to degenerative diseases and tumor invasion	Up-regulated	Hippocampus, cortex, choroids plexus
ELL2	Involved in the transcription rate	Up-regulated	Hippocampus
Kf-1	Related to the ubiquitin pathway; involved in many cell processes	Up-regulated	Frontal cortex, hippocampus
N-Myc downstream-regulated protein 2 (Ndrg2)	Involved in stress responses, cell proliferation, and differentiation	Down-regulated	Frontal cortex
Frizzled-3 (Frz3)	Involved in cell fate determination and behavior	Down-regulated	Frontal cortex
Vesicle-associated membrane protein 2 (VAMP2/synaptobrevin-2)	Involved in synaptic vesicle docking/fusion machinery	Up-regulated	Frontal cortex
Neuropeptide Y (NPY)	Involved in angiogenesis; related to antidepressant and anticonvulsant effects	Up-regulated	Frontal cortex, hippocampus
Neuroserpin	Involved in synaptic plasticity, learning, and memory; related to mood regulation	Up-regulated	Frontal cortex

Many genes in brain areas other than the hippocampus or the frontal cortex were found to be regulated by ECS. One of these brain areas is the choroid plexus, which has an important role in the synthesis of CSF as well as in the regulation of the blood–brain barrier. There is considerable evidence that depressed patients have reduced cerebral blood flow (CBF) and metabolism compared with that of normal subjects, although in some brain areas CBF and metabolism may be increased (Moretti et al., 2003). Some studies suggest that reduced CBF in depression is reversed by ECT, but others report a further reduction (Bonne et al., 1996; Nobler et al., 2000). The genes that were found to be regulated in the choroid plexus in response to chronic ECS are growth factor and angiogenesis signaling genes (such as insulin-like growth factor 2 [IGF2], insulin-like growth factor binding protein 2 [IGFBP2], fibronectin, and brain-derived neurotrophic factor [BDNF]) and other signaling genes (such as wint6 and somatostatin) (Newton et al., 2003).

Chromatin remodeling is also regulated by ECS. Chromatin, the physiological template of all eukaryotic genetic information, is subject to a diverse array of post-translational modifications that largely impinge on histone amino termini, thereby regulating access to the underlying DNA. The combinatorial nature of histone amino-terminal modifications reveals a "histone code" that considerably extends the information potential of the genetic code. The posttranslational modifications of histones were found to be altered at several gene promoters (such as c-fos, BDNF, and cAMP response element binding [CREB]) in rat hippocampus after acute or repeated ECS (Tsankova et al., 2004).

The BDNF/CREB pathway

The BDNF/CREB pathway is illustrated in Figure 3.2. The influence of chronic ECS on expression of BDNF and its receptor, tyrosine kinase B (trkB), is well established. BDNF is important in neuronal survival and protection from the damaging effects of stress. BDNF is one of the four genes that were found by Altar et al. (2004) to be codirectionally changed after acute and chronic ECS in the hippocampus and frontal cortex. More specifically, ECS was found to elevate 17 genes along the BDNF and trkB-stimulated mitogen-activated protein (MAP) kinase pathway, including Grb-2, Grb-2-like, RAS homolog, growth arrest and DNA-damage inducible gene (GADD153), neuritin, glypican, phosphotyrosine phosphatase, and Vesl/homer.

Consistent with these findings, acute and chronic ECS significantly increased BDNF mRNA in the frontal cortex. In the granule cell layer of the hippocampal dentate gyrus, acute and chronic ECS decreased the acute induction of BDNF and trkB mRNA, but chronic ECS prolonged their expression (Nibuya et al., 1995; Ploski et al., 2006). In the CA3 and CA1 pyramidal cell layers of the hippocampus and in layer 2 of the pyriform cortex, chronic ECS elevated the acute induction of BDNF, and prolonged the expression of BDNF and trkB mRNA. These changes after chronic ECS persisted up to 48 hours after the last shock (Zetterström et al.,

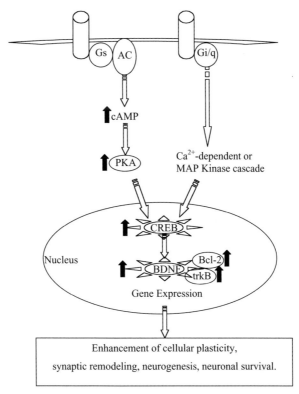

Figure 3.2   The brain-derived neurotrophic factor (BDNF) and cyclic adenosine monophosphate (cAMP) response element binding (CREB) pathway. Basically, receptor activation might cause an increase of adenylate cyclase and protein kinase A as well as an increase in the mitogen-activated protein (MAP) kinase cascade. These two processes increase the level of the CREB protein and the level of BDNF and its related proteins, tyrosine kinase B (trkB) and B-cell lymphoma 2 (Bcl-2). Activation of the BDNF pathway results in expression of many genes that enhance cellular plasticity, synaptic remodeling, neurogenesis, and neuronal survival. AC, adenylate cyclase; PKA, protein kinase A.

1998). In parallel measurements of BDNF mRNA and protein expression in the frontal cortex and hippocampus of the rat after chronic ECS, it was found that ECS increased BDNF mRNA and protein in the hippocampus and BDNF protein but not mRNA in the frontal cortex (Jacobsen and Mørk, 2004). Chronic ECS also blocked the down-regulation of BDNF mRNA in the hippocampus in response to environmental restraint stress. Administration of an N-methyl-D-aspartate (NMDA) antagonist (ketamine) was found to attenuate ECS-induced BDNF expression in the medial prefrontal cortex and the dentate gyrus (Chen et al., 2001). Similar results were found after chronic administration of several antidepressants but not after chronic administration of non-antidepressant psychotropic drugs. However, some studies demonstrated no change in BDNF concentration after ECS (Angelucci et al., 2003).

CREB is a transcription factor that is activated in the nervous system in response to a wide range of extracellular stimuli. CREB-dependent gene expression has been implicated in complex and diverse processes ranging from development to plasticity to disease. The CREB signaling pathway has been demonstrated to be a core component of the molecular switch that converts short- to long-term memory, and to be involved in many cognitive and psychiatric disorders such as depression, anxiety, and cognitive decline (Carlezon et al., 2005). In general, DNA-binding factors that activate gene transcription are thought to do so via reversible interaction with DNA. However, most studies suggest that the transcriptional activator, CREB, is exceptional in that it is constitutively bound to the promoter, where its phosphorylation leads to the recruitment of CREB-binding protein (CBP) to form a CREB/CBP/promoter complex. Ser-133 phosphorylation of the CREB protein is sufficient to induce cellular gene expression in response to cAMP, but additional promoter-bound factors are required for target gene activation by CREB in response to stress signals. Tanis et al. (2007) recently studied CREB–DNA interactions in the rat brain after ECS. They found 860 genomic CREB-binding sites and found that CREB-occupied transcripts interact extensively to promote cell proliferation, plasticity, and resiliency. CREB phosphorylation or occupancy was found to be changed acutely by ECS in the frontal cortex, hippocampus, and striatum, but not in the cerebellum.

ECS was found to regulate many immediate early genes in the CREB pathway. Whereas b-jun mRNA was found to be up-regulated in the cortex and hippocampus (Hsieh et al., 1998), c-jun mRNA was down-regulated or unchanged by chronic ECS (Winston et al., 1990). In the hippocampus, c-jun phosphorylation was found to be increased (Ahn et al., 2002). Another related transcription factor is delta-FosB. Members of the Fos family of proteins play physiological roles in the neuronal, electrophysiological, and behavioral plasticity associated with repeated seizures (Hiroi et al., 1998). Delta-FosB was found to be induced rapidly and transiently by acute ECS in the cortex, but not by chronic ECS in the hippocampus and the frontal cortex. It was found that c-fos mRNA was up-regulated by acute ECS in the cortex and hippocampus but down-regulated by chronic ECS in most cortical and hippocampal areas (except CA4 of the hippocampus) (Hsieh et al., 1998). In the hilar neurons of the hippocampus, prolonged induction of c-fos occurred mostly in NPY or somatostatin-containing cells. Delta-FosB was found to regulate many other genes that are related to ECS such as cyclin-dependent kinase 5 (cdk5), which has a role in regulating neuronal structure; CCAAT-enhancing binding protein-beta (C/EBPbeta), which has a role in behavioral conditioning models; or activator protein-1 (AP-1), which has a role in regulation of gene transcription (Chen et al., 2000, 2004).

One of the BDNF-related genes that are up-regulated by ECS is Vesl/homer. The homer protein binds to metabotropic glutamate receptors, and the homer gene is regulated as an immediate early gene and is dynamically responsive to physiological synaptic activity, particularly during cortical development. BDNF was found to promote the accumulation of Vesl/homer at synapses, and the extent of this accumulation was correlated with the level of activation of extracellular signal-regulated kinases (ERKs) following treatment with BDNF (Kato et al., 2003).

Another BDNF-related gene that is up-regulated by ECS is neuritin, an activity and neurotrophic factor-induced gene that encodes a glycosylphosphatidylinositol-anchored neuronal protein that enhances neurite outgrowth of cultured hippocampal and cortical neurons. The neuritin gene was found to be up-regulated after both acute and chronic ECS in the granule cell layer of the dentate gyrus as well as in the CA1 pyramidal cell layer of the hippocampus (Newton et al., 2003).

Growth arrest and DNA damage inducible gene 45-beta (Gadd45-beta) plays a role in blood cell development, in inflammatory responses to invading microorganisms, and in response to environmental stress and physiological stress, such as hypoxia, which results in ischemic tissue damage. Gadd45-beta has a protective role by inhibiting the apoptotic process and was found to be up-regulated by ECS in the dentate gyrus of the hippocampus (Ploski et al., 2006).

Growth factor receptor bound 2 (Grb2) is a protein that is related to the signaling pathway from tyrosine kinase receptors to G protein–coupled receptors (transactivation) such as epidermal growth factor (EGF), platelet-derived growth factor (PDGF), FGF, BDNF, and insulin receptors; thus, it regulates cell growth and differentiation (Newton et al., 2004). Grb2 was found to be up-regulated in the hippocampal dentate gyrus as well as superficial and deep layers of the cortex with both acute and chronic ECS (Newton et al., 2004).

Arachidonic acid cascade genes

Cytosolic phospholipase A2 (cPLA2) is the factor that releases arachidonate from phospholipids. The cPLA2 gene was found to be up-regulated after both acute and chronic ECS in the hippocampus. Cox-2 prostaglandin–endoperoxide synthase 2 is the inducible form of prostaglandin–endoperoxide synthase that catalyzes the rate-limiting step in converting arachidonic acid to prostaglandins. It is an immediate early gene that has an important role in cell proliferation, synaptic plasticity, angiogenesis, vasodilation, and inflammation. Cox-2 is involved in hippocampal neurogenesis: The administration of Cox inhibitors suppressed neurogenesis in the dentate gyrus of adult rodents and in heterozygous and homozygous Cox-2 knockout mice, and neurogenesis is significantly lower than in wild-type littermates. Cox-2–generated prostaglandin E2 regulates membrane excitability and long-term synaptic plasticity in hippocampal perforant path–dentate gyrus synapses. The Cox-2–induced increase in blood flow after ECS might supply essential nutrients and growth factors necessary for proliferation and neurogenesis. The Cox-2 gene was found to be up-regulated after both acute and chronic ECS in the granule cell layer of the dentate gyrus and the CA3 pyramidal cell layer of the hippocampus, in the outer layer of the cerebral cortex, and in the amygdala (Altar et al., 2004). Two related genes that were found to be down-regulated by chronic ECT in both the hippocampus and frontal cortex are prostaglandin D synthase, which is thought to be neurotoxic, and IGF2 (somatomedin A) (Altar et al., 2004).

Angiogenesis-, metabolism-, and homeostasis-regulating genes

The (VGF) gene encodes a neuronal and neuroendocrine polypeptide, VGF, which has a significant role in energy balance and the regulation of homeostasis. The VGF gene was found to be up-regulated after both acute and chronic ECS in the dentate gyrus and after chronic ECS in the CA3 pyramidal cell layer of the hippocampus (Newton et al., 2003).

VEGF is known for its angiogenesis stimulation. Lately it has been suggested that VEGF is also important in neurogenesis and neuroprotection, because angiogenesis co-occurs or even precedes neurogenesis. The VEGF gene was found to be up-regulated after an acute ECS in the dentate gyrus and after acute and chronic ECS in the CA1 and CA3 pyramidal cell layer of the hippocampus (Newton et al., 2003).

Other genes

FGF-2

FGF-2 is thought to have effects on angiogenesis and neurogenesis. The FGF-2 gene was found to be up-regulated after both acute and chronic ECS in many brain areas, including the hippocampus (Kondratyev et al., 2002). FGF-2 mRNA was found to be up-regulated after chronic ECS in the frontal cortex, but not after acute ECS (Gwinn et al., 2002).

Nerve growth factor

The nerve growth factor (NGF) gene was found, like FGF-2, to be up-regulated after both acute and chronic ECS in many brain areas, including the hippocampus (Kondratyev et al., 2002). In an animal model of depression, NGF was found to be up-regulated by ECS in the hippocampus in the "depressed" animals but not in the control animals (Angelucci et al., 2003). NGF was found to be down-regulated by ECS in the frontal cortex but up-regulated by ECS in the striatum in both depressed and control animals (Angelucci et al., 2003).

Activity regulated cytoskeleton gene

Activity regulated cytoskeleton (Arc) is an immediate early gene that might be related to the decline in memory consolidation seen in depressed patients subjected to ECT. Arc mRNA was found to be up-regulated after acute ECS in the dentate gyrus and CA1 of the hippocampus and in the parietal cortex, and then returned to baseline after 2 to 24 hours. Arc mRNA was found to be down-regulated after chronic ECS in the CA1 of the hippocampus (Larsen et al., 2005).

ERK5-MEF2C

ERK5, along with its downstream molecule MEF2C, has been implicated in many aspects of neuronal survival and neuroprotection. Increased phosphorylation of ERK5 was observed immediately after ECS in the frontal cortex and hippocampus, but was barely detectable 2 minutes after ECS in both the frontal cortex and the hippocampus. The level of MEF2C phosphorylation was decreased immediately after ECS in both regions. It was increased from 2 minutes until 10 minutes after ECS in the frontal cortex, but it returned to the basal level by 2 minutes after ECS in the hippocampus (Yoon et al., 2005).

Thyrotropin-releasing hormone

Thyrotropin-releasing hormone (TRH) is an essential hormone in regulating thyroid gland function. The thyroid hormone, triiodothyronine (T3), has been used to augment and accelerate the clinical effects of antidepressants. TRH had been demonstrated to have an antidepressant effect in rodents as well as in humans. TRH has also been suggested to have a neuroprotective effect against glutamate toxicity in primary hippocampal neuronal culture. The TRH gene was found to be up-regulated by chronic ECS in the hippocampus (Altar et al., 2004), and was found to be markedly up-regulated (by 16-fold) in the dentate gyrus of the hippocampus (Ploski et al., 2006).

Tissue inhibitors of metalloproteinases-1

Tissue inhibitors of metalloproteinases-1 (TIMP-1) is one of the four members of the tissue inhibitor of metalloproteinases (TIMP) family. TIMP-1 is a multifunctional protein that inhibits the activities of all known matrix metalloproteinases (MMPs) and as such plays a key role in maintaining the balance between extracellular matrix (ECM) deposition and degradation in different physiological processes. Accelerated breakdown of ECM occurs in various pathological processes, including inflammation, chronic degenerative diseases, and tumor invasion. TIMP-1 exhibits growth factor-like activity and can inhibit angiogenesis. It probably has a neuroprotective function following excitotoxic (glutamatergic) injury. TIMP-1 was found to be up-regulated by acute and chronic ECS in the dentate gyrus of the hippocampus, in the cortex, and in the choroid plexus (Newton et al., 2003). More specifically, TIMP-1 was found to be up-regulated in the granule cell layer of the hippocampus after acute ECS and in the molecular layer after chronic ECS.

ELL2

ELL2 is an RNA polymerase II elongation factor and thus increases the transcription rate in the cell. ELL2 was found to be up-regulated by ECS in the dentate gyrus of the hippocampus (Ploski et al., 2006).

Kf-1

Kf-1 is a gene with a RING-H2 nger motif that can facilitate E2 (ubiquitin-conjugating enzymes)–dependent ubiquitination. The Ub–proteasome system plays important roles in the control of numerous processes, including cell-cycle progression, signal transduction, transcriptional regulation, receptor down-regulation, endocytosis, long-term facilitation, and long-term memory in the brain. Kf-1 mRNA was found to be up-regulated after acute and chronic ECS in the frontal cortex and the hippocampus (Nishioka et al., 2003).

N-Myc downstream-regulated protein 2 gene

N-Myc downstream-regulated protein 2 (Ndrg2) is highly related to N-Myc downstream-regulated protein 1 (Ndrg1), which is linked to stress responses, cell proliferation, and dierentiation. Ndrg2 complementary DNA (cDNA) was found to be down-regulated after acute and chronic ECS in the frontal cortex (Takahashi et al., 2005).

Frizzled-3 gene

The frizzled protein (Frz) family is a group of receptor proteins with seven putative transmembrane helixes that bind wingless proteins (Wnts), a family of secreted cysteine-rich glycosylated ligands. The Frz/Wnt pathway is a highly conserved developmental pathway involved in cell fate determination in the CNS and in complex behavioral phenomena. Frizzled-3 (Frz3) cDNA was found to be down-regulated after acute and chronic ECS in the frontal cortex (Yamada et al., 2005).

Vesicle-associated membrane protein 2

Vesicle-associated membrane protein 2 (VAMP2/synaptobrevin-2) is a key component of the synaptic vesicle docking/fusion machinery that forms the soluble N-ethylmaleimide-sensitive fusion protein attachment protein receptor (SNARE) complex. VAMP2 cDNA was found to be up-regulated by chronic ECS in the frontal cortex (Yamada et al., 2002).

The effect of ECS on synaptic plasticity and neurogenesis

Recently there has been a great deal of interest in the effect of ECT on synaptic plasticity and neurogenesis. Brain plasticity refers to the ability of neural tissue to adapt to environmental as well as internal changes. Plastic changes in the brain occur at different levels, from molecular to structural and functional levels. One of the structural changes that underlies plastic adaptation of the brain is the generation of newly born neurons in the process of neurogenesis. Adult neurogenesis, the life-long addition of new neurons, was first documented in the rat hippocampus in 1965 by Altman and Das (Altman and Das, 1965). It is now well established that neurogenesis occurs in several different species, including humans, and that the newly generated cells mature into functional neurons. In the mammalian brain, neurogenesis is mainly confined to two regions, the subgranular zone (SGZ) of the hippocampal dentate gyrus and the subventricular zone (SVZ). Newly born SGZ neurons migrate into the granule cell layer and send axonal projections via mossy fiber pathways into hippocampal CA regions. These regions have high potential for long-term potentiation (LTP), a mechanism involved in learning and memory formation (reviewed by Bliss and Collingridge, 1993). Newborn cells from the SVZ migrate into the olfactory bulb. Hippocampal newborn neurons form synapses, integrate into preexisting neuronal circuits, and are functionally involved in memory formation and emotional learning.

Neurogenesis may be regulated and modulated by many different factors, suggesting that the process is an adaptive mechanism that helps the brain to adjust to internal and environmental demands. Enriched environment, physical exercise, and learning up-regulate adult hippocampal neurogenesis, whereas aging, social isolation, and drug administration (opiates, amphetamine, and cocaine), as well as alcohol exposure down-regulate neurogenesis. Internal states such as hormonal status may also affect cell proliferation. Ovariectomy and thyroidectomy inhibit cell proliferation, whereas estrogen and thyroid hormone administration, respectively, restore neurogenesis levels to normal. Adrenalectomy, in contrast, enhances neurogenesis, whereas corticosterone administration attenuates granule cell proliferation. Stressful events that may result in increased corticosterone levels were also found to attenuate neurogenesis, when the stress is physical or psychosocial.

It is well established that depression is associated with lower hippocampal volume, but not overall brain size. Furthermore, lifetime duration of untreated depression correlates with hippocampal volume loss. Antidepressant treatment, in contrast, may have neuroprotective properties in the hippocampus, although further clinical support is needed. Preclinical studies have shown that chronic but not acute antidepressant treatment with different classes of antidepressants enhances neurogenesis in the rodent hippocampus (Malberg et al., 2000), consistent with the clinical time course required for achieving therapeutic effects in humans. Antidepressant-induced enhancement of neurogenesis is required for the effect of the drug, because blocking antidepressant-induced neurogenesis enhancement also blocks the behavioral response to the drug in an animal model of depression

Table 3.2 Effects of electroconvulsive shock (ECS) on neurogenesis and synaptic plasticity

	Main finding
Neurogenesis	↑ hippocampal mossy fiber sprouting
	↑ cell proliferation in the hippocampus
	Blocks stress-induced cell proliferation attenuation
Neurotrophins in the hippocampus	↑ brain-derived neurotrophic factor (BDNF) messenger RNA (mRNA)
	↑ BDNF mRNA expression duration
	↑ BDNF protein
	Blocks stress-induced decrease in BDNF mRNA
	↑ nerve growth factor (NGF) mRNA
	↑ NGF protein
Hippocampal synaptic plasticity	↑ long-term potentiation-like synaptic activity

(Santarelli et al., 2003). Furthermore, antidepressant treatment reverses the effect of stress to reduce hippocampal neurogenesis (Malberg and Duman, 2003).

The first, although indirect, indication for possible effects of ECS on hippocampal neurogenesis was described by Gray and Sundstrom (1998). These authors showed that convulsions or seizures induced by intraventricular kainic acid administration enhanced hippocampal neurogenesis (Gray and Sundstrom, 1998). Immediately thereafter it was found that chronic ECS enhances hippocampal dentate gyrus granule cell axonal sprouting and synaptic organization in the rat brain (Lamont et al., 2001; Vaidya et al., 1999), and eventually it was shown that ECS enhances neurogenesis in the adult dentate gyrus (Madsen et al., 2000; Malberg et al., 2000; Scott et al., 2000). ECS has a dose-dependent and long-lasting effect on granule cell proliferation in the hippocampal dentate gyrus (Madsen et al., 2000). Furthermore, ECS reverses the effect of glucocorticoid (corticosterone) administration to reduce hippocampal granule cell proliferation, thereby restoring neurogenesis to normal levels (glucocorticoid administration mimics the endogenous enhancement of hypothalamic–pituitary–adrenal [HPA] axis function that occurs after exposure to stress) (Hellsten et al., 2002). Recently it was shown that ECS enhances hippocampal neurogenesis not only in rodents, but also in non-human primates (Perera et al., 2007). Major effects of ECS on neurogenesis and synaptic plasticity are summarized in Table 3.2.

Adult neurogenesis may be regulated by neurotrophic signaling. Intrahippocampal BDNF infusion up-regulates adult hippocampal neurogenesis whereas down-regulation of BDNF signaling, although it does not affect hippocampal cell proliferation, impairs antidepressant-induced newborn neuronal survival (Sairanen et al., 2005). As mentioned before, ECS increases the transcription of several genes in the rat hippocampus, among them BDNF, its receptor trkB, and the MAP kinase pathway genes (Altar et al., 2004). ECS increases BDNF protein level in the hippocampus, as well as the cortex and neostriatum, and the effect in the hippocampus lasts at least seven days after ECS administration (Li et al., 2007). Furthermore, ECS blocks stress-induced decrease in hippocampal BDNF mRNA level. A recent pilot study found that ECT increases plasma BDNF in depressed patients (Marano et al., 2007). ECS also increases the level of NGF mRNA in the rat hippocampus (Kondratyev et al., 2002), and NGF protein level in the hippocampus of a genetic animal model of depression, the Flinders Sensitive Line (FSL) (Angelucci et al., 2003).

Neurotrophic factors, such as BDNF, NGF, or Neurotrophin 3(NT-3), play a role in modulating synaptic transmission via a wide range of physiological actions at both presynaptic and postsynaptic sites (reviewed by Binder, 2007). Exposure of hippocampal tissue to BDNF or NG-3 produces a sustained enhancement of synaptic strength. When measured in hippocampal tissue from mice genetically impaired in BDNF signaling pathway, significantly reduced LTP is observed, whereas treatment of hippocampal slices from BDNF knockout mice with recombinant BDNF completely reverses LTP impairment. LTP is the process of activity-dependent long-lasting enhancement of efficacy of synaptic transmission, and it is one of the mechanisms that underlie several forms of memory formation and learning (reviewed by Bliss and Collingridge, 1993). Induction of LTP can be impaired by stress, whereas chronic (but not acute) antidepressant treatment reverses stress-induced LTP impairment. Stewart et al. (1994) showed that ECS induces LTP-like changes in synaptic activity. The same investigators later showed that the effect of ECS to induce LTP in rat hippocampus is similar to that of fluoxetine, a common pharmacological antidepressant, and suggested that this may be one of the mechanisms that underlies the antidepressant effect of ECT in humans. The paradox of this hypothesis is that ECS-induced synaptic plasticity could have been expected to enhance memory formation, whereas one of the side effects of ECT in depressed patients is memory impairment. Further study is crucial for a fuller understanding the role of synaptic plasticity in the antidepressant effect of ECT.

Conclusions

Seymour Kety, a pioneer of biological research in several areas of psychiatry, noted in 1974, in the first volume published on the mechanism of action of ECT: ECT "... involves massive discharge over wide areas of the brain, activation of the peripheral autonomic nervous system, release of the secretion of many endocrine glands; ... "; as a result "... the difficulty lies not in demonstrating such changes but in differentiating... which of the changes may be related to the important antidepressive and amnestic effects and which are quite irrelevant to these" (Kety, 1974). The extensive but nevertheless still incomplete review of neurochemical changes induced by ECS in rodent and human brain presented in this chapter highlights the accuracy of this statement. Another pioneer of biological psychiatry, Herman van Praag, drew the conclusion that only an "incorrigible optimist could hope to select from the numerous changes precisely those which determine the therapeutic effect" (van Praag, 1977).

In the 35 years that have elapsed since the publication of *Psychobiology of Convulsive Therapy* (Kety, 1974), neuroscience has undergone several technological revolutions yielding powerful methods to study the effect of treatments on brain function. These include high-throughput technologies that enable massively parallel study of genomic changes involving thousands of genes. At the same time, rapid advances in brain imaging increasingly permit the effects of ECT on brain function to be studied directly in humans and neurochemical changes to be evaluated in vivo. These developments have inevitably led to a further increase in the volume of data available on the neurochemical effects of ECT. Have comprehensive, testable theories regarding the neurochemical mechanisms of ECT emerged from the large volume of data generated? One of the most comprehensive is the brain plasticity/neurogenesis theory originally proposed by Duman et al. (1997), which takes into account a chain of effects from the level of neurotransmitter changes, through effects on gene expression, to alterations at the tissue level and the production of new brain cells (see section titled "The effect of ECS on synaptic plasticity and neurogenesis"). Inevitably the theory has several weaknesses and awaits proof that induction of neurogenesis in the dentate gyrus of the hippocampus (and other regions, if shown to be relevant) by means other than ECT or drugs with known antidepressant mechanisms has antidepressant effects in depressed patients.

Another development of pivotal importance to understanding the neurochemical mechanism of ECT is the rapidly progressing field of brain stimulation as applied to the treatment of depression. Several brain stimulation modalities are being tested experimentally with one (vagus nerve stimulation) already approved for clinical use (even though concerns remain regarding its efficacy). It is of great interest whether brain stimulation techniques that have antidepressant effects act via neurochemical mechanisms that are similar to or different from those of ECT. Studies in this regard are already in progress, and results are already available but not yet at a level of resolution to provide definitive answers. This is an important research approach because it provides the possibility to test theories regarding the neurochemical mechanisms of ECT in a focused, regionally specific way. At the same time, regionally specific effects of ECS, some of which have been outlined in this chapter, can inform the development of brain stimulation techniques by directing focus toward specific brain regions. Thus, the interplay between observed neurochemical effects of ECT and of novel brain stimulation techniques used to treat depression is likely to be a highly productive research area in the future.

References

Ahn, Y. M., Kang, U. G., Oh, S. W., et al. 2002. Region-specific phosphorylation of ATF-2, Elk-1 and c-Jun in rat hippocampus and cerebellum after electroconvulsive shock. Neurosci Lett 329: 9–12.

Altar, C. A., Laeng, P., Jurata, L. W., et al. 2004. Electroconvulsive seizures regulate gene expression of distinct neurotrophic signaling pathways. J Neurosci 24: 2667–77.

Altman, J. and Das, G. D. 1965. Autoradiographic and histological evidence of postnatal hippocampal neurogenesis in rats. J Comp Neurol 24(3): 319–35.

Angelucci, F., Aloe, L., Jiménez-Vasquez, P., and Mathé, A. A. 2003. Electroconvulsive stimuli alter nerve growth factor but not brain-derived neurotrophic factor concentrations in brains of a rat model of depression. Neuropeptides 37: 51–6.

Bijak, M., Zahorodna, A., and Tokarski, K. 2001. Opposite effects of antidepressants and corticosterone on the sensitivity of hippocampal CA1 neurons to 5-HT1A and 5-HT4 receptor activation. Naunyn Schmiedebergs Arch Pharmacol 363: 491–8.

Binder, D. K. 2007. Neurotrophins in the dentate gyrus. Prog Brain Res 163: 371–97.

Blier, P. and Bouchard, C. 1992. Effect of repeated electroconvulsive shocks on serotonergic neurons. Eur J Pharmacol 211: 365–73.

Bliss, T. V. and Collingridge, G. L. 1993. A synaptic model of memory: long-term potentiation in the hippocampus. Nature 361: 31–9.

Bolwig, T. G., Woldbye, D. P., and Mikkelsen, J. D. 1999. Electroconvulsive therapy as an anticonvulsant: a possible role of neuropeptide Y (NPY). J ECT 15: 93–101.

Bonne, O., Krausz, Y., Shapira, B., et al. 1996. Increased brain Tc-99m HMPAO uptake in depressed patients who have responded to electroconvulsive therapy. J Nucl Med 37: 1075–80.

Bowdler, J. M., Green, A. R., Minchin, M. C., and Nutt, D. J. 1983. Regional GABA concentration and [3H]-diazepam binding in rat brain following repeated electroconvulsive shock. J Neural Transm 56: 3–12.

Burnet, P. W., Sharp, T., LeCorre, S. M., and Harrison, P. J. 1999. Expression of 5-HT receptors and the 5-HT transporter in rat brain after electroconvulsive shock. Neurosci Lett 277: 79–82.

Carlezon, W. A. Jr, Duman, R. S., and Nestler, E. J. 2005. The many faces of CREB. Trends Neurosci 28: 436–45.

Chen, A. C., Shin, K. H., Duman, R. S., and Sanacora, G. 2001. ECS-induced mossy fiber sprouting and BDNF expression are attenuated by ketamine pretreatment. J ECT 17: 27–32.

Chen, J., Newton, S. S., Zeng, L., et al. 2004. Downregulation of the CCAAT-enhancer binding protein beta in deltaFosB transgenic mice and by electroconvulsive seizures. Neuropsychopharmacology 29: 23–31.

Chen, J., Zhang, Y., Kelz, M. B., et al. 2000. Induction of cyclin-dependent kinase 5 in the hippocampus by chronic electroconvulsive seizures: Role of [Delta]FosB. J Neurosci 20: 8965–71.

Christensen, D. Z., Olesen, M. V., Kristiansen, H., et al. 2006. Unaltered neuropeptide Y (NPY)-stimulated [35S]GTPgammaS binding suggests a net increase in NPY signalling after repeated electroconvulsive seizures in mice. J Neurosci Res 84: 1282–91.

Collier, D. A., Stober, G., Li, T., et al. 1996. A novel functional polymorphism within the promoter of the serotonin transporter gene: Possible role in susceptibility to affective disorders. Mol Psychiatry 1: 453–60.

Cupello, A., Patrone, A., Robello, M., et al. 1993. Electric shock convulsions in the rabbit and brain cortex GABAA receptor function. Neurochem Res 18: 883–6.

Devanand, D. P., Shapira, B., Petty, F., et al. 1995. Effects of electroconvulsive therapy on plasma GABA. Convuls Ther 11: 3–13.

Donati, R. J. and Rasenick, M. M. 2003. G protein signaling and the molecular basis of antidepressant action. Life Sci 73: 1–17.

Dremencov, E., Gur, E., Lerer, B., and Newman, M. E. 2002. Effects of chronic antidepressants and electroconvulsive shock on serotonergic neurotransmission in the rat hypothalamus. Prog Neuropsychopharmacol Biol Psychiatry 26: 1029–34.

Dremencov, E., Gur, E., Lerer, B., and Newman, M. E. 2003. Effects of chronic antidepressants and electroconvulsive shock on serotonergic neurotransmission in the rat hippocampus. Prog Neuropsychopharmacol Biol Psychiatry 27: 729–39.

Duman R. S., Heninger G. R., and Nestler E. J. 1997. A molecular and cellular theory of depression. Arch Gen Psychiatry. 54: 597–606.

Gartside, S. E., Ellis, P. M., Sharp, T., and Cowen, P. J. 1992. Selective 5-HT1A and 5-HT2 receptor-mediated adrenocorticotropin release in the rat: Effect of repeated antidepressant treatments. Eur J Pharmacol 221: 27–33.

Gray, W. P. and Sundstrom, L. E. 1998. Kainic acid increases the proliferation of granule cell progenitors in the dentate gyrus of the adult rat. Brain Res 790: 52–9.

Gwinn, R. P., Kondratyev, A., and Gale, K. 2002. Time-dependent increase in basic fibroblast growth factor protein in limbic regions following electroshock seizures. Neuroscience 114: 403–9.

Hellsten, J., Wennström, M., Mohapel, P., et al. 2002. Electroconvulsive seizures increase hippocampal neurogenesis after chronic corticosterone treatment. Eur J Neurosci 16: 283–90.

Hiroi, N., Marek, G. J., Brown, J. R., et al. 1998. Essential role of the fosB gene in molecular, cellular, and behavioral actions of chronic electroconvulsive seizures. J Neurosci 18: 6952–62.

Hsieh, T. F., Simler, S., Vergnes, M., et al. 1998. BDNF restores the expression of Jun and Fos inducible transcription factors in the rat brain following repetitive electroconvulsive seizures. Exp Neurol 149: 161–74.

Ishihara, K. and Sasa, M. 2001. Potentiation of 5-HT(3) receptor functions in the hippocampal CA1 region of rats following repeated electroconvulsive shock treatments. Neurosci Lett 307: 37–40.

Ishihara, K. and Sasa, M. 2004. Failure of repeated electroconvulsive shock treatment on 5-HT4-receptor-mediated depolarization due to protein kinase A system in young rat hippocampal CA1 neurons. J Pharmacol Sci 95: 329–34.

Jacobsen, J. P. and Mørk, A. 2004. The effect of escitalopram, desipramine, electroconvulsive seizures and lithium on brain-derived neurotrophic factor mRNA and protein expression in the rat brain and the correlation to 5-HT and 5-HIAA levels. Brain Res 1024: 183–92.

Jiménez-Vasquez, P. A., Diaz-Cabiale, Z., Caberlotto, L., et al. 2007. Electroconvulsive stimuli selectively affect behavior and neuropeptide Y (NPY) and NPY Y(1) receptor gene expressions in hippocampus and hypothalamus of Flinders Sensitive Line rat model of depression. Eur Neuropsychopharmacol 17: 298–308.

Kabbani, N., Negyessy, L., Lin, R., et al. 2002. Interaction with neuronal calcium sensor NCS-1 mediates desensitization of the D2 dopamine receptor. J Neurosci 22(19): 8476–86.

Kang, I., Miller, L. G., Moises, J., and Bazan, N. G. 1991. GABAA receptor mRNAs are increased after electroconvulsive shock. Psychopharmacol Bull 27: 359–63.

Kato, A., Fukazawa, Y., Ozawa, F., et al. 2003. Activation of ERK cascade promotes accumulation of Vesl-1S/Homer-1a immunoreactivity at synapses. Brain Res Mol Brain Res 118: 33–44.

Kety, S. 1974. Effects of repeated electroconvulsive shock on brain catecholamines. In Psychobiology of convulsive therapy (eds. Fink, M., Kety, S., McGaugh, J. W. T. A.). Washington, DC: Winston and Sons.

Kondratyev, A., Ved, R., and Gale, K. 2002. The effects of repeated minimal electroconvulsive shock exposure on levels of mRNA encoding fibroblast growth factor-2 and nerve growth factor in limbic regions. Neuroscience 114: 411–16.

Lammers, C. H., Diaz, J., Schwartz, J. C., and Sokoloff, P. 2000. Selective increase of dopamine D3 receptor gene expression as a common effect of chronic antidepressant treatments. Mol Psychiatry 5: 378–88.

Lamont, S. R., Paulls, A., and Stewart, C. A. 2001. Repeated electroconvulsive stimulation, but not antidepressant drugs, induces mossy fibre sprouting in the rat hippocampus. Brain Res 893: 53–8.

Larsen, M. H., Olesen, M., Woldbye, D. P., et al. 2005. Regulation of activity-regulated cytoskeleton protein (Arc) mRNA after acute and chronic electroconvulsive stimulation in the rat. Brain Res 1064: 161–5.

Lerer, B. 1987. Neurochemical and other neurobiological consequences of ECT: Implications for the pathogenesis and treatment of affective disorders. In Psychopharmacology: The third generation of progress (ed. Meltzer, H.). New York: Raven Press.

Li, B., Suemaru, K., Cui, R., and Araki, H. 2007. Repeated electroconvulsive stimuli have long-lasting effects on hippocampal BDNF and decrease immobility time in the rat forced swim test. Life Sci 80: 1539–43.

Lloyd, K. G., Thuret, F., and Pilc, A. 1985. Upregulation of gamma-aminobutyric acid (GABA) B binding sites in rat frontal cortex: A common action of repeated administration of different classes of antidepressants and electroshock. J Pharmacol Exp Ther 235: 191–9.

Madsen, T. M., Treschow, A., Bengzon, J., et al. 2000. Increased neurogenesis in a model of electroconvulsive therapy. Biol Psychiatry 47: 1043–9.

Malberg, J. E., Duman, R. S. 2003. Cell proliferation in adult hippocampus is decreased by inescapable stress: reversal by fluoxetine treatment. Neuropsychopharmacology 28: 1562–71.

Malberg, J. E., Eisch, A. J., Nestler, E. J., and Duman, R. S. 2000. Chronic antidepressant treatment increases neurogenesis in adult rat hippocampus. J Neurosci 20: 9104–10.

Mann, J. J. 1998. Neurobiological correlates of the antidepressant action of electroconvulsive therapy. J ECT 14: 172–80.

Marano, C. M., Phatak, P., Vemulapalli, U. R., et al. 2007. Increased plasma concentration of brain-derived neurotrophic factor with electroconvulsive therapy: A pilot study in patients with major depression. J Clin Psychiatry 68: 512–17.

Mathé, A. A. 1999. Neuropeptides and electroconvulsive treatment. J ECT 15: 60–75.

Mathé, A. A., Husum, H., El Khoury, A., et al. 2007. Search for biological correlates of depression and mechanisms of action of antidepressant treatment modalities. Do neuropeptides play a role? Physiol Behav 92: 226–31.

Meduna, L. 1936. New methods of medical treatment of schizophrenia. Arch Neurol Psychiat 35: 361–3.

Mikkelsen, J. D. and Woldbye, D. P. 2006. Accumulated increase in neuropeptide Y and somatostatin gene expression of the rat in response to repeated electroconvulsive stimulation. J Psychiatr Res 40: 153–9.

Mongeau, R., Blier, P., and de Montigny, C. 1997. The serotonergic and noradrenergic systems of the hippocampus: Their interactions and the effects of antidepressant treatments. Brain Res Brain Res Rev 23: 145–95.

Moretti, A., Gorini, A., and Villa, R. F. 2003. Affective disorders, antidepressant drugs and brain metabolism. Mol Psychiatry 8: 773–85.

Neumaier, J. F., Sexton, T. J., Yracheta, J., et al. 2001. Localization of 5-HT(7) receptors in rat brain by immunocytochemistry, in situ hybridization, and agonist stimulated cFos expression. J Chem Neuroanat 21: 63–73.

Newman, M. E., Gur, E., Shapira, B., and Lerer, B. 1998. Neurochemical mechanisms of action of ECS: Evidence from in vivo studies. J ECT 14: 153–71.

Newton, S. S., Collier, E. F., Bennett, A. H., et al. 2004. Regulation of growth factor receptor bound 2 by electroconvulsive seizure. Brain Res Mol Brain Res 129: 185–8.

Newton, S. S., Collier, E. F., Hunsberger, J., et al. 2003. Gene profile of electroconvulsive seizures: Induction of neurotrophic and angiogenic factors. J Neurosci 23: 10841–51.

Nibuya, M., Morinobu, S., and Duman, R. S. 1995. Regulation of BDNF and trkB mRNA in rat brain by chronic electroconvulsive seizure and antidepressant drug treatments. J Neurosci 15: 7539–47.

Nishioka, G., Yamada, M., Kudo, K., et al. 2003. Induction of kf-1 after repeated electroconvulsive treatment and chronic antidepressant treatment in rat frontal cortex and hippocampus. J Neural Transm 110: 277–85.

Nobler, M. S., Teneback, C. C., Nahas, Z., et al. 2000. Structural and functional neuroimaging of electroconvulsive therapy and transcranial magnetic stimulation. Depress Anxiety 12: 144–56.

Perera, T. D., Coplan, J. D., Lisanby, S. H., et al. 2007. Antidepressant-induced neurogenesis in the hippocampus of adult nonhuman primates. J Neurosci 27: 4894–901.

Pitra, P., Tokarski, K., Grzegorzewska, M., and Hess, G. 2007. Effects of repetitive administration of tianeptine, zinc hydroaspartate and electroconvulsive shock on the reactivity of 5-HT(7) receptors in rat hippocampus. Pharmacol Rep 59: 627–35.

Ploski, J. E., Newton, S. S., and Duman, R. S. 2006. Electroconvulsive seizure-induced gene expression profile of the hippocampus dentate gyrus granule cell layer. J Neurochem 99: 1122–32.

Rosa, D. V., Souza, R. P., Souza, B. R., et al. 2007. NCS-1 expression in rat brain after electroconvulsive stimulation. Neurochem Res 32: 81–5.

Sackeim, H. A., Devanand, D. P., and Nobler, M. S. 1995. Electroconvulsive therapy. In Psychopharmacology: The third generation of progress (eds. Bloom, F. E. and Kupfer, D. J.). New York: Raven Press.

Sairanen, M., Lucas, G., Ernfors, P., et al. 2005. Brain-derived neurotrophic factor and antidepressant drugs have different but coordinated effects on neuronal turnover, proliferation, and survival in the adult dentate gyrus. J Neurosci 25: 1089–94.

Santarelli, L., Saxe, M., Gross, C., et al. 2003. Requirement of hippocampal neurogenesis for the behavioral effects of antidepressants. Science 301: 805–9.

Scott, B. W., Wojtowicz, J. M., and Burnham, W. M. 2000. Neurogenesis in the dentate gyrus of the rat following electroconvulsive shock seizures. Exp Neurol 165: 231–6.

Serretti, A., Kato, M., De Ronchi, D., and Kinoshita, T. 2007. Meta-analysis of serotonin transporter gene promoter polymorphism (5-HTTLPR) association with selective serotonin reuptake inhibitor efficacy in depressed patients. Mol Psychiatry 12: 247–57.

Shapira, B., Lerer, B., Kindler, S., et al. 1992. Enhanced serotonergic responsivity following electroconvulsive therapy in patients with major depression. Br J Psychiatry 160: 223–9.

Shen, H., Numachi, Y., Yoshida, S., et al. 2001. Electroconvulsive shock regulates serotonin transporter mRNA expression in rat raphe nucleus. Psychiatry Clin Neurosci 55: 75–7.

Stewart, C., Jeffery, K., and Reid, I. 1994. LTP-like synaptic efficacy changes following electroconvulsive stimulation. Neuroreport 5: 1041–4.

Strome, E. M., Clark, C. M., Zis, A. P., and Doudet, D. J. 2005. Electroconvulsive shock decreases binding to 5-HT2 receptors in nonhuman primates: an in vivo positron emission tomography study with [18F]setoperone. Biol Psychiatry 57(9): 1004–10.

Strome, E. M., Zis, A. P., and Doudet, D. J. 2007. Electroconvulsive shock enhances striatal dopamine D1 and D3 receptor binding and improves motor performance in 6-OHDA-lesioned rats. J Psychiatry Neurosci 32: 193–202.

Takahashi, K., Yamada, M., Ohata, H., et al. 2005. Expression of Ndrg2 in the rat frontal cortex after antidepressant and electroconvulsive treatment. Int J Neuropsychopharmacol 8: 381–9.

Tanaka, S., Yamada, M., Kitahara, S., et al. 2006. Induction of neuroserpin expression in rat frontal cortex after chronic antidepressant treatment and electroconvulsive treatment. Nihon Shinkei Seishin Yakurigaku Zasshi 26: 51–6.

Tanis, K. Q., Duman, R. S., and Newton, S. S. 2007. CREB binding and activity in brain: Regional specificity and induction by electroconvulsive seizure. Biol Psychiatry [Epub ahead of print].

Tsankova, N. M., Kumar, A., and Nestler, E. J. 2004. Histone modifications at gene promoter regions in rat hippocampus after acute and chronic electroconvulsive seizures. J Neurosci 24: 5603–10.

Vaidya, V. A., Siuciak, J. A., Du, F., and Duman, R. S. 1999. Hippocampal mossy fiber sprouting induced by chronic electroconvulsive seizures. Neuroscience 89: 157–66.

van Praag, H. M. 1977. Depression and schizophrenia: A contribution on their chemical pathologies. New York: Spectrum, p. 119.

Wielosz, M., Stelmasiak, M., Ossowska, G., and Kleinrok, Z. 1985. Effects of electroconvulsive shock on central GABA-ergic mechanisms. Pol J Pharmacol Pharm 37: 113–22.

Winston, S. M., Hayward, M. D., Nestler, E. J., and Duman, R. S. 1990. Chronic electroconvulsive seizures down-regulate expression of the immediate-early genes c-fos and c-jun in rat cerebral cortex. J Neurochem 54: 1920–5.

Yamada, M., Iwabuchi, T., Takahashi, K., et al. 2005. Identification and expression of frizzled-3 protein in rat frontal cortex after antidepressant and electroconvulsive treatment. J Pharmacol Sci 99: 239–46.

Yamada, M., Takahashi, K., Tsunoda, M., et al. 2002. Differential expression of VAMP2/synaptobrevin-2 after antidepressant and electroconvulsive treatment in rat frontal cortex. Pharmacogenomics J 2: 377–82.

Yoon, S. C., Ahn, Y. M., Jun, S. J., et al. 2005. Region-specific phosphorylation of ERK5-MEF2C in the rat frontal cortex and hippocampus after electroconvulsive shock. Prog Neuropsychopharmacol Biol Psychiatry 29: 749–53.

Zetterström, T. S., Pei, Q., and Grahame-Smith, D. G. 1998. Repeated electroconvulsive shock extends the duration of enhanced gene expression for BDNF in rat brain compared with a single administration. Brain Res Mol Brain Res 57: 106–10.

Zis, A. P., Nomikos, G. G., Brown, E. E., et al. 1992. Neurochemical effects of electrically and chemically induced seizures: An in vivo microdialysis study in the rat hippocampus. Neuropsychopharmacology 7: 189–95.

4

Hypothesized mechanisms and sites of action of electroconvulsive therapy

Nikolaus Michael

Introduction

Hypothesized mechanisms of action concerning electroconvulsive therapy (ECT) are legion. There is a practical need to explain how ECT works to patients, and beyond it a theory of action should be of heuristic value to gain insight into the pathophysiology of disorders amenable to ECT.

Any formulation of mechanisms of ECT will encounter several difficulties: ECT is effective in different illnesses such as schizophrenia, depression, and mania. Have these different disorders a common pathophysiological basis, or has ECT multiple effects just exerting the relevant one with the actual disorder under treatment? A useful theory therefore should not be restricted to a single neurotransmitter or only to the antidepressant effect. Although innumerable discoveries have been made from applying modern molecular, neurochemical, neurophysiological, and neuroimaging techniques to the investigation of mental diseases, the etiology and pathophysiology of mood disorders and schizophrenia are far from being unraveled. Hence, a theory of ECT mechanism cannot be complete. But ECT may stimulate pathophysiological thinking independent of pharmacological research.

Current hypotheses

A few hypotheses gained importance and should be considered here (Table 4.1).

Neurochemical theories

Neurotransmitter theories

Concerning the action of psychotropic drugs, a disturbed neurotransmitter action has been claimed to constitute the pathophysiological basis of mental diseases. The serotonin hypothesis, for example, should explain mood disorders and the dopamine hypothesis of schizophrenia. However, no single-transmitter–based theory will meet all aspects of the complex neurochemistry of psychiatric disorders.

Table 4.1 Hypotheses of mechanisms of action

Hypothesis	Theory	Chemical	Physiological	Anatomical
Transmitter	Recovery of disturbed neurotransmitter action	+		
Molecular	Disturbed intracellular signaling, modifying genetic expression, e.g., neurotrophic action	+		
Neuroendocrine	"Centrencephalic" stimulation, especially of hypothalamus with hormonal reactions	+		(+)
Anticonvulsive	Anticonvulsive properties responsible for effect, combined with "kindling hypothesis"		+	
Seizure generalization	Generalized seizure necessary condition		+	(+)
Anatomical	Stimulation of prefrontal brain, i.e., critical regions for mood regulation			+
Combined anatomical/ictal	Combination: generalized seizures with effects on critical, especially prefrontal, brain regions		+	+

Therefore, the dopamine hypothesis (schizophrenia) and the monoamine hypothesis (mood disorders) have been extended to other neurotransmitter systems, for example, glutamate or gamma-aminobutyric acid (GABA). Additionally, intracellular signaling, neurotrophic factors, and theories of neuroplasticity have been included in pathophysiological models. Because ECT seems to alter virtually every neurotransmitter system (see Chapter 3), it is difficult to discern its essential effects. Briefly, the neurotransmitter theory supposes that ECT restores a disturbed transmitter function either by elevating transmitter concentrations or by activating receptors.

Intracellular signaling, gene transcription, and neurotrophic action

Recently, neuronal plasticity and resilience have gained much interest. It was supposed that severe depression is accompanied by increased neurotoxicity and diminished neurotrophic stimulation (Duman et al., 1997). Meanwhile, antidepressants, anticonvulsants, and lithium were shown to exert neurotrophic effects by modulating gene expression. It is suggested that ECT exerts neurotrophic effects, too (Bolwig and Madsen, 2007). Data from animal studies show that ECT stimulates neurogenesis and axonal sprouting (Lamont et al., 2001; Madsen et al., 2000). In severely depressed patients, ECT was demonstrated to increase *N*-acetylaspartate (NAA) in responding patients only. NAA is a marker of neuronal viability, and its increase indicates a neurotrophic effect (Michael et al., 2003c). The significance of these observations remains unclear but they point toward nurturing and regenerating effects of ECT and away from potential neurotoxicity (for further discussion, see Chapter 3). The neurotrophic theory focuses on the existence of structural abnormalities, for example, hippocampal atrophy in severely depressed patients (Sheline et al., 1999). Although the neurotrophic model of depression may well account for the time lag until the specific antidepressant effect occurs, it should be complemented by functional concepts to satisfactorily explain clinical observations such as abrupt switches in mood state, circadian mood fluctuations, and early response to ECT.

The diencephalic theory or neuroendocrine view

Severe depression is accompanied by disturbed hormonal secretion (Nemeroff et al., 1991), particularly of cortisol, and dysfunction of the hypothalamic–pituitary–adrenal (HPA) axis (Sapolsky, 2000). Cortisol and several other hormones (such as thyroxine and sex hormones) have psychotropic effects, and excesses or deficiencies of these hormones can induce states of depression or mania (Aihara et al., 2007). Furthermore, subcortical clinical symptoms of disturbed sleep, appetite, level of consciousness, and sexual drive during depression or mania suggest a central role of the hypothalamus. Some advocates of the neuroendocrine view of depression propose that severe mood disorders are caused by a deficiency of certain hormonal substances, and ECT would act via deep stimulation of centrencephalic structures to level out this deficiency. However, such hormonal substances have not been identified (Fink, 1990). It has been further argued that a close relationship exists between the success of ECT and the vegetative response to the induced seizure such as an increase of blood pressure and heart rate (Chapter 30; Swartz, 2000). Moreover, an increase of blood flow in the basal ganglia, brainstem, and diencephalon, as shown by positron emission tomography (PET), indicates that centrencephalic brain structures are stimulated by ECT (Takano et al., 2007). Unfortunately, it is still unsettled whether hormonal aberrations are central etiological factors or merely functional sequelae of the illness and the ECT seizure (Garlow et al., 1999). Symptoms thought to arise from disturbed hypothalamic function, such as disturbed libido, appetite, and sleep, are not specific to mood disorders, but can occur outside mood episodes. Although these symptoms are typical features of melancholic depression, they may be absent during mood episodes. Because a close interconnection exists between the limbic system and the hypothalamus, generalized seizures inevitably involve stimulation of the hypothalamus with massive activation of the sympathetic nervous system, including increased heart rate, blood pressure, and hormone levels. These effects may play a role in the process of recovery. Nevertheless, it remains controversial if ECT acts predominantly through such an indirect neurochemical mechanism or by direct stimulation of the frontal lobe.

Anticonvulsant theory

Typically, the seizure threshold increases across a treatment course, indicating an anticonvulsant action of ECT (Sackeim et al., 1987). Lack of increase in seizure threshold was postulated to be associated with worse clinical outcome (Sackeim, 1999), that is, ECT was suggested to act through antiepileptic mechanisms. This view claims support from the kindling hypothesis (Post and Weiss, 1999) that recurrence of mood episodes may be triggered by labile and facilitated neuronal excitability. Kindling may explain the clinical antimanic effect of anticonvulsants such as carbamazepine and valproate. According to this theory, a positive correlation should exist between the anticonvulsant action and therapeutic efficacy. However, the opposite was found: The greater the seizure threshold increase, the less favorable the clinical improvement (Krystal et al., 1998). Likewise, anticonvulsive drugs such as benzodiazepines impair the efficacy of ECT. The interdependency of seizures and anticonvulsant action could account for the inconsistency of the results. An increase of seizure threshold may indicate that the seizures are sufficient and at the same time interfere with effectiveness. Thus, ECT would be less effective in patients predisposed to develop rapid increase of seizure threshold, which may hamper seizure generalization. Therefore, it seems unlikely that anticonvulsant activity constitutes the therapeutic principle of ECT.

Anatomical theory or prefrontal model

An anatomically based model proposes that the prefrontal lobe, which is critically involved in the regulation of mood and cognition (Fuster, 2001; Gray et al., 2002), must be stimulated. It emphasizes the direct and vigorous stimulation of the prefrontal lobe in contrast to the indirect action via the monoaminergic transmitters or the diencephalon. This hypothesis of direct stimulation of the prefrontal cortex applies as well to transcranial magnetic stimulation (TMS). The notion of greater efficacy of bilateral (bifrontal and bitemporal) than unilateral stimulation treatment – except for high stimulus doses – is in line with this view, as is the reported association between clinical improvement and greater prefrontal slowing of electroencephalogram (EEG) activity (Sackeim et al., 1996). Because mental disorders do not affect only mood, thought, and cognition, but also somatic function, the anatomical model should include the limbic system and brainstem. Still, it remains obscure what exactly happens within these brain regions.

Seizure generalization theory

Seizure generalization seems to be essential for the efficacy of ECT (Ottosson, 1960). It can be estimated from ictal EEG amplitude, coherence, postictal suppression, and from physiologic responses such as increased heart rate or prolactin release (Chapters 8 and 30; Abrams, 1991). Near-threshold or low-dose unilateral stimulation seems to be less effective than unilateral high dose or bilateral seizure induction, and these methods are associated with weak seizure spread through the brain. The more extensively the seizure spreads through the brain, the greater the therapeutic effect. A more generalized seizure should correspond to more brainstem stimulation. In ECT the stimulus is applied to the cortex, not the brainstem. If the brainstem is involved in therapeutic mechanisms, greater generalization should correspond to greater efficacy. Furthermore, epileptological research has shown that extended activation of cortico-thalamo-cortical circuits seems to be critical for the efficacy of ECT (McNally and Blumenfeld, 2004). This theory likely meets the significant point of the unique principle of ECT. It covers aspects such as the stimulation of centrencephalic structures. This model relates more to the site than the physiological mechanism. Although Abrams (2002) approves this theory, he limits its value with respect to nonconvulsive treatment options such as TMS. As ECT far surpasses TMS in efficacy (Eranti et al., 2007), the seizure generalization theory seems a promising hypothesis. Still it leaves unexplained the nature of the therapeutic changes that occur as a result of the seizure.

Objections to the seizure generalization theory are that generalized seizures may not truly be generalized, and it is not necessary to involve the entire brain. In this respect it seems contradictory to combine the generalization theory with the (localized) prefrontal model suggested by Abrams ("anatomico-ictal theory").

In summary, generalized and repeated seizures affecting in particular prefrontal regions and centrencephalic structures seem to be a necessary condition for efficacy. Even if the actual consequences of these seizures await elucidation, stimulating prefrontal areas might produce more stimulation to the brainstem than to other cortical areas. Promoting seizure in cortical regions that funnel into centrencephalic structures is consistent with the seizure generalization hypothesis.

Developing a theory of ECT action – synthesis

Different organizational levels are involved in the pathophysiology of mental disorders

The brain is organized into several different functional levels (Figure 4.1), each forming an organizational unit interacting with other systems on higher or lower levels (Scott, 2002). On the highest level, the brain consists of complex assemblies of dynamically interconnected neuronal systems regulating their own and each other's activity. Lower levels extend down to the organizational units of cells, neurons,

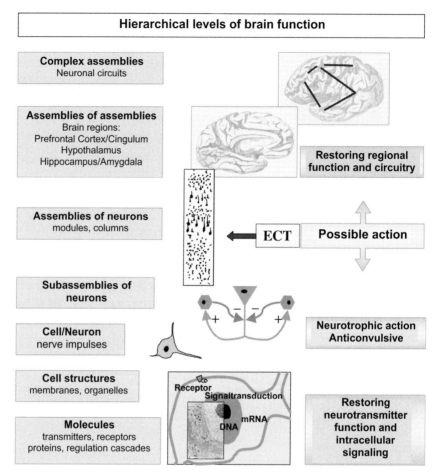

Figure 4.1   The brain is organized in different hierarchical levels, and electroconvulsive therapy (ECT) is likely to affect functions on every level. mRNA, messenger RNA. (See Color Plate I.)

and supporting glial cells, and, finally, subcellular structures and molecules (Figure 4.1). Mental disorders seem to involve neuronal function on every level. They are accompanied by molecular, neurochemical, and regional dysfunction (assemblies of neurons) up to macrofunctioning abnormalities within neuronal circuits (complex assemblies).

Mental disorders arise from the complex interaction of multiple genes and environmental factors during the brain's development and later in life (Figure 4.2). Structural abnormalities occur before (as well as a result of) a disease. They may underlie particular symptoms and influence the course of illness. For example, structural abnormalities may account for clinically stable (trait) signs whereas acute (state) symptoms emerge from functional disturbances. The nervous system is provided with a large compensatory capacity for structural aberrations. If these

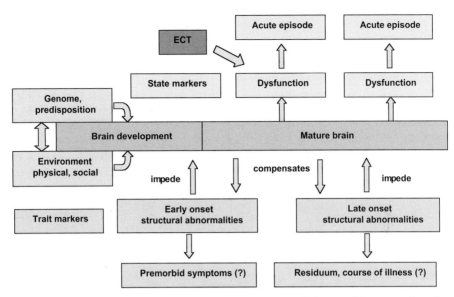

Figure 4.2   Hypothesized relationship between structural and functional abnormalities. Genetic and environmental factors interact during brain development; both can cause early onset structural abnormalities. An abnormal neuronal architecture may underlie some premorbid symptoms. Structural abnormalities can also be acquired as a consequence of illness and in this way contribute to the development of residual symptoms or influence the course of illness. The brain is equipped with a large capacity to compensate for structural abnormalities. Acute mental symptoms finally emerge from a specific pattern of disordered brain function. Electroconvulsive therapy (ECT) helps to restore proper brain function.

capacities are exceeded, dysfunction of neural networks develops and produces acute neuropsychiatric symptoms (Figure 4.2).

Mental disorders are accompanied by nonspecific functional abnormalities, for example, decreased frontal activity with schizophrenia or depression (Baxter et al., 1989) or increased frontal activity with mania (Blumberg et al., 2000; Drevets et al., 1997). Structural abnormalities may also be associated with mental disorders, for example, neuronal atrophy of prefrontal brain areas with mood disorder (Harrison, 2002) or abnormalities of neuronal architecture, probably acquired during early development, with schizophrenia (Lewis and Levitt, 2002). Structural aberrations sometimes develop in the course of illness such as greater hippocampal atrophy with increased time spent depressed (Sheline et al., 1999). Neurochemically, mental illnesses correlate with abnormalities of different transmitter systems; for instance, catecholamines and GABA as discussed for mood disorders or dopamine and glutamate for schizophrenia. Finally, mental illnesses are accompanied by abnormalities on the molecular level of intracellular signaling and genetic expression (Manji et al., 2001). All these different levels of neuronal function and structure seem to participate in the pathogenesis of severe mental diseases. Therefore, it seems implausible to restrict a mechanism of action to any one of these levels, and it should be expected that ECT produces effects within each organizational level and in several different regions of pathology.

What happens during electrical stimulation?

Eliciting a seizure by overcoming surrounding inhibition

For the central nervous system (CNS) to ensure proper functioning and avoid damage, it is extremely important to prevent any synchronous and rhythmic depolarization of larger populations of neurons. Prevention is achieved by maintaining a delicate balance of inhibitory (mainly GABA) and excitatory (mainly glutamate) synaptic activity. Thus the brain is well prepared to obstruct any spreading of uncontrolled electrical activity through inhibitory mechanisms such as feedforward, feedback, and surrounding inhibition provided mainly by GABAergic inhibitory neurons.

These mechanisms, in particular the inhibitory counterbalance of GABAergic neurons, are overcome by ECT seizure induction, which is achieved by a calculated stimulation resulting in rapid-onset synchronization of electrical activity of large populations of neurons (see Chapter 1). In contrast to TMS, which affects only a small cortical region near the surface, or drugs, which act indirectly via enhancing or blunting the effectiveness of transmitter action, ECT directly stimulates large populations of cortical neurons – and consequently multiple subcortical structures – by spreading synchronized neuronal activity throughout the brain (Figure 4.3).

Relatively small amounts of electrical charge are needed to elicit a seizure. Seizure induction is achieved by applying brief (0.5- to 1-ms) pulses to the scalp (see Chapter 1). The total time of current flowing when aggregating all pulses of the stimulation is less than 1 second (Figure 4.4). The remaining work of propagating the seizure and then limiting it takes about 1 minute, and this sets off a series of physiological reactions following the ECT session (Figure 4.4). Among these reactions are effects that ultimately lead to remission of the illness. In simplistic terms, ECT assists the brain to help itself and, remarkably, the brain needs no further support or guidance besides the seizures to regain normal function.

There are fundamental differences between ECT and spontaneous epileptic seizures (Table 4.2). An ECT seizure occurs under controlled conditions, in other words, anesthesia, muscle relaxation, and oxygenation. Seizure duration is limited by the administering physician to ensure a desirable risk–benefit relationship. In contrast, epileptic seizures can be prolonged and consequently cause injury from derangements of metabolism (hypoglycemia, hypoxia, acidemia, hypotension, and

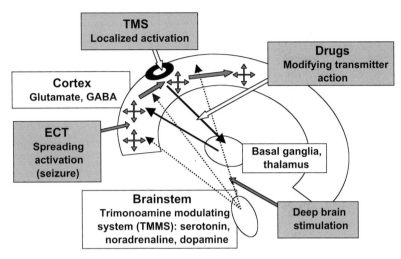

Figure 4.3   Targets of electroconvulsive, neuromodulational, and pharmacological therapy.
Electroconvulsive therapy (ECT) induces the spreading of excessive neuronal activity,
transcranial magnetic stimulation (TMS) stimulates nonconvulsively a small area of the
cortical surface, and drugs act enhancingly or bluntingly on the effectiveness of synaptic
transmitter action. GABA, gamma-aminobutyric acid.

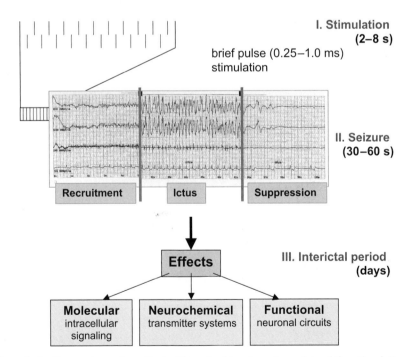

Figure 4.4   Seizure induction and ensuing effects. The actual treatment consists of the stimulation,
which takes a few seconds (I). The seizure (II), its limitation, and the resulting effects (III)
are the brain's work. (See Color Plate II.)

Table 4.2 Differences between epileptic and electrically induced seizures

Seizure	Electroconvulsive seizure	Epileptic seizure
Occurrence	Calculated	Spontaneous
Duration	30 to 60 s	Often longer
Beginning/Termination	Abrupt	Gradually
Oxygenation	Yes	No
Hyperexcitability	No	Proneness
Brain damage	No	Sometimes
Epileptogenesis	No, anticonvulsant	Probably yes, kindling

intracellular exhaustion of energy) (Chamberlin and Tsai, 1998). An instantly achieved generalization of seizure activity may favor the immediate anticonvulsant action of ECT. In this respect, ECT seizures resemble the generalized epilepsies – for example, juvenile myoclonic epilepsy – that are less toxic epilepsies. Finally, the induction of ECT seizure is achieved by stimulating large frontal brain volumes, from which the epileptic activity spreads over the brain. In comparison, epileptic seizures start from specific small foci, often within the temporal lobe, with surrounding inhibition (Table 4.2).

It is not likely the seizure, but various ensuing reactions of the brain that lead to benefit in psychiatric illness (Figure 4.4). If the seizure itself were curative, a dose dependency should be expected in such a way that increasing length or frequency of seizures should improve the efficacy of ECT. The multiple monitored ECT (MMECT) technique has shown that this is not the case (Maletzky, 1986); moreover, long seizures are not more effective than short ones (Shapira et al., 1996). Rather the quality of the seizure determines the therapeutic result. The efficacy of ECT does not follow a simple all-or-none or the-more-the-better pattern. A therapeutic range exists between too short to be effective and too long to be harmless (Figure 4.5); in other words, there is an optimal range of seizure duration

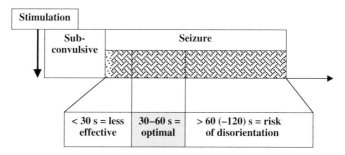

Figure 4.5   The optimal seizure duration. If the seizure duration is too short, it will be less effective; if it is too long, the risk of adverse effects increases.

for obtaining desirable efficacy and minimizing adverse effects. The assessment of seizure quality comprises its onset, termination, generalization, intensity, and duration. However, there exists only an indirect relationship between a seizure and its efficacy; thus, good seizure quality does not necessarily perfectly predict good clinical response and vice versa.

Functional consequences in response to ECT

In particular, single photon emission computed tomography (SPECT) and PET have been applied to elucidate the functional reactions to ECT. In addition, magnetic resonance spectroscopy (MRS) provides insight into metabolism. These techniques have yielded interesting although contradictory results (see Chapter 5).

Major depression seems to be accompanied by decreased metabolic activity of prefrontal brain regions, especially dorsolateral prefrontal cortex (DLPFC) and anterior cingulate cortex (ACC) (Baxter et al., 1989; Bench et al., 1993). This abnormality fades with successful treatment, including with ECT (Blumenfeld et al., 2003; Bonne et al., 1996; Galynker et al., 1997; Henry et al., 2001; Milo et al., 2001). Preliminary observations indicate that acute mania may be associated with abnormalities in the opposite direction, that is, hypermetabolism of frontocortical regions (Blumberg et al., 1999; Drevets et al., 1997).

Abnormal metabolism as observed by SPECT or PET mainly follows alterations in glutamatergic neurotransmission. As the major excitatory neurotransmitter in the CNS, glutamate is used by up to 60% to 80% of brain synapses (Braitenberg and Schüz, 1998). Similarly, glutamatergic neurotransmitter circulation expends up to 80% of brain metabolic energy consumption (Rothman et al., 2003). Glutamate/glutamine (Glx) as measured by MRS may serve as a marker for neuronal activity. Glx levels as measured by MRS should correspond to the results of neuroimaging studies. In fact, severely depressed patients revealed decreased Glx levels prior to ECT, and Glx levels normalized in patients responding to ECT but not in nonresponders within the DLPFC (Michael et al., 2003a) and the ACC (Pfleiderer et al., 2003). By contrast, acute mania is apparently accompanied by elevated Glx levels, presumably correlating with increased activation (Michael et al., 2003b).

Interestingly, GABA concentrations seem to change parallel to Glx levels, so they are reduced in major depression (Hasler et al., 2007) and they normalize after ECT (Sanacora et al., 2003). In a small subgroup of depressed patients, an increased uptake of iomazenil, a GABA receptor ligand detectable by SPECT, has been demonstrated after successful ECT, indicating increased GABA sensitivity (Mervaala et al., 2001). A similar pattern has already been observed with simultaneously increased serotonin and its receptor (5-HT_2 receptor) after ECT. Perhaps

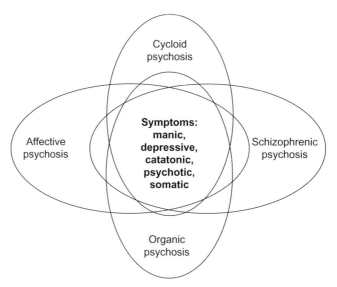

Figure 4.6   Syndromal overlap among psychotic illnesses: Manic, depressive, catatonic, and psychotic (hallucinations, delusions) symptoms may occur with all psychotic diseases.

the strong excitatory activity of ECT enhances GABA neurotransmission, which then contributes to normalizing neuronal function (see Chapter 3).

From a psychopathological perspective, schizophrenia and affective disorders (as well as organic and cycloid psychoses) show similar affective (depressive, manic), psychotic (delusions, hallucinations), catatonic, and somatic symptoms (vegetative dysfunction), all of which diminish as the illness responds to ECT (Figure 4.6). Comparable pathophysiological mechanisms may underlie a particular affective or psychotic symptom, irrespective of whether the basic illness is schizophrenia or bipolar disorder. Decreased frontal activity ("hypofrontality") may likewise reflect a depressive state, whereas elevated Glx levels may occur with manic or acute psychotic symptoms (Thiéberge et al., 2002) in patients with schizophrenia. ECT presumably ameliorates particular symptoms by restoring balanced function. Preliminary results of a PET study on acute psychotic patients with schizophrenia indicate that frontal hypermetabolism decreases with successful ECT (Uesugi et al., 1995). Presumably acute affective and psychotic symptoms emerge from functional abnormalities, whereas residual chronic symptoms such as flat affect, cognitive impairment, and passive patterns of thinking correspond to structural changes. The difference between functional and structural basis may explain why ECT effectively improves acute symptoms more than negative symptoms occurring with schizophrenia. Because of substantial diagnostic uncertainties in differentiating among chronic psychotic disorders (including schizoaffective disorder and psychotic mood disorders), it remains unclear how well ECT treats schizophrenia. Yet it seems reasonable to expect that ECT is effective in a variety of psychiatric diagnoses with similar acute symptoms (see Chapters 7 and 22).

Restoring balanced neuronal network function after repeated seizures

The seizure marks the beginning of the healing process. It produces an instantaneous and profound disruption of ordinary brain function. After the hypersynchronous – mainly glutamatergic excitatory – excessive activity of widespread cortical and subcortical neurons, the brain ordinarily limits the seizure by strong – mainly GABAergic – inhibition. The result is a hyperpolarization, discernible as suppression on the EEG. Diminished neuronal activity after repeated seizures may account for some findings of decreased brain metabolism after ECT (Conca et al., 2003; Nobler et al., 1994, 2001). Function recovers along with the gradual reappearance of normal EEG activity and, clinically, consciousness. The process of recovering function involves neuronal systems of all sizes, from single neurons to network assemblies (Figure 4.1). Repeated seizures modulate functions on the molecular level as seen, for example, from increased protein syntheses revealed by PET using the labeled amino acid methionine, $[^{11}C]MET$ (Sermet et al., 1998), as well as on the complex level of neuronal circuits as depicted by PET (Kohn et al., 2007; Navarro et al., 2004). The particular mechanisms of recovering neuronal function are largely unknown. They may be of particular interest to elucidate the mechanisms of action of ECT. Perhaps it is the brain's ability to restore balanced function after convulsive activity that leads to recovered homeostasis and restoration of function (Figure 4.7). This capability – restoring balanced function – constitutes a general feature of complex biological systems and does not differ in principle, but only in complexity, from cardiac arrhythmia converted to normal heart action by defibrillation.

As mentioned earlier, ECT seems to normalize pathologically up- or down-regulated neuronal function, for example, regional hyperactivity with mania or acute psychosis or regional hypoactivity with depression or perhaps catatonia. It is reasonable to suppose that multiple interconnected neuronal systems (e.g., prefrontal cortex, ACC, thalamus, hippocampus, amygdala, hypothalamus, and brainstem) subserve mood, affect, and behavior. Then affective or psychotic symptoms may emerge from specific patterns of activation in neuronal networks that are distributed across the brain. ECT probably restores a normal functional balance within complex neuronal networks (Figure 4.8). However, such a model remains somewhat speculative because of the paucity of available data concerning the underlying mechanisms of these different mood states and their reactions to ECT.

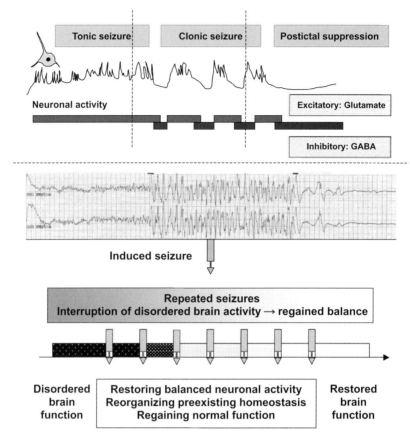

Figure 4.7   Induced seizures disrupt neuronal activity, followed by reorganization and restoration of normal function. It is perhaps the repeated disruption of disordered activity and the rebuilding of ordinary balanced neuronal activity from postictal suppression that are essential for efficacy. GABA, gamma-aminobutyric acid. (See Color Plate III.)

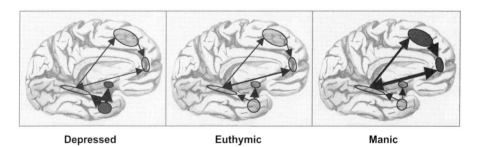

Figure 4.8   Sketch (hypothetical) of imbalanced activity within a neuronal circuit. Clinical syndromes may result from distinct patterns of dysregulated (= imbalanced) neuronal circuitry, in other words, overactivated as well as underactivated regions contribute to a complex constellation of symptoms (e.g., manic, depressive, catatonic, and psychotic symptoms). Gray intensity and thickness of arrows indicate disordered activity. (See Color Plate IV.)

The neuronal mechanisms underlying this process, the roadmaps to ordinary function, remain unknown. For elucidating the mechanisms of action of ECT, it will be important to look at the neuronal reactions immediately following seizure.

Overall view

Neither the pathophysiology of severe mental disorders (such as affective disorders or schizophrenia) nor the mechanisms of action of antidepressant, antimanic, and antipsychotic therapies have yet been elucidated, including drug treatments. Therefore, any theory of ECT mechanism of action is hypothetical. Still, a theory of action is helpful to explain the intent of ECT to patients. It may also contribute to understanding the pathophysiology of disorders treatable by ECT.

ECT is used to treat several very different conditions, for example depressive, manic, delusional, hallucinatory, catatonic, and associated somatic (vegetative) syndromes. These syndromes are not specific but can occur with schizophrenic, affective, or organic psychoses. Each syndrome may be caused by distinctly different pathophysiologic mechanisms, for instance, a characteristic pattern of dysfunction within complex neuronal circuits. Malfunction concerns particular neuronal circuits including prefrontal brain regions, the limbic system, the hypothalamus, the brainstem, as well as neurotransmission and intracellular chemistry.

Eliciting a generalized seizure seems crucial for efficacy. Subconvulsive or less widely spread seizures may have some effect, but the more that large-scale neuronal networks get stimulated, the better the clinical response. The primary site of action seems to be the excitable cortex, preferably the frontal lobe, although it seems essential to stimulate subcortical structures such as the hypothalamus and brainstem.

Severe mental disorders are accompanied by functional disturbance of large-scale neuronal networks, but it seems unlikely that the whole brain is pathologically involved. Therefore, whole brain stimulation presumably is not required for successful treatment. Nevertheless, if prefrontal regions must undergo seizure, it will be impossible to decide whether the inevitable stimulation of interconnected deep brain structures is necessary for efficacy. However, the manifold physical signs of subcortical dysfunction imply that stimulation of the hypothalamus and brainstem play an essential role in the treatment process.

Finally, it is not the seizure that cures but the brain that restores function by unknown mechanisms as a result of a series of ECT seizures. There must exist an essential capability for rebuilding balanced function in response to repeated seizures. Biological systems in general seem to be equipped with mechanisms to restore homeostasis. Neuronal tissue in particular restores balanced function after repeated seizures, which consist of excessive excitation followed by profound inhibition. These processes demand further investigation. However, a broad set of basic and clinical investigations is needed before we can step forward from preclinical intuition to clinical evidence about the mechanisms of action of ECT.

References

Abrams, R. 1991. Seizure generalization and the efficacy of unilateral electroconvulsive therapy. Convuls Ther 7: 213–17.

Abrams, R. 2002. Electroconvulsive therapy, 4th edn. Oxford: Oxford University Press.

Aihara, M., Ida, I., Yuuki, N., et al. 2007. HPA axis dysfunction in unmedicated major depressive disorder and its normalization by pharmacotherapy correlates with alteration of neural activity in prefrontal cortex and limbic/paralimbic regions. Psychiatry Res 155: 245–56.

Baxter, L. R., Schwartz, J. M., Phelps, M. E., et al. 1989. Reduction of prefrontal cortex glucose metabolism common to three types of depression. Arch Gen Psychiatry 46: 243–50.

Bench, C. J., Friston, K. J., Brown, R. G., et al. 1993. Regional cerebral blood flow in depression measured by positron emission tomography: The relationship with clinical dimensions. Psychol Med 23: 579–90.

Blumberg, H. P., Stern, E., Ricketts, S., et al. 1999. Rostral and orbital prefrontal dysfunction in the manic state of bipolar disorder. Am J Psychiatry 156: 1986–88.

Blumberg, H. P., Stern, E., Martinez, D., et al. 2000. Increased anterior cingulate and caudate activity in bipolar mania. Biol Psychiatry 48: 1045–52.

Blumenfeld, H., McNally, K. A., Ostroff, R. B., and Zubal, I. G. 2003. Targeted prefrontal cortical activation with bifrontal ECT. Psychiatry Res 123(3): 165–70.

Bolwig, T. G. and Madsen, T. M. 2007. Electroconvulsive therapy in melancholia: The role of hippocampal neurogenesis. Acta Psychiatr Scand Suppl (433): 130–5.

Bonne, O., Krausz, Y., Shapira, B., et al. 1996. Increased cerebral blood flow in depressed patients responding to electroconvulsive therapy. J Nucl Med 37(7): 1075–80.

Braitenberg, V. and Schüz, A. 1998. Cortex: Statistics and geometry of neuronal connectivity, 2nd edn. Berlin: Springer.

Chamberlin, E. and Tsai, G. E. 1998. A glutamatergic model of ECT-induced memory dysfunction. Harv Rev Psychiatry 5: 307–17.

Conca, A., Prapotnik, M., Peschina, W., and König, P. 2003. Simultaneous pattern of rCBF and rCMRGlu in continuation ECT: Case reports. Psychiatry Res 124(3): 191–8.

Drevets, W. C., Price, J. L., Simpson, J. R., et al. 1997. Subgenual prefrontal cortex abnormalities in mood disorders. Nature 386: 824–7.

Duman, R. S., Heniger, G. R., and Nestler, E. J. 1997. A molecular and cellular theory of depression. Arch Gen Psychiatry 54: 597–606.

Eranti, S., et al. 2007. A randomized, controlled trial with 6-month follow-up of repetitive transcranial magnetic stimulation and electroconvulsive therapy for severe depression. Am J Psychiatry 164(1): 73–81.

Fink, M. 1990. How does convulsive therapy work? Neuropsychopharmacology 3: 73–82.

Fuster, J. M. 2001. The prefrontal cortex – an update: Time is of the essence. Neuron 30(2): 319–33.

Galynker, I. I., Weiss, J., Ongseng, F., and Finestone, H. 1997. ECT treatment and cerebral perfusion in catatonia. J Nucl Med 38(2): 251–4.

Garlow, S. J., Musselman, D. L., and Nemeroff, C. B. 1999. The neurochemistry of mood disorders: Clinical studies. In Neurobiology of mental illness (eds. Charney, D. S., Nestler, E. J., and Bunney, B. S.). New York: Oxford University Press, pp. 348–64.

Gray, J. R., Braver, T. S., and Raichle, M. E. 2002. Integration of emotion and cognition in the lateral prefrontal cortex. Proc Natl Acad Sci USA 99(6): 4115–20.

Harrison, P. J. 2002. The neuropathology of primary mood disorder. Brain 125: 1428–49.

Hasler, G., Van Der Veen, J. W., Tumonis, T., Meyers, N., et al. 2007. Reduced prefrontal glutamate/glutamine and GABA levels in major depression determined using proton magnetic resonance spectroscopy. Arch Gen Psychiatry 64: 193–200.

Henry, M. E., Schmidt, M. E., Matochik, J. A., et al. 2001. The effects of ECT on brain glucose: A pilot FDG PET study. J ECT 17(1): 33–40.

Kohn, Y., Freedman, N., Lester, H., et al. 2007. 99mTc-HMPAO SPECT study of cerebral perfusion after treatment with medication and electroconvulsive therapy in major depression. J Nucl Med 48(8): 1273–8.

Krystal, A. D., Coffey, C. E., Weiner, R. D., and Holsinger, T. 1998. Changes in seizure threshold over the course of electroconvulsive therapy affect therapeutic response and are detected by ictal EEG ratings. J Neuropsychiatry Clin Neurosci 10(2): 178–86.

Lamont, S. R., Pauls, A., and Stewart, C. A. 2001. Repeated electroconvulsive stimulation, but not antidepressant drugs, induces mossy fibre sprouting in the rat hippocampus. Brain Res 893: 53–58.

Lewis, D. A. and Levitt, P. 2002. Schizophrenia as a disorder of neurodevelopment. Annu Rev Neurosci 25: 409–32.

Madsen, T. M., Treschow, A., Bengzon, J., et al. 2000. Increased neurogenesis in a model of electroconvulsive therapy. Biol Psychiatry 47: 1043–9.

Maletzky, B. M. 1986. Conventional and multiple-monitored electroconvulsive therapy. A comparison in major depressive episodes. J Nerv Ment Dis 174(5): 257–64.

Manji, H. K., Drevets, W. C., and Charney, D. 2001. The cellular neurobiology of depression. Nat Med 5: 541–7.

McNally, K. A. and Blumenfeld, H. 2004. Focal network involvement in generalized seizures: New insights from electroconvulsive therapy. Epilepsy Behav 5(1): 3–12.

Mervaala, E., Könönen, M., Föhr, J., et al. 2001. SPECT and neuropsychological performance in severe depression treated with ECT. J Affect Disord 66(1): 47–58.

Michael, N., Erfurth, A., Ohrmann, P., et al. 2003a. Metabolic changes within the left dorsolateral prefrontal cortex occurring with electroconvulsive therapy in patients with treatment resistant unipolar depression. Psychol Med 33(7): 1277–84.

Michael, N., Erfurth, A., Ohrmann, P., et al. 2003b. Acute mania is accompanied by elevated glutamate/glutamine levels within the left dorsolateral prefrontal cortex. Psychopharmacology 168: 344–6.

Michael, N., Erfurth, A., Ohrmann, P., et al. 2003c. Neurotrophic effect of electroconvulsive therapy: A proton magnetic resonance study of the left amygdalar region in severely depressed elderly patients. Neuropsychopharmacology 28: 720–5.

Milo, T. J., Kaufman, G. E., Barnes, W. E., et al. 2001. Changes in regional cerebral blood flow after electroconvulsive therapy for depression. J ECT 17(1): 15–21.

Navarro, V., Gastó, C., Lomeña, F., et al. 2004. Frontal cerebral perfusion after antidepressant drug treatment versus ECT in elderly patients with major depression: A 12-month follow-up control study. J Clin Psychiatry 65(5): 656–61.

Nemeroff, C. B., Bissette, G., Akil, H., and Fink, M. 1991. Neuropeptide concentrations in the cerebrospinal fluid of depressed patients treated with electroconvulsive therapy. Br J Psychiatry 158: 59–63.

Nobler, M. S., Sackeim, H. A., Prohovnik, I., et al. 1994. Regional cerebral blood flow in mood disorders, III. Treatment and clinical response. Arch Gen Psychiatry 51(11): 884–97.

Nobler, M. S., Oquendo, M. A., Kegeles, L. S., et al. 2001. Decreased regional brain metabolism after ECT. Am J Psychiatry 158(2): 305–8.

Ottosson, J. O. 1960. Experimental studies of the mode of action of electroconvulsive therapy: Introduction. Acta Psychiatr Scand Suppl 35(145): 5–6.

Pfleiderer, B., Michael, N., Erfurth, A., et al. 2003. Effective electroconvulsive therapy reverses glutamate/glutamine deficit in the left anterior cingulum of unipolar depressed patients. Psychiatry Res 122(3): 185–92.

Post, R. M. and Weiss, S. R. B. 1999. Neurobiological models of recurrence of mood disorder. In Neurobiology of mental illness (eds. Charney, D. S., Nestler, E. J., and Bunney, B. S.). New York: Oxford University Press, pp. 365–84.

Rothman, D. L., Behar, K. L., Hyder, F., and Shulman, R. G. 2003. In vivo NMR studies of the glutamate neurotransmitter flux and neuroenergetics: Implications for brain function. Annu Rev Physiol 65: 401–27.

Sackeim, H. A. 1999. The anticonvulsant hypothesis of the mechanisms of action of ECT: Current status. J ECT 15(1): 5–26.

Sackeim, H. A., Decina, P., Portnoy, S., et al. 1987. Studies of dosage, seizure threshold, and seizure duration in ECT. Biol Psychiatry 22(3): 249–68.

Sackeim, H. A., Luber, B., Katzman, G. P., et al. 1996. The effects of electroconvulsive therapy on quantitative electroencephalograms. Relationship to clinical outcome. Arch Gen Psychiatry 53(9): 814–24.

Sanacora, G., Mason, G. F., Rothman, D. L., et al. 2003. Increased cortical GABA concentrations in depressed patients receiving ECT. Am J Psychiatry 160: 577–9.

Sapolsky, R. M. 2000. Glucocorticoids and hippocampal atrophy in neuropsychiatric disorders. Arch Gen Psychiatry 57: 925–35.

Scott, A. 2002. Neuroscience. A mathematical primer. New York/Berlin/Heidelberg: Springer-Verlag, p. 352.

Sermet, E., Grégoire, M. D., Galy, G., et al. 1998. Paradoxical metabolic response of the human brain to a single electroconvulsive shock. Neurosci Lett 254(1): 41–4.

Shapira, B., Lidsky, D., Gorfine, M., and Lerer, B. 1996. Electroconvulsive therapy and resistant depression: Clinical implications of seizure threshold. J Clin Psychiatry 57(1): 32–8.

Sheline, Y. I., Sanghavi, M., Mintun, M. A., and Gado, M. D. 1999. Depression duration but not age predicts hippocampal volume loss in medically healthy women with recurrent major depression. J Neurosci 19: 5034–43.

Swartz, C. M. 2000. Physiological response to ECT stimulus dose. Psychiatry Res 97(2–3): 229–35.

Takano, H., Motohashi, N., Uema, T., et al. 2007. Changes in regional cerebral blood flow during acute electroconvulsive therapy in patients with depression: Positron emission tomographic study. Br J Psychiatry 190: 63–8.

Thiéberge, J., Bartha, R., Drost, D. J., et al. 2002. Glutamate and glutamine measured with 4.0T proton MRS in never-treated patients with schizophrenia and healthy volunteers. Am J Psychiatry 159: 1944–6.

Uesugi, H., Toyoda, J., and Iio, M. 1995. Positron emission tomography and plasma biochemistry findings in schizophrenic patients before and after electroconvulsive therapy. Psychiatry Clin Neurosci 49(2): 131–5.

5

Brain imaging and electroconvulsive therapy

Kathy Peng and Hal Blumenfeld

Introduction

To more fully investigate the mechanisms of electroconvulsive therapy (ECT), techniques are needed to noninvasively measure brain structure and function during and following the course of ECT treatment. Neuroimaging offers the opportunity to noninvasively measure changes throughout the brain both during and following ECT-induced seizures. In this chapter, we review recent work by using a variety of neuroimaging methods including single photon emission computed tomography (SPECT), positron emission tomography (PET), and a variety of magnetic resonance imaging- (MRI-) based techniques. We discuss changes found to occur acutely during ECT-induced seizures, changes found in the immediate postictal period shortly following seizures, as well as longer-lasting changes found after the course of ECT treatment. We hope, with further investigation, that these techniques will shed light on ECT mechanisms, allowing improved treatment methods to be developed.

The mechanisms of ECT should be related to the pathophysiology of depression. A variety of neuroimaging evidence points to both neurophysiological and structural abnormalities in patients with depression. For example, early xenon-133 inhalation studies found reduced global cerebral blood flow (CBF) in addition to reduced regional CBF (rCBF) in selective frontal, central, superior temporal, and anterior parietal regions in patients with major depressive disorder compared with that of healthy controls, reflecting a dysfunction in fronto–temporo–parietal cortical networks (Sackeim et al., 1990). Magnetic resonance spectroscopy (MRS) studies detected increased glutamate levels, decreased occipital cortex gamma-aminobutyric acid (GABA) concentrations, and changes in white matter of patients with major depressive disorder compared with that of healthy controls (Sanacora et al., 2004). MRI diffusion tensor imaging (DTI) in patients with major depressive disorder, both young and elderly, showed microstructural abnormalities in prefrontal white matter that may be linked to the neuropathology of depression (Li et al., 2007).

Neuroimaging studies have been used to study ECT for a variety of purposes. Some investigators have used neuroimaging primarily to elucidate the morphology and neurophysiology of the ECT-induced "generalized" tonic-clonic seizures. Others not only hope to mechanistically understand the benefits and side effects of ECT-induced seizures, but more optimistically aim to investigate how ECT methods can be improved.

Effects of ECT can both occur during the induced seizures and persist into the period of time between ECT treatments. In this chapter, we briefly describe the definitions of the ictal (during seizures) and interictal (between seizures) periods, summarize the main neuroimaging techniques being actively used, and, finally, discuss the neuroimaging research that has been done on ECT effects on the brain, both ictally and interictally.

Definition of the ictal and interictal periods

The ictal, postictal, and interictal periods are defined as the periods during seizure, immediately after seizure, and otherwise between seizures. The boundaries between the postictal and interictal periods are vague and arbitrary because the postictal period is theoretically continuous with the interictal period. Continual changes occur after seizures, making the demarcation difficult to judge. In this review, we refer to the postictal period as defined by acute ECT effects and transient changes that reverse within a few hours of treatment. The interictal period is characterized by more enduring changes from ECT-induced seizures.

Established biological changes during seizures are characterized by a general increase in neuronal electrical activity, neurotransmitter release, neuronal metabolism, and CBF in focal regions of the brain, with some focal decreases (Engel and Pedley, 2008). Postictal changes are mostly a reversal of the changes seen in the ictal period, with general decreases in neuronal electrical activity, neurotransmitter release, neuronal metabolism, and CBF, with some focal increases. Long after seizures, certain interictal changes in physiology have been documented that may characterize the patient's new "baseline," and these can last for hours, weeks, or months before changing again.

What does neuroimaging measure?

When we want to understand the brain, the most intuitive way is to construct a visual representation. Modern neuroimaging techniques can measure the anatomy or function of the brain, and some have been used extensively for investigating the effects and neurological mechanisms of ECT.

Anatomy is best measured with MRI, which has a spatial resolution of 1 to 2 mm. MRI can also be coupled with other techniques to measure function. Brain functions, being more diverse and numerous, can be measured by a host of different techniques. Glucose metabolism is often measured by fluorine-18 (F-18) fluorodeoxyglucose-PET (FDG-PET) with 8- to 12-mm spatial resolution and 30-minute temporal resolution. CBF is commonly measured by SPECT with 6- to 8-mm spatial resolution and 30-second temporal resolution or by ^{15}O ($H_2{}^{15}O$) PET with 10-second temporal resolution. Blood oxygen level dependent (BOLD) functional MRI (fMRI) is indirectly coupled to neuronal activity through changes in brain blood flow and metabolism, with 2- to 3-mm spatial resolution and 1-second temporal resolution. The older xenon-133 inhalation technique and transcranial Doppler (TCD) have also been used to measure CBF, and near-infrared spectrophotometry has been used to measure brain blood flow and oxygenation. Another older method is measurement of electrical activity by electroencephalography (EEG) with high temporal but low spatial resolution. Maps of electrical activity can be derived from EEG with a variety of techniques, including low-resolution brain electromagnetic tomography (LORETA). More recently, additional MRI techniques have been used, including the investigation of white matter pathways by DTI, neuronal damage by diffusion-weighted imaging (DWI), brain water content by T1 or T2 relaxometry, resting functional connectivity by functional connectivity MRI (fcMRI), and neurotransmitter and neurometabolite levels and turnover by MRS.

Ictal neuroimaging in ECT

Now we approach a basic question: What is ECT doing to the brain, both ictally and interictally? Ictal imaging is interesting because it tells us what is happening during the actual ECT-induced seizure and what therapeutic or harmful changes may be taking place. Although some investigators have found no significant difference between neuroimaging measurements before and during treatment (Pridmore et al., 2001), the consensus is that there is a general increase in brain activity (increased neuronal firing, blood flow, metabolite turnover, oxygen and glucose consumption) during ECT-induced generalized seizures with certain regions having a decrease in activity as well (Bajc et al., 1989; Blumenfeld et al., 2003a, 2003b; Engel et al., 1982; Sestoft et al., 1993; Takano et al., 2007).

An early neuroimaging study measured rCBF using the xenon clearance method and glucose and oxygen uptake using blood sample analysis during ECT-induced seizures showed an ictal doubling of rCBF, glucose metabolism, and oxygen consumption (Brodersen et al., 1973). Prohovnik and colleagues later used this technique to discover that bilateral and unilateral electrode placement resulted in lateralized differences in rCBF (Prohovnik et al., 1986).

Very few other ictal imaging studies were done in early studies, but with the advent of SPECT, researchers and physicians have a reliable method for studying the ictal phase. In this method, the patient can be injected with the radioactive ^{99m}Tc-labeled SPECT tracer at some delay or immediately after a seizure begins. The radiotracer does not redistribute to other areas of the brain, so imaging done 60 to 90 minutes postseizure accurately captures a snapshot of CBF at the time of the seizure, and avoids possible movement artifacts.

Work from our laboratory has shown that selective focal networks in the brain involving the frontal and parietal association cortices experience increased CBF during ECT-induced generalized seizures, regardless of bilateral or unilateral electrode placement, and that increased dominant temporal lobe activity is correlated with impaired retrograde verbal memory (Blumenfeld et al., 2003b). Interestingly, increased ictal CBF was not found when merely global signal changes were inspected (Blumenfeld et al., 2003b).

This research was later extended to examine the differences between different electrode placements (Figure 5.1). Although bifrontal electrode placement is less commonly used than is bitemporal electrode placement, it produces different patterns of seizure activation than does bitemporal placement (Blumenfeld et al., 2003a). Bifrontal electrode placement resulted in increased rCBF in the prefrontal cortex and anterior cingulate while sparing the temporal lobes, whereas bitemporal electrode placement resulted in increased rCBF in lateral frontal cortex and anterior temporal cortex, an area thought to be critical for verbal memory (Blumenfeld et al., 2003a). Unilateral electrode placement, in contrast, produced asymmetrical seizures with greater rCBF increases on the side of stimulation and that were less disruptive of verbal retrograde memory compared to bitemporal placement (Blumenfeld et al., 2003b; McNally and Blumenfeld, 2004) (Figure 5.1).

Increased ictal CBF has also been seen in the temporal lobe (Elizagarate et al., 2001), cerebellum, brainstem, midbrain tegmentum, and other subcortical structures such as thalamus and basal ganglia (Blumenfeld et al., 2003b; Elizagarate et al., 2001; Enev et al., 2007; McNally and Blumenfeld, 2004) (Figure 5.2). Cortical and subcortical seizure propagation in ECT has also been studied by neuroimaging (Enev et al., 2007). Injection of SPECT radiotracer at two times (0 s and 30 s) after ECT stimulation was used to track the spatial progression of rCBF changes during ECT-induced generalized seizures (Figure 5.3). It was found that seizures initially cause increased rCBF in the regions of stimulation in the anterior fronto-temporal cortex and in subcortical structures such as the thalamus and basal ganglia, whereas later increases appear in the bilateral parietal and occipital lobes (Enev et al., 2007).

PET studies also show that ictal rCBF increases in basal ganglia, brainstem, diencephalon, amygdala, vermis, and the frontal, temporal, and parietal cortices compared with rCBF before ECT (Takano et al., 2007). With PET, cerebral metabolism

A. Bitemporal ECT

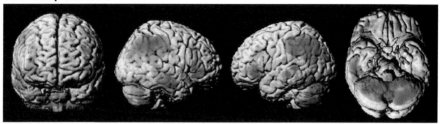

B. Right Unilateral ECT

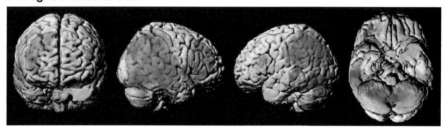

C. Bifrontal ECT

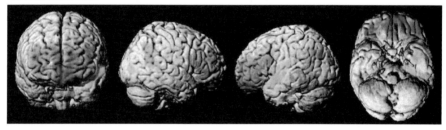

Figure 5.1   Ictal cerebral blood flow changes during bitemporal, right unilateral, and bifrontal electroconvulsive therapy (ECT-) induced seizures. (A) Bitemporal ECT-induced seizures ($n = 10$). (B) Right unilateral ECT-induced seizures ($n = 8$). (C) Bifrontal ECT-induced seizures ($n = 4$). For (A) – (C), ictal images were compared with interictal images using SPM99. Focal single photon emission computed tomography increases (**red**) and decreases (**green**) were seen during ECT-induced seizures compared with baseline scans done under the same conditions. SPM extent threshold, $k = 125$ voxels and height threshold, $p = .02$ (equivalent to a z score > 2.05), using a two-sample t-test model. For further details of methods, see Blumenfeld et al. (2003a, 2003b). (A) and (B) modified with permission from Blumenfeld et al. (2003b); (C) modified with permission from Blumenfeld et al. (2003a). (See Color Plate V.)

can be measured by injection of FDG, a radioactive sugar tracer, and rCBF can be measured by injection of radioactive water $(O^{15})H_2O$.

Future work should further illuminate, in greater detail, exactly what changes occur during and after ECT, how these seizures produce benefits and side effects, and how ECT can be modified to increase therapeutic benefits and minimize side effects.

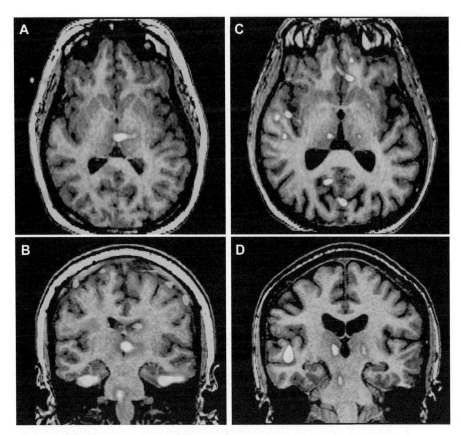

Figure 5.2   Focal ictal subcortical cerebral blood flow (CBF) increases in bitemporal and right
unilateral electroconvulsive therapy (ECT-) induced seizures. (A) and (B) single photon
emission computed tomography (SPECT) ictal–interictal difference imaging in a bilateral
ECT-induced seizure, axial and coronal images, showing bilateral medial, thalamic, CBF
increases. (C) and (D) SPECT ictal–interictal difference imaging in a right unilateral
ECT-induced seizure, axial and coronal images, showing asymmetric involvement of the
medial thalamus. CBF increases are displayed on each patient's high-resolution
T1-weighted magnetic resonance imaging scan. **Orange:** Increases of 55%; **purple:**
increases of 35% relative to interictal scan. The right side of each image corresponds to
the left side of the brain. Reproduced with permission from Blumenfeld et al. (2003a).
(See Color Plate VI.)

Interictal neuroimaging in ECT

Postictal neuroimaging studies show the short-term effects in patients immediately
after ECT, whereas true interictal neuroimaging studies show longer-term, longer-
lasting effects of ECT after patients have returned to a steady baseline. Although
not truly ictal or interictal, postictal imaging still provides valuable information
about the transition between acute treatment conditions and return to baseline (or

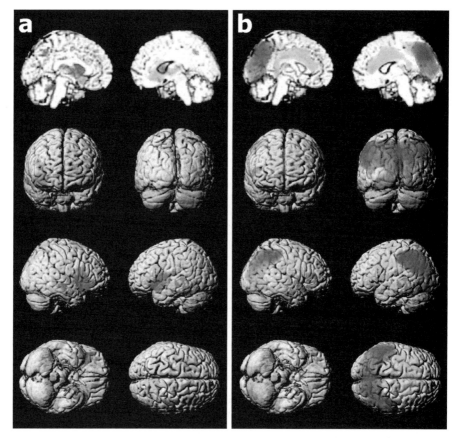

Figure 5.3   Evidence for ictal propagation: Early cerebral blood flow (CBF) increases in frontal cortex
and late CBF increases in parietal cortex with bitemporal electroconvulsive therapy (ECT).
Single photon emission computed tomography (SPECT) images of significant CBF changes
during bitemporal ECT-induced seizures. Statistical parametric maps depict CBF increases
(hyperperfusion) in **red** and decreases (hypoperfusion) in **green**. (a) CBF changes in
patients with ictal injections at onset (0 s after ECT stimulus). Increases occur in the
bilateral inferior frontal gyrus, anterior insula, putamen, and thalamus. No significant
decreases were found ($n = 4$). (b) Changes in patients with ictal injections 30 s after ECT
stimulus. Increases occur in bilateral parietal and occipital cortex, whereas decreases occur
in the bilateral cingulate gyrus and left dorsolateral frontal cortex ($n = 7$). For (a) and (b),
extent threshold, $k = 125$ voxels (voxel size $= 2 \times 2 \times 2$ mm). Height threshold, $p = .01$.
Equivalently, only voxel clusters > 1 cm^3 in volume and with z scores > 2.33 are
displayed. Reproduced with permission from Enev et al. (2007). (See Color Plate VII.)

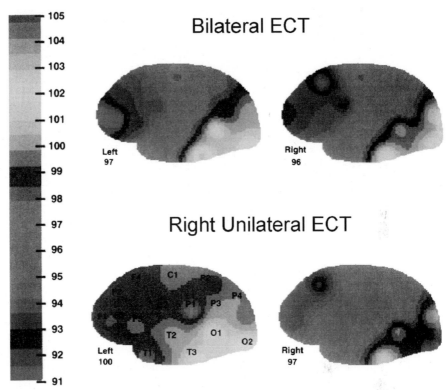

Figure 5.4   Interictal (postictal) cerebral blood flow (CBF) patterns following bitemporal and right unilateral electroconvulsive therapy (ECT). Xenon-133 regional CBF (rCBF) 50 minutes after ECT compared with 30 minutes before ECT. Values of 100 indicate no change. The ratio scores were color coded so that **purple** and **blue** correspond to postictal CBF reductions, whereas **orange** and **red** correspond to postictal CBF increases (scale on left). Mean CBF percent changes are indicated next to each hemisphere. Positions of the rCBF detectors are labeled at bottom left. Reproduced with permission from Nobler et al. (1994). (See Color Plate VIII.)

adjusted baseline) conditions. Postictal imaging studies have used several methods: the xenon inhalation technique, TCD sonography, the SPECT methods introduced earlier, and PET.

Most studies have shown a general decrease in rCBF and brain glucose metabolism in several distinct brain regions (including the anterior cingulate and medial frontal cortex) immediately postictally (Nobler et al., 1994; Prohovnik et al., 1986a; Scott et al., 1994). In anatomical agreement with ictal studies (Figure 5.1, A and B), bilateral ECT was found to cause bilateral frontal hypoperfusion in the postictal period, whereas right unilateral ECT caused asymmetrical right greater than left frontal postictal hypoperfusion (Figure 5.4) (Nobler et al., 1994). This finding suggests that regions showing greatest hyperperfusion ictally will show the greatest hypoperfusion postically, in both cases likely reflecting the anatomical regions where ECT exerts its strongest effects.

TCD studies have shown increases in CBF velocity postically, especially in the left middle cerebral artery (MCA) (Saito et al., 1995; Vollmer-Haase et al., 1998). Increases in rCBF to other regions after ECT may be linked to antidepressive effects, especially because patients with depression have lower than "normal" rCBF to the frontal lobe and limbic regions, and these increases bring their rCBF to a closer-to-normal baseline after ECT (Milo et al., 2001; Takano et al., 2006). The size of these CBF changes from pre-ECT baseline to a more normal post-ECT baseline seem to be correlated with severity of depression, antidepressive effects, and post-ECT memory impairment (Scott et al., 1990, 1994).

PET imaging studies show increased rCBF in the thalamus and decreased rCBF in the anterior cingulate and medial frontal cortex postictally, compared with pre-ECT measurements (Takano et al., 2007) and decreased cerebral glucose metabolism postictally in both prefrontal regions, which is speculated to be related to the therapeutic effects of ECT for treating depression (Conca et al., 2003).

True interictal neuroimaging captures the longer-term effects of ECT and how patients' baselines change after therapy. Depending on ECT dosage, characteristics of the individual patient, amount of time elapsed after ECT before neuroimaging, and method of analysis, results of interictal neuroimaging in ECT patients are harder to generalize than are ictal and postictal study results. However, studies have found that there is a general depression of brain activity interictally and that ECT does not produce measurable long-term neuroanatomical damage.

Early studies used a variety of methods that have since been replaced with SPECT, PET, and MRI. These early techniques included the nitrous oxide (NO) method, the xenon clearance method, the xenon inhalation technique, TCD sonography, and EEG with LORETA.

One of the earliest CBF measures used the NO method, in which the inert gas is inhaled and delivered to the brain via arterial blood, and the brain's blood concentrations are measured (Kety and Schmidt, 1948). However, there were no observable CBF changes in ECT patients as measured by this technique (Wilson et al., 1952).

The earliest xenon clearance studies done in the 1970s to measure rCBF showed that rCBF returns to baseline about 15 minutes after ECT for most patients (Brodersen et al., 1973). Xenon-133, which is capable of crossing the blood–brain barrier, can be given intravenously or by inhalation. The former technique measures the external washout of xenon that is injected into the internal carotid artery (Brodersen et al., 1973). Although technically easier than the inhalation technique, it allows measurement of rCBF only in one hemisphere. The xenon inhalation technique was popular in the late 1980s and early 1990s and can measure rCBF simultaneously in both hemispheres as gamma rays emitted near the head are collimated and analyzed. This allows for a less invasive, bihemispheric rCBF measure that can be performed multiple times per day because of rapid clearance from the brain. Studies with the inhalation technique found substantial regional differences between unilateral and bilateral ECT (Prohovnik et al., 1986), that bilateral electrode placement resulted in larger interictal decreases in rCBF than did unilateral placement (Silfverskiold et al., 1987a), that EEG and rCBF changes do not always correlate (Silfverskiold et al., 1987a), and that interictal rCBF decreases are correlated with improvements in symptoms of depression (Nobler et al., 1994; Silfverskiold et al., 1987b).

TCD can noninvasively measure the dynamics of CBF at relatively high time resolution, although spatial resolution and sampling are poor compared with other neuroimaging methods. In this technique, a high-frequency ultrasonic wave is used to produce Doppler signals from which the pulsatility index (PI) is calculated as (systolic–diastolic) / mean velocities in the MCA or other arteries. Saito et al. (1995) measured CBF velocity in the MCA and found dramatic increases postictally, but a return to normal 10 minutes after ECT-induced seizures in depressed patients. Vollmer-Haase and colleagues (1998) found return to baseline 2 to 6 minutes after ECT.

LORETA is a technique applied to EEG as a popular solution to the "inverse problem," in which EEG information about seizure morphology is difficult to localize to specific brain regions. In one study, researchers found that slow-wave theta activity comes from the left temporal lobe during the interictal state, localizing an area of dysfunction interictally associated with memory impairment, a common ECT side effect (Neuhaus et al., 2005).

Interictal SPECT imaging gives us more information about CBF after ECT-induced seizures, although findings from different studies do not always agree. One study of preictal, ictal, and interictal ECT with SPECT showed that CBF "normalization" (convergence toward CBF patterns of normal control subjects) takes place interictally (Rosenberg et al., 1988). Another showed increased perfusion in the right temporal and bilateral parietal lobes (Mervaala et al., 2001), but such interictal increases in CBF are considered to be signs of remission rather than treatment effect by some researchers (Bonne and Krausz, 1997). However, more recent research found significant negative correlations between changes in Hamilton Rating Scale for Depression (HRSD) scores and rCBF changes 5 to 10 minutes after ECT in the left frontopolar gyrus, left amygdala, globus pallidus, nucleus accumbens, and left superior temporal gyrus. This finding suggests that increased interictal perfusion to certain regions is related to the antidepressive effects of ECT

(Segawa et al., 2006). Long-term interictal frontal and limbic decreases in CBF even one month after ECT treatment have been observed This highlights that brain changes continue to occur after ECT and that patients should be monitored for at least a month after a course of ECT (Takano et al., 2006).

Interictal FDG-PET imaging captures the effects of ECT on brain glucose metabolism. Most studies indicate that many regions of the brain show decreased cerebral metabolic rates for glucose (CMRglu) after ECT. These include frontal and parietal cortex, anterior and posterior cingulate gyri, and left temporal cortex (Nobler et al., 2001; Volkow et al., 1988), right anterior frontal, and left posterior frontal lobes (Henry et al., 2001). Decreased CMRglu also seem to be significantly correlated with decreases in HRSD scores (Henry et al., 2001). Such depression in neuronal activity in selected cortical regions may be causally linked to the anticonvulsant and antidepressant effects of ECT (Nobler et al., 2001). Other PET studies have shown that long-term ECT does not permanently alter metabolism in the brain (Anghelescu et al., 2001) and that changes in CMRglu seem to subside after one week (Yatham et al., 2000).

Interictal MRI methods, including MRS, DWI, T2 relaxometry, DTI, and computed tomography combined with MRI, can give us more anatomically precise insight into the effects (anatomical, physiological, and functional) of ECT and how it can produce both therapeutic effects and cognitive impairment posttreatment.

MRS combines principles of MRI and nuclear magnetic resonance to obtain spatial and temporal information about brain neurochemistry. In ECT research, MRS has been used to look at changes in metabolite turnover, including glutamate, glutamine, GABA, N-acetylaspartate (NAA), choline-containing compounds (Cho), creatine and phosphocreatine (tCr), lactate, and lipids. Sanacora and colleagues (2003) found that ECT leads to increased cortical GABA concentrations measured by MRS, possibly explaining both antidepressant and anticonvulsant effects of ECT treatment. In addition, studies have found that ECT patients demonstrate interictal increases in lipids, glucose, tCr, NAA, and Cho (Sartorius et al., 2006), with NAA increases specifically found in the left amygdala region (Michael et al., 2003).

MRI studies suggest that the breakdown of the blood–brain barrier is implicated in both therapeutic and side effects of ECT. One MRI-based study of brain water content showed peak increases from baseline at 2 hours post-ECT, followed by a return to baseline within 6 hours (Scott et al., 1990). This finding has been interpreted as supporting the "neuroendocrine theory" of ECT, which hypothesizes that ECT-induced seizures break down the blood–brain barrier, allowing crucial peptides into the central nervous system. Significant interictal increases in T2 relaxation times have also been observed in right and left thalamus following ECT (Diehl et al., 1994). These findings are consistent with a post-ECT increase in brain water content (perhaps secondary to a breakdown of the blood–brain barrier) and suggest that this process may be related to the characteristic post-ECT memory impairment (Diehl et al., 1994).

DTI studies measuring white matter fractional anisotropy (FA) in patients with depression before and after ECT provide another indicator of the antidepressant action of ECT. In one study, researchers found that depressed patients referred to ECT had a significantly lower white matter FA over much of the frontal and temporal regions, compared with that of healthy controls, and that this white matter FA increased significantly after bilateral ECT (Nobuhara et al., 2004).

Recent work with DWI provides evidence that ECT does not cause obvious strokelike damage to the brain. In their study, Szabo and colleagues (2007) measured focal tissue DWI changes associated in other settings with abnormal metabolism, cerebral ischemia, and extended seizures. They found that in ECT patients after treatment, there were no significant brain abnormalities in both qualitative MRI and quantitative DWI analyses (Szabo et al., 2007). Further studies will be needed to determine whether more subtle DWI changes in the hippocampus may be related to short-term memory impairments following ECT.

Future research on interictal imaging may see more work with new techniques like DTI, DWI, MRS, and resting fcMRI, which can detect coupled neural networks by measuring interregional temporal correlations of BOLD signal fluctuations (Biswal et al., 1995; Castellanos et al., 2008; Greicius et al., 2003). These methods may become increasingly important with additional study to monitor the long-term effects of ECT.

Conclusions and future directions

Neuroimaging has greatly enhanced our understanding of what ECT does to the brain, how it may treat depression, and how it causes cognitive side effects. Neuroimaging allows us to measure changes in neurometabolite turnover, blood flow, oxygen levels, brain water content, network connectivity, and anatomical integrity before, during, and after ECT. ECT neuroimaging research with older techniques (such as the NO method, xenon inhalation, TCD, and EEG) has now been overtaken by newer methods including SPECT, PET, and, most recently, a variety of MRI-based techniques. Currently, SPECT imaging is the best option for ictal imaging because of its ability to capture the rCBF at the time of the ECT-induced seizure, free of movement artifacts from the patient. However, it is limited in its lower spatial and temporal resolution compared with fMRI and ^{15}O-PET. Furthermore, it relies on relative signal changes, which can be difficult to correctly interpret, and there is only an indirect relationship between CBF and neuronal firing that is not fully understood. Nonetheless, SPECT studies have shed light on optimal electrode placement and patterns of seizure propagation. PET is valuable for interictal imaging because of its ability to take absolute measurement in vivo, in real time. MRI combined with newer techniques like DTI and MRS provides functional and biochemical data with high spatial resolution.

There is still much to be discovered about ECT. Ideally, new technologies will be developed to allow us to fully measure ictal and interictal brain activity in high spatiotemporal resolution, and with this to illuminate mechanism and site of action and facilitate clinical improvements.

References

Anghelescu, I., Klawe, C. J., Bartenstein, P., and Szegedi, A. 2001. Normal PET after long-term ECT. Am J Psychiatry 158: 1527.

Bajc, M., Medved, V., Basic, M., et al. 1989. Acute effect of electroconvulsive therapy on brain perfusion assessed by ^{99m}Tc-hexamethylpropyleneamineoxim and single photon emission computed tomography. Acta Psychiatr Scand 80: 421–6.

Biswal, B., Yetkin, F. Z., Haughton, V. M., and Hyde, J. S. 1995. Functional connectivity in the motor cortex of resting human brain using echo-planar MRI. Magn Reson Med 34: 537–41.

Blumenfeld, H., McNally, K. A., Ostroff, R. B., and Zubal, I. G. 2003a. Targeted prefrontal cortical activation with bifrontal ECT. Psychiatry Res 123: 165–70.

Blumenfeld, H., Westerveld, M., Ostroff, R. B., et al. 2003b. Selective frontal, parietal, and temporal networks in generalized seizures. Neuroimage 19: 1556–66.

Bonne, O. and Krausz, Y. 1997. Pathophysiological significance of cerebral perfusion abnormalities in major depression-trait or state marker? Eur Neuropsychopharmacol 7: 225–33.

Brodersen, P., Paulson, O. B., Bolwig, T. G., et al. 1973. Cerebral hyperemia in electrically induced epileptic seizures. Arch Neurol 28: 334–8.

Castellanos, F. X., Margulies, D. S., Kelly, C., et al. 2008. Cingulate-precuneus interactions: A new locus of dysfunction in adult attention-deficit/hyperactivity disorder. Biol Psychiatry 63: 332–7.

Conca, A., Prapotnik, M., Peschina, W., and Konig, P. 2003. Simultaneous pattern of rCBF and rCMRGlu in continuation ECT: Case reports. Psychiatry Res 124: 191–8.

Diehl, D. J., Keshavan, M. S., Kanal, E., et al. 1994. Post-ECT increases in MRI regional T2 relaxation times and their relationship to cognitive side effects: A pilot study. Psychiatry Res 54: 177–84.

Elizagarate, E., Cortes, J., Gonzalez Pinto, A., et al. 2001. Study of the influence of electroconvulsive therapy on the regional cerebral blood flow by HMPAO-SPECT. J Affect Disord 65: 55–9.

Enev, M., McNally, K. A., Varghese, G., et al. 2007. Imaging onset and propagation of ECT-induced seizures. Epilepsia 48: 238–44.

Engel, J. Jr., Kuhl, D. E., and Phelps, M. E. 1982. Patterns of human local cerebral glucose metabolism during epileptic seizures. Science 218: 64–6.

Engel, J. Jr. and Pedley, T. A. 2008. Epilepsy: A comprehensive textbook, 2nd edn. Philadelphia: Lippincott Williams & Wilkins.

Greicius, M. D., Krasnow, B., Reiss, A. L., and Menon, V. 2003. Functional connectivity in the resting brain: A network analysis of the default mode hypothesis. Proc Natl Acad Sci USA 100: 253–8.

Henry, M. E., Schmidt, M. E., Matochik, J. A., et al. 2001. The effects of ECT on brain glucose: A pilot FDG PET study. J ECT 17: 33–40.

Kety, S. S. and Schmidt, C. F. 1948. The nitrous oxide method for the quantitative determination of cerebral blood flow in man: Theory, procedure and normal values. J Clin Invest 27: 476–83.

Li, L., Ma, N., Li, Z., et al. 2007. Prefrontal white matter abnormalities in young adult with major depressive disorder: A diffusion tensor imaging study. Brain Res 1168: 124–8.

McNally, K. A. and Blumenfeld, H. 2004. Focal network involvement in generalized seizures: New insights from electroconvulsive therapy. Epilepsy Behav 5: 3–12.

Mervaala, E., Kononen, M., Fohr, J., et al. 2001. SPECT and neuropsychological performance in severe depression treated with ECT. J Affect Disord 66: 47–58.

Michael, N., Erfurth, A., Ohrmann, P., et al. 2003. Neurotrophic effects of electroconvulsive therapy: A proton magnetic resonance study of the left amygdalar region in patients with treatment-resistant depression. Neuropsychopharmacology 28: 720–5.

Milo, T. J., Kaufman, G. E., Barnes, W. E., et al. 2001. Changes in regional cerebral blood flow after electroconvulsive therapy for depression. J ECT 17: 15–21.

Neuhaus, A. H., Gallinat, J., Bajbouj, M., and Reischies, F. M. 2005. Interictal slow-wave focus in left medial temporal lobe during bilateral electroconvulsive therapy. Neuropsychobiology 52: 183–9.

Nobler, M. S., Oquendo, M. A., Kegeles, L. S., et al. 2001. Decreased regional brain metabolism after ECT. Am J Psychiatry 158: 305–8.

Nobler, M. S., Sackeim, H. A., Prohovnik, I., et al. 1994. Regional cerebral blood flow in mood disorders, III. Treatment and clinical response. Arch Gen Psychiatry 51: 884–97.

Nobuhara, K., Okugawa, G., Minami, T., et al. 2004. Effects of electroconvulsive therapy on frontal white matter in late-life depression: A diffusion tensor imaging study. Neuropsychobiology 50: 48–53.

Pridmore, S., Burke, G., Tivendale, N., and Batt, G. 2001. A failure to find large visible effects of ECT-induced seizures on SPECT scans. J ECT 17: 155–6.

Prohovnik, I., Sackeim, H. A., Decina, P., and Malitz, S. 1986. Acute reductions of regional cerebral blood flow following electroconvulsive therapy. Interactions with modality and time. Ann N Y Acad Sci 462: 249–62.

Rosenberg, R., Vorstrup, S., Andersen, A., and Bolwig, T. G. 1988. Effect of ECT on cerebral blood flow in melancholia assessed with SPECT. Convuls Ther 4: 62–73.

Sackeim, H. A., Prohovnik, I., Moeller, J. R., et al. 1990. Regional cerebral blood flow in mood disorders. I. Comparison of major depressives and normal controls at rest. Arch Gen Psychiatry 47: 60–70.

Saito, S., Yoshikawa, D., Nishihara, F., et al. 1995. The cerebral hemodynamic response to electrically induced seizures in man. Brain Res 673: 93–100.

Sanacora, G., Gueorguieva, R., Epperson, C. N., et al. 2004. Subtype-specific alterations of gamma-aminobutyric acid and glutamate in patients with major depression. Arch Gen Psychiatry 61: 705–13.

Sanacora, G., Mason, G. F., Rothman, D. L., et al. 2003. Increased cortical GABA concentrations in depressed patients receiving ECT. Am J Psychiatry 160: 577–9.

Sartorius, A., Henn, F. A., and Ende, G. 2006. Proton magnetic resonance spectroscopy as a monitoring tool for electroconvulsive therapy effects on the brain. Curr Psychiatry Rev 2: 39–49.

Scott, A. I., Dougall, N., Ross, M., et al. 1994. Short-term effects of electroconvulsive treatment on the uptake of ^{99m}Tc-exametazime into brain in major depression shown with single photon emission tomography. J Affect Disord 30: 27–34.

Scott, A. I., Douglas, R. H., Whitfield, A., and Kendell, R. E. 1990. Time course of cerebra; Magnetic resonance changes after electroconvulsive therapy. Br J Psychiatry 156: 551–3.

Segawa, K., Azuma, H., Sato, K., et al. 2006. Regional cerebral blood flow changes in depression after electroconvulsive therapy. Psychiatry Res 147: 135–43.

Sestoft, D., Meden, P., Hemmingsen, R., et al. 1993. Disparity in regional cerebral blood flow during electrically induced seizure. Acta Psychiatr Scand 88: 140–3.

Silfverskiold, P., Rosen, I., and Risberg, J. 1987a. Effects of electroconvulsive therapy on EEG and cerebral blood flow in depression. Eur Arch Psychiatry Neurol Sci 236: 202–8.

Silfverskiold, P., Rosen, I., Risberg, J., and Gustafson, L. 1987b. Changes in psychiatric symptoms related to EEG and cerebral blood flow following electroconvulsive therapy in depression. Eur Arch Psychiatry Neurol Sci 236: 195–201.

Szabo, K., Hirsch, J. G., Krause, M., et al. 2007. Diffusion weighted MRI in the early phase after electroconvulsive therapy. Neurol Res 29: 256–9.

Takano, H., Kato, M., Inagaki, A., et al. 2006. Time course of cerebral blood flow changes following electroconvulsive therapy in depressive patients – measured at 3 time points using single photon emission computed tomography. Keio J Med 55: 153–60.

Takano, H., Motohashi, N., Uema, T., et al. 2007. Changes in regional cerebral blood flow during acute electroconvulsive therapy in patients with depression: Positron emission tomographic study. Br J Psychiatry 190: 63–8.

Volkow, N. D., Bellar, S., Mullani, N., et al. 1988. Effects of electroconvulsive therapy on brain glucose metabolism: A preliminary study. Convuls Ther 4: 199–205.

Vollmer-Haase, J., Folkerts, H. W., Haase, C. G., et al. 1998. Cerebral hemodynamics during electrically induced seizures. Neuroreport 9: 407–10.

Wilson, W. P., Schieve, J. F., and Scheinberg, P. 1952. Effect of series of electric shock treatments on cerebral blood flow and metabolism. AMA Arch Neurol Psychiatry 68: 651–4.

Yatham, L. N., Clark, C. C., and Zis, A. P. 2000. A preliminary study of the effects of electro-convulsive therapy on regional brain glucose metabolism in patients with major depression. J ECT 16: 171–6.

6

Evidence for electroconvulsive therapy efficacy in mood disorders

Keith G. Rasmussen

Introduction

There are several questions pertinent to the issue of the efficacy of electroconvulsive therapy (ECT), most notably in depression. What is the evidence that ECT is effective for depression? Is this efficacy related to the inherent neurobiological effects of electrically induced seizures or could it be placebo effect? How does ECT compare with antidepressant medications? Do different forms of ECT have different efficacy? Do different subtypes of depression respond differently to ECT? Finally, is ECT effective in manic states?

How effective is ECT for depression?

We will consider data from modern, well-designed studies using the strongest form of ECT, bitemporal. Other placements may have equal efficacy in some circumstances, but none have proven to be superior. During the past two decades there have been six large studies using structured diagnostic evaluation, systematic outcome assessment, the Hamilton Rating Scale for Depression (HRSD) (Williams, 2001), and brief-pulse, square wave stimuli with stated dosage (Abrams et al., 1991; Kellner et al., 2006; McCall et al., 2002; Sackeim et al., 1987, 1993, 2000). Table 6.1 presents only the response (or remission) rates in the bitemporal groups for each. These vary from 70% to 87.8%, overall 83.7%. Thus ECT is a highly efficacious treatment for depression. The next question concerns whether this efficacy is based on inherent neurobiological features of the treatment or some component of placebo phenomena.

Is ECT more effective than placebo procedure?

Twelve sham-controlled studies for depressed patients have been reported, providing enough information to infer outcomes in depressed patients (Table 6.2). Sham

Table 6.1 Modern data on response rates with bitemporal electroconvulsive therapy

Study	Sample size	No. of responders	Response[2] rate[a] (%)
Kellner et al., 2006	394[b]	346	87.8
McCall et al., 2002	37	27	73
Abrams et al., 1991	18	14	77.8
Sackeim et al., 1987	27	19	70.4
Sackeim et al., 1993	50	35	70
Sackeim et al., 2000	20	16	80
Total	546	457	83.7

[a] "Response" refers either to response or remission, depending on the terminology of the paper.
[b] Excludes dropouts; if one assumes all dropouts would have been nonresponders, response rate becomes 64.2%.

ECT consisted of anesthesia alone in 11 studies, whereas in 1 study a subconvulsive electrical current was also applied (Brill et al., 1959). All meta-analytic reports of this literature conclude that, in the aggregate, ECT is more effective than sham ECT for depression (Janicak et al., 1985; Kho et al., 2003; Pagnin et al., 2004; UK ECT Review Group, 2003).

There are several methodological shortcomings. Only 2 of the 12 studies involved diagnosis with structured interviews (Brandon et al., 1984; Johnstone et al., 1980); both used the Present State Exam (Wing et al., 1974). Other studies mentioned diagnostic criteria (Gregory et al., 1985; West, 1981), but apparently the patients were diagnosed according to routine clinical examination. None used the most current diagnostic nosology (American Psychiatric Association, 2000). We might question whether all 12 studies involved patients with the same illness, as needed for meta-analysis.

None of the 12 studies used brief-pulse square wave stimuli; all used sine wave or chopped sine wave stimuli. None of the studies reported electrical dosing in units of charge, recently the standard method. Two studies used right unilateral electrode placement (Gregory et al., 1985; Lambourn and Gill, 1978), but this was with the now-outdated Lancaster placement (Lancaster et al., 1958) vis-à-vis the d'Elia placement (d'Elia and Widepalm, 1974).

In two studies, sham group responding was quite high. The Lambourn and Gill (1978) study is instructive. Patients were randomly assigned to receive either right unilateral (Lancaster placement) ECT or sham treatments. The groups did not differ in outcome. Abrams (2002) explained that this is because their use of right unilateral ECT has low efficacy. Close inspection of the data reveals that the active ECT group showed a 25-point reduction in HRSD scores. This is a large improvement. The sham group had a similar mean reduction of 23 points. This result does

Table 6.2 Sham electroconvulsive therapy (ECT) studies

Study	No. of patients	Diagnostic method	Diagnostic subtypes	Outcome assessment	ECT waveform	Placement	Active group response	Sham response	#Tx's	ECT schedule	Masking of patients?
Ulett et al., 1956	42	Clinical impression	DSM-I, II	Rating scale	Sine wave	Unknown	17/21 "recovered"	9/21 "recovered"	12–15	Thrice weekly	Not mentioned
Brill et al., 1959	30	Clinical impression	DSM-I, II	Rating scale	Sine wave	Bitemporal	76.2% "recovered"	4/9 "recovered"	21	Thrice weekly	Not mentioned
Sainz, 1959	20	Clinical impression	DSM-I, II	Clinical impression	Not specified	Unknown	9/10 "recovered"	1/10 "recovered"	12	Thrice weekly	Not mentioned
Harris and Robin, 1960	8	Clinical impression	Depressive reaction	Clinical impression	Not specified	Unknown	2 "slight," 2 "great" improvement	1 "slight," 3 "no" improvement	4	Twice weekly	Not mentioned
Wilson et al., 1963	12	Clinical impression	DSM-I, II	Rating scale	Not specified	Unknown	All 6 "much improved"	2/6 "much," 1/6 "modest" improvement	10	Twice weekly	Not mentioned
Fahy et al., 1963	34	Clinical impression	None	Clinical impression	Not specified	Unknown	6 recovered 6 improved 5 no change or worse	2 recovered 6 improved 9 no change or worse	6	Twice weekly	Yes
Lambourn and Gill, 1978	32	Clinical impression	Depressive psychosis	Rating scale	Chopped sine wave	Lancaster	25-point mean drop in Hamilton ratings	23-point mean drop in Hamilton ratings	6	Thrice weekly	Yes

(continued)

Table 6.2 (*continued*)

Study	No. of patients	Diagnostic method	Diagnostic subtypes	Outcome assessment	ECT waveform	Placement	Active group response	Sham response	#Tx's	ECT schedule	Masking of patients?
Freeman et al., 1978	40	Clinical impression	None	Rating scale	Chopped sine wave	Bitemporal	Better at one week than sham	Equal to active ECT at end of week 2	2 sham	Twice weekly	Yes
Johnstone et al., 1980	70	PSE[a]	Delusional; retarded; agitated	Rating scale	Chopped sine wave	Bifrontal	Approx. 37-point drop in Hamilton ratings	Approx. 20-point drop in Hamilton ratings	8	Twice weekly	Yes
West, 1981	22	RDC[b]	None	Visual analog; self-rating scale	Sine wave	Bitemporal	15.8-point drop in BDI[d]	1.9-point drop in BDI[d]	6	Twice weekly	Yes
Brandon et al., 1984	95	PSE	Delusional; retarded; neurotic	Rating scale	Chopped sine wave	Bitemporal	Approx. 30-point drop in Hamilton ratings	Approx. 10-point drop in Hamilton ratings	8	Twice weekly	Yes
Gregory et al., 1985	69	ICD-9[c]	None	Rating scale	Chopped sine wave	Bitemporal or Lancaster	Approx. 24-point drop in MADRS[e] ratings for both ECT groups	Approx. 8.7-point drop in MADRS[e] ratings	6	Twice weekly	Yes

Note: DSM I, II, *Diagnostic and Statistical Manual of Mental Disorders*, 1st and 2nd editions.

[a] PSE, Present State Exam (Wing et al., 1974).

[b] RDC, Research Diagnostic Criteria (Spitzer et al., 1978).

[c] ICD-9, *International Classification of Diseases*, Ninth Revision.

[d] BDI, Beck Depression Inventory (Beck et al., 1988).

[e] MADRS, Montgomery Asberg Depression Rating Scale (Montgomery and Asberg, 1979).

not point to low unilateral efficacy but to puzzling high efficacy for sham *and* for unilateral ECT. The patients were described as having "depressive psychosis," so were apparently severely ill.

In the Northwick Park trial (Johnstone et al., 1980), HRSD scores in sham ECT patients decreased about 25 points on average according to the figure, again a large improvement. Only patients with psychotic depression had reductions significantly greater than sham ECT. Meeting research criteria for endogeneity was required, so again, one may assume that "neurotic" patients with depression (with high placebo responses) were excluded. Thus, in two well-controlled sham ECT studies, substantial proportions of apparently severely ill patients responded to sham treatment, and equally to ECT.

In the Freeman et al. (1978) study, patients were randomly assigned to twice-weekly active ECT or to two sham treatments in one week followed by twice-weekly active treatments. At the end of one week (thus, a comparison of two active vs. two sham treatments), the active ECT patients had lower rating scale scores than the sham-treated patients, the latter having HRSD scores essentially unchanged from baseline. This is often cited as evidence in favor of real versus sham ECT (Abrams, 2002). However, inspection of the graphically displayed HRSD scores over time in that trial reveals that at the end of week two (thus, two sham plus two real vs. four real treatments), the two groups have identical depression scores. That is, the initially sham-treated patients had dramatic reductions in HRSD scores with just two real treatments. Again, it is enigmatic that two ECTs plus two sham treatments appear equal in effectiveness to four ECTs.

Perhaps the relative contributions of placebo and nonplacebo effects in ECT practice could be separated more clearly if outcome research focused on verifiable observable measures of depressive psychopathology rather than just subjectively reported symptoms. Quantified measures of psychomotor retardation or agitation, observer-based assessments of affective expression, and the disappearance of delusion-related behavior might escape self-report scales. A related problem is that the most severely ill patients (e.g., profoundly slowed melancholia, catatonia, psychosis, delirious mania) are unable to participate in studies requiring informed consent or provide reflective self-judgments. In other words, the patients who most clearly and observably respond to ECT are the least likely to be studied. A further issue clouding diagnostic specificity is the lack of attempt to establish other (comorbid) primary psychiatric diagnoses after the patient has remitted from depression with ECT. The severely depressed state can mask underlying anxiety or other disorders that are later revealed as substantially affecting the patient's quality of life.

A final methodological issue regarding sham ECT trials is the adequacy of anesthesia induction alone as a "believable" placebo condition. A prerequisite for placebo-controlled trials is that each patient must believe there is a chance that he or she is receiving an active treatment. This prerequisite is easy to achieve in pharmacologic trials, in which placebo pills identical to the active drug can be developed. In procedural trials such as ECT, it is more difficult to develop a placebo condition that is sufficiently close to the active treatment so that patients do not know which one they are receiving. Is the mere induction of anesthesia for a few minutes similar enough to the real ECT experience for patients not to know what treatment they are receiving? In none of the sham ECT trials was there an attempt to determine if patients correctly guessed to which group they had been randomized.

In summary, based on several meta-analyses, it appears that the sham-controlled evidence for ECT efficacy in depression is strong and solid. However, methodological problems exist and are related mainly to diagnostic heterogeneity across studies, outmoded treatment technique, and concerns about the adequacy of anesthesia induction alone as an "ECT placebo." Finally, some of the studies indicate an unexpectedly high rate of response in the sham groups. Accordingly it remains highly relevant how ECT compares with antidepressant medications.

Is ECT more effective than antidepressant medications?

There are 22 trials in which a group of depressed patients was randomly assigned to at least one form of ECT or at least one type of psychotropic medication (Bruce et al., 1960; Davidson et al., 1978; Dinan and Barry, 1989; Fahy et al., 1963; Folkerts et al., 1997; Gangadhar et al., 1982; Greenblatt et al., 1964; Harris and Robin, 1960; Herrington et al., 1974; Hutchinson and Smedberg, 1963; Janakiramaiah et al., 2000; Kiloh et al., 1960; MacSweeney, 1975; McDonald et al., 1966; Medical Research Council, 1965; Panneer Selvan et al., 1999; Robin and Harris, 1962; Stanley and Fleming, 1962; Steiner et al., 1978; Wilson et al., 1963; Wittenborn et al., 1961, 1962). Table 6.3 lists the studies and some of the aspects of the methodology. One publication, by Greenblatt et al. (1962), appears to be a preliminary data set for the publication in 1964 by the same group (Greenblatt et al., 1964) and will not be counted as separate. All four meta-analyses comparing medications versus ECT report greater efficacy for ECT than for medications (Janicak et al., 1985; Kho et al., 2003; Pagnin et al., 2004; UK ECT Review Group, 2003). However, closer inspection of the data reveals some methodological problems. The first is the consideration of all psychotropic drugs as a single class of treatment. Variations in comparison medications are shown in Table 6.3.

A second methodological problem is that almost all studies were nonblinded. Differences between ECT and medication may simply indicate that ECT is a better placebo than medications. Three studies were blinded (Gangadhar et al., 1982; Harris and Robin, 1960; Robin and Harris, 1962). The Harris and Robin (1960) study, in which depressed patients were randomly assigned to ECT, sham ECT plus placebo pill, or sham ECT plus phenelzine, would have been an excellent test

Table 6.3 Electroconvulsive therapy (ECT)/Medication comparison studies

Study	Medication	Dosage (mg)	Duration	ECT technique
Kiloh et al., 1960	Iproniazid	150	3 weeks	?
Bruce et al., 1960	Imipramine	$\leq$150	4 weeks	?
Harris and Robin, 1960	Phenelzine	$\leq$150	2 weeks	?
Wittenborn et al., 1961	Iproniazid	mean = 125	10 weeks	?
Wittenborn et al., 1962	Imipramine	$\leq$200	10 weeks	?
Stanley and Fleming, 1962	Phenelzine	90	4 weeks	?
Robin and Harris, 1962	Imipramine	?	?	?
Hutchinson and Smedberg, 1963	Multiple[a]	Multiple[a]	3 weeks	?
Fahy et al., 1963	Imipramine	100	3 weeks	?
Wilson et al., 1963	Imipramine	?	5 weeks	?
Greenblatt et al., 1964	Imipramine	200 or 250	8 weeks	?
	Phenelzine	60 or 75		
	Isocarboxazid	40 or 50		
Medical Research Council, 1965	Imipramine	$\leq$ 200	4–8 weeks	?
	Phenelzine	$\leq$ 60		
McDonald et al., 1966	Amitriptyline	150	4 weeks	?
Herrington et al., 1974	Tryptophan	8,000	4 weeks	?
MacSweeney, 1975	Tryptophan	3,000	4 weeks	?
Davidson et al., 1978	Amitriptyline/ phenelzine combination	Mean[b] = 71/34	3–5 weeks	Bilateral; ?waveform
Steiner et al., 1978	Imipramine[c]	150	5 weeks	Bilateral; ?waveform
Gangadhar et al., 1982	Imipramine	150	12 weeks	Bilateral; ?waveform
Dinan and Barry, 1989	Tricyclic/lithium combination[d]	Variable[d] Li = 0.5–0.7	3 weeks	Bilateral; ?waveform
Folkerts et al., 1997	Paroxetine	Mean 44	4 weeks	Unilateral; brief pulse
Panneer Selvan et al., 1999	Imipramine	Variable[e]	4 weeks	Bilateral; brief pulse
Janakiramaiah et al., 2000	Imipramine	150	4 weeks	Bilateral; brief pulse

Note: NS, not specified.

[a] Phenelzine 45 mg/d; chlorprothixene 120–180 mg/d; tranylcypromine/trifluoperazine 30/3 mg/d; amitriptyline $\leq$225 mg/d; pheniprazine 12 mg/d; imipramine $\leq$250 mg/d.

[b] Mean amitriptyline/nortriptyline blood level = 52.5 ng/mL; range of platelet monoamine oxidase inhibition = 64%–97% with one value increased.

[c] Imipramine with or without T_3 augmentation.

[d] TCAs (tricyclic antidepressants) were amitriptyline ($N = 8$), desipramine ($N = 5$), or prothiaden ($N = 2$). Doses not specified.

[e] For patients older than 50 years, dose = 150 mg/d. For those 50 years old or younger, dose = 225 mg/d.

of the possible placebo effects of ECT or medications, but the sample sizes were extremely small (i.e., four patients per group), so the data are not helpful. The Robin and Harris (1962) study compared ECT with placebo pill against sham ECT with imipramine. Imipramine doses, ECT technique, and treatment duration were not mentioned, and again group sizes were quite small. The Gangadhar et al. (1982) study involved comparing imipramine 150 mg + sham ECT versus bilateral ECT + placebo pill for 12 weeks. The patients were all endogenously depressed according to modern research criteria and were blindly assessed for outcome with the HRSD (Williams, 2001). Despite the apparently low imipramine dose, outcomes were the same for the two groups, albeit improvement arrived somewhat faster for the ECT group.

A third methodological problem is that most studies used outmoded ECT techniques. Most study publications made no mention of ECT technique (see Table 6.3). Similar problems are encountered in the sham ECT literature previously cited. In only one of the trials comparing ECT and medication was electrical dose properly specified and seizure threshold determined (Folkerts et al., 1997). In that trial, moderately suprathreshold (i.e., 2.5 times threshold) right unilateral ECT was more effective than a mean dose of 44 mg per day of paroxetine.

A fourth methodological weakness is inadequate dosage and duration of medication. In the imipramine studies, drug blood levels were not reported. In two of these studies doses are not specified, and in most others only a maximum possible dose is listed. A maximum dose is hard to interpret because not all study patients reach that dose (see Table 6.3). In the Davidson et al. (1978) study, in which the medication-treated patients received a combination of amitriptyline and tranylcypromine, the tricyclic blood levels were markedly subtherapeutic, and in one case, blood monoamine oxidase activity was increased, not decreased as expected. In the one study in which drug blood levels appear therapeutic (i.e., serum lithium exceeded 0.5 mEq/L), the medication-treated group fared as well as the ECT group (Dinan and Barry, 1989). Besides adequate dosage, sufficient duration is essential. Table 6.3 lists the dosages and durations of pharmacotherapy for the 22 studies. For many studies the duration was short.

A fifth problem with the ECT-medication literature concerns use of medications that are not clearly antidepressant (e.g., tryptophan and chlorprothixene) or are archaic (e.g., pheniprazine, iproniazid, and isocarboxazid). In modern psychiatry, newer agents have virtually replaced monoamine oxidase inhibitors and somewhat replaced tricyclics. There is only one trial of a selective serotonin reuptake inhibitor (SSRI) (Folkerts et al., 1997) and no trial of many other commonly used medications (i.e., other SSRIs, venlafaxine, mirtazapine, bupropion, or duloxetine).

Variability in diagnosis, as in the sham studies, is also a methodological problem in the ECT-medication literature. Older studies involve patients whose psychopathology is only vaguely described. This lack of diagnostic specificity obstructs generalizability to modern clinical practice and research. Additionally, small samples are typical in this literature. Meta-analyses, by treating all patients in all studies as part of one data set, are primarily influenced by the few large-scale studies (Greenblatt et al., 1964; Medical Research Council, 1965), but these are old and they use outmoded diagnostic assessment and depression subtyping methods.

Finally, failure in the meta-analyses to distinguish psychotic from nonpsychotic depression is a very substantial shortcoming. In some studies, psychotic patients were included in the medication groups (e.g., Davidson et al., 1978; Greenblatt et al., 1964; Medical Research Council, 1965). Antidepressant pharmacotherapy alone is insufficient for most patients with psychotic depression, whereas ECT is highly effective for this population (Petrides et al., 2001).

In summary, merely to say that patients randomized to ECT fare better than those randomized to medications is not sufficient if one is postulating that ECT is an inherently superior medical treatment, because placebo phenomena may explain the greater efficacy. A relevant example is the Janakiramaiah et al. (2000) study of patients who met research criteria for melancholic depression. There was therapeutic equivalence among bilateral ECT, imipramine, and a form of yoga consisting of nothing more than paced breathing exercises. It is hard not to suppose that placebo effects would rate high in such a trial.

Do various forms of ECT differ in therapeutic efficacy?

ECT should not be conceptualized as a unitary treatment, because several technical variations can strongly affect clinical outcomes. These variations include stimulus waveform and other stimulus characteristics, electrode placement, stimulus dosing, treatment session frequency, total course length, concurrent benzodiazepine use, and prophylaxis medication choice. Several studies have shown that one type of ECT is superior to another (Heshe et al., 1978). If one assumes that a sham ECT group would fare no better than the least effective form of ECT in a comparison study, by implication the more effective forms of ECT are better than sham.

Relevant studies are discussed in Chapters 27 and 28 here on electrode placement and on stimulus dosing. It is sufficient to say here that, for unilateral electrode placement effectiveness, the stimulus dose must be well above the minimum required to elicit a seizure (Sackeim et al., 1987, 1993, 2000). This relationship between electrical dose and efficacy represents strong evidence that the efficacy of ECT results from its neurobiology and is not merely placebo related.

Do subtypes of depression respond differently to ECT?

Modern nosology characterizes several subtypes of broadly defined depression, such as psychotic, melancholic (endogenous), and atypical. It has long been clinical lore in the ECT field that melancholic and psychotic depressed patients respond particularly well and that neurotic, "reactive," or atypical depressed patients do not. The very early sham ECT studies are unhelpful largely because of depressive terminology that is no longer used. Additionally, those studies were not statistically powered to tease out differential response rates of the various forms of depression studied.

Many of the sham studies did not use any diagnostic criteria but did mention subtypes, although the latter were often outdated (e.g., "involutional melancholia" or "depressive reaction"). In only two of these studies were the patients specifically stratified according to psychosis status using modern concepts of psychotic depression (Brandon et al., 1984; Johnstone et al., 1980). The Northwick Park trial (Clinical Research Centre, 1984; Johnstone et al., 1980) found that only patients with psychotic depression enjoy a substantially greater response to ECT, as compared with that of sham treatment. Interestingly, only patients meeting criteria for endogenous depression were entered into the trial. Thus, there could be no endogenous versus nonendogenous comparison. It is puzzling that, among the nonpsychotic patients with endogenous depression, there was an equal response rate between real and sham ECT. This runs counter to the widely held belief that melancholic depression is poorly responsive to placebo treatment.

The Leicestershire Trial (Brandon et al., 1984) compared ECT versus sham response rates among psychotic, "retarded," and neurotic patients with depression. In the latter group, which was very small, there was no difference in response rates between real and sham ECT. For the other two groups, real ECT emerged as more effective acutely than sham ECT. If retarded depression represents melancholia, these data imply that melancholic depression does respond better to ECT than do nonmelancholic depressions. Some data do corroborate that psychomotor retardation in depression predicts good response to ECT (Parker and Hadzi-Pavlovic, 1996).

In the Lambourn and Gill (1978) report, all patients were described as suffering "depressive psychosis," but no structured diagnostic assessment or criteria were used, nor was any further description given of what was meant by the term. The modern reader of that study is left wondering if the patients truly suffered from delusions or hallucinations or if the term "depressive psychosis" was used loosely by modern standards. If in fact the patients were psychotic, then it is a most interesting finding that sham ECT resulted in a mean reduction of 23 points on the HRSD.

Some lessons regarding differential ECT responsivity in depressive subtypes can be gleaned from the non–sham-controlled literature. Petrides et al. (2001), in a large trial of bitemporal electrode placement ECT in psychotic and nonpsychotic unipolar patients with depression, found that the psychotic group had a higher remission rate than did the nonpsychotic group. In a separate report from the same study, the melancholic patients showed a slightly lower acute remission rate with ECT than did the nonmelancholic patients (Fink et al., 2007). Additionally, melancholic features as defined by abstraction from certain items of the HSRD were not found to predict substantially better ECT response in another large modern trial (Prudic et al., 1989). This outcome runs counter to some of the older non–sham-controlled ECT literature, which does support the contention that melancholic (or endogenous) depression responds better to ECT than nonmelancholic depression does (Carney et al., 1965; Rose, 1963). This may relate to numerous methodologic changes over the decades in studying melancholia (such as the use of highly structured, blindly administered rating scales in modern trials as opposed to extensive mental status examination and collateral information obtained in the older studies) as well as to changes in diagnostic terminology (Rasmussen, 2007). Undiagnosed comorbid anxiety disorders may have influenced the outcome. A final depressive typology question concerns whether unipolar and bipolar depressions respond differently to ECT. In two trials, overall remission rates were the same (Daly et al., 2001; Grunhaus et al., 2002).

ECT in mania

A wealth of uncontrolled, retrospective data point to strong efficacy of ECT in manic states (Mukherjee et al., 1994). However, only four randomized controlled trials exist (Langsley et al., 1959; Mukherjee et al., 1988; Mukherjee, 1989; Sikdar et al., 1994; Small et al., 1988). Langsley et al. (1959) randomly assigned 106 patients with mania or schizophrenia to ECT or chlorpromazine but did not report data for the two diagnostic groups separately.

Small et al. (1988) compared bitemporal brief-pulse ECT with lithium carbonate for acute mania in 34 patients. The ECT-treated patients improved more quickly for the first 8 weeks of the trial; thereafter, the two groups fared equally well. All ECT patients met research criteria for response.

In a study at Columbia University (Mukherjee, 1989; Mukherjee et al., 1988), patients with mania were randomized in the first phase of the study to right or left unilateral ECT and in the second phase to lithium–haloperidol treatment or to right unilateral, left unilateral, or bitemporal ECT. There were no differences in outcome among the ECT groups, but the total ECT-treated patients numbered only 22. Fifty-nine percent of these patients remitted from mania whereas none of the five medication-treated patients remitted.

Sikdar et al. (1994) compared bitemporal ECT with sham ECT in patients with mania, both in addition to 600 mg per day of chlorpromazine. There were 15 patients per group. This trial found real ECT superior to sham ECT, although ECT was delivered with a sine wave current. At the end of eight treatments, 12 of 15 real ECT-treated patients remitted whereas only 1 of 15 in the sham-treated group did. Thus, at least in the short term, augmentation of chlorpromazine with ECT resulted in quicker improvement than use of the medication alone.

Concluding remarks

Hundreds of published data collections, prospective or retrospective in design, conducted over the past seven decades attest to the high efficacy that can be achieved with ECT for patients with mood disorders, especially major depression. There are several variants of ECT and concepts of depression that add complexity to the literature. The gold standard efficacy study in clinical medicine is the randomized, placebo-controlled trial, and such trials relevant to ECT are lacking, for reasons cited earlier. Of course this does not mean that ECT is no better than placebo treatment, but it does mean that definitive studies without major flaws have not been done. Furthermore, in comparing ECT with psychotropic medications, published study methods are problematic. It is unlikely that well-controlled sham or medication-controlled studies will ever be done. As newer methods of "brain stimulation" are increasingly studied (e.g., transcranial magnetic stimulation, vagus nerve stimulation, deep brain stimulation), we should keep in mind the desirability of properly designed studies comparing these newer methods with sham forms of treatment.

References

Abrams, R. 2002. Electroconvulsive therapy, 4th edn. New York: Oxford University Press.

Abrams, R., Swartz, C. M., and Vedak, C. 1991. Antidepressant effects of high-dose right unilateral electroconvulsive therapy. Arch Gen Psychiatry 48: 746–8.

American Psychiatric Association. 2000. Diagnostic and statistical manual of mental disorders, 4th edn-text revision. Washington, DC: American Psychiatric Association.

Beck, A. T., Steer, R. A., and Garbin, M. G. 1988. Psychometric properties of the Beck Depression Inventory: Twenty-five years of evaluation. Clin Psychol Rev 8: 77–100.

Brandon, S., Cowley, P., McDonald, C., et al. 1984. Electroconvulsive therapy: Results in depressive illness from the Leicestershire trial. BMJ 288: 22–25.

Brill, N. Q., Crumpton, E., Eiduson, S., et al. 1959. Relative effectiveness of various components of electroconvulsive therapy. Arch Neurol Psychiatry 81: 627–35.

Bruce, E. M., Crone, N., Fitzpatrick, G., et al. 1960. A comparative trial of ECT and tofranil. Am J Psychiatry 117: 76.

Carney, M. W. P., Roth, M., and Garside, R. F. 1965. The diagnosis of depressive syndromes and the prediction of ECT response. Br J Psychiatry 111: 659–74.

Clinical Research Centre, Division of Psychiatry. 1984. The Northwick Park ECT trial. Predictors of response to real and simulated ECT. Br J Psychiatry 144: 227–37.

Daly, J. J., Prudic, J., Devanand, D. P., et al. 2001. ECT in bipolar and unipolar depression: Differences in speed of response. Bipolar Disord 3: 95–104.

Davidson, J., McLeod, M., Law-Yeone, B., et al. 1978. A comparison of electroconvulsive therapy and combined phenelzine-amitriptyline in refractory depression. Arch Gen Psychiatry 35: 639–42.

d'Elia, G. and Widepalm, K. 1974. Comparison of frontoparietal and temporoparietal unilateral electroconvulsive therapy. Acta Psychiatr Scand 50: 225–32.

Dinan, T. G. and Barry, S. 1989. A comparison of electroconvulsive therapy with a combined lithium and tricyclic combination among depressed tricyclic nonresponders. Acta Psychiatr Scand 80: 97–100.

Fahy, P., Imlah, N., and Harrington, J. 1963. A controlled comparison of electroconvulsive therapy, imipramine, and thiopentone sleep in depression. J Neuropsychiatr 4: 310–14.

Fink, M., Rush, A. J., Knapp, R. G., et al. 2007. DSM melancholic features are unreliable predictors of ECT response. A CORE publication. J ECT 23(3): 139–46.

Folkerts, H. W., Michael, N., Tolle, R., et al. 1997. Electroconvulsive therapy vs. paroxetine in treatment-resistant depression – a randomized study. Acta Psychiatr Scand 96: 334–42.

Freeman, C. P. L., Basson, J. V., and Crighton, A. 1978. Double-blind controlled trial of electro-convulsive therapy (E.C.T.) and simulated E.C.T. in depressive illness. Lancet 1: 738–40.

Gangadhar, B. N., Kapur, R. L., Kalyanasundaram, S. 1982. Comparison of electroconvulsive therapy with imipramine in endogenous depression: A double blind study. Br J Psychiatry 141: 367–71.

Greenblatt, M., Grosser, G. H., and Wechsler, H. 1962. A comparative study of selected antide-pressant medications and EST. Am J Psychiatry 119: 144–153.

Greenblatt, M., Grosser, G. H., and Wechsler, H. 1964. Differential response of hospitalized depressed patients to somatic therapy. Am J Psychiatry 120: 935–43.

Gregory, S., Shawcross, C. R., and Gill, D. 1985. The Nottingham ECT study. A double-blind comparison of bilateral, unilateral, and simulated ECT in depressive illness. Br J Psychiatry 146: 520–4.

Grunhaus, L., Schreiber, S., Dolberg, O. T., et al. 2002. Response to ECT in major depression: Are there differences between unipolar and bipolar depression? Bipolar Disord 4(Suppl. 1): 91–3.

Harris, J. A. and Robin, A. A. 1960. A controlled trial of phenelzine in depressive reactions. J Ment Sci 106: 1432–7.

Herrington, R. N., Bruce, A., and Johnstone, E. C. 1974. Comparative trial of L-tryptophan and E.C.T. in severe depressive illness. Lancet 2: 731–4.

Heshe, J., Roeder, E., and Theilgaard, A. 1978. Unilateral and bilateral ECT. A psychiatric and psychological study of therapeutic effect and side effects. Acta Psychiatr Scand Suppl 275: 1–180.

Hutchinson, J. and Smedberg, D. 1963. Treatment of depression: A comparative study of ECT and six drugs. Br J Psychiatry 109: 536–8.

Janakiramaiah, N., Gangadhar, B. N., Naga Venkatesha Murthy, P. J., et al. 2000. Antidepressant efficacy of Sudarshan Kriya Yoga (SKY) in melancholia: A randomized comparison with electroconvulsive therapy (ECT) and imipramine. J Affect Disord 57: 255–9.

Janicak, P. G., Davis, J. M., Gibbons, R. D., et al. 1985. Efficacy of ECT: A meta-analysis. Am J Psychiatry 142(3): 297–302.

Johnstone E. C., Deakin, J. F. W., Lawler, P., et al. 1980. The Northwick Park electroconvulsive therapy trial. Lancet 2: 1317–20.

Kellner, C. H., Knapp, R. G., Petrides, G., et al. 2006. Continuation electroconvulsive therapy versus pharmacotherapy for relapse prevention in major depression: A multi-site study from the Consortium for Research in Electroconvulsive Therapy (CORE). Arch Gen Psychiatry 63(12): 1337–44.

Kho, K. H., van Vreeswijk, M. F., Simpson, S., et al. 2003. A meta-analysis of electroconvulsive therapy efficacy in depression. J ECT 19(3): 139–47.

Kiloh, L. J., Child, J. P., and Latner, G. 1960. A controlled trial of iproniazid in the treatment of endogenous depression. J Ment Sci 106: 1139–44.

Lambourn, J. and Gill, D. 1978. A controlled comparison of simulated and real ECT. Br J Psychiatry 133: 514–19.

Lancaster, N. P., Steinert, R. R., and Frost, I. 1958. Unilateral electro-convulsive therapy. J Ment Sci 104: 221–7.

Langsley, D. G., Enterline, J. D., and Hickerson, G. X. 1959. A comparison of chlorpromazine and ECT in treatment of acute schizophrenic and manic patients. Arch Neurol Psychiatry 81: 384–91.

MacSweeney, D. A. 1975. Treatment of unipolar depression (letter). Lancet 2: 510–11.

McCall, W. V., Dunn, A., Rosenquist, P. B., et al. 2002. Markedly suprathreshold right unilateral ECT versus minimally suprathreshold bilateral ECT: Antidepressant and memory effects. J ECT 18(3): 126–9.

McDonald, I. M., Perkins, M., Marjerrison, G., et al. 1966. A controlled comparison of amitriptyline and electroconvulsive therapy in the treatment of depression. Am J Psychiatry 122: 1427–31.

Medical Research Council. 1965. Clinical trial of the treatment of depressive illness. BMJ 1: 881–6.

Montgomery, S. A. and Asberg, M. 1979. A new depression scale designed to be sensitive to change. Br J Psychiatry 134: 382–9.

Mukherjee, S. 1989. Mechanisms of the antimanic effect of electroconvulsive therapy. Convuls Ther 5(3): 227–43.

Mukherjee, S., Sackeim, H. A., and Lee, C. 1988. Unilateral ECT in the treatment of manic states. Convuls Ther 4: 74–80.

Mukherjee, S., Sackeim, H. A., and Schnur, D. A. 1994. Electroconvulsive therapy of acute manic episodes: A review of 50 years' experience. Am J Psychiatry 151(2): 169–76.

Pagnin, D., de Queiroz, V., Pini, S., et al. 2004. Efficacy of ECT in depression: A meta-analytic review. J ECT 20(1): 13–20.

Panneer Selvan, C., Mayur, P. M., Gangadhar, B. N., et al. 1999. Comparison of therapeutic efficacy of ECT and imipramine: A randomized controlled trial. Indian J Psychiatry 41(3): 228–35.

Parker, G. and Hadzi-Pavlovic, D., eds. 1996. Melancholia: A disorder of movement and mood. Cambridge: Cambridge University Press.

Petrides, G., Fink, M., Husain, M., et al. 2001. ECT remission rates in psychotic versus non-psychotic depressed patients. J ECT 17: 244–53.

Prudic, J., Devanand, D. P., Sackeim, H. A., et al. 1989. Relative response of endogenous and non-endogenous symptoms to electroconvulsive therapy. J Affect Disord 16: 59–64.

Rasmussen, K. G. 2007. Attempts to validate melancholic depression: Some observations on modern research methodology. Bull Menninger Clin 71(2): 150–63.

Robin, A. A. and Harris, J. A. 1962. A controlled comparison of imipramine and electroplexy. J Ment Sci 108: 217–19.

Rose, J. T. 1963. Reactive and endogenous depression – Response to ECT. Br J Psychiatry 109: 213–17.

Sackeim, H. A., Decina, P., Kanzler, M., et al. 1987. Effects of electrode placement on the efficacy of titrated, low dosage ECT. Am J Psychiatry 144: 1449–55.

Sackeim, H. A., Prudic, J., Devanand, D. P., et al. 1993. Effects of stimulus intensity and electrode placement on the efficacy and cognitive effects of electroconvulsive therapy. N Engl J Med 328: 839–46.

Sackeim, H. A., Prudic, J., Devanand, D. P., et al. 2000. A prospective, randomized, double-blind comparison of bilateral and right unilateral electroconvulsive therapy at different stimulus intensities. Arch Gen Psychiatry 57: 425–34.

Sainz, A. 1959. Clarification of the action of successful treatment in the depressions. Dis Nerv Syst (Suppl.) 20: 53–7.

Sikdar, S., Kulhara, P., Avasthi, A., et al. 1994. Combined chlorpromazine and electroconvulsive therapy in mania. Br J Psychiatry 164: 806–10.

Small, J. G., Klapper, M. H., Kellams, J. J., et al. 1988. Electroconvulsive treatment compared with lithium in the management of manic states. Arch Gen Psychiatry 45(8): 727–32.

Spitzer, R. L., Endicott, J., and Robins, E. 1978. Research diagnostic criteria: Rationale and reliability. Arch Gen Psychiatry 35(6): 773–82.

Stanley, W. J. and Fleming, H. 1962. A clinical comparison of phenelzine and electro-convulsive therapy in the treatment of depressive illness. Br J Psychiatry 108: 708–10.

Steiner, M., Radwan, M., Elizur, A., et al. 1978. Failure of L-triiodothyronine (T3) to potentiate tricyclic antidepressant response. Curr Ther Res Clin Exp 23(5): 655–9.

UK ECT Review Group. 2003. Efficacy and safety of electroconvulsive therapy in depressive disorders: A systematic review and meta-analysis. Lancet 361: 799–808.

Ulett, G. A., Smith, K., and Gleser, G. C. 1956. Evaluation of convulsive and subconvulsive shock therapies utilizing a control group. Am J Psychiatry 112: 795–802.

West, E. D. 1981. Electric convulsion therapy in depression: A double-blind controlled trial. BMJ 282: 355–7.

Williams, J. B. W. 2001. Standardizing the Hamilton Depression Rating Scale: Past, present, and future. Eur Arch Psychiatry Clin Neurosci 251 (Suppl. 2): II/6–II/12.

Wilson, I. C., Vernon, J. T., Guin, T., et al. 1963. A controlled study of treatments of depression. J Neuropsychiatr 4: 331–7.

Wing, J. K., Cooper, J. E., and Sartorius, N. 1974. The measurement and classification of psychiatric symptoms. London: Cambridge University Press.

Wittenborn, J. R., Plante, M., Burgess, F., et al. 1961. The efficacy of electroconvulsive therapy, iproniazid and placebo in the treatment of young depressed women. J Nerv Ment Dis 133: 316–32.

Wittenborn, J. R., Plante, M., Burgess, F., et al. 1962. A comparison of imipramine, electroconvulsive therapy and placebo in the treatment of depressions. J Nerv Ment Dis 135: 131–7.

7

Clinical evidence for the efficacy of electroconvulsive therapy in the treatment of catatonia and psychoses

Gabor Gazdag, Stephan C. Mann, Gabor S. Ungvari, and Stanley N. Caroff

Introduction

Although Kahlbaum (1874) initially described catatonia as a separate disease entity, its association with a diversity of psychiatric and neuromedical conditions attests to its syndromal nature. Kraepelin (1919) acknowledged that catatonic symptoms occurred in other conditions, but the poor prognosis he observed in longitudinal studies led him to classify catatonia as a subtype of dementia praecox. This exclusive link between catatonia and schizophrenia remained fixed in English diagnostic systems until Abrams and Taylor (1976) and Gelenberg (1976) refocused attention on catatonia as a syndrome. This effort to broaden recognition of catatonia is reflected in *The Diagnostic and Statistical Manual of Mental Disorders*, 4th edition (DSM-IV; American Psychiatric Association [APA], 1994) and *International Classification of Diseases*, 10th Revision (ICD-10; World Health Organization [WHO], 1992), where catatonia now can be associated with mood disorders or medical conditions. Catatonia continues to be recognized as a subtype of schizophrenia with uncertain therapeutic and prognostic implications.

Two patients recovered from catatonia following epileptic seizures (Muller, 1930), an early link to convulsive therapy. The first successful electroconvulsive therapy (ECT) was performed on a patient thought to have catatonic schizophrenia (Cerletti and Bini, 1938). In the subsequent two decades, schizophrenia was one of the main indications for ECT (Kalinowsky and Worthing, 1943). By the 1960s, however, it became clear that such optimism was exaggerated, and the therapeutic effects of ECT in schizophrenia were often transitory. Later studies found its efficacy in schizophrenia inferior to antipsychotic treatment (Fink and Sackeim, 1996; Tharyan and Adams, 2005). With the exception of a few centers in the developing world and Eastern Europe (e.g., Gazdag et al., 2004), ECT is rarely used in the treatment of schizophrenia (APA, 2001; Scott, 2005). Although interest in ECT as a treatment for schizophrenia in general has waned, increasing awareness of catatonia as a syndrome in conditions apart from schizophrenia has rekindled interest and research in ECT as one of its most effective treatments.

The aim of this chapter is to review the role of ECT in the treatment of catatonia associated with mood disorders, nonaffective psychoses, and medical conditions.

Methodological limitations

There are numerous methodological shortcomings in studies of ECT in treating catatonia and schizophrenia. First, there are diagnostic difficulties. Since the introduction of ECT 70 years ago, the concept of schizophrenia has fluctuated considerably, becoming more precise and narrow. As a consequence, studies conducted before 1980 include patients who would now be diagnosed with mood disorders. In addition, during the past century the catatonic subtype of schizophrenia has averaged a 59% decline across studies repeated at single sites (Caroff et al., 2004), although underrecognition of catatonic symptoms may be partly responsible for this decline (van der Heijden et al., 2005). Potentially, both of these trends have exerted a major negative impact on the treatment response of schizophrenia to ECT. That is, fewer cases of schizophrenia have acute catatonic or mood-related symptoms, which predict good response to ECT. Another problem complicating comparisons across studies is that ECT was used in different stages of schizophrenia; frequently, the boundaries between the acute and chronic phases became blurred or the two phases of illness were combined in patient samples.

There are also conceptual and diagnostic problems with catatonia. Its boundaries are imprecise, and the number and definitions of individual symptoms vary greatly as reflected in the published rating scales (Caroff and Ungvari, 2007). The symptomatological diversity of catatonia is rarely addressed in the literature. Attention is centered on the acute, retarded type of catatonia. Only rarely studied are the excited and chronic forms and qualitative peculiarities of movement.

An important confounding factor is the heterogeneity of psychotropic drugs and drug doses co-prescribed with ECT in most investigations after the late 1950s. Furthermore, ECT technique has been significantly refined through the decades, making the comparison of results from different eras problematic. Standardized assessment tools were rarely used before the 1980s, and, apart from retrospective chart reviews, most prospective studies have small sample sizes. The preponderance of the relevant modern literature consists of case reports or small case series because collecting large samples is impractical, informed consent for research is particularly difficult, and random allocation to standardized treatment protocols can be hard to justify or accomplish.

Certain methodological limitations are inherent in ECT. Transient cognitive dysfunction can undermine the double-blind method. Patient hesitance to ECT consent inevitably biases the selection of potential study subjects. Ethical and sometimes legal constraints, particularly in the last 30 years, preclude designing controlled studies using sham ECT or placebo. Less cumbersome pharmacological treatments for acute catatonia (benzodiazepines) and schizophrenia (antipsychotics) typically seem more desirable than ECT to patients and their relatives (see Chapter 23).

To date, no large-scale randomized, controlled double-blind trial (RCT) of ECT with sophisticated assessment tools meeting rigorous methodological criteria has been conducted in schizophrenia or catatonia. Although catatonia rating scales are available, they have never been used as outcome measures in studies of ECT in schizophrenia. However, there have been several sufficiently well-designed trials of ECT in schizophrenia that are reviewed here. As for catatonic schizophrenia specifically, only one study met the methodological criteria for inclusion in the Cochrane database (Miller et al., 1953).

Because of methodological shortcomings and the scarcity of published trials, most of the results and recommendations referred to in this chapter reflect accumulated clinical evidence rather than conclusions of rigorous scientific studies. Yet, the existing body of knowledge should not be understated. It is remarkable that, despite difficulties conducting well-designed treatment trials, there are a number of catatonic syndromes (e.g., acute retarded catatonia and malignant or lethal catatonia) and certain types or phases of schizophrenia (e.g., acute or catatonic schizophrenia) for which the efficacy of ECT appears to be supported. We focus primarily on reviewing the few studies that meet basic methodological standards, with additional references to case reports.

ECT in schizophreniform disorder

Data are very limited on using ECT in schizophreniform disorder. Two RCTs using sham ECT in a control group have addressed this issue. In one trial, 78 patients with schizophreniform illness were randomized to ECT with placebo or sham ECT with chlorpromazine over 4 weeks (Bagadia et al., 1983). There was no significant difference in outcome between the groups. More ECT-treated patients complained of memory impairment, and extrapyramidal side effects were more frequent in the chlorpromazine-sham ECT group.

Sarkar et al. (1994) randomized 30 patients with first-episode psychosis to six bitemporal ECTs or six sham sessions, both with 15 mg/day haloperidol. No differences were found between the two groups after six weeks and six months of treatment. The findings of these two RCTs suggest that ECT given with antipsychotic drugs is not more effective than antipsychotic drugs alone in schizophreniform disorder, or that these drugs obscure the effects of ECT.

Suzuki et al. (2006e) argued that ECT improves the outcome of first-episode schizophreniform disorder by shortening the psychotic episode, preventing significant disruption in vocational and social functioning and limiting exposure to the neurological complications of antipsychotic drugs. In support of this notion, 13 of 90 patients with schizophreniform disorder, most with catatonic symptoms, were treated with ECT because of violent behavior and nonresponse to antipsychotic drugs (Ücok and Cakir, 2006). These ECT patients showed significantly greater reductions in psychotic symptoms compared with patients receiving antipsychotics. However, at one-year follow-up, patients treated with ECT had relapsed more frequently and sooner than the others, despite use of maintenance antipsychotic medication in both groups. Increased relapses in ECT-treated patients may reflect their already established refractory history with antipsychotic drugs. The use of lithium or other types of medications in post-ECT maintenance treatment of schizophreniform illness may be more effective and is an important unstudied issue.

In view of conflicting evidence from these few reports, the role of ECT in acute schizophreniform psychoses remains uncertain. Because current recommendations (APA, 2001; Scott, 2005) do not provide guidance, the decision to use ECT in schizophreniform disorder should be individualized and based on psychopathology and treatment history.

ECT in the acute phase of schizophrenia

The majority of studies of ECT in schizophrenia published during the past few decades have addressed acute schizophrenic conditions. However, the term "acute" appears poorly defined in these investigations, sometimes denoting newly emerging, intensifying, or recurrent positive symptoms occurring within the first 5 years of the illness.

In an early, large-scale survey of the treatment of acute schizophrenia (Meduna and Friedman, 1939), convulsive treatment helped to achieve full short-term remission in 60% of 210 acutely ill patients in the United States and 53.5% of 590 European patients. Subsequent reports claimed success in up to 80% of acute episodes of schizophrenia (Kelly and Sargant, 1965). Presumably, these studies included a sizable proportion of patients who would have been diagnosed with psychotic mood disorders under current criteria.

Eventually, antipsychotic drugs proved to be at least as efficacious as ECT and by the 1970s had become the mainstay in treating acute schizophrenia. However, it became increasingly clear that antipsychotic drugs not only have serious side effects (see Chapter 23) but are not effective for all patients or for all conditions diagnosable as schizophrenia (Lieberman, 2007). Consequently, the role of ECT in the management of acute schizophrenia is being reexamined, as exemplified by five recent comprehensive reviews of this topic (Braga and Petrides, 2005; Caroff et al., 2007; Painuly and Chakrabarti, 2006; Tharyan and Adams, 2005).

Because of variations among trials in research design, patient selection, diagnostic criteria, outcome measures, methodologies, and number of ECT treatments administered, the findings of all four meta-analyses are similarly inconclusive. One potential bias in these meta-analyses is that they aggregated all acute, chronic, and treatment-resistant patient groups. Although no definitive conclusion can be reached on the role of ECT in schizophrenia, it appears safe and remains both a treatment choice and a subject for further investigation.

In the English-language literature, we found six RCTs of ECT in acute schizophrenia using a sham ECT control group (Table 7.1). Even though the findings were inconsistent across studies and are not robust enough to serve as the basis for firm recommendations, they are promising enough to foster further research.

The comparison between real versus sham ECT with concurrent antipsychotic drugs was compromised in all studies by such factors as wide variation in antipsychotic drug dosages, small numbers of subjects, and limited numbers of ECT sessions likely rendering the additional therapeutic effect of ECT marginal and undetectable. All studies randomly allocated patients to bitemporal ECT or sham ECT groups; two studies also included a right unilateral ECT group. The studies were of short duration lasting four weeks each, with only three (Abraham and Kulhara, 1987; Brandon et al., 1985; Taylor and Fleminger, 1980) having a longer follow-up phase of up to six months. Three studies failed to show any difference between the two treatment methods (Agarwal and Vinny, 1985; Sarita et al., 1998; Ukpong et al., 2002), and another three (Abraham and Kulhara, 1987; Brandon et al., 1985; Taylor and Fleminger, 1980) found the ECT–antipsychotic combination more efficacious during the first four to eight weeks of treatment, but noted no differences between groups at follow-up. Agarwal and Vinny (1985) observed, in line with the findings of open studies, a significant reduction of depressive symptoms when ECT was added to the antipsychotic medication. ECT was generally well tolerated in these studies, with only one study (Sarita et al., 1998) reporting more cognitive deficits in the bitemporal ECT group.

Other investigations using less rigorous methodology had the advantage of considerably larger sample sizes. The majority of these studies favored complementing antipsychotic drugs with ECT in acute schizophrenia during the acute phase of treatment only. The ECT–antipsychotic combination was superior to the use of antipsychotic drugs alone, particularly during the first few weeks of treatment in six single-blind and open Indian studies comprising 498 patients (Painuly and

Table 7.1 Studies using sham electroconvulsive therapy (ECT) as control group in schizophrenia

Author	Method	Sample size	Diagnosis	Interventions	Outcome measures	Results
Miller et al., 1953	Random, not blinded	3 × 10 pts	Catatonic Sch. (all chronic, average hospitalization 10 years)	1. Unmodified ECT 2. Anesthesia + subconvulsive ECT 3. Sham ECT	Employment	ECT group showed better outcomes but not significantly
Brill et al.,1959	Random, double blind	97 pts 1–19; 2–20; 3–20; 4–20; 5–18	Sch. (mainly chronic, ill < 1 month to 10 years)	1. Unmodified ECT 2. ECT and muscle relaxant 3. ECT and anesthesia 4. Sham ECT and anesthesia 5. Sham ECT without anesthesia	Global impression; early termination	No significant difference in global impression
Taylor and Fleminger, 1980	Random, double blind	2 × 10 pts	Sch. (ill > 6 months, nonresponsive to antipsychotics)	1. ECT + 300 mg chlorpromazine equivalent (CPZeq) 2. Sham ECT + 300 mg CPZeq	Global impression; relapse; early termination	Significantly higher improvement, but also higher relapse rate in the ECT group
Bagadia et al., 1981	Random, double blind	78 pts 1. 40 2. 38	Sch. (ill > 1 month)	1. ECT + placebo 2. Sham ECT + CPZ	CGI, BPRS, early termination	No significant difference between the two groups
Agarwal and Vinny, 1985	Random, double blind	2 × 15 pts	Sch. (ill 1 month < and < 2 years)	1. ECT + CPA 2. Sham ECT + CPZ	BPRS; early termination	No difference in the number of subjects leaving the study early; higher improvement on BPRS in ECT group
Brandon et al., 1985	Random, double blind	19 pts. 1–9; 2–10	Sch. (ill < 6 months: 5 in each group)	1- ECT + unchanged antipsychotics (317 mg/day CPZeq) 2- Sham ECT + unchanged antipsychotics (273 mg/day CPZeq)	Global impression; relapse; early termination	Significantly higher improvement rate and less relapse in ECT group

(continued)

Table 7.1 (*cont.*)

Author	Method	Sample size	Diagnosis	Interventions	Outcome measures	Results
Abraham and Kulhara, 1987	Random, double blind	2 × 11 pts	Sch.	1. ECT + 20 mg trifluoperazine 2. Sham ECT + 20 mg trifluoperazine	Relapse; BPRS, CGI; early termination	No significant difference in relapse rate/early termination of treatment; higher improvement on BPRS in ECT group
Sarita et al., 1998	Random, double blind	3 × 12 pts	ICD-10 Sch. 78% of pts ill > 2 years	1. Unilateral ECT + haloperidol (14.2 ± 8.2mg) 2. Bilateral ECT + haloperidol (14.6 ± 5.8 mg) 3. Sham ECT + haloperidol (18.3 ± 7.2mg)	CGI, BPRS; adverse effects	No significant difference in improvement between the groups, although control group showed a bit higher improvement on BPRS with less memory impairment; no difference in termination of treatment early
Goswami et al., 2003	Random, double blind	31 pts	Sch. (DSM-IV, treatment resistant, mean duration of illness 7 years)	1. Bilateral ECT + CPZ 2. Sham ECT + CPZ	BPRS, CGI, early termination	No significant difference in improvement. Worse results on BPRS in ECT-treated group. More patients left the study early from control group; lower rehospitalization rate in ECT group
Ukpong et al., 2002	Random, double blind	16 pts 1. 9 2. 7	ICD-10 Sch. (ill < 2 years)	1. ECT + CPZ 2. Sham ECT + CPZ	BPRS, SANS, CGIS	No significant difference in BPRS and SANS between the groups

Notes: pts, patients; Sch., schizophrenia; CGI, Clinical Global Impression ; BPRS, Brief Psychiatric Rating Scale; DSM-IV, *The Diagnostic and Statistical Manual of Mental Disorders*, 4th edition; ICD-10, *International Classification of Diseases*, 10th Revision; SANS, Scale for the Assessment of Negative Symptoms.

Chakrabarti, 2006). Having pooled together more than 1,000 patients from 34 single-blind and open studies, Braga and Petrides (2005) came to a similar conclusion. They emphasized the value of ECT–antipsychotic drug combinations, particularly ECT with clozapine, for treatment-resistant patients.

Of the single-blind studies, the large-scale investigation of May et al. (1981) deserves mention because of its scope and thorough design. Two hundred twenty-eight first-admission schizophrenia patients were randomly assigned to one of five treatments: psychotherapy, antipsychotic drugs, the combination of these two, ECT, or milieu therapy. Patients were followed for two to five years with assessments performed by blind raters. Initial successful outcome was defined as discharge within one year of admission. The initial results were that antipsychotics and antipsychotics with psychotherapy (96% and 95%, respectively) had better outcomes than ECT (79%), followed by psychotherapy (65%) and milieu therapy (59%). Over longer follow-up, the ECT group did not differ significantly from the antipsychotic groups (May et al., 1981).

Probably the most informative of the several retrospective chart reviews is Wells' study (1973) covering 10 years. The files of 276 schizophrenia patients who received a course of ECT were scrutinized. The main indication for ECT was lack of improvement with pharmacotherapy and prominent depressive or catatonic symptoms. Full and partial symptomatic relief was achieved in 36% and 38%, respectively. The catatonic subtype (55%) showed the best response to ECT followed by the schizoaffective (40%), paranoid (34%), and undifferentiated (32%) subtypes. Ninety-two percent of the patients were discharged home, but 46% had relapses two years later. Besides first-episode psychosis, depressive features were significant predictors of response to ECT. This reasonably good response to ECT raises the possibility that some psychotic depressive patients were misdiagnosed as having schizophrenia.

Taking into consideration the current guidelines (APA, 2001; Scott, 2005), only a cautious conclusion can be drawn from these studies. Some but not all studies provide support for ECT augmenting the effect of antipsychotic drugs in the short-term treatment of patients with acute schizophrenia. This effect is strongest in patients with catatonic and depressive symptoms, but is not sustained on long-term follow-up. The combined antipsychotic–ECT treatment combination is well tolerated and does not increase the likelihood of adverse effects (Nothdurfter et al., 2006).

ECT in the acute phase of catatonic schizophrenia

With two recent studies (Girish and Gill, 2003; Hatta et al., 2007) excepted, limited data are available on the role of ECT in the acute phase of catatonic schizophrenia. Girish and Gill's (2003) RCT started by giving lorazepam (6–8 mg/day) for a maximum of 5 days to 68 mainly stuporous young psychotic patients. The 14 nonaffective patients who failed to respond to lorazepam were randomized to either ECT with oral placebo or sham ECT with risperidone (4–6 mg) in a three-week trial. Bitemporal ECT (8.8 sessions on average) was administered three times a week. Outcome measures were the Bush-Francis Catatonia Rating Scale (BFCRS) and the Positive and Negative Syndrome Scale (PANSS). The ECT-treated subjects showed significantly greater improvement on both the BFCRS and PANSS total scores. Apart from the small sample size and the relatively short study period, the main limitation of the study was the significant difference between the two treatment groups in duration of catatonia prior to the study treatment.

In a series of 586 Japanese patients in an intensive care unit, 50 presented with catatonic symptoms; 23 were diagnosed with schizophrenia (Hatta et al., 2007). Catatonic patients received either ECT or a benzodiazepine first guided by clinical decision. If benzodiazepines were ineffective, the next step was either ECT or an antipsychotic drug; if the latter failed, ECT was the last resort. As benzodiazepine doses were low, only 1 of the 41 patients who received benzodiazepines responded fully and 19 responded partially. In contrast, all 17 patients who received ECT achieved remission from their catatonic state. All five schizophrenia patients who received ECT became symptom free, whereas none of the 18 schizophrenia patients who were given benzodiazepines responded to these drugs.

During an 18-month period, 20 patients were diagnosed with catatonic schizophrenia in a German university department. Only five patients received ECT, all of whom experienced complete resolution of catatonia and improvement in psychotic condition (Finkbeiner, 1995). Another prospective study compared the response to ECT of five patients with catatonic schizophrenia and that of four patients with catatonic depression (Escobar et al., 2000). Catatonic symptoms associated with depression remitted faster and more completely than those associated with schizophrenia.

In a chart review of 250 catatonic schizophrenia patients (Morrison, 1974), remission in both psychopathology and social function from a single episode was judged blind to the type of treatment. Of the 250 patients, 214 were followed for a median of 2 years. Eighty-five (40%) patients remitted overall; the rate of remission was 53% for those who had received ECT. Recovery correlated with the symptoms of "denudativeness" and "stereotypy" and with the use of ECT; these were identified from 26 factors examined for predicting recovery.

In some studies, catatonic symptoms accompanying acute schizophrenia were less responsive to ECT than was catatonia associated with mood disorders. The retrospective chart review by Rohland et al. (1993) identified 28 episodes in 22 catatonic patients receiving ECT for 3.5 years; seven had schizophrenia, two had organic catatonia, and the rest had mood disorders. Twenty-six of the 28 catatonic episodes resolved or significantly improved after ECT, but mood disorder patients showed a higher rate of reduction in catatonic signs than did patients with schizophrenia (93% vs. 42%).

In an attempt to identify factors predictive of a favorable response to ECT in schizophrenia, Dodwell and Goldberg (1989) found an association with perplexity. Perplexity may represent catatonic semistupor.

Clinical evidence suggests that ECT may be more effective than benzodiazepines in the treatment of acute catatonic symptoms in general and schizophrenia in particular, leading some authors to suggest that ECT should be a first-line treatment for catatonia, regardless of the associated psychiatric disorder (Fink, 1990). Only a few clinical reports support the superiority of ECT over benzodiazepines. Waller et al. (2000) observed full response to three bilateral ECT sessions in one patient after the failure of 23-mg lorazepam; the response to ECT was excellent even after 45 days of unsuccessful benzodiazepine treatment. Boyarsky et al. (1999) reported that ECT led to the resolution of catatonia after 32 days of benzodiazepine treatment. When ECT and lorazepam were administered concurrently, the combination appeared to be superior to monotherapy in five consecutively identified cases (Petrides et al., 1997).

ECT in malignant catatonia

Stauder (1934) described "lethal catatonia" as characterized by extreme motor excitement, followed by stuporous exhaustion, cardiovascular collapse, coma, and death. The entire course involved progressive hyperthermia, autonomic dysfunction, clouding of consciousness, and prominent catatonic features (Mann et al., 2004). Although the incidence of lethal catatonia, or malignant catatonia, appears to have declined following the introduction of modern psychopharmacologic agents, it remains the subject of frequent case reports. Malignant catatonia represents a syndrome rather than a specific disease and can develop in association with diverse neuromedical illnesses as well as with the major psychoses. From this perspective, neuroleptic malignant syndrome (NMS), a potentially fatal complication of antipsychotic drug treatment, can be conceptualized as a drug-induced form of malignant catatonia.

The evidence that antipsychotic drugs are of benefit in the treatment of malignant catatonia is limited to anecdotal reports. However, the bulk of evidence indicates that the dopamine receptor-blocking effects of antipsychotic drugs are likely to aggravate episodes of malignant catatonia, as in NMS. In view of their questionably efficacy and their clear potential to aggravate malignant catatonia episodes, antipsychotic drugs should be withheld whenever malignant catatonia is suspected.

Although controlled studies are lacking, findings from case reports and series of consecutive cases indicate that ECT represents a safe and effective treatment for malignant catatonia when it occurs as an outgrowth of a major psychotic disorder (Mann et al., 1986, 1990, 2004). Arnold and Stepan (1952) used a "shock-block" method in the treatment of malignant catatonia. Sixteen (84%) of their 18 patients receiving ECT within the first five days after the onset of malignant catatonia survived. However, Arnold and Stepan (1952) stressed that early identification and prompt initiation of treatment are critical; none of the 14 patients starting ECT more than five days after the onset of malignant catatonia survived. Treatment began with a "block" of three bilateral "electroshocks" spaced at 15-minute intervals. The fourth "electroshock" was given 8 to 24 hours later, depending on the clinical condition. Following this, one to two "electroshocks" were given daily for the next two to three days, followed by treatment on alternate days or twice weekly to a total of 12 to 15 treatments.

Tolsma (1967) administered ECT to 20 malignant catatonia patients using an even more aggressive shock-block schedule: three to five bilateral "electroshocks" at 15-minute intervals followed by three additional "electroshocks" spaced at four-hour intervals, with the interval between shock blocks then gradually increased as the patient's mental condition improved. Eighteen patients (90%) survived. The majority of patients received 25 to 40 treatments, although one patient required a total of 200. Such extreme measures are rarely, if ever, necessary.

More recent publications have reported response with far fewer ECT sessions. These reports underscore that ECT appears far more effective if initiated before severe progression of malignant catatonia has occurred. Sedivec (1981) discussed eight cases of malignant catatonia treated with ECT. In seven cases, malignant catatonia remitted after five to seven treatments. An eighth patient, who was comatose on admission, died despite receiving ECT. Sedivec (1981) stressed that the development of a comatose state or a temperature in excess of 41°C augurs poorly for malignant catatonia even with ECT. Hafner and Kasper (1982) treated nine malignant catatonia patients. Seven patients were treated with unilateral ECT and attained remission following 2 to 14 treatments. Treatments were given once daily for two to five days and then administered two to three times per week. Gabris and Muller (1983) reported on 13 malignant catatonia cases. Each patient was treated with antipsychotic drugs, and six received concurrent ECT. All six patients treated with ECT survived, whereas two of seven treated with only antipsychotics died.

Among 50 patients reported in four large series, 40 of 41 patients treated with ECT survived (Mann et al., 2003). In contrast, just five of nine patients who received only antipsychotics and supportive care recovered. Similarly, in a review by Philbrick and Rummans (1994), 11 of 13 patients treated with ECT survived, compared with only one of five patients who did not receive ECT.

When malignant catatonia occurs as an outgrowth of a neuromedical illness or is substance induced, treatment must obviously be directed at the underlying disorder. Nevertheless, anecdotal evidence suggests that ECT can be dramatically effective, and at times lifesaving, in suppressing the symptoms of severe malignant catatonialike delirious states complicating a wide variety of neuromedical illnesses and intoxications. Along these lines, ECT has been used effectively in the treatment of NMS, as a drug-induced form of malignant catatonia.

ECT in schizoaffective disorders

Schizoaffective disorder is a heterogeneous condition with questionable validity and uncertain nosological position (Vollmer-Larsen et al., 2006). It might be supposed that patients with schizoaffective disorders frequently receive ECT because of the prominent affective symptoms. Yet, the literature on ECT in the acute treatment of schizoaffective illness is limited to a case series (Ries et al., 1981) and case reports (Lapensée, 1992).

A retrospective study by Ries et al. (1981) involved nine schizoaffective patients (per Research Diagnostic Criteria) who had not responded to antipsychotic medication. Patients received a mean of eight unilateral treatments. During a 1- to 18-month-long follow up, seven maintained an excellent, moderate, or good response to the initial course of ECT.

In the only prospective controlled open investigation on the effects of maintenance ECT (MECT) in schizoaffective disorder, the outcome of a one-year-long MECT in eight patients with ICD-10 schizoaffective patients was compared with that of a well-matched control group on maintenance drug therapy (Swoboda et al., 2001). All subjects were resistant to drug treatment. Outcome measures included relapse measured by the rehospitalization rate, the length of time spent in hospital, and survival in the community. The MECT group showed less rehospitalization (4 vs. 7), spent less time in hospital when hospitalized (106 ± 118 vs. 121 ± 76 weeks), and survived longer in the community (7.6 vs. 2.8 months) than controls. Because of the small sample size these results can be regarded only as preliminary.

A number of questions arise: Are affective or psychotic symptoms responsive to ECT? Do affective and schizophrenic symptoms respond in the same way? Is ECT efficacy in the manic episode the same as in the depressive episode? It has been reported that patients with depressive type schizoaffective disorder respond favorably to ECT, as patients with psychotic depression do (Lapensée, 1992). Perhaps the improvement noted in case reports results from a short-term response of affective symptoms whereas the chronic schizoaffective disorder itself remains unchanged.

ECT in the chronic phase of schizophrenia

As with acute schizophrenia, there is lack of consensus regarding the definition of chronic schizophrenia. In the early literature it generally referred to cases characterized by duration longer than five years, persistent positive and negative symptoms, and functional impairment despite adequate treatment. Modern studies approach the issue of chronicity from a different perspective, focusing on medication-resistant schizophrenia.

Five RCTs have examined the efficacy of ECT in chronic schizophrenia (Table 7.1). A controlled, nonblind study by Miller et al. (1953) compared unmodified ECT with nonconvulsive stimulation and sham ECT in patients with chronic catatonic schizophrenia. The sample size was small, and employment was the sole outcome measure. There were no significant differences among the three treatment methods.

Naidoo (1956) conducted a 12-week, double-blind trial comparing ECT, reserpine, and placebo in patients with chronic schizophrenia. ECT was administered weekly for six weeks and biweekly thereafter. Assessment was based on global clinical impression. Both ECT and reserpine proved superior to placebo, but reserpine was significantly better than ECT. Brill et al. (1959) compared unmodified ECT, modified ECT, and sham ECT administered three times a week for a total of 20 sessions in each group. No differences were observed among the groups.

Goswami et al. (2003) conducted the only modern RCT comparing ECT versus sham ECT in the treatment of treatment-resistant chronic schizophrenia patients. During the four-week trial, patients and controls received 8 to 12 ECT and sham ECT and equal doses of antipsychotics. At the endpoint, no significant difference in Brief Psychiatric Rating Scale (BPRS) scores was observed between patients and controls.

Chanpattana and his coworkers (2000) studied the efficacy of short-term ECT, continuation ECT, and MECT in patients with treatment-resistant schizophrenia. They investigated the effects of electrical stimulus dose on the speed of response and efficacy of ECT. Sixty-two schizophrenia patients received combination treatment with bitemporal ECT and flupenthixol, a very long-acting oral antipsychotic that strongly blocks dopamine. Using a randomized, double-blind design, the effects of three doses of the ECT stimulus were compared. The ECT stimulus doses were just above the seizure threshold, two times the threshold, and four times the threshold. The three groups were equivalent in number of patients who met criteria of remission, but remission was achieved more rapidly and with fewer ECT sessions in the two higher-dose groups. There was no difference in change of global cognitive status on the Mini-Mental State Examination (MMSE).

This same group reported several additional randomized open trials combining ECT with flupenthixol. The most robust study (Chanpattana and Chakrabhand, 2001) involved a large sample of 293 patients unresponsive to a mean of three trials of high-dose antipsychotics. One hundred sixty patients (54.6%) met response criteria. Responders were younger, had shorter duration of illness and current episode, more admissions, and less family history of schizophrenia. Duration of current illness, baseline Global Assessment of Functioning (GAF) scores, duration of illness, baseline MMSE scores, duration of previously failed antipsychotic drug trials, family history of schizophrenia, and paranoid type predicted the therapeutic outcome. Treatment resulted in marked improvement only in positive symptoms.

Several other open-label prospective and retrospective studies have examined the role of ECT–first generation antipsychotic drug combinations in drug-resistant schizophrenia. Because of the disparate ECT techniques used and the diversity of sampling methods, results of these studies do not lend themselves to meta-analysis. The conclusion drawn from 17 studies comprising 822 patients clearly favors the ECT-antipsychotic drug combination over ECT or antipsychotic drugs alone in the short-term treatment of schizophrenia (Braga and Petrides, 2005). No data are available regarding the long-term effects of combined treatment. Whereas all studies found the ECT–antipsychotic combination safe, its impact on short- and long-term cognitive performances remains uncertain.

A retrospective chart review by Nothdurfter et al. (2006) of 5,482 ECT sessions in 455 patients evaluated the effects of antipsychotic drugs on neurophysiological ECT parameters. Combining ECT with antipsychotic drugs did not increase the likelihood of ECT-related adverse effects. Postictal suppression was highest in treatments with second generation antipsychotics; the same group showed the lowest convulsive energy and convulsive concordance indices, but these indices are less meaningful. Effectiveness of combined treatment was also better with the ECT–second generation antipsychotic combinations.

The ECT–clozapine combination has been reported as safe and effective in more than 20 case reports as well as several retrospective and prospective open-label studies. In the review by Kupchik et al. (2000) of 36 treatment-resistant patients, 67% improved significantly on the ECT–clozapine combination. The 2006 review of the world literature by Havaki-Kontaxaki et al. (2006) identified 21 clozapine-resistant schizophrenia patients, 16 of whom showed marked short-term improvement with the ECT–clozapine combination. However, post-ECT improvement persisted beyond four months in only five patients.

The largest chart review studying the ECT–clozapine combination (Gazdag et al., 2006) involved 43 subjects and concluded that schizoaffective patients responded significantly better than catatonic or hebephrenic patients. Furthermore, this study demonstrated that ancillary augmentation strategies added to the ECT–clozapine combination conferred no benefit but increased the rate and severity of side effects.

The most thorough study to date on the efficacy of ECT combined with clozapine (Kho et al., 2004) followed 11 patients with schizophrenia who were nonresponsive to clozapine. If by the sixth ECT session there was insufficient response, placement was switched to bilateral. If the patient showed no response after six bilateral sessions, treatment was stopped. Of the nine completing patients, eight were considered responders. After initial response, five patients showed relapse; three of them had a second successful ECT course and remained well with MECT and clozapine. No significant adverse effect complicated the ECT–clozapine combination, with only two patients reporting transient memory problems.

Effect of catatonic features on response to ECT in chronic schizophrenia

Beyond the positive–negative symptom distinction, the response of other schizophrenia subtypes to ECT has rarely been explored (Chanpattana and Chakrabhand, 2001; Gazdag et al., 2006), and very few studies addressed the ECT response of catatonic symptoms in chronic schizophrenia.

In a series of studies involving the same cohort of patients, Suzuki et al. investigated the efficacy of ECT in nonacute, antipsychotic-resistant middle-aged and elderly patients with catatonic schizophrenia. Eleven patients were enrolled in the short-term study of acute ECT and received ECT sessions three times weekly in combination with antipsychotic drugs (Suzuki et al., 2003). All 11 patients completed this phase of the study, and the acute ECT response rate (measured on BPRS and GAF) was 100%. All 11 patients also completed the long-term study in which they were evaluated weekly for one year or until relapse. Seven patients relapsed, all within the first three months (Suzuki et al., 2004). These seven patients underwent a second course of ECT followed by continuation ECT-MECT for one year, and four patients remained in remission (Suzuki et al., 2005). Meanwhile, those three who again relapsed were treated successfully with more frequent continuation ECT and subsequent MECT (Suzuki et al., 2006a). The authors report that no patient experienced severe adverse effects from continuation ECT or MECT, but cognitive assessments were not performed. Small sample size and failure to use a standardized rating instrument to assess catatonia are additional limitations of these studies.

Continuation ECT and MECT

Chanpattana et al. systematically studied the efficacy of continuation ECT and MECT in the treatment of drug-resistant schizophrenia. One hundred fourteen patients received acute treatment with bilateral ECT and flupenthixol. Fifty-eight met remitter criteria, including clinical stability during a three-week stabilization period, and were eligible for the continuation treatment study of six-month duration. Fifty-one of these enrolled in the continuation trial and were randomized to one of three treatment groups: continuation flupenthixol alone, continuation ECT alone, or combined continuation ECT–flupenthixol. Forty-five patients finished the continuation phase of the study, and six dropped out. Among completers, 6 of 15 (40%) patients relapsed in the combined ECT–flupenthixol group. In the groups treated with ECT alone and flupenthixol alone, the relapse rate was 93%. An extension of this study (Chanpattana, 2000) followed 21 patients receiving the ECT–flupenthixol combination for one year. No patient experienced a relapse, and there were marked improvements in BPRS and GAF scores. No significant adverse effects were reported. These findings were further replicated in 46 additional patients (Chanpattana and Kramer, 2003). Robust decreases on the BPRS total and positive symptom scores were achieved during the acute phase and maintained for the one-year duration of the study. A limitation of these studies is the absence of a thorough cognitive assessment.

ECT in catatonia associated with depression

Catatonic signs occur in 13%–31% of patients with mood disorders (Caroff et al., 2004), and their presence is an important predictor of good clinical response to ECT (Fink, 1979). Several earlier studies (Habson, 1953; Mendels, 1967; Weckowicz et al., 1971) concluded that psychomotor retardation is an independent predictor of favorable response to ECT. Subsequent studies of ECT in depression (Dombrovski et al., 2005; Husain et al., 2004; Petrides et al., 2001) have either failed to address the role of psychomotor dysfunction, or yielded inconsistent results. Maletzky (2004) reported the results of first line ECT treatment in 13 depressive patients whose clinical presentation was characterized by catatonic signs. After five to seven bilateral treatments all patients showed marked improvement. Finally, there is a unique follow-up study (Swartz et al., 2001) that reviewed the case histories of 19 patients with major depression and catatonic signs who were followed up for 3 to 7 years. All patients responded to ECT with left anterior right temporal electrode placement (described in Chapter 27).

ECT in catatonia associated with mania

The antimanic properties of ECT proved to be equal or superior compared with pharmacotherapy (APA, 2001; Rudorfer et al., 2003). Catatonic signs are also frequently associated with mania (Caroff et al., 2004). Catatonic mania states were found responsive to ECT in 56% to 100% of cases (Mukherjee et al., 1994). ECT can be life-saving in cases of mania complicated by exhaustion, inanition, or extreme catatonic excitement. In a comprehensive early review (Morrison, 1973), 67 patients who presented with severe agitation had a significantly higher chance to receive ECT than "retarded" patients and had a better outcome. Abrams and Taylor (1976) reported 62% prevalence rate of mania among patients with catatonia; 67% of these patients responded well to ECT. Unfortunately, later ECT studies involving manic patients (Mukherjee et al., 1988; Sikdar et al., 1994; Small et al., 1988) failed to evaluate catatonic signs or psychomotor function in the assessment of treatment response.

ECT in catatonia associated with medical conditions ("organic" catatonia)

Catatonia due to general medical conditions (organic catatonia) as a diagnostic category first appeared in the DSM-IV (APA, 1994). It oftentimes goes undetected. This probably explains why only single case reports have been published about its treatment with ECT. As catatonic symptoms are usually associated with grave medical conditions, clinicians inexperienced with ECT are reluctant to administer it. Yet, anecdotal evidence suggests that ECT is a safe and effective treatment in organic catatonia, although treatment failures are also reported. Swartz et al. (2003) described four patients with a variety of neurological impairments who showed only transient and partial improvement to ECT as well as to benzodiazepines. There have been a few other case reports with similar conclusions (e.g., Kaestner et al., 2007; Malur et al., 2001). Organic catatonia may be less responsive to therapeutic interventions because of the advanced pathological changes of the central nervous system, or these states might require particularly intensive treatment (Swartz et al., 2003).

Catatonia is a well-known concomitant of medical and infectious diseases and toxic conditions. Successful ECT of the associated catatonic syndrome was reported in a patient with encephalitis lethargica (Dekleva and Husain, 1995), in 12 patients suffering from typhoid fever (Breakey and Kala, 1977), in a patient suffering from toxic epidermal necrolysis (Weller et al., 1992), in a case of ziconotide-induced delirium with associated pneumonia and respiratory failure (Levin et al., 2002), in two cases of lysergic acid diethylamide (LSD)-induced stupor (Kessing et al., 1994; Perera et al., 1995), and in a patient with severe depression complicated by cardiac and respiratory insufficiency (Geretsegger and Rochowanski, 1987).

Several neurological diseases that present with symptoms that are clinically indistinguishable from catatonia are also responsive to ECT. Partial (Malur et al., 2001) or good (Ditmore et al., 1992; Fricchione et al., 1990) clinical response to treatment was reported in patients with neurological complications of lupus erythematosus. ECT proved useful in alleviating catatonic syndromes following a cerebrovascular insult (Spear et al., 1997) or associated with dementia (Perry, 1983), hereditary cerebellar ataxia (Folkerts et al., 1998), Parkinson's disease (Suzuki et al., 2006b), epilepsy (Suzuki et al., 2006c), hereditary spinocerebellar degeneration (Suzuki et al., 2006d), or testicular cancer–induced paraneoplastic encephalitis (Kaestner et al., 2007). Organic catatonia showed only limited (Mattingly et al., 1992) improvement in cases of multiple sclerosis, and no effect in a case of kernicterus-induced learning disability (Brasic et al., 2000).

ECT in childhood and adolescent psychoses associated with catatonia

The role of ECT in children and adolescents has been controversial since Hemphill and Walter (1941) first detailed its use in a 3-year-old child with epilepsy. That report was followed by a case series including patients with a variety of conditions (Heuyer et al., 1943) treated with this new procedure. Since the introduction of antipsychotic and antidepressant drugs, ECT has been administered infrequently in this age group. Nevertheless, available information suggests that it is well tolerated, effective, and not associated with long-term cognitive impairment (Cohen et al., 1999; Rey and Walter, 1997).

The data on the efficacy of ECT in the nonaffective psychoses of childhood and adolescence remain limited to reports of single cases, series of patients, and literature reviews. There have been no controlled trials of ECT for psychosis in this age group. Apparently differing from that in adults, catatonia in children seems most frequently associated with schizophrenia (Bloch et al., 2001; Cohen et al., 2005).

In their systematic overview, Rey and Walter (1997) summarized the results of ECT administered to patients younger than 18 years for whom adequate information about diagnosis and outcome could be identified. Of the 154 patients, 24 were diagnosed with catatonia; ECT induced remission or marked improvement in 18 (75%). This response was surpassed only by patients with mania (80%). ECT was effective in 42% of schizophrenia patients, 50% of schizoaffective disorder patients, and 43% of patients with psychotic depression. At a six-month follow-up, 10% of the schizophrenia patients, 46% of the catatonia patients, and all remitted mania patients were functioning satisfactorily.

A more recent article by Cohen et al. (1999) reviewed 38 patients with childhood or adolescent catatonia reported between 1977 and 1997, in addition to nine consecutive cases seen at the authors' own institution. ECT was effective in 21 of 25 cases of catatonia due to mood disorders and schizophrenia.

Another brief review reported the treatment of 29 children and adolescents with DSM-IV catatonia due to a variety of psychiatric and medical conditions. Of the seven cases receiving ECT, only one did not improve significantly within days (Dhossche and Bouman, 1997).

Two retrospective chart reviews compared the ECT response between child/adolescent and adult patients. Bloch et al. (2001) analyzed the charts of 24 adolescent and 33 adult patients; 19 of the 24 adolescents were diagnosed with schizophrenia, 4 having catatonic features. The majority of adults suffered from affective psychoses. The number of ECT sessions and the stimulus intensity did not differ significantly between the two groups. Fifty-eight percent of both groups achieved symptomatic remission from the index episode. However, at one year the rehospitalization rate was 33% for adolescents and only 10% for adults. No major adverse effects of ECT were reported. A study by Stein et al. (2004) compared 36 adolescent with 57 adult patients. The rates of improvement and rehospitalization at one year were 61% and 53% for the adolescent and 83% and 49% for the adult patients. The main indications for ECT in adolescents were catatonia and high suicidal risk irrespective of the nosological status.

In their review of the literature, Lahutte et al. (2008) reported on 38 children and adolescents who presented with catatonia occurring in the context of a severe medical condition that included intoxication ($n = 12$), infection and neurological diseases ($n = 10$), and genetic conditions ($n = 6$). ECT was the treatment of choice in 11 cases and resulted in substantial, albeit transient, remission of catatonia in more than 80% of the cases.

It is important to emphasize again that there is no international consensus regarding the use of ECT in this age group. The role of ECT in childhood and adolescent psychoses remains poorly defined, as is the legal status of ECT in this age group. When administering ECT with children and adolescents, attention must be paid to their lower seizure threshold necessitating low initial stimulus dose during an ECT course (APA, 2001; see Chapter 32).

References

Abraham, K. R. and Kulhara, P. 1987. The efficacy of electroconvulsive therapy in the treatment of schizophrenia. A comparative study. Br J Psychiatry 151: 152–7.

Abrams, R. and Taylor, M. A. 1976. Catatonia: A prospective clinical study. Arch Gen Psychiatry 33: 579–81.

Agarwal, A. and Vinny, G. C. 1985. Role of ECT-phenothiazines combination in schizophrenia. Indian J Psychiatry 27: 233–6.

American Psychiatric Association (APA). 1994. Diagnostic and statistical manual of mental disorders, 4th edn. Washington, DC: American Psychiatric Press.

American Psychiatric Association (APA). 2001. The practice of ECT: Recommendations for treatment, training and privileging. Washington, DC: American Psychiatric Press.

Arnold, O. H. and Stepan, H. 1952. Untersuchungen zur Frage der akuten todlicken Katatonie. Wien Z Nervenheilkd Grenzgeb 4: 235–58.

Bagadia, V. N., Abhyankar, R. R., Doshi, J., et al. 1983. A double blind controlled study of ECT vs. chlorpromazine in schizophrenia. J Assoc Phys of India 31: 637–40.

Bloch, Y., Levcovitch, Y., Bloch, A. M., et al. 2001. Electroconvulsive therapy in adolescents: Similarities to and differences from adults. J Am Acad Child Adolesc Psychiatry 40: 1332–6.

Boyarsky, B. K., Fuller, M., and Early, T. 1999. Malignant catatonia-induced respiratory failure with response to ECT. J ECT 15: 232–6.

Braga, R. J. and Petrides, G. 2005. The combined use of electroconvulsive therapy and antipsychotics in patients with schizophrenia. J ECT 21: 75–83.

Brandon, S., Cowley, P., McDonald, C., et al. 1985. Leicester ECT trial: Results in schizophrenia. Br J Psychiatry 146: 177–83.

Brasic, J. R., Zagzag, D., Kowalik, S., et al. 2000. Clinical manifestations of progressive catatonia. German J Psychiatry 3: 13–24.

Breakey, W. R. and Kala, A. K. 1977. Typhoid catatonia responsive to ECT. BMJ 2: 357–9.

Brill, N. Q., Crumpton, E., Eiduson, S., et al. 1959. Predictive and concomitant variables related to improvement with actual and simulated ECT. Arch Gen Psychiatry 1: 263–72.

Caroff, S. N., Mann, S. C., Campbell, E. C., and Sullivan, K. A. 2004. Epidemiology. In Catatonia: From psychopathology to neurobiology (eds. Caroff, S. N., Mann, S. C., Francis, A., and Fricchione, G. L.). Washington, DC: American Psychiatric Press, pp. 15–31.

Caroff, S. N. and Ungvari, G. S. 2007. Expanding horizons in catatonia research. Psychiatr Ann 37: 7–9.

Caroff, S. N., Ungvari, G. S., Bhati, M. T., et al. 2007. Catatonia and prediction of response to electroconvulsive therapy. Psychiatr Ann 37: 57–64.

Cerletti, U. and Bini, L. 1938. Un nuevo metodo di shockterapie "l'elettro-shock." Bollettino Accademia Medica Roma 64: 136–8.

Chanpattana, W. 2000. Maintenance ECT in treatment-resistant schizophrenia. J Med Assoc Thai 83: 657–62.

Chanpattana, W., Chakrabhand, M. L., Buppanharun, W., and Sackeim, H. A. 2000. Effects of stimulus intensity on the efficacy of bilateral ECT in schizophrenia: a preliminary study. Biol Psychiatry 48: 222–8.

Chanpattana, W. and Chakrabhand, M. L. S. 2001. Combined ECT and neuroleptic therapy in treatment-refractory schizophrenia: Prediction of outcome. Psychiatry Res 105: 107–15.

Chanpattana, W. and Kramer, B. A. 2003. Acute and maintenance ECT with flupenthixol in refractory schizophrenia: Sustained improvements in psychopathology, quality of life, and social outcomes. Schizophr Res 63: 189–93.

Cohen, D., Flament, M., Dubos, P.-F., and Basquin, M. 1999. Case series: Catatonic syndrome in young people. J Am Acad Child Adolesc Psychiatry 38: 1040–6.

Cohen, D., Nicolas, J. D., Flament, M., et al. 2005. Clinical relevance of chronic catatonic schizophrenia in children and adolescents: Evidence from a prospective naturalistic study. Schizophr Res 76: 301–8.

Dekleva, K. B. and Husain, M. M. 1995. Sporadic encephalitis lethargica: A case treated successfully with ECT. J Neuropsychiatry Clin Neurosci 7: 237–9.

Dhossche, D. M. and Bouman, N. H. 1997. Catatonia in an adolescent with Prader-Willi syndrome. Ann Clin Psychiatry 9: 247–53.

Ditmore, B. G., Malek-Ahmadi, P., Mills, D. M., and Wediger, R. L. 1992. Manic psychosis and catatonia stemming from systemic lupus erythematosus: Response to ECT. Convuls Ther 8: 33–7.

Dodwell, D. and Goldberg, D. 1989. A study of factors associated with response to electroconvulsive therapy in patients with schizophrenic symptoms. Br J Psychiatry 154: 635–9.

Dombrovski, A. Y., Mulsant, B. H., Haskett, R. P., et al. 2005. Predictors of remission after electroconvulsive therapy in unipolar major depression. J Clin Psychiatry 66: 1043–9.

Escobar, R., Rios, A., Montoya, I. D., et al. 2000. Clinical and cerebral blood flow changes in catatonic patients treated with ECT. J Psychosom Res 49: 423–9.

Fink, M. 1979. Convulsive therapy: Theory and practice. Raven Press New York.

Fink, M. 1990. Is catatonia a primary indication for ECT? J ECT 6: 1–4.

Fink, M. and Sackeim, H. A. 1996. Convulsive therapy in schizophrenia? Schizophr Bull 22: 27–39.

Finkbeiner, T. EKT-behandlung katatoner Psychosen: Indikation und Praktische durchfuhrung. 1995. In Differnzierung katatoner und neuroleptika-induzierter Bewegungsstorungen (ed. Braunig, P.). Stuttgart/New York: Thieme, pp. 98–104.

Folkerts, H. W., Stadtland, C., and Reker, T. 1998. ECT for organic catatonia due to hereditary cerebellar ataxia. J ECT 14: 53–5.

Fricchione, G. L., Kaufman, L. D., Gruber, B. L., and Fink, M. 1990. Electroconvulsive therapy and cyclophosphamide in combination for severe neuropsychiatric lupus with catatonia. Am J Med 88: 442–3.

Gabris, G. and Muller, C. 1983. La catatonie dite "pernicieuse." Encephale 9: 365–85.

Gazdag, G., Kocsis, N., and Lipcsey, A. 2004. Rates of electroconvulsive therapy use in Hungary in 2002. J ECT 20: 42–4.

Gazdag, G., Kocsis-Ficzere, N., and Tolna, J. 2006. The augmentation of clozapine treatment with electroconvulsive therapy. Ideggyogy Sz 59: 261–7.

Gelenberg, A. J. 1976. The catatonic syndrome. Lancet 1: 1339–41.

Geretsegger, C. and Rochowanski, E. 1987. Electroconvulsive therapy in acute life-threatening catatonia associated with cardiac and respiratory decompensation. Convuls Ther 3: 291–5.

Girish, K. and Gill, N. S. 2003. Electroconvulsive therapy in lorazepam non-responsive catatonia. Indian Journal of Psychiatry 45: 21–5.

Goswami, U., Kumar, U., and Singh, B. 2003. Efficacy of electroconvulsive therapy in treatment-resistant schizophrenia: A double blind study. Indian J Psychiatry 45: 26–9.

Habson, B. 1953. Prognostic factors in electric convulsive therapy. J Neurol Neurosurg Psychiatry 16: 275–81.

Hafner, H. and Kasper, S. 1982. Akute lebensbedrohilche Katatonie: Epidemiologische und klinische Befunde. Nervenzart 53: 385–94.

Hatta, K., Miyakawa, K., Ota, T., et al. 2007. Maximal response to electroconvulsive therapy for the treatment of catatonic symptoms. J ECT 23: 233–5.

Havaki-Kontaxaki, B, J., Ferentinos, P. P., Kontaxikis, V. P., et al. 2006. Concurrent administration of clozapine and electroconvulsive therapy in clozapine-resistant schizophrenia. Clin Neuropharmacol 29: 52–6.

Hemphill, R. E. and Walter, W. G. 1941. The treatment of mental disorders by electrically induced convulsions. J Ment Sci 87: 256–75.

Heuyer, G., Bour, K. and Leroy, R. 1943. L' électrochoc chez les enfants. Ann Med Psychol (Paris) 2: 402–7.

Husain, M. M., Rush, A. J., Fink, M. et al. 2004. Speed of response and remission in major depressive disorder with acute electroconvulsive therapy (ECT): A consortium for research in ECT (CORE) report. J Clin Psychiatry 65: 485–91.

Kaestner, F., Mostert, C., Behnken, A., et al. 2007. Therapeutic strategies for catatonia in paraneoplastic encephalitis. World J Biol Psychiatry 12: 1–5 (Epub ahead of print).

Kahlbaum, K. L. 1874. Die Katatonie oder das Spannungsirresein. Eine klinische Form psychischer Krankheit. Berlin: Hischwald.

Kalinowsky, L. B. and Worthing H. J. 1943. Results with electric convulsive treatment in 200 cases of schizophrenia. Psychiatr Q 17: 144–53.

Kelly, D. H. W. and Sargant, W. 1965. Present treatment of schizophrenia – a controlled follow-up study. BMJ 1: 147–50.

Kessing, L., LaBianca, J. H., and Bolwig, T. 1994. HIV-induced stupor treated with ECT. Convuls Ther 10: 232–5.

Kho, K. H., Blansjaar, B. A., De Vries, S., et al. 2004. Electroconvulsive therapy for the treatment of clozapine nonresponders suffering from schizophrenia – an open label study. Eur Arch Psychiatry Clin Neurosci 254: 372–9.

Kraepelin, E. 1919. Dementia praecox and paraphrenia. Translated by Barclay, R. M. Edinburgh: Livingstone.

Kupchik, M., Spivak, B., Mester, R., et al. 2000. Combined electroconvulsive-clozapine therapy. Clin Neuropharmacol 23: 14–16.

Lahutte, B., Cornic, F., Bonnot, O., et al. 2008. Multidisciplinary approach of organic catatonia in children and adolescents may improve treatment decision making. Prog Neuropsychopharm Biol Psychiatry 32: 1393–8.

Lapensée, M. A. 1992. A review of schizoaffective disorder: II. Somatic treatment. Can J Psychiatry 37: 347–9.

Levin, T., Petrides, G., Weiner, J., et al. 2002. Intractable delirium associated with ziconotide successfully treated by electroconvulsive therapy. Psychosomatics 43: 63–6.

Lieberman, J. A. 2007. Effectiveness of antipsychotic drugs in chronic schizophrenia; efficacy, safety and cost outcomes of CATIE and other trials. J Clin Psychiatry 68: e04.

Maletzky, B. M. 2004. The first-line use of electroconvulsive therapy in major affective disorders. J ECT 20: 112–17.

Malur, C., Pasol, E., and Francis, A. 2001. ECT for prolonged catatonia. J ECT 17: 55–9.

Mann, S. C., Caroff, S. N., Bleier, H. R., et al. 1986. Lethal catatonia. Am J Psychiatry 143: 1374–81.

Mann, S. C., Caroff, S. N., Bleier, H. R., et al. 1990. Electroconvulsive therapy of the lethal catatonia syndrome: case report and review. Convuls Ther 6: 239–47.

Mann, S. C., Caroff, S. N., Keck, P. E. Jr., et al. 2003. The neuroleptic malignant syndrome and related conditions, 2nd edn. Washington, DC: American Psychiatric Publishing.

Mann, S. C., Caroff, S. N., Fricchione, G., et al. 2004. Malignant catatonia. In Catatonia: From psychopathology to neurobiology (eds. Caroff, S. N., Mann, S. C., Francis, A., and Fricchione, G.). Washington, DC: American Psychiatric Publishing, pp. 105–19.

Mattingly, G., Baker, K., Zorumski, C. F., and Figiel, G. S. 1992. Multiple sclerosis and ECT: Possible value of gadolinium-enhanced magnetic resonance scans for identifying high-risk patients. J Neuropsychiatry Clin Neurosci 4: 145–51.

May, P. R., Tuma, A. H., and Dixon, W. J. 1981. Schizophrenia. A follow-up study of the results of five forms of treatment. Arch Gen Psychiatry 38: 776–84.

Meduna, L. and Friedman, G. 1939. The convulsive-irritative therapy of the psychoses. Survey of more than 3,000 cases. JAMA 112: 501–9.

Mendels, J. 1967. The prediction of response to electroconvulsive therapy. Am J Psychiatry 124: 153–9.

Miller, D. H., Clancy, J., and Cumming, E. 1953. A comparison between unidirectional current nonconvulsive electrical stimulation given with Reiters machine, standard alternating current electroshock (Cerletti method), and penthotal in chronic schizophrenia. Am J Psychiatry 109: 617–20.

Morrison, J. R. 1973. Catatonia: retarded and excited types. Arch Gen Psychiatry 28: 39–41.

Morrison, J. R. 1974. Catatonia: Prediction of outcome. Compr Psychiatry 15: 317–24.

Mukherjee, S., Sackeim, H. A., and Lee, C. 1988. Unilateral ECT in the treatment of manic episodes. Convuls Ther 4: 74–80.

Mukherjee, S., Sackeim, H. A., and Schnur, D. B. 1994. Electroconvulsive therapy of acute mania episodes: A review of 50 years experience. Am J Psychiatry 151: 169–76.

Muller, G. 1930. Anfalle bei schizophrenen Erkrankungen. Allg Z Psychiatr 83: 235–40.

Naidoo, N. 1956. The effects of reserpine (Serpasil) on the chronic disturbed schizophrenic: A comparative study of rauwolfia alkaloids and electroconvulsive therapy. J Nerv Ment Dis 123: 1–13.

Nothdurfter, C., Eser, D., Schule, C. et al. 2006. The influence of concomitant neuroleptic medication on safety, tolerability and clinical effectiveness of electroconvulsive therapy. World J Biol Psychiatry 7: 162–70.

Painuly, N. and Chakrabarti, S. 2006. Combined use of electroconvulsive therapy and antipsychotics in schizophrenia: The Indian evidence. A review and a meta-analysis. J ECT 22: 59–66.

Perera, K. M., Ferraro, A., and Pinto, M. R. 1995. Catatonia LSD-induced? Aust NZ J Psychiatry 29: 324–7.

Perry, G. F. 1983. ECT for dementia and catatonia. J Clin Psychiatry 44: 117.

Petrides, G., Divadeenam, K., Bush, G., and Francis, A. 1997. Synergism of lorazepam and electroconvulsive therapy in the treatment of catatonia. Biol Psychiatry 42: 375–81.

Petrides, G., Fink, M., Husain, M. M., et al. 2001. ECT remission rates in psychotic versus non-psychotic depressed patients: a report from CORE. J ECT 17: 244–53.

Philbrick, K. and Rummans, T. A. 1994. Malignant catatonia. J Neuropsychiatry Clin Neurosci 6: 1–13.

Rey, J. M. and Walter, G. 1997. Half a century of ECT use in young people. Am J Psychiatry 154: 595–602.

Ries, R. K., Wilson, L., Bokan, J. A., and Chiles, J. A. 1981. ECT in medication resistant schizoaffective disorder. Compr Psychiatry 22: 167–73.

Rohland, B. M., Carroll, B. T., and Jacoby, R. G. 1993. ECT in the treatment of the catatonic syndrome. J Affective Disorders 29: 255–61.

Rudorfer, M. V., Henry, M. E., and Sackeim, H. A. 2003. Electroconvulsive therapy in psychiatry, 2nd edn. (eds. Tasman A., Kay J., and Leiberman J.). New York: Wiley.

Sarita, E. P., Janakiramaiah, N., Gangadhar, B. N., et al. 1998. Efficacy of combined ECT after two weeks of neuroleptics in schizophrenia: A double-blind controlled study. NIMHANS J 16: 243–51.

Sarkar, P., Andrade, C., Kapur B., et al. 1994. An exploratory evaluation of ECT in haloperidol-treated DSM-IIIR schizophreniform disorder. Convuls Ther 10: 271–8.

Scott, A. I. F. (ed). 2005. The ECT handbook, 2nd edn. London: Royal College of Psychiatrists (RCP).

Sedivec, V. 1981. Psychoses endangering life (in Czech). Cesk Psychiatr 77: 38–41.

Sikdar, S., Kulhara, P., Avasthi, A. and Singh, H. 1994. Combined chlorpromazine and electroconvulsive therapy in mania. Br J Psychiatry 164: 806–10.

Small, J. G., Klapper, M. H., Kellams, J. J. et al. 1988. Electroconvulsive treatment compared with lithium in the management of manic states. Arch Gen Psychiatry 45: 727–57.

Spear, J., Ranger, M., and Herzberg J. 1997. The treatment of stupor associated with MRI evidence of cerebrovascular disease. Int J Geriatr Psychiatry 12: 791–4.

Stauder, K. H. 1934. Die todliche Katatonie. Arch Psychiatr Nervenkr 102: 614–34.

Stein, D., Kurtsman, L., Stier, S., et al. 2004. Electroconvulsive therapy in adolescent and adult psychiatric inpatients – a retrospective chart design. J Affect Disord 82: 335–42.

Suzuki, K., Awata, S., and Matsuoka, H. 2003. Short-term effect of ECT in middle-aged and elderly patients with intractable catatonic schizophrenia. J ECT 19: 73–80.

Suzuki, K., Awata, S., and Matsuoka, H. 2004. One-year outcome after response to ECT in middle aged and elderly patients with intractable catatonic schizophrenia. J ECT 20: 99–106.

Suzuki, K., Awata, S., Takano, T., et al. 2005. Continuation electroconvulsive therapy for relapse prevention in middle-aged and elderly patients with intractable catatonic schizophrenia. Psychiatry Clin Neurosci 59: 481–9.

Suzuki, K., Awata, S., Takano, T., et al. 2006a. Adjusting the frequency of continuation and maintenance electroconvulsive therapy to prevent relapse of catatonic schizophrenia in middle-aged and elderly patients who are relapse-prone. Psychiatry Clin Neurosci 60: 486–92.

Suzuki, K., Awata, S., Nakagawa, K., et al. 2006b. Catatonic stupor during the course of Parkinson's disease resolved with electroconvulsive therapy. Mov Disord 21: 123–4.

Suzuki, K., Miura, N., Awata, S., et al. 2006c. Epileptic seizures superimposed on catatonic stupor. Epilepsia 47: 793–98.

Suzuki, K., Itou, K., Takana, T., et al. 2006d. Catatonic stupor superimposed on hereditary spinocerebellar degeneration resolved with electroconvulsive therapy. Prog Neuropsychopharmacol Biol Psychiatry 30: 1179–81.

Suzuki, K., Awata, S., Takano, T., et al. 2006e. Improvement of psychiatric symptoms after electroconvulsive therapy in young adults with intractable first-episode schizophrenia and schizophreniform disorder. Tohoku J Exp Med 210: 213–20.

Swartz, C. M., Morrow, V., Surles, L. and James, J. F. 2001. Long-term outcome after ECT for catatonic depression. J ECT 17: 180–3.

Swartz, C. M., Acosta, D., and Bashir, A. 2003. Diminished ECT response in catatonia due to chronic neurological conditions. J ECT 19: 110–14.

Swoboda, E., Conca, A., König, P., et al. 2001. Maintenance electroconvulsive therapy in affective and schizoaffective disorder. Neuropsychobiology 43: 23–8.

Taylor, P. and Fleminger, J. J. 1980. ECT for schizophrenia. Lancet 1: 1380–3.

Tharyan, P. and Adams, C. E. 2005. Electroconvulsive therapy for schizophrenia. Cochrane Database of Systematic Reviews. Issue 2. Art. No: CD 000076.

Tolsma, F. J. 1967. The syndrome of acute pernicious psychosis. Psychiatr Neurol Neurochir 70: 1–21.

Üçok, A. and Cakir, S. 2006. Electroconvulsive therapy in first-episode schizophrenia. J ECT 22: 38–42.

Ukpong, D. I., Makanjuola, R. O., and Morakinyo, O. 2002. A controlled trial of modified electroconvulsive therapy in schizophrenia in a Nigerian teaching hospital. West Afr J Med 21: 237–40.

van der Heijden, F. M., Tuinier, S., Arts, N. J., et al. 2005. Catatonia: Disappeared or under-diagnosed? Psychopathology 38: 3–8.

Vollmer-Larsen, A., Jacobsen, T. B., Hemmingsenn, R., and Parnas, J. 2006. Schizoaffective disorder – the reliability of its clinical diagnostic use. Acta Psychiatr Scand 113: 402–7.

Waller, K., Borik, A., and Choi, C. 2000. Breast cancer, bipolar disorder, catatonia, and life-preserving electroconvulsive therapy. Psychosomatics 41: 442–5.

Weckowicz, T. E., Yonge, K. A., Crapley, A. J., Muir W. 1971. Objective therapy predictors in depression: A multivariate approach. J Clin Psychopathology. 27: 4–29.

Weller, M., Kornhuber, J., and Beckmann, H. 1992. Electroconvulsive therapy in the treatment of toxic epidermal necrolysis [Lyell syndrome]. Nervenarzt 63: 308–10.

Wells, D. A. 1973. Electroconvulsive treatment for schizophrenia. A ten-year survey in a university hospital psychiatric department. Compr Psychiatry 14: 291–8.

World Health Organization (WHO). 1992. The ICD-10 classification of mental and behavioural disorders. Geneva: WHO.

8

Hormonal effects of electroconvulsive therapy

Conrad M. Swartz

Introduction

Electroconvulsive therapy (ECT)-induced changes in hormone levels have promise in illuminating the pathophysiology of depression, the therapeutic mechanism of ECT, and the causes of ECT side effects because these changes reflect seizure-driven neurochemical changes in the brain. However, because they are mediated by the pituitary, these reflections are indirect.

Still, hormonal changes or abnormalities might correspond to psychiatric diagnoses, selection of patients for ECT, or severity of illness. Less ambitiously, hormonal measurements might reflect therapeutic benefits of ECT and then serve as a proxy for them, or for side effects. The value of a proxy is indicating progress in therapy, such as when sufficient ECT sessions have been given, when the interval between maintenance treatments is sufficiently short, or when relapse is impending. Still more humbly, hormone changes might correlate with treatment intensity and reflect the quality of the ECT method, such as the therapeutic impact of the combination of electrode placement and stimulus dose.

Only a small amount of this promise has been fulfilled, even within the least ambitious last group of expectations. The literature describing ECT hormonal effects includes a few useful and potentially useful findings, much redundant verification, and many reports in which artifacts and typical large interpatient variations overwhelm trends and obscure results. This chapter reviews useful findings and how artifacts can be reduced.

ECT is not known to have lasting effects on hormone levels or function except by correcting minor abnormalities in corticosteroid regulation that occur during psychiatric episodes. Then again, ECT is not known to cause persisting effects of any kind except for quelling illness episodes, analogous to terminating an infection by antibiotic therapy. The hormonal effects of ECT last variously for minutes to weeks.

Presented first are close relationships between ECT-induced hormone release and physiology. These relationships are the consequences of ECT-induced hormone release. Then I present how ECT-induced hormone release can reflect ECT treatment intensity and psychiatric illness severity. This review is introduced by a discussion of methods of measuring and interpreting hormone release. These methods are not difficult but have many different steps and aspects, analogous to an income tax return.

Consequences of ECT-induced hormone release

Postictal excitement and uterine contractions are distinct medical consequences of ECT-induced hormone release. Although they concern a small percentage of patients, they are important in managing these patients.

About 5% of ECT patients experience postictal excitement, also called emergence agitation. The vast majority of patients recover calmly and quietly after the ECT treatment. Patients with postictal excitement typically start showing agitation even before they awaken, with utterances and undirected movements of arms or legs. On awakening, they are usually not oriented to circumstances and they need to lie down while the effects of anesthesia wear off. They move agitatedly, speak loudly or yell, and make restless demands to stand or walk. Their discomfort and agitation resist verbal guidance. Many strike out physically at the staff. Despite their enthusiastic protestations, these patients cannot stand or walk stably and are very likely to fall if they try. When they become oriented, agitation usually decreases or disappears, but these patients feel akathisia and show restlessness for several hours. The unpleasant experience of these symptoms leads some patients to avoid further ECT.

Postictal excitement can be calmed with benzodiazepines but it can also be prevented without tranquilization. The prevention method was deduced from reports of greater elevations of epinephrine and norepinephrine accompanying ECT without anesthesia than with it (Griswold, 1958; Pina-Cabral and Rodrigues, 1974) and from vigorous lactate elevations accompanying unanesthetized ECT (Vigas et al., 1975). Postictal agitation might be the same phenomenon as lactate-induced panic and carbon dioxide-induced panic (Pitts and McClure, 1967). Lactate and carbon dioxide are generated by muscle metabolism, presumably more so with unanesthetized ECT, and it was expected that higher doses of succinylcholine should decrease lactate and carbon dioxide further. A trial showed that higher succinylcholine doses, 1.1 mg/kg, prevented postictal excitement when lower doses, typically 0.7 mg/kg, did not (Swartz, 1990). Because succinylcholine does not cross the blood–brain barrier it demonstrated the mechanism. Confirmatory evidence was provided by serum lactate measurements, which increased by 175% in patients with postictal excitement but by only 50% in patients without it (Auriacombe et al., 2000). Some patients require more than the ordinary maximum dose of 1.1 mg/kg succinylcholine. They can be clinically managed by administering a (second) dose of methohexital immediately after the motor seizure (Swartz, 1993). Apparently this methohexital dose lessens their sensitivity to lactate and carbon dioxide, but any delay in administration diminishes its effect.

Late-stage pregnant females who undergo ECT can experience uterine contractions or abruptio placenta shortly after the seizure (Walker and Swartz, 1994). This is probably a direct result of the oxytocin released by ECT seizure; it is not a contraindication, but preventive steps can be taken.

Comparing hormone changes

Unfortunately, hormones released from the brain (e.g., the hypothalamus) are too dilute for reliable assay in the bloodstream. Attempts to study them (e.g., Widerlov et al., 1989) have not been productive. Hormone release from the pituitary produces much higher hormone concentrations in the bloodstream.

A universal problem with measurements of hormones (indeed any physiology) in psychiatric patients is that these measurements vary enormously in ways unrelated to psychiatric conditions. These patient-to-patient variations in hormone concentrations are typically vastly larger than hormone changes attributable to neuropsychiatric effects. So, to observe neuropsychiatric effects on hormone levels, the study method must somehow remove these artifactual patient-to-patient variations or compensate for them. Compensation by the statistical techniques of linear regression (such as analysis of variance or covariance) is usually inadequate because of the nonlinear nature and enormous size of these variations. These variations are so large that deviations from linearity exceed the sought-after effects, and ranges of normal values for ECT-induced hormone elevations have never been identified.

To illustrate, consider an ordinary report describing serum prolactin levels 20 min after the ECT seizure in three groups of patients (Robin and De Tissera, 1982). Usually ECT induces a large increase in serum prolactin levels, in the range of 3 to 20 times the resting baseline level. Twenty minutes happens to be the optimal sampling time for serum prolactin. Nevertheless, the prolactin results were chaotic and unrelated to the clinical results. Clinically, patients receiving low-energy pulse stimuli improved less with each treatment and required more treatments than did patients receiving other stimuli. However, their post-ECT serum prolactin was not lower than that of the other two groups. It averaged 1,821 (standard deviation [SD] 1,306) mU/L. Patients receiving medium-energy pulse stimuli improved faster, and their average prolactin level was 1,514 (SD 1,079) mU/L. Patients receiving high-energy sine wave stimuli improved at the same rate as those receiving medium-energy pulse stimuli, and their average serum prolactin was 1,664 (SD 618) mU/L. It makes no sense that the weakest clinical response corresponds to the highest prolactin levels. The SD values for prolactin levels were very large, corresponding to large variations from patient to patient. Indeed, it indicates that, among patients who received low-energy stimuli, one sixth showed a prolactin level that was less than one third of the group mean prolactin level (i.e., ≤500 mU/L) and another one sixth had a prolactin level that was more than six times that.

There is no reason to suppose a relationship between psychiatric illness and the amount of prolactin in either the bloodstream or the pituitary. Prolactin functions only to stimulate milk production. That seizure liberates prolactin from the pituitary into the bloodstream does not provide a rationale for this release to reflect the presence or severity of psychiatric illness. Indeed, cases of vigorous clinical response to ECT with no prolactin release, because of pituitary prolactin deficiency, are noted (e.g., Swartz, 1985a), so it should be no surprise that studies examining relationships between psychiatric illness and elevated prolactin levels have found none, regardless of whether prolactin levels were elevated by antipsychotic drugs or ECT (e.g., Lisanby et al., 1998). The lack of relationship does not address the possibility that diencephalic seizure activity is involved in the therapeutic mechanism of ECT; it is simply not relevant.

There is a fundamental difference between measuring hormone changes in medical conditions that directly affect those hormones (e.g., hypothyroidism, Cushing disease) and hormone changes in psychiatric conditions. This difference must be recognized and incorporated in the study method. However, this is rarely done, so results of hormone testing for psychiatric illness or treatments are clinically unreliable if not chaotic, and then they are discarded.

One way to compensate for interpatient variations is to use the repeated-measures method. Each patient receives each of the treatments to be compared. For each patient, only one value representing each treatment is taken; this value may be an average, a median, or any systematic, impartially selected representation. These values are then statistically analyzed by a repeated-measures analysis of variance. If there are two treatments, the difference can be taken and statistically compared with zero (as in a paired *t* test). There are still many pitfalls.

There are several pitfalls in using baseline hormone levels in expressing hormone release – that is, subtracting baseline levels from elevated hormone levels. Typically there are large random variations in baseline hormone levels from one day to the next. Perhaps the simplest perspective is that these baseline variations will contribute to hormone levels observed after the seizure according to their size, and the baseline effect can be removed by subtracting the baseline from the post-ECT hormone level. This is the usually reasonable approach. However, the influence of the baseline level might fade after the seizure. That is, hormone-release processes that contributed to the baseline level might be interrupted by the ECT seizure. This is a real possibility, and it has not been disproven. Its occurrence would be demonstrated by a post-ECT hormone level that decreases below baseline.

In describing ECT-induced hormone release, some investigators have reported the ratio between post-ECT and baseline hormone concentrations as the result (e.g., Robin et al., 1985). This ratio can magnify the effects of random variation of the baseline, particularly if the baseline level is much smaller than the highest post-ECT hormone level, as is usually (and ideally) the case. If the highest post-ECT level is 50 units it should matter little if the baseline level is 3 or 6 units, but using the ratio produces a huge (100%) effect if the baseline decreases from 6 to 3. This huge effect shows the inappropriateness of using the ratio; moreover, the ratio has no specific physiological meaning.

Subtracting the baseline hormone level from the post-ECT hormone level does not remove all the effects that are associated with the baseline. Indeed, peak prolactin elevations above baseline correlate ($r = 0.6$, $p < .001$) with baseline prolactin levels (Swartz, 1985a). This correlation apparently reflects prolactin release sensitivity, which surely varies far more among patients than among sessions within individual patients. Fortunately, this correlation does not invalidate (or validate) subtracting the baseline hormone level from post-ECT hormone levels.

Another way to compensate for interpatient variations – and baseline variations – is the Benchmark Method. This is a variation of the repeated-measures method. It applies also to monitoring and using heart rate elevations during the ECT seizure and is described in the chapter here on heart rate and ECT (Chapter 30). In the Benchmark Method, a particular peak hormone value is used as a point for reference and comparison. This hormone value might be found by giving a high-dose ECT stimulus, to produce what is assuredly an intense ECT seizure, and measuring the peak hormone level associated with that treatment. It may appear desirable to identify the benchmark by administering a drug that induces hormone release; however, until proven otherwise, drug-induced hormone release has no relevance to ECT-induced release of the same hormone.

Prolactin release, an archetype

The potential for ECT to induce adrenocorticotropic hormone (ACTH) release was so evident that the study introducing radioimmunoassay (RIA) to medicine measured it, to help establish credibility for the RIA method (Berson and Yalow, 1968). Nevertheless, for several reasons, the most frequently reported ECT-induced hormone release is prolactin.

Prolactin release is vigorous, peaking typically threefold to tenfold higher than baseline. The serum prolactin assay is reliable, inexpensive, more precise, and more easily performed than for ACTH, and is widely available. Serum prolactin level changes are fast enough to be conveniently measured but slow enough to show a smooth increase to a peak at 15 to 20 minutes and a return to baseline without overshoot within two hours (Swartz et al., 1985b). Most pituitary hormones show negligible change with ECT; these include thyroid-stimulating hormone (TSH), growth hormone, follicle-stimulating hormone, and luteinizing hormone. Levels of other hormones increase and decrease so rapidly that reasonably precise determinations of the peak and total amount of hormone released by the seizure are not feasible from venous blood sampling. These hormones include vasopressin, oxytocin, ACTH, and catecholamines. For these, the time elapsed between the seizure end point and the occurrence of the peak is comparable to the circulation time; likewise for the return to baseline after the peak. This brevity prevents precision. Comparatively, measuring serum prolactin is practical.

ECT-induced prolactin release does not appear to correspond to any specific change in brain neurochemistry (Swartz, 1991b). Although the mechanism underlying ECT-induced prolactin release is not proven, several lines of evidence suggest that it begins with seizure-induced release of dopamine from the posterior pituitary into the bloodstream. This release diverts the dopamine from its previous path into the anterior pituitary, where it acts to inhibit prolactin release. Likewise, in the hypothalamus the seizure interrupts dopamine synthesis and flow directly into the anterior pituitary. As the effect of dopamine on the prolactin-secreting cells in the anterior pituitary wears off, they release prolactin into the bloodstream. With recovery from the seizure, dopamine is synthesized in the hypothalamus and travels down the pituitary stalk to shut off prolactin release. In this mechanism, ECT-induced prolactin release primarily reflects depletion of dopamine in the pituitary, and it does not correspond to any change in the central nervous system itself (Swartz, 1991b). Alternatively but very similarly, ECT-induced oxytocin release from the posterior pituitary might mediate ECT-induced prolactin release. Oxytocin receptors in the anterior pituitary stimulate prolactin release (Chadio and Antoni, 1993). This makes sense physiologically as oxytocin stimulates milk ejection whereas prolactin promotes milk production, and the milk ejection mechanism should logically induce prolactin release.

Although the mechanisms of prolactin release are largely peripheral to the central nervous system, total prolactin release appears to represent a summation of seizure activity. It is analogous to the total amount of gasoline used during an automobile trip as a representation of the distance traveled. Variability in miles-per-gallon fuel efficiency corresponds to patient-to-patient variations in prolactin release sensitivity.

Prolactin release is an archetype of ECT-induced pituitary hormone release. The amounts of the other pituitary hormones released by ECT (vasopressin, oxytocin, their neurophysins, and ACTH) probably similarly reflect pituitary hormone stores and general seizure intensity rather than seizure-induced changes in brain neurochemistry. The result of measuring serum prolactin is a time series of hormone blood levels. To derive physiological meaning from these levels, they need to be used within a description of the physiology of prolactin release. Resemblances between ECT-induced prolactin release and the Thyrotropin Releasing Hormone (TRH) test for hypothyroidism suggest that the results be interpreted similarly. In the TRH test there is a single brief stimulus for TSH release, an intravenous infusion of TRH; this is analogous to ECT. Several minutes after this infusion, the blood TSH concentration starts rising at a rate that increases, slows, and then stops. There is a single peak in TSH concentration. It is severalfold larger than the baseline concentration. Near its peak, the TSH concentration changes much more slowly than before or after the peak. After this peak the TSH concentration decreases more slowly than it had increased before the peak, and it returns to baseline within about two hours.

The time course of blood prolactin levels after ECT has this same course, with faster release and elimination and an earlier peak. Deviation from the expected shape indicates artifact (and invalid results) unless proven otherwise. Examples of deviation include more than one prolactin peak, an abnormally high baseline prolactin level, a blood prolactin level below baseline, a peak prolactin level about the same as baseline, prolactin levels decreasing faster than they increased, and elevation of the blood prolactin level after 90 minutes. Deviations are common (Swartz, 1989). A second peak indicates a second hormone-releasing process, something besides ECT seizure-producing prolactin release. If the peak prolactin level is close to baseline, the amount of prolactin released is negligible. An abnormally high baseline speaks for itself. ECT-induced prolactin is always released more quickly than it is eliminated from the bloodstream; nonconforming results should be artifactual. There are many artifactual influences on prolactin release, including cigarette smoking, protein intake, hypoglycemia, and use of birth control pharmaceuticals. Dopamine-blocking agents such as metoclopramide and antipsychotic drugs powerfully raise prolactin levels. If given in repeated doses, antipsychotics continue to influence prolactin release for a month after the last dose. Even after prolactin levels return to baseline, prolactin release is hypersensitive for several weeks after antipsychotic use (Swartz, 1985a, 1991b). Most published studies of ECT-induced prolactin release are contaminated by exposure of the patients to antipsychotics.

In the TRH test the course of TSH blood levels – the result – is routinely summarized into a single number, the largest observed TSH elevation over baseline, called "delta." However, delta is unnecessarily inaccurate. It overlooks hormone release after the peak and hormone elimination before the peak. There is no consideration for the time of occurrence of the peak, whether early or late, even though slower release of the same hormone quantity produces a later and smaller peak. Moreover, the blood sampling schedule that is routinely used does not include the best time to measure the peak TSH level (Swartz et al., 1986). The same concerns apply to ECT-induced prolactin release. For a system with one temporary stimulus for hormone release (such as ECT or TRH) there are four basic and separate characteristics of hormone release: (a) total amount of hormone release, (b) latency for onset of hormone release, (c) hormone-release rate, and (d) hormone elimination rate. The time of occurrence of the peak can be calculated from these four hormone-release characteristics; it is not mathematically independent.

Just as in algebra, mathematically determining these four "unknowns" requires four simultaneous equations, corresponding to at least four blood samples during the period of substantial hormone release, besides a baseline sample. These results are then used with a kinetic model of hormone release, just as in pharmacokinetics (see equation below), in computerized calculation of the values of the four characteristics (Swartz, 1985b, 1991a). The blood samples should be drawn at times that well illuminate these four characteristics to be determined.

Regarding these specific times, the effects from latency and rate of release are largest before the peak and after hormone levels have started to increase. Therefore, two blood samples are needed during this period. For prolactin these should be at 5 and 10 minutes (after seizure end). Another sample is needed near the peak, to accurately reflect the total amount of prolactin released. Prolactin levels change much more rapidly before the peak than after, so the best routine sampling time is not the average time that the peak appears but slightly later. For prolactin, the average peak time is 15 minutes, so a good sampling time is 20 minutes. Describing the rate of elimination requires another blood sample after the peak and about halfway back to baseline. For prolactin, this is 45 minutes (Swartz, 1985b). These sampling times of 5, 10, 20, and 45 minutes are for males (and probably postmenopausal females). For premenopausal females, blood sampling times for prolactin should be 30% earlier, that is, 4, 7, 15, and 35 minutes.

Missing or rescheduling even one of these measurements undermines the determination of all the characteristics of hormone release. There is no known valid shortcut. Unfortunately, studies have typically reported the first serum prolactin level at 15, 20, or 30 minutes. For half of male patients, the peak occurs after more than 15 minutes, so a 15-minute prolactin level is often substantially below the peak.

Some investigators report the "area under the curve" as if it is the total hormone response, but it is not. Rather, it is the average hormone level over the period of measurement, multiplied by the duration of measurement. It is the body's exposure to the hormone, that is, the amount of physiological effect by this hormone. The area under the curve of prolactin concentration against time represents the stimulus for milk production. This is fundamentally different from the amount of effect by the seizure on the pituitary, which is the total amount of prolactin released.

The time course of hormone levels in the bloodstream can be modeled by the methods of chemical kinetics (Swartz 1985b, 1989, 1991a). Perhaps the most basic model of hormone release has these components:

There is a single temporary process of hormone release, that is, any other simultaneous processes are negligible.

There may be a latency period before this process begins to deliver hormone to the bloodstream.

The rate of hormone release decays proportionally to its intensity, or is instantaneous.

Hormone elimination from the bloodstream is proportional to its concentration.

The hormone concentration changes more slowly than the time taken to distribute the hormone through the bloodstream (the circulation time).

The hormone is distributed through a single compartment.

This model is represented by the equation:

$$C = P \left(e^{-E(T-L)} - e^{-R(T-L)} \right).$$

In this equation, $T =$ time elapsed, $C =$ hormone concentration elevation above baseline, $P =$ total hormone release into the bloodstream (divided by bloodstream volume), $E =$ fractional elimination rate, $R =$ fractional release rate, and $L =$ latency. The total amount of prolactin released is $P(1 - E/R)$.

Still more complicated systems can be described, such as by including several compartments, several simultaneous hormone-release processes, and interruption of baseline steady hormone release so that blood hormone levels might fall below baseline. However, each additional complication introduces more unknown characteristics, requires more blood samples to determine these characteristics, increases the number of simultaneous equations, and increases opportunities for artifactual and uncontrolled influences.

In contrast, less complicated systems are possible. If every patient had the same hormone-release rate, elimination rate, and latency there would be no need to measure these because all variability would be in the total hormone release. However, this is not the case for prolactin (Swartz, 1985b) or TSH (Swartz et al., 1986). Specifically, on average the total prolactin release is 80% higher than the actual peak prolactin level, and their shared variance is 74% (Swartz, 1985b, 1991a). Still, latency and the rates of release and elimination should vary little within individual patients from one ECT to another. This expected lack of variation within patients implies that hormone peaks can be compared among different sessions within individual patients, according to paired or repeated-measures analysis. This intraindividual comparison method also controls for variations among patients in total releasable prolactin pool and prolactin release sensitivity.

Indeed, several studies have reported paired measurements (on the same patients and different treatment days) and found that post-ECT prolactin levels were higher with a more intense ECT method. They were higher after bitemporal ECT than after unilateral ECT in male patients (Swartz and Abrams, 1984). This result was significant (at $p = .02$) although there were only six patients. The same result and statistical significance were also seen in a study of six female patients (Swartz, 1985a). Similarly, right unilateral ECT given at minimal dose and three times minimal dose produced significantly higher prolactin levels with the latter (Zis et al., 1996). The results of these three reports are in the same direction as results from studies comparing clinical outcome (see Chapters 27 and 28).

Several investigators have reported a progressive decrease in the prolactin peak along the course of ECT in about half of patients. This too is a repeated-measures observation. This decrease has not been examined further to see if it corresponds to the progressive increase in seizure threshold along the course of ECT, which also occurs in about half of patients (Coffey et al., 1995).

However, studies of prolactin release that did not use the repeated-measures (or paired) method and did not determine at least the actual peak prolactin level can have positive results only if the effect on prolactin release or the number of patients studied is particularly large. The effect must be visible, despite variations in the other characteristics and in total releasable prolactin pool and prolactin release sensitivity as well. There are many other reports of ECT-induced prolactin release, but their findings do not add to those reviewed here.

Clinically, measurement of seizure-induced prolactin elevation has been used in distinguishing among grand mal seizure, pseudoseizure, complex partial seizure, focal seizure, and seizure aura (Dana-Haeri et al., 1983; Hoppener et al., 1982; Sperling et al., 1985; Trimble, 1978). In one patient, ECT-induced prolactin elevation occurred without observable motor activity (Abrams and Swartz, 1985). Analogously, I have clinically used prolactin measurements to establish the presence of nonconvulsive seizures undetectable by electroencephalography (EEG) and previously incorrectly dismissed as pseudoseizures.

Posterior pituitary hormone release

ECT-induced release of vasopressin, oxytocin, and their neurophysins occurs much faster than prolactin release. Peak levels are reached in about 2 min, and vasopressin and oxytocin return to baseline within a few minutes (e.g., McGuire et al., 1989). These changes progress so quickly (relative to the blood circulation time) that it is not possible to obtain reasonable precision in measuring total hormone release.

Moreover, dopaminergic (and therefore antidopaminergic) drugs affect oxytocin release (Uvnas et al., 1995), so antipsychotic drugs can change ECT-induced oxytocin release. There is no reason to suppose any relationship between depression severity or remission on one hand and the pituitary content of oxytocin or vasopressin or its release by ECT on the other. Between this lack of expectation and the enormous obstacles to measuring the release of these hormones, it is no surprise that studies of ECT-induced release of vasopressin and oxytocin have found no relationship to psychiatric status (e.g., Smith et al., 1994). Some earlier reports claimed such relationships, but antipsychotic drugs were given, total hormone release was not determined, and ECT nonresponse was excessively high at 68% (Scott et al., 1991). There are other reports of ECT-induced pituitary hormone release, but their findings do not add to those reviewed here.

Cortisol release

Serum cortisol levels increase after ECT by a much smaller percentage of baseline than the 300% to 1000% seen with prolactin. ECT-induced cortisol elevations in depressed patients vary from none (Deakin et al., 1983) to 20% to 50% more than baseline (Arato et al., 1980; Zis et al., 1996). The smaller percentage increase leaves the cortisol elevation less clear-cut and subject to greater influence by random variations of the baseline. Nevertheless, higher stimulus dose with unilateral ECT produced greater postictal cortisol levels than with lower dose (Zis et al., 1996).

The smaller percentage increase probably results from elevated resting cortisol levels associated with major depression of ECT-quality severity (Rush et al., 1996). Moreover, the pituitary ACTH depletion that accompanies these high cortisol levels (Gold and Chrousos, 1985) should also attenuate ECT-induced cortisol elevation. In effect, depression obscures the effect of ECT seizure on cortisol release.

The high pre-ECT cortisol levels in ECT patients, and presumably some ACTH depletion, were decreased by administering 2 mg of dexamethasone 9 hours prior to ECT (Swartz, 1992; Swartz and Chen, 1985). ECT seizure then increased serum cortisol by 800% on average, a percentage similar to ECT-induced prolactin elevation.

Under dexamethasone pretreatment, cortisol levels 30 minutes post-ECT increased 575% above baseline with the initial ECT, but only 180% above baseline with the final treatment in a course of bitemporal ECT with good clinical response (Swartz and Chen, 1985). A second study with dexamethasone pretreatment found that ECT-induced cortisol elevation decreased more with unilateral ECT than with bitemporal ECT, using a fixed stimulus dose (Swartz, 1992). This finding suggests that unilateral ECT might lose some efficacy along the course of treatment when the dose is not increased.

It is not clear how to relate postictal cortisol levels to physiological processes associated with the seizure, as described earlier for ECT-induced prolactin release. ECT-induced cortisol release is of course consequent to ECT-induced ACTH release, which itself follows CRH release in the hypothalamus, and so is at least one step further removed from the brain than prolactin release is.

Resting hypercortisolism

Endogenous major depression but not atypical (reactive) depression is associated with mild hypersecretion of cortisol, about 10% above normal, as reflected by dexamethasone nonsuppression of cortisol levels (Rush et al., 1996). Cortisol hypersecretion is particularly high in hospitalized patients with depression. Patients who respond to tricyclic antidepressants show normalization of cortisol levels (Nemeroff and Evans, 1984). Seemingly in contradiction with this, patients who respond to ECT do not show normalization of the dexamethasone suppression test, and some showed increasing cortisol levels (e.g., Coryell, 1986; Decina et al., 1983; Devanand et al., 1987; Fink et al., 1987; Palmer et al., 1990).

However, this contradictory pattern occurs only with a dexamethasone dose of 1 mg and not with 2 mg. With 2-mg doses, average cortisol levels decreased from 4 μg/dL pre-ECT to 1.8 μg/dL after the course, but with 1-mg doses in the same patients they increased from 6.0 μg/dL to 6.6 μg/dL (Swartz and Saheba, 1990). Apparently an aspect of the ECT procedure accelerates dexamethasone metabolism. As these studies were conducted under barbiturate anesthesia, barbiturate induction of hepatic metabolism is a likely explanation.

Resting hypercortisolism may be associated with larger temporary cognitive side effects. Higher pre-ECT salivary cortisol levels were associated with mild decreases in executive function, speed of visuospatial processing, and verbal memory (Neylan et al., 2001). These changes are more subtle than are changes in orientation and global cognitive functioning. The ECT method was medium-dose right unilateral ECT for six sessions. This method rarely produces substantial cognitive side effects, so the cognitive effects studied do not seem to be the ones that are clinically important. Moreover, the post-ECT Hamilton Rating Scale for Depression rating averaged 25, which does not approach the high efficacy expected for ECT. This means that the study method does not correspond to standard clinical ECT practices and its results do not apply to them.

Future clinical applications

Ideally, hormone testing should help assess the adequacy of the ECT course for individual patients, that is, the severity of illness. We would like to know if a sufficient number of ECT sessions have been provided so that a stable clinical response is obtained. Periodically after the course we would like to know if clinical decompensation is impending. For patients taking maintenance ECT, we'd like to know if the frequency of treatment is sufficient or needs to be increased. Candidate measurements for these seem to be resting cortisol levels and ECT-induced cortisol release, after pretreatment with 1.5 to 2 mg of dexamethasone at least 8 hours prior. Perhaps 1 mg of dexamethasone can be used if nonbarbiturate ECT anesthesia (e.g., etomidate) is given.

Clinically using prolactin measurements to describe the therapeutic adequacy or impact of single ECT treatments by the Benchmark Method (noted earlier) is also possible. This might be helpful in individual cases when the usual methods of monitoring ECT physiology (e.g., EEG, peak heart rate) are not able to show signs of an intense seizure, as happens occasionally in elderly patients.

References

Abrams, R. and Swartz, C. M. 1985. ECT and prolactin release: Relation to treatment response in melancholia. Convulsive Ther 1: 38–42.

Arato, M., Erdos, A., Kurcz, M., et al. 1980. Studies on the prolactin response induced by electroconvulsive therapy in schizophrenics. Acta Psychiatr Scand 61: 239–44.

Auriacombe, M., Rénéric, J. P., Usandizaga, D., et al. 2000. Post-ECT agitation and plasma lactate concentrations. J ECT 16: 263–7.

Berson, S. A. and Yalow, R. S. 1968. Radioimmunoassay of ACTH in plasma. J Clin Invest 47: 2725–51.

Chadio, S. E. and Antoni, F. A. 1993. Specific oxytocin agonist stimulates prolactin release but has no effect on inositol phosphate accumulation in isolated rat anterior pituitary cells. J Mol Endocrinol 10: 107–12.

Coffey, C. E., Lucke, J., Weiner, R. D., et al. 1995. Seizure threshold in electroconvulsive therapy (ECT) II. The anticonvulsant effect of ECT. Biol Psychiatry 37: 777–88.

Coryell, W. 1986. Are serial dexamethasone suppression tests useful in electroconvulsive therapy? J Affect Disord 10: 59–66.

Dana-Haeri, J., Trimble, M. R., and Oxley, J. 1983. Prolactin and gonadotropin changes following generalized and partial seizures. J Neurol Neurosurg Psychiatry 46: 331–5.

Deakin, J. W. F., Ferrier, I. N., Crow, T. J., et al. 1983. Effects of ECT on pituitary hormone release: Relationship to seizure, clinical variables, and outcome. Br J Psychiatry 143: 618–24.

Decina, P., Sackeim, H. A., and Malitz, S. 1983. Prognostic value of serial dexamethasone suppression tests during and following ECT. Psychopharm Bull 19: 85–7.

Devanand, D. P., Decina, P., Sackeim, H. A., et al. 1987. Serial dexamethasone suppression tests in initial suppressors and nonsuppressors treated with electroconvulsive therapy. Biol Psychiatry 22: 463–72.

Fink, M., Gujavarty, K., and Greenberg, L. 1987. Serial dexamethasone suppression tests and clinical outcome in ECT. Convulsive Ther 3: 111–20.

Gold, P. W. and Chrousos, G. P. 1985. Clinical studies with corticotropin releasing factor: Implications for the diagnosis and pathophysiology of depression, Cushing's disease, and adrenal insufficiency. Psychoneuroendocrinology 10: 401–19.

Griswold, R. L. 1958. Plasma adrenaline and noradrenaline in electroshock therapy in man and rats. J Appl Physiol 12: 117–20.

Hoppener, R. J. E., Rentmeester, T. H., Arnoldussen, W., et al. 1982. The changes in serum prolactin level following partial and generalized seizures. Br J Clin Pract Suppl 18: 193–5.

Lisanby, S. H., Devanand, D. P., Prudic, J., et al. 1998. Prolactin response to electroconvulsive therapy: Effects of electrode placement and stimulus dosage. Biol Psychiatry 43: 146–55.

McGuire, R. J., Scott, A. I., Bennie, J., and Watts, G. S. 1989. Reliability of the application of a kinetic model of hormone release: Prolactin and oestrogen-stimulated neurophysin after electroconvulsive therapy. Convuls Ther 5: 131–9.

Nemeroff, C. B. and Evans, D. L. 1984. Correlation between the dexamethasone suppression test in depressed patients and clinical response. Am J Psychiatry 141: 247–94.

Neylan, T. C., Canick, J. D., Hall, S. E., et al. 2001. Cortisol levels predict cognitive impairment induced by electroconvulsive therapy. Biol Psychiatry 50: 331–6.

Palmer, R. L., Mani, C., Abdel-Kariem, M. A. A., and Brandon, S. 1990. Dexamethasone suppression tests in the context of a double-blind trial of electroconvulsive therapy and simulated ECT. Convuls Ther 6: 13–8.

Pina-Cabral, J. M. and Rodrigues, C. 1974. Blood catecholamine levels, factor VIII and fibrinolysis after electroshock. Br J Hematol 28: 371–80.

Pitts, F. N. and McClure, J. N. 1967. Lactate metabolism in anxiety neurosis. N Engl J Med 277: 1329–36.

Robin, A., Binnie, C. D., and Copas J. B. 1985. Electrophysiological and hormonal responses to three types of electroconvulsive therapy. Br J Psychiatry 147: 707–12.

Robin, A. and De Tissera, S. 1982. A double-blind controlled comparison of the therapeutic effects of low and high energy electroconvulsive therapies. Br J Psychiatr 141: 357–66.

Rush, A. J., Giles, D. E., Schlesser, M. A., et al. 1996. The dexamethasone suppression test in patients with mood disorders. J Clin Psychiatry 57: 470–84.

Scott, A. I., Shering, P. A., Lightman, S. L., and Legros, J. J. 1991. The release of oxytocin, vasopressin and associated neurophysins after electroconvulsive therapy. Hum Psychopharmacol 6: 161–4.

Smith, J., Williams, K., Birkett, S., et al. 1994. Neuroendocrine and clinical effects of electroconvulsive therapy and their relationship to treatment outcome. Psychol Med 24: 547–55.

Sperling, M. R., Pritchard, P. B., Engel, J., et al. 1985. Limbic seizures and prolactin. Epilepsia 26: 529.

Swartz, C. M. 1985a. The time course of post-ECT prolactin levels. Convuls Ther 1: 81–9.

Swartz, C. M. 1985b. Characterization of the total amount of prolactin released by electroconvulsive therapy. Convuls Ther 1: 252–7.

Swartz, C. M. 1989. Anomalous patterns of ECT-induced hormone release. Convuls Ther 5: 185–9.

Swartz, C. M. 1990. ECT emergence agitation and succinylcholine dose. J Nerv Mental Dis 178: 455–7.

Swartz, C. M. 1991a. Quantity of prolactin released by ECT seizure. Convuls Ther 7: 62.

Swartz, C. M. 1991b. ECT-induced prolactin release as an epiphenomenon. Convuls Ther 7: 85–91.

Swartz, C. M. 1992. Electroconvulsive therapy-induced cortisol release after dexamethasone in depression. Neuropsychobiology 25: 130–3.

Swartz, C. M. 1993. ECT emergence agitation and methohexital-succinylcholine interaction. Gen Hosp Psychiatry 15: 339–41.

Swartz, C. M. and Abrams, R. 1984. Prolactin levels after bilateral and unilateral ECT. Br J Psychiatry 144: 643–5.

Swartz, C. M. and Chen, J. J. 1985. ECT-induced cortisol release: Changes with depressive state. Convuls Ther 1: 15–21.

Swartz, C. M. and Saheba, N. C. 1990. Dose effect on dexamethasone suppression testing with ECT. Ann Clin Psychiatry 2: 183–8.

Swartz, C. M., Wahby, V. S., and Vacha, R. 1986. Characterization of the pituitary response in the TRH test by kinetic modeling. Acta Endocrinol 112: 43–8.

Trimble, M. R. 1978. Serum prolactin in epilepsy and hysteria. Br Med J 2: 1682.

Uvnas, M. K., Alster, P., Hillegaart, V., and Ahlenius, S. 1995. Suggestive evidence for a DA D3 receptor-mediated increase in the release of oxytocin in the male rat. Neuroreport 6: 1338–40.

Vigas, M., Stowasserova, N., Nemeth, S., and Jurcovicova, J. 1975. Effect of electroconvulsive therapy without anticonvulsive premedication on serum growth hormone in man. Horm Res 6: 65–70.

Walker, W. R. and Swartz, C. M. 1994. ECT during high-risk pregnancy. Gen Hosp Psychiatry 16: 348–53.

Widerlov, E., Ekman, R., Jensen, L., et al. 1989. Arginine vasopressin, but not corticotropin releasing factor, is a potent stimulator of adrenocorticotropic hormone following electroconvulsive treatment. J Neural Transm 75: 101–9.

Zis, A. P., Yatham, L. N., Lam, R. W., et al. 1996. Effect of stimulus intensity on prolactin and cortisol release induced by unilateral electroconvulsive therapy. Neuropsychopharmacology 15: 263–70.

Part II

Historical, societal, and geographic perspectives

9

History of electroconvulsive therapy

Edward Shorter

Introduction

Electroconvulsive therapy (ECT) arose in the context of the so-called "physical therapies" of the first third of the 20th century. The physical therapies included treatments such as the malarial-fever therapy of neurosyphilis, insulin shock for schizophrenia, and chemical convulsive therapy and ECT for mood disorders. These treatments addressed the physical substance of the brain itself, not just the mind. They have also been called "shock therapies" because they were thought to jolt the brain. They represented a dramatic departure from the previous custodialism of psychiatry – and from the psychotherapy of private practice – because they promised genuine hope in serious psychiatric illness. It was this promise of hope that gave wing to these new treatments. At the dawn of the 21st century this promise has been increasingly fulfilled. The history of shock therapy has been addressed in detail by Shorter and Healy (2007) and by Dukakis and Tye (2006).

Origin of concept

The concept of shock therapy arose in France in the 1920s. In 1926, Paris psychiatrist Constance Pascal introduced the term "shock" to psychiatry, understanding by it "mental anaphylactic reactions" that might be induced by the injection of such substances as colloidal gold, milk, or vaccines. The treatments she proposed aroused little enthusiasm, but she implanted the notion of resetting the brain with some kind of chemical shock (Pascal and Davesne, 1926).

Insulin coma and early convulsive therapies

A trio of physical therapies emerged in the 1930s: insulin coma (insulin shock), pentylenetetrazol convulsive therapy, and ECT. Of these three, only ECT has survived.

In 1930 Manfred Sakel, a recent medical graduate of the University of Vienna employed in a private psychiatric clinic in Berlin, announced that he was using insulin to treat addiction to morphine (Sakel, 1930). In this report he said nothing about comas, although he was undoubtedly inducing them. Three years later, in 1933, Sakel said that the insulin treatment was a frank coma therapy and that it was useful in schizophrenia (Sakel, 1933). Insulin therapy involved inducing deep comas with injections of insulin. Several hours after the beginning of a coma session, the coma would be terminated with infusions of glucose, to be repeated the following day, for a series of up to 20 or 30 comas. One tenth to one third of the comas entailed convulsions, and it is possible that the convulsions were actually the curative agent in the procedure. Sakel's insulin coma lingered on for decades as the treatment of choice for what was then termed "schizophrenia." It was finally extinguished in the early 1960s with the belief that antipsychotic drugs were safer and easier to administer than coma therapy (Fink et al., 1958). Doubts linger even today about whether insulin coma did not possess some valuable (but never quite specified) principle of action (Healy, 2002).

Meanwhile, the young Budapest psychiatrist Ladislaus Meduna was developing the first explicit convulsive therapy. Inspired by the idea of an antagonism between epilepsy and schizophrenia, he reasoned that inducing convulsions might represent a treatment for schizophrenia. His first patients probably had acute catatonic episodes, and convulsive therapy is indeed effective in catatonia. After experimenting with camphor as a convulsive agent, Meduna hit on pentylenetetrazol, marketed in Europe as Cardiazol and in the United States as Metrazol. Meduna's 1935 report marked the true beginning of convulsive therapy in psychiatry (Meduna, 1935).

Yet Meduna's chemical convulsive therapy was not an entire success. The patients disliked it because of a panicky feeling that overcame them as they lay waiting for the onset of the convulsion. It was not without risk and was complex to administer. In 1938 Ugo Cerletti, professor of psychiatry in Rome, conceived the idea of initiating the convulsions with electricity, which had the advantage of instant unconsciousness, was safer, and was straightforward in its application. Patients were willing to return for subsequent treatments. Cerletti's assistant Luigi Bini designed the apparatus for the treatment and administered it clinically (Cerletti and Bini, 1938). From the beginning the treatment was a big success. This was the origin of ECT. In 1940 Cerletti reported that ECT was even more effective in the treatment of depressive illness than in schizophrenia (Cerletti, 1940). What people called schizophrenia in those days was often heavily infiltrated by mood disorders – hence the considerable success of these early treatments of "schizophrenia."

The technique of ECT has changed little since Cerletti initiated it in 1938, with the exception of the addition of muscle relaxants and anesthesia, necessary to relieve patients' anxiety about being unable to catch their breath as the muscle relaxant takes hold. Cerletti and Bini administered around 120 volts of alternating sine wave current, from the wall sockets, for about one tenth of a second with the electrodes in a bitemporal position. These investigators were clear that a complete grand mal seizure was necessary. Complications were negligible, and only later was the frequency of spinal fractures in unmodified seizures apparent (Bini, 1940). Their efficacy was virtually the same as today – 80% of their hospitalized patients with affective illness improved. Indeed, the rule prevails today that if at least 80% of one's patients do not improve, one is doing something wrong (Little et al., 2003).

As for the vexed question of memory loss, none of the early electrotherapists saw this as a significant issue. After questioning the patients closely, one of Cerletti's assistants did report that a substantial number had significant, usually brief, memory loss around the time of the procedure (Flescher, 1941), but in the early ECT literature, memory loss is really a nontheme. This raises the question: Were these skilled veteran clinicians simply imperceptive, or was a shibboleth later made of the memory issue that has unnecessarily caused public anxiety and limited the use of the procedure?

ECT in the United States

With the displacement of many psychiatrists during the Second World War, the United States soon established itself as the international center of gravity of ECT research. The leading figures were mainly European émigré physicians. From the American literature it became apparent that unmodified ECT treatment was feasible, providing the patients were properly restrained. Although there is some dispute about who was first to practice ECT in the United States, a reasonable candidate for the title is Chicago electrotherapist Victor Gonda – formerly of Budapest – who in 1941 described preparation of the patient: "To prevent injury to the vertebrae he is placed in bed with a blanket-covered firm wooden base placed under his back. This wooden base is merely a stave from a large barrel, and is so placed that the maximum convexity is under the middorsal spine. This hyperextension separates the anterior vertebral edges, which are most vulnerable to compression injuries" (Gonda, 1941).

The gray eminence of early ECT in the United States was Lothar Kalinowsky, a German émigré who had retrained in psychiatry at Cerletti's clinic in Rome before making his way to New York in 1940. In 1942, Kalinowsky described how his patients at Pilgrim State Hospital on Long Island in New York were restrained: "Three large sand bags are placed beneath the patient's middorsal spine. The shoulders and hips are then manually applied to the table with some force, producing hyperextension to the greatest degree that this relatively rigid section of the spine will permit." Postseizure x-rays in the first 60 ECT cases of Worthing and Kalinowsky (1942) showed no vertebral fractures.

It soon became apparent that, if patients were given proper restraint, office-practice ECT was feasible. William Karliner, a New York psychiatrist trained in Vienna who escaped in 1938, was a principal American advocate of office-practice ECT. "Office electroshock therapy has become an accepted psychiatric procedure," he wrote in 1952. "There have been fewer objections to it in the last few years" (Karliner and Savitsky, 1952). These historical remarks about office practice and proper restraint in unmodified ECT are important because the impression has arisen – to the detriment of patients in countries where an anesthetist is not readily available – that the only safe and effective form of ECT is in hospitals under conditions of full anesthesia and muscle relaxation. Historical experience makes clear that this generalization must be qualified.

A turning point in the history of ECT was the introduction of muscle relaxants in 1952. To be sure, curare had been attempted as a muscle relaxant previously, yet the agent was highly dangerous and results often unsatisfactory. In 1952 Carl Gunnar Holmberg, of the department of psychiatry of the Karolinska Institute in Stockholm, and Stephen Thesleff, of the departments of anesthesia and pharmacology, proposed the use of succinylcholine iodide as a short-acting blocker at the neuromuscular junction (Holmberg and Thesleff, 1952). Succinylcholine chloride was marketed in the United States by Burroughs Wellcome and Company under the brand name Anectine. At one fell swoop, the problem of muscular convulsions in ECT was abolished. Holmberg and Thesleff themselves initiated the use of a barbiturate anesthesia in the procedure, although they were not necessarily the first to use anesthesia in ECT.

The debate over technique

The form of current in ECT and the placement of the electrodes have produced a half-century debate that has not been resolved to this day. Concerns over memory brought about the first departure from Cerletti's alternating-current bitemporal placement technique. In 1942, Emerick Friedman and Paul H. Wilcox at the Metropolitan State Hospital in Waltham, Massachusetts, proposed unidirectional waveforms for a gentler seizure. Using half sine waves (unidirectional direct current, also called rectified sine wave) greatly reduced the amount of electricity flowing into the body, they claimed. They also suggested placing the electrodes in a so-called unilateral position, one on the vertex of the skull, the other just above one of the temples. This was suggested because they thought that the current would pass in a straight line through the motor cortex only, sparing the rest of the brain (Friedman and Wilcox, 1942). This, of course, was simplistic, as the electrical current diffuses in space.

In a second innovation in waveform, in 1944 Wladimir ("Ted") Liberson at the Institute of Living in Hartford, Connecticut, proposed "brief stimulus therapy"

(BST). He reduced the application of electricity to one thirtieth of the Cerletti dose by greatly shortening the individual impulses, separating them by long, energy-free gaps referred to as "square waves." Liberson developed a device that could generate up to 250 of them per second (Liberson, 1944). By 1948, using a machine designed by Franklin Offner, owner of Offner Electronics of Chicago, Liberson increased the size of the pulses (stimulus amplitude) progressively with every cycle. The responses of depressed patients were said to be excellent (Liberson, 1948). This was the true birth of BST.

BST was combined with right unilateral therapy electrode placement the following year, 1949, in the hands of Douglas Goldman at the Longview State Hospital in Cincinnati, Ohio. Using BST, Goldman placed one electrode on the vertex and the other on the right temporal area, "to avoid excessive application of current to the important areas of speech." He claimed it to be at least as effective as the Cerletti technique and that it resulted in a "marked diminution and, at times, complete absence of confusion associated with the electric shock therapy." As with all unidirectional therapies at these minimal currents, the patients were often not immediately unconscious and first had to be given a barbiturate anesthetic (Goldman, 1949).

The next 20 years produced much backing and forthing over unidirectional right unilateral placement versus the Cerletti bitemporal technique (Shorter and Healy, 2007, pp. 119–22). In 1991 Richard Abrams, Conrad Swartz, and Chandra Vedak established that a high-dose right unilateral ECT works the same as bilateral ECT, perhaps taking slightly longer (Abrams et al., 1991). McCall et al. (2000) confirmed expectations that higher stimulus doses increased efficacy and side effects of right unilateral ECT. Their confirmation suggests that, at very high doses, right unilateral would be the same as bitemporal ECT. So differences between right unilateral and bitemporal ECT are largest at low stimulus doses.

Since at least 1971 all ECT devices in the United States have used alternating current, whether they were brief pulse or sine wave; there has been no more unidirectional stimulus. The common medical impression now is that sine wave ECT is unnecessarily harmful compared with brief-pulse ECT. The cognitive side effects of brief-pulse ECT are vastly fewer than those from sine wave ECT, and sine wave ECT is actually banned in England. Any U.S. hospital that gives sine wave ECT is begging for a lawsuit.

Nevertheless, still today in many areas of the world sine wave stimuli remain in use; so does unmodified ECT. Both provide benefit and receive appreciation, as their shortcomings are small compared with the clinical benefits received by patients.

In 1953, Holmberg introduced oxygenation in the hope of reducing immediate cognitive effects. Yet adding oxygen and monitoring the seizures with electrocardiogram and electroencephalogram (EEG), although praiseworthy, added little clinically to the outcome. Moreover, the usual barbiturate anesthetic interferes with a proper treatment by increasing the convulsive threshold. The Rome clinic could not afford an EEG apparatus, but Cerletti and Bini did not need one to tell if their patients were having a grand mal seizure. Ironically, Italy, the birthplace of ECT, has virtually banned it outside a few university clinics, the only country to do so.

Research on these issues trickled slowly away in the 1960s. The last major contribution was the 1960 study of Jan-Otto Ottosson of the Karolinska Institute in Stockholm, who found that "the therapeutic effect and the disorganization of cerebral function . . . both are determined by the seizure" (Ottosson, 1960).

Stigmatization and the decline of ECT

During the 1960s ECT began to suffer from a media-induced stigma so oppressive that ECT almost disappeared. Hollywood was partly to blame. There had been previous anti-ECT movies and novels, such as *The Snake Pit* (1949), featuring Olivia de Haviland, based on Mary Jane Ward's 1946 novel of that title (Ward, 1946). Yet the media event that curdled public opinion definitively on ECT was Ken Kesey's 1962 novel *One Flew over the Cuckoo's Nest*. Milos Forman's 1975 film of that title, which garnered for United Artists all of the five main Oscars in that year, was a signal public health disaster: For the public, the movie associated ECT with torture and psychiatric abuse.

The antipsychiatry *Zeitgeist* of the 1960s and 1970s was a hook on which to hang these black Hollywood fantasies. Thanks to a series of antipsychiatric media bubbles, beginning with Thomas Szasz's *Myth of Mental Illness* in 1961 and Michel Foucault's *The History of Madness*, translated into English in 1965 as *Madness and Civilization*, the intellectual class – mesmerized by psychoanalysis – began to believe the physical therapies in psychiatry to be instruments of oppression (Shorter, 2005).

Finally contributing to the desuetude of ECT was the initial success of psychopharmacology. Chlorpromazine (Thorazine, Largactil), the first antipsychotic, entered clinical trials in 1952; imipramine (Tofranil), the first tricyclic antidepressant, was launched in Switzerland in 1957 and in the United States in 1959 (Shorter, 1997). The success of psychopharmacology in the 1960s seemed so ascertained that many believed convulsive therapy – increasingly seen as a barbarous remnant of an earlier and outdated epoch in psychiatry – could be entirely discontinued.

Yet the pendulum quickly turned back. The problem of "treatment-resistant depression" was quickly on the radar of the discipline. In 1962 Kurt Witton, an émigré psychiatrist at the Veterans Administration (VA) hospital in Fort Meade, South Dakota (he had studied at Bologna at the same time that Kalinowsky was in Rome), found that ECT improved significantly the thought processes of patients who had done poorly on neuroleptic drugs: "I have noted that in many cases refractory to drugs but following a rather prolonged use of phenothiazine derivatives a series of ECT (usually 20 treatments) will obtain a striking unexpected improvement or remission of the active psychotic, mainly schizophrenic, process" (Witton, 1962). This finding was the initial notice that the new drugs were not as effective as publicized. Then, in a landmark article in 1975, Alexander Glassman at the New York State Psychiatric Institute discovered that patients with psychotic depression who were unresponsive to antidepressant medication did well on ECT (Glassman, 1975).

The road back begins

Within the psychiatric profession, a small core of physicians, who knew of the efficacy and safety of ECT because they had experienced it in their practices, spearheaded a comeback of the much vilified treatment. In the wake of anti-ECT legislation looming in many states, on the model of California's harshly repressive legislation, in 1975 the American Psychiatric Association (APA) formed a task force to study ECT. The driving piston on the task force was Max Fink, who in the year before, 1974, had edited a volume assessing ECT from a scientific viewpoint, a volume that represented the first step in the scientific rehabilitation of the procedure (Fink et al., 1974). The task force's 1978 report was cautiously positive (APA, 1978). Fink, however, found the indecisiveness of the task force so vexing that in 1979 he published his own manual on ECT, the first in decades (Fink, 1979).

In 1990 another task force of the APA, chaired by Richard Weiner of Duke University and including Fink, Donald Hammersley, Iver Small, Louis Moench, and Harold Sackeim, brought out a second report, much more broad-minded than the first, making it clear that ECT had an essential role not just in treatment but in psychiatric training (APA, 1990). It was this report that swayed opinion within psychiatry on behalf of ECT.

The placement debate resurfaces

At this point a heated dispute over electrode placement and memory broke out within psychiatry that to the present day has not been fully resolved. The background is that clinical opinion in the field as a whole had a decided preference for bilateral placement, whereas the few research studies favored unilateral placement. Unilateral was given a decisive boost in 1958 by Neville Lancaster at Barrow Hospital in Bristol, England, and associates who delivered a plaidoyer for unilateral placement in, as they put it, "patients of very superior intelligence, and especially those who have to earn their livelihood with retained knowledge," which, in short order, became understood as everyone (Lancaster et al., 1958). A careful study by Richard Abrams and collaborators at Gracie Square Hospital in New York in 1972 expressed a preference for unilateral placement except for patients for whom rapid effective treatment was paramount (Abrams et al., 1972) – for this has always been the virtue of bilateral placement – even though it causes more memory impairment, it works.

In 1993, psychologist Harold Sackeim at the New York State Psychiatric Institute reopened the debate with the statement that high dose was preferable to low dose in either form of electrode placement. But high-dose bilateral placement caused three times more retrograde amnesia than did unilateral placement (Sackeim et al., 1993). The implication was that bilateral placement precipitated such apparently unnecessary memory loss that it was not even to be contemplated. I must observe as an aside that, in any event, most clinicians in private practice in the United States have always preferred bitemporal ECT, now, then, and before then.

The Sackeim study was, however, not the last word. At this writing, the advocates of bilateral placement have the upper hand, especially of bifrontal placement as opposed to bitemporal placement. In 2003 an ECT Review Group in England, led by John Geddes of Oxford, undertook a systematic overview and meta-analysis of all trials permitting comparison of unilateral and bilateral ECT, among other objectives. They concluded, "There is . . . a trade-off between making ECT optimally effective in terms of amelioration of depressive symptoms and limitation of cognitive impairment. . . . If there is a need to achieve rapid response of symptoms, and this is more important than minimisation of cognitive impairment, then the most effective form of ECT seems to be bilateral high-dose ECT" (UK ECT, 2003).

In the United States, two large multicenter studies – the Columbia University Consortium (CUC) and the Consortium for Research in ECT (CORE) – permit a direct comparison of the two electrode placements. The CORE study used bilateral ECT and energy doses 50% more than the seizure threshold. The CUC used unilateral ECT with much higher-energy dosing. The CORE study had a remission rate of 86%, the CUC study 55% (Fink and Taylor, 2007).

Yet today the debate continues. In November 2007, in the *New England Journal of Medicine*, Sarah H. Lisanby of the New York State Psychiatric Institute argued that "it would be appropriate to consider starting with right unilateral ECT at an adequate dosage." Only after nonresponse would one consider bilateral placement (Lisanby, 2007). In contrast, Max Fink argues, "RUL ECT is not as effective as BT ECT; we have fiddled with this placement for more than 40 years, and no credible way has been found to make its application effective" (Fink, 2002). Others argue that right unilateral placement is made as effective as bitemporal placement by giving a high-stimulus dose, but this modification simultaneously removes its cognitive advantages.

Electrode placement: Recent innovations

In terms of electrode placement, there have been two recent innovations. One is bifrontal placement instead of bitemporal. In 1969, James Inglis, in the Department of Psychology at Queen's University in Kingston, Ontario, Canada, reviewed previous electrode placement studies, concluding that bitemporal placement produced great cognitive disruption and that "the more frontally placed the electrodes, the less drastic the effects of shock are likely to be on learning and memory" (Inglis, 1969). In 1973, Richard Abrams and Michael Taylor undertook a clinical study of comparative placements and found that "bifrontal," to use their term, was optimal (Abrams and Taylor, 1973). In 1990, a large trial led by J. S. Lawson at the Kingston Psychiatric Hospital – and including Inglis and Felix Letemendia as senior members of the team – established that bifrontal placement was indeed superior to bitemporal and right unilateral in "sparing both verbal and nonverbal functions" (Lawson et al., 1990). But was bifrontal superior in efficacy? Yes was the answer, as the Kingston group determined three years later: "Because BF ECT causes fewer cognitive side effects than either RU or BT, and is independently more effective, it should be considered as the first choice of electrode position in ECT" (Letemendia et al., 1993).

Samuel Bailine at Hillside Hospital in 2000 had similar good results with bifrontal versus bitemporal placement, adding weight to the growing shift away from right unilateral placement as ineffective (Bailine et al., 2000).

A second innovation is Conrad Swartz's proposal in 1994 of left anterior right temporal (LART) placement, a bilateral technique attracting growing endorsement on the basis of neurobiological principles designed to reduce disorientation (Swartz, 1994). In a later article, Swartz, director of research in psychiatry at Southern Illinois University in Springfield, and Alexander Nelson, at Russia's Peoples' Friendship University in Moscow, hypothesized, "The neurobiology particular to the LART placement is primarily its asymmetry and the fully anterior location of the left electrode. It should interfere less with cognitive behavior than symmetrical placements do" (Swartz and Nelson, 2005).

The revival of ECT

In the first decade of the 21st century, the big news about convulsive therapy is its return. ECT has passed from a stigmatized procedure for last-ditch efforts to save personalities from disintegration, to a new prominence on the radar of the average community psychiatrist and general hospital. Although one third of the metropolitan areas in the United States do not offer ECT, the good news is that two thirds do (Hermann, 1995). In training programs and professional meetings across the country, convulsive therapy is once again in play. It is a belated but nonetheless welcome recognition of the triumph of scientific thinking within psychiatry.

More than 70 years after the introduction of convulsive therapy in 1935, it is interesting today to review what we know and what we do not know. The academics have scrapped mightily over electrode placement, a relatively minor issue in view of what is *not* known about ECT. Consider what has not been studied over the past 40 years, given that scientific research into the mechanisms of ECT virtually came to an end in the 1960s.

We know almost nothing about the neurobiological mechanisms of ECT. It remains a black-box empirical treatment, used because it works. But, as once was the case with aspirin, we do not know why it works. In melancholic depression, ECT seems to have a powerful effect on hypercortisolemia in the neuroendocrine system, normalizing the dexamethasone suppression test (Fink, 2000), but initially ECT increases cortisol levels: Although the seizure increases cortisol levels for about two hours, resting cortisol levels progressively decrease along the ECT course (Swartz and Chen, 1985). High serum cortisol is a phenomenon associated with worsening of depressive illness (Abrams, 2002).

As for continuation therapy after ECT, little is known. Continuation with ECT? With pharmacotherapy? With a combination? And for how long? These questions are addressed in other chapters of this book.

There have been almost no recent trials of ECT versus psychopharmacology. No drug company would risk its precious agent going head to head in a trial against ECT that the drug would almost certainly lose. We know that convulsive therapy represents a superior treatment in melancholia, catatonia, and mania, over virtually all pharmacological agents. But why? What is the neurochemical profile of ECT, its effect on second messengers, its role in nonsynaptic neurotransmission? None of these things had even been discovered at the time that basic research in convulsive therapy came to an end.

Finally, what agents might permit us to replace ECT with a pharmacological convulsive treatment, or nonconvulsive treatment, with the same safety and efficacy but less feared by patients and their families? In the early 1940s, Ugo Cerletti believed he had found such a drug, a pharmacological replacement for ECT that he called acroagonine (Cerletti, 1947). Alas, it did not work out. But the almost magical squiggle on the EEG indicating that a cerebral seizure has occurred is a powerful indicator of therapeutic efficacy, more powerful than any other in psychiatry. Replacing that squiggle with a drug is a task of the future.

Acknowledgment

The author is grateful for comments on an earlier version by Dr. Max Fink.

References

Abrams, R. 2002. Electroconvulsive therapy, 4th edn. New York: Oxford University Press.

Abrams, R., Dornbush, R. L., Feldstein, S., et al. 1972. Unilateral and bilateral electroconvulsive therapy: Effects of on depression, memory, and the electroencephalogram. Arch Gen Psychiatry 27(1): 88–91.

Abrams, R. and Taylor, M. A. 1973. Anterior bifrontal ECT: A clinical trial. Br J Psychiatry 122: 587–90.

Abrams, R., Swartz, C. M., and Vedak, C. 1991. Antidepressant effects of high-dose right unilateral electroconvulsive therapy. Arch Gen Psychiatry 48: 746–8.

American Psychiatric Association (APA). 1978. Report of the task force on electroconvulsive therapy. Washington, DC: APA.

American Psychiatric Association (APA). 1990. The practice of electroconvulsive therapy: Recommendations for treatment, training, and privileging: A task force report. Washington, DC: APA.

Bailine, S. H., Rifkin, A., Kayne, E., et al. 2000. Comparison of bifrontal and bitemporal ECT for major depression. Am J Psychiatry 157: 121–3.

Bini, L. 1940. La tecnica e le manifestazioni dell'elettroshock. Riv Sper Freniatr Med Leg Alien Ment 64: 361–458.

Cerletti U. 1940. l'Elettroshock. Riv Sper Freniatr Med Leg Alien Ment 64: 209–310.

Cerletti, U. 1947. Sostanze di estrema difesa prodotte dall'elettroshock(acroagonine). Il Lavoro Neuropsichiatrico 1: 367–99.

Cerletti, U. and Bini, L. 1938. Un nuovo metodo di shockterapie: 'l'elettroshock' (riassunto). Communicazione alla seduta del 28 maggio 1938–XVI della Reale Accademia Medica di Roma. Rome: Reale Accademia Medica.

Dukakis, K. and Tye, L. 2006. Shock: The healing power of electroconvulsive therapy. New York: Penguin.

Fink, M. 1979. Convulsive therapy: Theory and practice. New York: Raven.

Fink, M. 2000. Electroshock revisited. Am Sci 88: 162–7.

Fink, M. 2002. Stimulus titration and ECT dosing: Move on! J ECT 18: 11–13.

Fink, M., Kety, S., McGaugh, J., Williams, T. A., eds. 1974. Psychobiology of convulsive therapy. New York: Wiley.

Fink, M., Shaw, R., Gross, G. E., et al. 1958. Comparative study of chlorpromazine and insulin coma in therapy of psychosis. JAMA 166: 1846–50.

Fink, M. and Taylor, M. A. 2007. Electroconvulsive therapy: Evidence and challenges. JAMA 298: 330–2.

Flescher, G. 1941. L'amnesia retrograda dopo l'elettroshock: Contributo allo studio della patogenesi delle amnesie in genere. Schweiz Arch Neurol Psychiatr 48: 1–28.

Friedman, E. and Wilcox, P. H. 1942. Electrostimulated convulsive doses in intact humans by means of unidirectional currents. J Nerv Ment Dis 96: 56–63.

Glassman, A. 1975. Depression, delusions, and drug response. Am J Psychiatry 132: 716–19.

Goldman, D. 1949. Brief stimulus electric shock therapy. J Nerv Ment Dis 110: 36–45.

Gonda, V. 1941. Treatment of mental disorders with electrically induced convulsions. Dis Nerv Syst 2: 84–92.

Healy, D. 2002. The creation of psychopharmacology. Cambridge, MA: Harvard University Press, pp. 50–6.

Hermann, R. C. 1995. Variation in ECT use in the United States. Am J Psychiatry 152: 869–75.

Holmberg, G. 1953. The influence of oxygen administration on electrically induced convulsions in man. Acta Psychiatr Neurol Scand 28: 365–86.

Holmberg, G. and Thesleff, S. 1952. Succinyl-choline-iodide as a muscular relaxant in electroshock therapy. Am J Psychiatry 108: 842–6.

Inglis, J. 1969. Electrode placement and the effect of E. C. T. on mood and memory in depression. Can Psychiatr Assoc J 14: 463–71.

Karliner, W. and Savitsky, N. 1952. Office electroshock therapy. J Hillside Hosp 1: 131–44.

Lancaster, N. P., Steinert, R. R., and Frost, I. 1958. Unilateral electro-convulsive therapy. J Ment Sci 104: 221–7.

Lawson, J. S., Inglis, J., Delva N. J., et al. 1990. Electrode placement in ECT: Cognitive effects. Psychol Med 20: 335–44.

Letemendia, J. F., Delva, N. J., Rodenburg, J. S., et al. 1993. Therapeutic advantage of bifrontal electrode placement in ECT. Psychol Med 23: 349–60.

Liberson, W T. 1944. New possibilities in electric convulsive therapy: "Brief stimuli" technique. Institute of Living, Abstracts and Translations 12: 368–9.

Liberson, W T. 1948. Brief stimulus therapy. Am J Psychiatry 105: 28–39.

Lisanby, S. H. 2007. Electroconvulsive therapy for depression. N Engl J Med 357: 1939–45.

Little, J. D., Munday, J., Lyall, G., et al. 2003. Right unilateral electroconvulsive therapy at six times seizure threshold. Aust N Z J Psychiatry 37: 715–19.

McCall, W. V., Reboussin, D. M., Weiner, R. D., and Sackeim, H. A. 2000. Titrated, moderately suprathreshold versus fixed high dose right unilateral ECT: Acute antidepressant and cognitive effects. Arch Gen Psychiatry 57: 438–44.

Meduna, L. 1935. Versuche über die biologische Beeinflussung des ablaufes der Schizophrenie: Camphor und Cardiazol. Zeits Gesamte Neurologie Psychiatrie 152: 235–62.

Ottosson, J. O. 1960. Experimental studies of the mode of action of convulsive therapy. Copenhagen: Munksgaard.

Pascal, C. and Davesne, J. 1926. Traitement des maladies mentales par les chocs. Paris: Masson.

Sackeim, H. A., Prudic, J., Devanand, D. P., et al. 1993. Effects of stimulus intensity and electrode placement on the efficacy and cognitive effects of electroconvulsive therapy. N Engl J Med 328: 839–46.

Sakel, M. 1930. Neue Behandlung der Morphinsucht. Zeits Gesamte Neurologie Psychiatrie 56: 1777–8.

Sakel, M. 1933. Neue Behandlungsart schizophreniker und verwirrter erregter. Wien Klin Wochenschr 46: 1372.

Shorter, E. 1997. A history of psychiatry from the era of the asylum to the age of prozac. New York: Wiley.

Shorter, E. 2005. Historical dictionary of psychiatry. New York: Oxford University Press, pp. 22–6.

Shorter, E. and Healy, D. 2007. Shock therapy: A history of electroconvulsive treatment in mental illness. New Brunswick, NJ: Rutgers University Press.

Swartz, C. M. 1994. Asymmetric bilateral right frontotemporal left frontal stimulus electrode placement. Neuropsychobiology 29: 174–8.

Swartz, C. M. and Chen, J. J. 1985. ECT-induced cortisol release: Changes with depressive state. Convuls Ther 1: 15–21.

Swartz, C. M. and Nelson, A. I. 2005. Rational electroconvulsive therapy electrode placement. Psychiatry 2(7): 37–43.

UK ECT Review Group. 2003. Efficacy and safety of electroconvulsive therapy in depressive disorders: A systematic review and meta-analysis. Lancet 361: 799–808.

Ward, M. J. 1946. The snake pit. New York: Random House.

Witton, K. 1962. Efficacy of ECT following prolonged use of psychotropic drugs. Am J Psychiatry 119: 79.

Worthing, H. J. and Kalinowsky, L. B. 1942. The question of vertebral fractures in convulsive therapy and in epilepsy. Am J Psychiatry 98: 533–7.

10

Electroconvulsive therapy in biographical books and movies

Andrew McDonald and Garry Walter

"What is the sense of ruining my head and erasing my memory, which is my capital, and putting me out of business? It was a brilliant cure but we lost the patient."

(Hotchner, 1966)

"In my case, ECT was miraculous. My wife was dubious, but when she came into my room afterward, I sat up and said, 'Look who's back among the living.' It was like a magic wand."

(Cavett, 1992)

Introduction

With these vivid and widely quoted words, Ernest Hemingway and Dick Cavett describe their diametrically opposed experiences of electroconvulsive therapy (ECT). Often these quotations appear without explanation or analysis – at face value, they speak for themselves, but, other than further polarizing opinions of ECT, achieve little else. Looking behind the rhetorical phrases and examining the circumstances in which they were made reveals a far more complex picture, with many shades between unblemished cure and devastating failure. Recovery sometimes comes at a cost. For some people and the doctors who treat them, this is considered a fair trade. For others, it is too high a price to pay.

Readers will draw their own conclusions – two practicing psychiatrists will likely see matters differently than a disgruntled former recipient or a disinterested layperson, but these conclusions will be based not only on personal beliefs or experience, but on a series of filters through which such accounts are viewed: the remoteness of past events, the reliability of sources, the demands of narrative, the motives of the authors, and the perils of retrospective judgement.

The first part of this chapter explores these filters by presenting accounts from biographical books in which ECT is described in some detail: the context in which the treatment was given, the subject's preparation and experience of ECT, and its immediate and long-term effects. Where possible, we present contrasting interpretations by different authors of the same events and argue that their own sympathies toward physical fixes for psychic pain have a strong bearing on how they portray ECT. We then discuss how, in the small number of movies based (at times loosely) on true stories, the conventions of the genre often take precedence over reasoned analysis.

What we do not attempt to provide is a comprehensive list of every famous or notable recipient of the treatment – such lists are available on anti-ECT Web sites (www.ect.org and www.tmcrew.org/stopshock/post.htm to name but two) – nor do we mention, in this first section, every book that describes ECT. In particular, we do not discuss books in which only passing reference is made to ECT, but recommend biographies of poet Robert Lowell (Mariani, 1994) and pianist Vladimir Horowitz (Plaskin, 1983) for detailed accounts of the often desperate circumstances in which such treatment was given. Importantly, we do not try to use positive portrayals to refute the negative accounts nor, a priori, to provide an overall balance of positive and negative descriptions – to do so would be to follow the same practice as some of the more vehement opponents of the treatment and to run the risk of significant bias. We do not discuss in any depth the profusion of personal testimonies that now appear on internet Web sites and blogs, both positive and negative, as they are generally brief, decontextualized, and unverifiable, and often have a transparent agenda that has more to do with politics than with personal reflection.

The accounts of early treatment

One of the first individuals who publicly declared what he felt about the new electrical treatment was French actor, writer, and theatrical pioneer Antonin Artaud. His biography (Barber, 1993) shares much in common with other accounts of early ECT: a hostile recipient, doctors who assert that the ends justify the means, and a biographer who does not hide his skepticism of the treatment. Artaud suffered a major psychotic breakdown in the late 1930s. He was deported from Ireland in 1937 after traveling there to return a cane he believed had belonged to St. Patrick. On arrival in France (in a straitjacket), he was immediately hospitalized and would remain so until 1946, being considered incurably insane until his transfer in June 1943 to the Sainte-Marie Hospital in Cayssiol, Rodez, where over the next 18 months he received 51 unmodified ECTs. Artaud's biographer, Stephen Barber, writing in 1993, describes ECT as "*now generally discredited,*" but much in vogue in 1943 when "*many psychiatrists stubbornly believed that the temporary and clinically ungaugeable effects of the dangerous treatment were not due solely to the patient's stunned terror at the prospect of its next application.*" Dr. Latrémolière, who administered the treatments, described Artaud in his 1944 doctoral thesis, Incidents and Accidents Observed in the Course of 1,200 Electroshocks, as "*suffering from chronic hallucinatory psychosis, with luxuriant, polymorphous, delirious ideas."* Latrémolière states that, after three treatments, Artaud complained of violent back pain and spent two months recovering from a fractured vertebra, but he felt the treatment had *"very clearly diminished the bizarre and theatrical reactions of the subject in the face of his hallucinations . . . and the patient can now lead a normal life in the asylum, and devote himself to intellectual works which he would have been incapable of before the shocks."* There is no dispute that Artaud did return to writing and that the final years of his life were highly prolific, but there is also no doubt that he became vehemently and vociferously opposed to the treatment. After his first three shocks, Artaud had written to his psychiatrist, Dr. Ferdière, urging him to stop the treatment which *"has had an undeniable effect . . . in order not to risk more dangerous incidents."* His pleas went unanswered, and after 48 further treatments, his opposition hardened. Until his death from cancer in 1948, he maintained an intense rage against his perceived persecutors and what he believed to be their instrument of torture, ECT (Porter, 1987). Artaud declared: *"The mind, the brain, the consciousness and above all the body of Antonin Artaud are paralysed, held, garrotted by methods amongst which electric shock is a mechanical application and prussic acid or potassium cyanide or insulin a botanical or physiological transposition."*

In *An Angel at My Table*, the second of her three autobiographical volumes, the New Zealand writer Janet Frame describes (Frame, 1990), her years of institutionalization between 1947 and 1954 during which she received more than 200 unmodified ECTs. She paints herself as a pathologically shy and socially awkward young woman, more comfortable with books than with social discourse, who finds that *"the only way of arousing interest in those whose help I believed I needed"* is in colluding with the diagnosis she is wrongly given after an overdose – *"I again turned on my 'schizophrenia' at full flow."* She sees a counselor who persuades her to accept *"a new electric treatment, which, in her opinion, would help me. I therefore signed the necessary papers . . . I was given the new electric treatment, and suddenly my life was thrown out of focus. I could not remember. I was terrified. I behaved as others around me behaved . . . I grieved for everything lost – my career as a teacher, my past, my home . . . my sisters, my friends, my teeth, that is, myself as a person."* She does not describe the details of the ECT, but this is dramatically portrayed in the Jane Campion movie, also titled *An Angel at My Table* (1990), in which we see Janet receive her first shock. She lies on a bed in a dormitory ward surrounded by patients wailing and rocking, with one literally climbing the walls. Two trolleys move from bed to bed, the first collecting patients' dentures and the second carrying the ECT machine. A nurse comments, *"You're a newy, aren't you? Get yourself comfy."* The nurse adjusts her pillow and swabs her forehead. The treatment trolley arrives with a doctor who curtly declares, *"Good morning. Well then, we know what this is about."* Without anesthetic or further ado, she is told to close her eyes, electrodes are placed on her temples, the switch is flicked, Janet lets out a scream, a gag is placed in her mouth and she convulses violently for 15 seconds. Her voiceover declares, "*Over the next eight years, I received more than two hundred applications of electric shock treatments, each one equivalent in fear to an execution*" (Walter, 1998). Janet eventually escapes the institution, narrowly avoiding a lobotomy, after she wins a literary prize and the medical superintendent takes an interest in her.

Oscar Levant, the American pianist and actor, in his wisecracking and egomaniacal autobiography, *Memoirs of an Amnesiac* (Levant, 1965), describes a decade from 1953 onward of wildly unstable moods and addiction to barbiturates and painkillers. Along the way, he disparages every one of the many clinics and doctors with which he comes into contact. Around 1956, he consents to an eight-week course of 18 ECTs: "*There were no noticeable results. My life was that of a zombie. I couldn't participate . . . What worried me most was my loss of memory . . . My career depended on my memory and it was temporarily impaired . . . a doctor told me that my shock treatments caused some of my memory loss but that in addition I would always castrate whatever I needed. He explained, 'You depend on your memory. That's why it's betraying you.' That gave me small solace. I was a fractional amnesiac. Some lacunae in my memory remain to this day.*" It is only many years later, when his wife takes to locking him into his bedroom at night to block his access to dodgy doctors and pills, that he achieves any stability.

Hollywood actress Gene Tierney wrote in her autobiography (Tierney and Herskowitz, 1979) of a prolonged depressive breakdown in the mid-1950s. She becomes psychotically depressed, convinced she is being poisoned. She agrees to go into a sanatorium in New York City, where "*to my eternal regret I received my first electric shock treatments.*" Her mother signs the consent papers, but later says she hadn't read them, and Tierney states she was given no warning of aftereffects. She concedes that shock treatments help some people – "*In a sense, they chased the snakes from your mind. They chased everything from your mind.*" Despite her subsequent amnesia, she gives a detailed description of her first session of modified ECT. "*I woke up as if out of a dream, the kind that has no shape or detail but you know it was bad. I was confused, weak and disoriented. I recognized no-one.*" The following day, her family tell her she looks better and sounds brighter and she has an appetite. Her mother says, "*I don't understand how Gene got better so quickly. It was like the twinkling of an eye.*" She has seven further treatments, but only a week after the last treatment "*the fears and depression came back.*" She is later admitted to the Institute for the Living, where she receives a total of 32 shock treatments with what she describes as ever-diminishing returns, but mounting fear and memory loss: "*Pieces of my life just disappeared. A mental patient once said it must have been what Eve felt, having been created full grown out of somebody's rib, born without a history. . . . After a time the shock treatments left me physically ill, nauseated, and I came to dread and fear them. . . . The horror of that experience I cannot fully recapture. One feels, yes, like a lab rat."* She reaches a temporary plateau and is able to return home, but after threatening to jump from a New York window ledge, she ends up in the Menninger Clinic. She is relieved to be spared further ECT and eventually recovers with a combination of tablets, cold packs, and psychotherapy.

One of the staples of movie ECT is the nameless man in a white uniform who holds patients down while they are administered treatment. Gene Wilder was such a man, after he was drafted into the army in 1956 and stationed at an army hospital (Wilder, 2005): *"My main job on the day shift was to help administer electroshock therapy, which meant holding the patient down while the doctor induced a grand mal seizure. I had a terrible time emotionally for three or four weeks, until I started to see the good that often came from it – perhaps only temporarily. The analogy the doctors gave us was that it was like lifting up a car that was stuck in the snow because its wheels kept spinning, digging the car in deeper. When the troubled mind is no longer in the same rut, maybe it will take a new path."*

The two figures who appear most frequently in the publications of groups opposed to ECT are Sylvia Plath and Ernest Hemingway, their rhetorical words quoted with little context or explanation. Plath's vivid description of unmodified ECT from her novel *The Bell Jar* is widely quoted: *"Then something bent down and took hold of me and shook me like the end of the world. Whee-ee-ee-ee-ee, it shrilled, through an air crackling with blue light, and with each flash a great jolt drubbed me till I thought my bones would break and the sap fly out of me like a split plant. / I wondered what terrible thing it was that I had done"* (Plath, 1963).

Plath herself experienced a severe crisis in the summer of 1956 that culminated in a near-successful suicide attempt and eventual recovery following a hospitalization of several months. After becoming suicidal, she was referred to a psychiatrist who prescribed a course of unmodified ECT. According to Ronald Hayman, *"It's hard to calculate how much damage the treatment did . . . It helped to demoralise her, and death seemed preferable to a life in which she was regularly submitted to this terrifying, painful and humiliating experience"* (Hayman, 1991). Many years later, her husband Ted Hughes would disparage her treatment in his poem, *The Tender Place: "Somebody wired you up. / Somebody pushed the lever. They crashed / The thunderbolt into your skull. / . . . Terror / Was the cloud for you / Waiting for these lightnings"* (Hughes, 1998; Walter et al., 2002). It is unclear how many treatments she had before her suicide attempt, in which she swallowed a bottle full of sleeping tablets and hid in the cellar of her house, only to be found by sheer luck two days later, near to death. She was eventually admitted to the McLean Hospital. There she formed a close bond with a female psychiatrist who treated her with insulin therapy. Plath gained weight but stayed depressed and finally was persuaded to accept a second course of ECT, this time with apparent effect (Wagner-Martin, 1987).

It is worthwhile referring to *The Bell Jar* because, although a work of fiction, the fate of its central character Esther closely parallels Plath's, and it provides a much more complex reading of that much-quoted excerpt. It refers to her first dose of ECT, a terrifying experience Plath anticipates on the first page of the novel when Esther talks of the impending execution of the Rosenbergs: "*I couldn't help wondering what it would be like, being burned alive all along your nerves.*" Esther paints a vivid picture of her slide into depression – she feels like a zombie, can't sleep, wash, write, or read, and becomes fixated with death: "*Wherever I sat – on the deck of a ship or at a street café in Paris or Bangkok – I would be sitting under the same glass bell jar, stewing in my own sour air.*" Esther instantly dislikes her first psychiatrist. He rushes into ECT and treats her without explanation, anesthetic, or her consent. Later, when interviewed by her new, more sympathetic psychiatrist, Esther tells Dr. Nolan "*about the machine, and the blue flashes, and the jolting and the noise. While I was telling her she went very still. / 'That was a mistake,' she said then. 'It's not supposed to be like that. . . . If it's done properly . . . it's like going to sleep.'*" However, Esther remains terrified of the prospect of ECT, and very reluctantly consents to a further course. She approaches this with much trepidation, but afterwards, "*All the heat and fear had purged itself. I felt surprisingly at peace. The bell jar hung, suspended, a few feet above my head. I was open to the circulating air.*" She willingly submits to four further ECT treatments, grows ever stronger, and, with the aid of Dr. Nolan, who appears to have supplanted Esther's own "bad mother," makes a full recovery. Elaine Showalter (1987) argues that, after initially trying to bury the memories of her own illness and treatment, Plath later came to see her deliverance from madness by ECT as a poetic rebirth, a ritualistic casting off of her feminine vulnerability that emancipated her from a woman's traditional roles and allowed her to be ambitious and creative. In her poem, *The Hanging Man*, Plath wrote, "*By the roots of my hair some god got hold of me. / I sizzled in his blue volts like a desert prophet*" (Plath, 1981).

When two accounts of Ernest Hemingway's final months are read, the influence of the biographer becomes clear. The basic facts are not in dispute – by late 1960, Hemingway was severely depressed and beset with fears that various federal agencies were after him. He had lost the ability to write or even function in everyday life. His friends and family were increasingly desperate about his condition, finally persuading him to enter the Mayo Clinic in Rochester, Minnesota, where he then received a series of between 12 and 15 ECT treatments. These appeared to improve Hemingway's mood and general functioning, but his paranoid fears stayed intact and he complained bitterly of the effects on his brain and ability to work. He was discharged in late January 1961, but within three months had deteriorated. In late April, he twice had to be disarmed of shotguns and, after reluctantly consenting to a return to the Mayo Clinic, attempted to walk into a moving propeller while in transit. He received a second course of 10 ECTs before persuading his doctors to stop and convincing them he was better despite the fears of his wife and close friends that he was feigning recovery to achieve discharge. On July 2, several days following his second discharge, he died of a self-inflicted gunshot wound at his house in Ketchum. Although the coroner left an open verdict and his wife claimed it was an accident, there is little doubt he committed suicide.

Jeffrey Meyers (1985) and A. E. Hotchner (1966) interpret these events very differently. In Meyers' biography, we are left in no doubt of his own views on ECT, which he describes in emotive and at times inaccurate detail – for instance, he tops the list of most common aftereffects with "death." He appears to frame Hemingway's suicide as the final act of a heroic narrative, describing it as "a careful and courageous act" after outlining its literary and personal pedigree. Although acknowledging the numerous physical and mental problems besetting Hemingway, he discounts his paranoia by presenting evidence that the FBI was indeed monitoring events. In a questionable display of priorities, he observes, "*Now, in the most tragic moment of his life (far more so than his suicide), he realized that his memory had been virtually destroyed.*"

A. E. Hotchner, a close friend of Hemingway, has a quite different take on events. Having witnessed events firsthand, he provides a greater sense of the turmoil of the situation, the horror felt by family and friends at Hemingway's clearly deranged mental state, their uncertainty as to how to respond, the difficulty in shepherding such an overwhelmingly powerful if wounded personality into accepting treatment, and the dubious outcome of his treatment. Hotchner is not an uncritical advocate of Hemingway's doctors, who he believed were seduced by force of charm, Hemingway bestowing "pal status" on them and concealing the tenacity of his persecutory delusions: "*He had been to their houses for meals, and one of the doctors told me they had shot skeets in back of his house the previous Sunday.*" He paraphrases in some detail his discussion with Hemingway's psychiatrist, who describes the rationale for the continued ECT treatments. He acknowledges what improvements he sees, while giving credence to Hemingway's statements on the effects on his cognition and ability to write: "*What these shock doctors don't know is about writers and such things as remorse and contrition and what they do to them.*" Nevertheless, he appears to endorse the impression of Hemingway's family doctor and wife that the second course of ECT was terminated prematurely. He recounts his last visit to Hemingway, and despite the chilling nature of their conversation in which Hemingway more than hints that he intends to take his life – "*Hotch, if I can't exist on my own terms, then existence is impossible. Do you understand?*" – Hotchner finds hope that

Hemingway "*could be reached*" and that with further treatment he could be helped to adjust to a life in which his literary and physical "*prowesses were not so important.*"

So what does one make of these differing accounts? Was Hemingway overdosed or underdosed with electricity? It may seem self-evident that the perspectives and priorities of a close friend would differ from those of a biographer writing 30 years after Hemingway's death, and that neither account necessarily trumps the other, but what this highlights is the need to be cautious about any conclusions one draws and to acknowledge that these conclusions will be flavored by the attitudes the reader brings to the table. This caution is clearly not shared by the many anti-ECT Web sites that table Hemingway's fate as indisputably damning evidence for the prosecution of the treatment. According to the Citizens Commission on Human Rights, a lobby group founded by the Church of Scientology in 1969, "*Tricked into a visit to the Mayo psychiatric clinic, Nobel Prize winning author Ernest Hemingway found himself subjected to a series of brutal shock treatments that destroyed his writing career and his life*" (www.cchr.org).

In 1959, American rock star Lou Reed was treated, with his parents' consent, for depression and to overcome his homosexuality with eight weeks of three-weekly modified ECT treatments (Bockris, 1995). Bockris gives a surprisingly detailed account of the treatment, describing the still unconscious Reed's appearance – "*a deathly pallor clung to his mouth, he was spitting, and his eyes were tearing red*" – and makes issue of the unadjusted dose of electricity – "*the vulnerable seventeen year old received the same degree of electricity as would have been given to a heavyweight axe-murderer.*" The treatment seems to have had only bad outcomes for Reed, and he told his biographer he thought he had "*become a vegetable.*" The extent of his subsequent rage at his doctors and parents and the effects of the treatment are clear in the lyrics of his song *Kill Your Sons*: "*All your two-bit psychiatrists are / giving you electric shock / They say, they let you live at home, with mom and dad / Instead of mental hospital / But everytime you tried to read a book / You couldn't get past page 17 / 'Cause you forgot, where you were / . . . Don't you know, they're going to kill, kill your sons / Until they run run run run run run run run away.*"

Little is published of the reactions of family or caregivers, which makes English writer Alan Bennett's (2005) moving account of his mother's treatment for late-onset recurrent psychotic depression so valuable. Admitted with her first depressive episode, she is treated with ECT with the family's consent: "*We had no thought then that ECT was particularly invasive, an interference with the mental make-up of the personality. . . . I do not, then or now, see it as torture or punishment and no more routinely decreed or callously administered than any other treatment, though these were the objections to it at the time as they are objections to it now. . . . Given her first bout of ECT in the morning, by the afternoon Mam was walking and talking with my father as she hadn't for months. He saw it as a miracle, as I did too. . . . Successive treatments consolidated the improvement and soon she was her old self, confused a little as to how this terrible visitation had come about and over what period, but that and other short-term memory loss could be put down to the treatment."* Bennett also recalls watching the Ken Loach film *Family Life* in a cinema: When a doctor recommends ECT, the audience *"roundly hissed the supposed villain. Unable to join in or share the general indignation, I felt rather out of it. Faced with a loved one who is mute with misery and immobilised with depression and despair, what was to be done?"* Some years later, when Bennett's mother begins to lose her memory, he ponders what contribution the ECT may have made. He reflects whether he was wrong to sanction the treatment, but concludes that in the same circumstances, he would have done so again and still thinks *"when the controversy periodically surfaces that the opponents of ECT don't really know the half of it."*

Later accounts

There are surprisingly few available accounts of individuals having ECT in the 1960s and 1970s, the height of the antipsychiatry movement during which the treatment may have reached its lowest ebb in public acceptability and clinical use. One could argue that the release of *One Flew over the Cuckoo's Nest* (Forman, 1975) loosened the shackles and prompted those on both sides of the debate to air their views in public. Of the accounts already discussed, only those of Oscar Levant, Hemingway (Hotchner's account), and Sylvia Plath (*The Bell Jar*) precede the release of this seminal antipsychiatry film, and of the five biographies discussed here that chronologically follow the film, each discusses *Cuckoo's Nest*. Some of these books endorse the film's depiction of the treatment, but others seem determined to directly oppose its arguments, and the film *Frances* seems to go so far as adopting its narrative arc, sacrificing historical accuracy for theatrical effect.

Holiday of Darkness, in which the Canadian psychology professor Norman Endler recounts his treatment for two depressive episodes of bipolar disorder in 1977 through 1978 with two courses of ECT, appears to have a demagogic and demythologizing mission (Endler, 1982). Details of his own experiences alternate with expositions on depression, ECT, medications, and stigma, and one is left with the impression of a learned man deploying his intellect in an effort to overwhelm the illness that has temporarily derailed his life. He describes his slide into melancholia and a series of failed trials of medication before his psychiatrist suggests ECT. He explains his initial aversion to the treatment, a combination of a traumatic observation of unmodified ECT during his training and a professional bias against such poorly targeted and ill-understood methods, and tells of the 11th-hour efforts of a psychologist colleague to dissuade him from going ahead with the treatment – *"he wanted to know why I was willing to 'get half my brains burned out.'"* He has a course of seven ECT treatments with dramatic effect, such that after months of personal and work paralysis he returns to his head of department role after two weeks. However, he has been tipped into hypomania, which continues for the next two to three months before his mood settles. A year after his first depressive episode started, his mood again declines and he accepts a second course of treatment, this time with some but not dramatic improvement – it takes several more months and escalating medication regimens to return his mood to normal. Despite the partial effect of this second course, he has overcome his preconceptions and ultimately endorses the treatment as safe, humane, and effective on the basis of his own experience as well as his reading of the literature. His only other notable side effect is transient confusion during the second course, and he avoids any significant memory loss – he accepts medical assurances that such side effects are only short term. The book also contains an interesting discussion of how the ongoing demarcation dispute between psychologists and psychiatrists introduces unhelpful heat into the assessment of physical treatments.

Another clinical psychologist, Martha Manning, wrote of her experience of ECT during a severe depressive episode in 1990 (Manning, 1994). In many ways, this has a more intimate tone than Endler's work and is presented as a two-year diary with the evolution of a melancholic depression and the profound effects this has on her marriage, family, and work. Despite the efforts of thorough and sympathetic clinicians, therapy and medication fail to arrest or reverse her decline to the point where her thoughts turn to suicide – "*I can't sleep. I can't eat. I can't read or talk or concentrate for more than several seconds. The force of gravity around me has tripled. It takes so much effort to lift an arm or take a step. When I am not curled up in a ball on the couch, I pace. I rock desperately in my rocking chair. I wring my hands.*" She reluctantly consents to ECT, which she had previously opposed for professional reasons similar to Endler's. She recounts each of her six doses, describing fear at the first treatment – "*This is my nightmare . . . In my terror, I am frozen. I cannot run, or move, or scream. The waves slam me down and take me with them. I am drowning.*" By ECT number three, she expects to be desensitized, but the treatments become more difficult to endure over time. "*The hands seem rougher, the needles sharper, the band around my head tighter, the hangover longer.*" By her fifth treatment, her mood has definitely lifted; she is less agitated, and is sleeping and eating more. She initially feigns imperviousness to ill effects, spurning the advice of nursing staff to prepare for memory loss, but she becomes aware in future months of gaps in her memory, some for recent events, but others for far remoter memories she had expected to be immune. For instance, driving to a friend's house, she freezes at a set of traffic lights and realizes she has no idea where to go. Her diary continues for a year after her ECT course. This proves to be a difficult period of adjustment. When she reveals to friends that she has had ECT, some react with horror – "*How could you let them do that to you?"* but she becomes increasingly assertive – "*. . . lately I've been thinking, 'Damn it. I didn't rob a bank. I didn't kill anybody. I have nothing to be ashamed of. In choosing the hospital and ECT I chose to fight for my life.'*"

Andy Behrman, self-confessed narcissist and eponymous hero of *Electroboy* (2002) has written a dizzying account of his struggle with bipolar disorder, multiple substance abuse, and the excesses of his character. A dodgy art dealer by day and hustler by night, Behrman wonders why no tablet works and every therapist fails to fix him while after hours he leads the life of a drug- and alcohol-fueled hedonist. Depressed while serving home arrest for fraud, he reluctantly consents to a course of ECT. Waking from the first treatment, "*My head feels as if I've just downed a frozen margarita too quickly. My jaw and limbs ache. But I am elated. . . . Someone finally repaired my brain this morning.*" His mood appears to stabilize but he experiences confusion, disorientation, and memory loss, which reveals itself gradually in coming weeks but does not appear permanent. He is discharged after four ECT treatments, but within two months his mood is again swinging wildly and he commences weekly maintenance ECT that continues for four months and 19 treatments. All this time he maintains his hectic recreational substance use. Eventually, he decides the ECT is not working and calls a halt – "*the last year of ECT has sucked every bit of life from me.*" Only several months later when he finds a resilient therapist and due attention is paid to his substance abuse does his life seem to stabilize. By the end of the book, he has constructed a narrative in which manic depression has been the architect of his downfall and ECT has helped a little but, like much else, ultimately let him down. One could argue that his assessment of his treatment has suffered from unrealistic expectations that ECT, or any magic bullet, could deliver him unscathed from the chaos in which he finds himself. Behrman appears to have become something of a survivor celebrity, his memoirs being optioned for a film starring *Spiderman*'s Tobey Maguire and his Web site (www.electroboy.com) providing mental health information.

On the Sea of Memory, by *Rolling Stone* journalist and author Jonathan Cott (2005), is a very different kettle of fish. Initially stating the catastrophic effects of his course of ECT, most of the book is an exploration of memory through the lenses of science, the arts, and spirituality. From 1998 through 1999, Cott was treated at four New York hospitals for major depression and suicidal thoughts. In the first two, he received 36 ECT treatments. We learn nothing of his circumstances before, during, or after his treatment, other than his almost total amnesia for the previous 15 years of his life. He meets friends and fails to recognize them. Photos and mementos are all that remain of his many travels. He has no memory of world events or his work. Other cognitive domains are also affected: His IQ is diminished, and he has deficits in word-finding and abstract reasoning. He feels that the benefits of ECT are overstated and its ill effects grossly downplayed, and he briefly reviews both scientific evidence and the testimony of survivors. He calls for the treatment to be restricted and its complications more openly acknowledged – "*The pact with the devil that is ECT requires that one trade certain memory loss (short-term, long-term or both), possible brain damage, and cognitive dysfunction for the temporary relief of depression.*"

If Cott is quietly pressing the case against ECT, Kitty Dukakis is vehemently fighting in its defense. This very public figure writes with a campaigning zeal in *Shock: The Healing Power of Electroconvulsive Therapy* (Dukakis and Tye, 2006a). The book alternates between her candid retelling of her protracted struggles with amphetamine and alcohol dependence and recurrent major depression, and a balanced and well-researched summary of the rise, fall, and rise again of ECT by medical journalist Larry Tye. Excerpts have been republished in *Newsweek* magazine (Dukakis and Tye, 2006b), taking them to a far wider audience. After withdrawing from diet pills in the early 1980s, then seeking treatment for alcohol dependence following her husband's grueling presidential campaign of 1988, Dukakis continues to experience episodes of depression that would initially respond to antidepressants and lithium but invariably recur. In 2001, she commences her first course of unilateral ECT, which she describes in detail. The speed of her response surprises her family, her doctors, and possibly her readers. The night after her first treatment she is able to go out and celebrate her wedding anniversary. She has now become a "*fully-fledged member of the mental health family*" and subsequently returns for seven further courses of treatment. She suffers some long-term memory loss, which she describes as "*real but manageable.*" She forgets long-remembered phone numbers and does not recognize the faces of acquaintances. She states that her memory losses become less severe as time goes on. Her advocacy seems almost too good to be true, and one is left wondering how prescient is the comment of one of her psychiatrists 13 years before her first miraculous treatment: "*. . . she saw herself as having a disease for which a specific treatment would mechanically cure her of and that she would otherwise be exactly the same person that she had always been. The shallowness of that approach is surprising, if not shocking.*"

The movies

Given the evergreen popularity of the biopic and the dramatic potential of convulsive therapy, it is surprising that there are relatively few movies that portray the genuine experiences of historical characters, and some of these are of doubtful provenance. One can trace the development of a cinematic shorthand in the depiction of ECT in film, with *One Flew over the Cuckoo's Nest* exerting a dominant influence on the movies that followed. For this reason, the movies are discussed in order of production.

Fear Strikes Out (Mulligan, 1956) tells the story of baseball player Jimmy Piersall who, at the high point of his career when he makes the Boston Red Sox team, suffers a catatonic breakdown. He has a course of ECT to draw him out of his catatonia and enable psychoanalysis to begin. Shortly after Jimmy is admitted, his sage and saintly psychiatrist seeks consent for ECT from Jimmy's wife: "*I can't promise anything and I won't minimize the risk,*" he declares, and leaves it at that. This first "based on a true story" reference to ECT on celluloid is without a doubt its most unconditionally positive, and perhaps to preserve the audience's sympathy, the treatment is in fact not portrayed, with the camera stopping at the doors marked "Electrotherapy Room," through which we see Jimmy emerge unconscious on a gurney following his first treatment. The psychiatrist proves better than his word, and an unscathed and unlocked Jimmy has soon benefited from his talking cure.

A social rebel is sent to the madhouse, where oppressive and misguided doctors apply ever more radical methods of social control. Both medication and electroshocks fail to work, but finally the beast is brutally tamed by lobotomy. If this reads like the fate of Randle P. McMurphy, Jack Nicholson's star turn in *One Flew over the Cuckoo's Nest* (Forman, 1975), it also describes that of Hollywood actress Frances Farmer, at least according to the 1982 movie *Frances* (Clifford, 1982). This plot mirrors William Arnold's 1978 book *Shadowland,* which has now largely been discredited as a work of nonfiction. Arnold admitted, during a trial in which he sued the filmmakers for royalties, that he had "fictionalized" large sections of the book, most sensationally the claim that Farmer received a lobotomy (Kaufmann, 1999). In the movie, the strong-willed and hedonistic actress fights the Hollywood studios, the police, and the law, and loses. An arrest for drunk driving leads to her admission to a private psychiatric clinic where a well-meaning but misguided shrink prescribes "vitamin injections" and insulin therapy. She escapes, but is captured and is sent in a straitjacket to a county asylum where ECT saps her will to fight. At her discharge review, the chief clinician proclaims, "*I think this case demonstrates just how successfully anti-social behaviour can be modified . . . a significant victory for the mental hygiene movement.*" Her cure is, alas, short lived and she is soon back in the hospital where her last starring role before invited guests is as recipient of an ice-pick lobotomy. The once vital and vivacious beauty is reduced to a dowdy, impassive hulk (McDonald and Walter, 2001).

Not only does *Frances* appear to trace the narrative arc of *Cuckoo's Nest,* but its shock therapy scene is strikingly similar. The seamlessly choreographed sequence is thus: shackled patient is led into ECT suite (McMurphy sanguinely in restraints / Farmer struggling in straitjacket); white-clad assistant swabs forehead and inserts mouth guard; doctor applies pincer electrodes to temples of fully conscious subject; and button is pressed with immediate (but shorter lived and less convincing in the case of *Frances*) clonic seizure. Not only did *Cuckoo's Nest* act as a cinematic template for the depiction of ECT – *An Angel at My Table*, discussed earlier, does not substantially stray from this sequence – it provided a code. Thereafter in movies, the following can be read as axiomatic: ECT is bad, it is brutal, it does no good and only harm, it misreads distress or suppresses the individual, it is the tool of the misguided or the malevolent.

Shine, which depicts the triumph over adversity of Australian pianist David Helfgott, follows this pattern neatly (Hicks, 1996). As in *Fear Strikes Out*, the hero's father is the source of his suffering, but now, 40 years later, ECT does not help uncover the truth but willfully ignores it. The film's version of events has been contested by Helfgott's sister Margaret, who published her own account in *Out of Tune* (Helfgott and Gross, 1998) and accused the filmmakers of unjustly demonizing her father – they in turn staunchly defended their account (Rosen and Walter, 2000). The young Helfgott suffers at the hands of his tyrannical father. He escapes to London to study piano, but after publicly conquering the "Rach 3," he collapses, and in the next scene receives convulsive therapy. We see only the hands of those treating him. A close-up of the ECT machine reveals the voltage setting (80) and phone dial, which is rotated, delivering the dose. The camera pans to David, with bilateral electrodes secured by a rubber band and a mouth guard in situ as he gently convulses for 14 seconds, his trembling hand parodying his piano playing. A phone rings in the background throughout this scene and continues ringing into the next. His father answers but hangs up after David identifies himself. The answer to young David's problems, the filmmakers seem to suggest as the film progresses, will not be found in dialing up heavy doses of electricity, but in understanding his relationship with his father.

Discussion

Most of the accounts discussed above are of famous or wealthy individuals treated in exclusive private clinics, and – notwithstanding the many surveys that have been conducted of patients' views of ECT – it is difficult to know how much these accounts represent the experiences of people treated in large state institutions where historically the majority of ECT treatments took place. What can be said is that early biographical accounts of ECT, with *Fear Strikes Out* and possibly *The Bell Jar* as exceptions, are invariably negative. One could argue that this negativity reflects the poorer targeting and more traumatic nature of the treatment in the early days, but despite all the examples in which doctors may have overreached and patients suffered significant complications, ECT took off and spread internationally with such speed because it was then the most effective treatment available. It is fair to assume that many patients benefited from it. Even considering examples such as that of Artaud from which recipients may draw very different conclusions regarding the benefits and ill effects of treatment, the question is still raised: Where are the positive accounts? Possibly the popularity of such frank disclosures of personal crises is a more modern phenomenon and that earlier social norms and the weight of stigma may have constrained such self-revelation, but accounts such as that of Oscar Levant somewhat put lie to that. One could argue that those early accounts that remain in the public domain have been kept there by antipsychiatry and anti-ECT lobby groups and therefore overwhelmingly describe negative experiences of the treatment. The review by Braslow (1997) of the clinical interviews at Stockton Hospital in California indicates that at least some patients, especially those treated for internal distress rather than disordered behavior, spoke positively about the outcome of their treatment.

The accounts of those persons treated in the last 30 years are generally more positive, and even those individuals who are ultimately critical of the treatment (such as Jonathan Cott) are more measured and reasoned in their criticisms. In contrast to the earlier biographies in which ECT is often just one incident in a long life, albeit often at a central point of crisis or change, many of the later examples focus on the circumstances that led to ECT and its aftermath, and therefore provide greater detail and nuance. Invariably in these later accounts, the individuals emerge from the crises that prompted the prescription of ECT. All acknowledge varying degrees of benefit from the treatment, but for some the clinical outcomes their doctors consider desirable have come at too high a cost. The most common cost, and the subject on which the supporters and opponents of ECT find common ground, is memory loss. There seems a consensus that long-term memory loss is worse than doctors say, from patchy and tolerable losses, such as that which Kitty Dukakis experiences, to the severe and catastrophic, like Jonathan Cott's. When Alan Bennett's mother shows early signs of dementia, he is told that her past ECT is totally unrelated: "*I am not wholly convinced of this, if only because the proponents of ECT must nowadays feel themselves so blamed and beleaguered that they are forced into demanding from its opponents evidence of its ill effects that is hard and fast and, in the nature of things, impossible to provide.*" Some portray the "official line" as benign medical shortsightedness, whereas others are less charitable. This latter stance is best argued by American lawyer Anne B. Donahue who, although crediting the 33 ECT treatments she received in the mid-1990s as life saving, decries her severe memory loss and now campaigns for more stringent informed consent and preparation for patients receiving ECT: "*There is an aura of dishonesty about side effects: discrepancies between official positions and numerous personal testimonies of more severe problems that are discounted or left unexplained*" (Donahue, 2000).

It is impossible to read the biographies, or view the films, without imposing something of one's own beliefs and prejudices on how they are interpreted, but one must also take into account the ideas or agendas of the writers/filmmakers and the period in which their works were generated, both of which shape the way in which these stories are retold. To read of, or witness in the cinema, the often desperate circumstances in which individuals found themselves and to wonder whether, in that time and place with what was known and what was available, things would have been done any differently, is a powerful remedy to the modern conceit of moral and intellectual superiority.

References

Arnold, W. 1978. Shadowland. New York: McGraw-Hill Education.

Barber, S. 1993. Antonin Artaud, blows and bombs. London: Faber & Faber.

Behrman, A. 2002. Electroboy. New York: Penguin.

Bennett, A. 2005. Untold stories. London: Faber & Faber, pp. 32–109.

Bockris, V. 1995. Transformer, the Lou Reed story. New York: Simon & Schuster.

Braslow, J. 1997. Mental ills and bodily cures, psychiatric treatment in the first half of the twentieth century. Berkeley: University of California Press, pp. 95–124.

Campion, J. (Director). 1990. Angel at my table. [Motion picture]. UK: Australian Broadcasting Corporation.

Cavett, D. 1992, August 3. Goodbye, Darkness. People.

Clifford, G. (Director). 1982. Frances [Motion picture]. United States: Brooksfilms.

Cott, J. 2005. On the sea of memory, a journey from forgetting to remembering. New York: Random House.

Donahue, A. B. 2000. Electroconvulsive therapy and memory loss: A personal journey. J ECT 16(2): 133–43.

Dukakis, K. and Tye, L. 2006a. Shock, the healing power of electroconvulsive therapy. New York: Avery.

Dukakis, K. and Tye, L. 2006b, September 18. 'I Feel Good, I Feel Alive'. Newsweek.

Endler, N. S. 1982. Holiday of darkness, a psychologist's personal journey out of his depression. New York: Wiley.

Forman, M. (Director). 1975. One flew over the cuckoo's nest [Motion picture]. United States: Fantasy Films.

Frame, J. 1990. An autobiography, Vol 2: An angel at my table. London: The Women's Press.

Hayman, R. 1991. The death and life of Sylvia Plath. Stroud, UK: Sutton Publishing, pp. 59–87.

Helfgott, M. and Gross, T. 1998. Out of tune, David Helfgott and the myth of Shine. Boston: Time Warner Inc.

Hicks, S. (Director). 1996. Shine [Motion picture]. Australia: Australian Film Finance Corporation.

Hotchner, A. E. 1966. Papa Hemingway. London: Weidenfeld and Nicholson, pp. 260–99.

Hughes, T. 1998. The tender place. In Birthday letters. London: Faber & Faber.

Kaufmann, J. 1999. Shedding light on Shadowland. Available at http://jeffreykauffman.net/francesfarmer/sheddinglight.html.

Levant, O. 1965. Memoirs of an amnesiac. New York: G. P. Putnam's Sons, pp. 253–311.

Manning, M. 1994. Undercurrents, a life beneath the surface. HarperSanFrancisco.

Mariani, P. 1994. Lost puritan, a life of Robert Lowell. New York: Norton.

McDonald, A. and Walter, G. 2001. The portrayal of ECT in American movies. J ECT 17(4): 264–74.

Meyers, J. 1985. Hemingway, a biography. New York: Macmillan, pp. 538–63.

Mulligan, R. (Director). 1956. Fear strikes out [Motion picture]. United States: Paramount Pictures.

Plaskin, G. 1983. Horowitz, a biography of Vladimir Horowitz. UK: Macdonald and Co.

Plath, S. 1963. The bell jar. London: Faber & Faber.

Plath, S. 1981. The hanging man. In Collected poems. London: Faber & Faber.

Porter, R. 1987. A social history of madness: Stories of the insane. UK: Weidenfeld & Nicolson, pp. 141–5.

Rosen, A. and Walter, G. 2000. Way out of tune: Lessons from Shine and its expose. Aust N Z J Psychiatry 34: 237–44.

Showalter, E. 1987. The female malady, women, madness and English culture, 1830–1980. UK: Virago Press, pp. 216–19.

Tierney, G. and Herskowitz, M. 1979. Self-portrait. New York: Wyden Books, pp. 191–214.

Wagner-Martin, L. W. 1987. Sylvia Plath, a biography. London: Chatto and Windus, pp. 86–119.

Walter, G. 1998. Portrayal of ECT in movies from Australia and New Zealand. J ECT 14(1): 56–60.

Walter, G., Fisher, K., and Harte, A. 2002. ECT in poetry. J ECT 18(1): pp. 47–53.

Wilder, G. 2005. Kiss me like a stranger. New York: St. Martin's Press, pp. 42–3.

11

Professional barriers to providing electroconvulsive therapy

William H. Reid

Introduction

Readers of this chapter already know that the nonclinician public has, as a group, a substantial misunderstanding of electroconvulsive therapy (ECT).[1] That misunderstanding appears primarily related to unfortunate stereotypes, fueled by the entertainment media (not unlike some stereotypes about mental illness and psychiatric patients). One expects, however, that psychiatrists and, to some extent, other physicians and mental health professionals will transcend stereotypes in favor of clinical education and research. After all, surgeons are not reticent about performing necessary surgery, and nonsurgical clinicians are not particularly biased against surgical procedures that their colleagues may recommend or perform. In short, no one thinks twice about recommending the flaying of skin and tissue, cutting into vital organs, and probing the very heart and brain with sharp instruments so long as it is done by qualified specialists in the name of needed medical treatment.

Another medical treatment, ECT, is among the most studied clinical procedures in modern medical practice. Its relative effectiveness and safety in patients for whom it is indicated, compared with other biological and psychotherapeutic treatments, is virtually incontrovertible in objective research (see Chapters 6 and 7 in this book; UK ECT Review Group, 2003). Most patients tolerate ECT well. The great majority of persons who have experienced it report therapeutic satisfaction and few side or adverse effects (Pagnin et al., 2004; UK ECT Review Group, 2003). The author observed ECT as a child, studied it in residency, and has provided it to patients, overseen its availability in clinical settings, studied patterns of ECT use,

---

[1] This chapter will avoid the archaic and misleading terms "electroshock" and "shock treatment," even though some older clinicians use these terms. ECT is based on the effects of a neurological seizure, which may or may not be accompanied by a "convulsion" and is quite unrelated to the common concept of "shock." In fact, as most practitioners know, the amount of electrical current that actually reaches the surface of the brain in ECT is tiny (a few volts) compared with what lay readers commonly view as a "shock."

dealt with social and political concerns and barriers (discussed elsewhere in this book), and has seen at least three family members respond positively to it over the years.

Why, then, are so many eligible patients in the United States never even offered ECT? Why do so many U.S. psychiatrists and other mental health professionals fail to mention it to patients? Why are others seemingly unaware of its potential for clinical usefulness? There are professional barriers to qualified patients' being offered ECT, and those barriers are largely indefensible by informed psychiatrists.

This chapter addresses the above questions in terms of psychiatrists' training, their practice settings, common psychiatric practice patterns, malpractice liability concerns, and informal "mindset." Public and patient perceptions about ECT are addressed elsewhere in this book. Clinicians are members of the "public," too, and their attitudes as medical students and trainees often contribute to a foundation of professional barriers to good patient care. In fact, a number of studies indicate a great negative influence of movies and television (even clearly fictional accounts in comedy skits and daytime dramas) on trainees' attitudes toward ECT (Walter et al., 2002).

I have become convinced that the undeserved social stigma attached to ECT by antipsychiatry opponents and media sensationalists cannot be adequately addressed through public education or debate. Two points appear important as we try to make this and other good treatments available to the patients who need them: First, being certain that psychiatrists understand and work with ECT just as they do with other safe and effective treatments, and, second, relying on psychiatrists to make certain that ECT – and appropriate patient information and advocacy concerning it – is available to patients when it is indicated.

Barriers to care

Practicing psychiatrists, psychiatry residents, and other clinical trainees have often been surveyed about their views with respect to ECT. Medical students, psychotherapy students, and nurses in the United States and elsewhere have generally negative to very negative stereotypes concerning ECT (Andrade and Rao, 1996; Byrne et al., 2006; Gazdag et al., 2005; Walter et al., 2002; Warnell et al., 2005), which sometimes (Andrews and Hasking, 2004), but not always (Walter et al., 2002), are mitigated by education.

Although ECT is underused in many parts of the world in addition to the United States (Bertolín-Guillén et al., 2006; Sienaert et al., 2005), psychiatrists in the United States and Canada are often found to be less knowledgeable about ECT, and less willing to recommend it, than are those in many other countries (even those countries where the treatment is given without anesthesia or muscle relaxants

[Nelson, 2005]). Demographic and training issues strongly affect whether or not ECT is available to patients (Hermann et al., 1998).

Training issues

Nonpsychiatric physicians

Medical students and residents in nonpsychiatric clinical programs are unlikely to receive any exposure to ECT, even from teachers who are psychiatrists. Their psychiatric and other clinical teachers often have little knowledge about ECT, and their lack of knowledge, or, worse, their ill-founded negative bias, is passed to the student. The student then carries what he or she has learned into specialty training and later medical practice. It is not unusual to mention ECT to a primary care physician and receive a curious look and a comment such as "do they still do that?"

Medical students' attitudes may be changeable, but the available studies differ on the subject. Some studies find that increasing knowledge about ECT is associated with lessening anti-ECT bias (Oldewening et al., 2007; Szuba et al., 1992). Other studies suggest that the prejudice inculcated by years of misinformation and inaccurate media portrayals is not overcome simply through information, even in a medical school (Clothier et al., 2001).

Psychiatry residency

The Accreditation Council on Graduate Medical Education (ACGME) promulgates the official requirements for post-M.D. training in all fully recognized specialties, including psychiatry. It is noteworthy that in the entire 34-page detailed list of ACGME psychiatry residency requirements, there is only one very brief (eight-word) expectation for residents regarding ECT:

"understanding the indications and uses of electroconvulsive therapy"

– from ACGME Competencies in Psychiatry Programs, a), 3, (d)

(ACGME, 2007)

There is no clarification and no requirement to actually perform ECT, receive clinical or didactic training in it, or even observe it.

In contrast to the mere "understanding" requirement for indications and uses for ECT, all other treatment modalities and clinical ACGME requirements are described using verbs such as (underlining mine)

"using pharmacological regimens, including concurrent use of medications and psychotherapy";

"applying supportive, psychodynamic, and cognitive-behavioral psychotherapies to both brief and long-term individual practice, as well as to assuring exposure to family, couples, group and other individual evidence-based psychotherapies";

"providing psychiatric consultation in a variety of medical and surgical settings";

"providing appropriate psychopharmacologic, psychotherapeutic, and social rehabilitative interventions (for the chronically mentally ill";

"participating in psychiatric administration."

(ACGME, 2007)

There is broad variety in the extent of ECT experience provided (when there is any) in psychiatry residencies. A few programs include hands-on rotations as part of routine clinical training. Others merely offer brief, elective observations (when ECT is done at all at one of the training sites) (Dolenc and Philbrick, 2007). A "fully trained" psychiatrist ready to take his or her certifying board exams thus may have very little real knowledge of one of the basic treatments needed by many severely ill psychiatric patients.

Many psychiatric organization recommendations for increasing knowledge of ECT in psychiatry residency training have been less than ambitious. A 1999 "teaching guide for electroconvulsive therapy" (Kramer, 1999) suggests covering

"preconceptions, history, patient selection, conditions of increased risk, medical and neurological side effects, memory issues, technical aspects, electrode placement, clinical problems, management of the post-ECT course, legal and ethical issues, mechanisms of action, and educational issues"

with psychiatry residents in only six hours (admittedly more than currently provided in many U.S. psychiatry training programs). The American Psychiatric Association (APA) published ECT Task Force reports in 1991 and 2001 that included more robust training recommendations.

It is interesting that psychiatry residents themselves seem to want more education and training in ECT. Yuzda et al. (2002) found that, in Canada at least, 88% of senior residents surveyed thought "theoretical and practical" ECT training should be a mandatory part of residency. Unfortunately, Canadian psychiatry, like that in the United States, has decried the paucity of training and promulgated guidelines over the past decade or two, but little has been done to implement them. In the fairly large Canadian resident sample (91 respondents), "few (18%) feel competent to administer ECT after completing their training," and "the publication of training guidelines has made little impact on training in and attitudes toward ECT in senior psychiatric residents."

Interference from practice patterns and settings

When referral sources, consultants, and direct-care psychiatrists do not think about ECT, they do not look for it for their patients. If no one is looking for the treatment, facilities and practitioners have little motivation to offer it. Many effective treatments become better available because practitioners know they are effective (or see an opportunity to develop a market) and work to develop referral sources. This works in large population centers, but the practice opportunity is limited in smaller communities and markets, just as is specialty surgery. In some cases, it is reasonable for patients to go to a central place for hospitalization and ECT, but it is difficult to generate interest for outpatient ECT when someone must drive the patient 50 to 200 miles up to three times a week (and many communities are not even within 200 miles of available ECT).

Psychiatrists who do not practice in a community in which ECT is readily visible tend not to think of it, or not to consider that it should be a routine resource for one part of their practices. If the psychiatrist is not thinking of ECT, patients who should be considered for ECT far earlier are forced to endure painful, often dangerous, symptoms while months of unsuccessful medication trials drag on (see the subsequent section on "Malpractice and other liability concerns").

Sociopolitical barriers

An ECT suite requires a substantial – but far from overwhelming – investment in staffing and equipment (see Chapter 20). Inpatient facilities, particularly, expect to recover their investments in a reasonable way. This recovery is usually not a problem if nearby psychiatrists are aware of the service and of the potential usefulness of ECT. Unlike hospital programs that are highlighted in the popular press, such as those for eating disorders or women's issues, it is unusual for a facility administrator to think of offering ECT unless a local psychiatrist informs him or her of the patient and economic benefits.

Sociopolitical barriers can become professional ones, for example, when hospitals withdraw their support or legislatures bend to pressure from antipsychiatry groups. Some hospitals that offer ECT must deal with protests from small, but vocal and often well-financed, anti-ECT or antipsychiatry organizations.

Hospital A, a psychiatric hospital in a midwestern city medical center, provided ECT to patients via contracts with psychiatrists who performed the treatment with a local anesthesia group. The ECT suite served severely and chronically ill public-sector patients as well as private referrals from more than a dozen psychiatrists in the region. In the decade that the service had been open, it had helped thousands of patients without serious adverse reactions or malpractice lawsuits.

The facility was eventually targeted by an antipsychiatry group, which organized protests and gave local media interviews in which protesters alleged terrible damage from ECT received elsewhere. Although the number of protesters was small, the undeserved adverse publicity was substantial. The hospital administrators and board decided that an eating disorders clinic would be a less controversial use of the facility space and staff. The closing of the unit left a metropolitan area of 450,000 people with no access to ECT for more than 300 miles in any direction. Nearly a decade later, the same group used its success to protest plans for a new ECT suite in another state. The unit never opened.

Some hospitals have acted differently under similar threats of protest. Hospital B, a freestanding psychiatric hospital that offered ECT in a community of more than 700,000 people, became aware that an anti-ECT, anti-Hospital B protest was being planned by the same group. The chief medical officer called several colleagues, including the author, to discuss how best to deal with the upcoming issue.

The hospital was advised to refrain from reacting defensively, to play down any artificially created "controversy," and to refuse to be drawn into the media-manufactured "fray." When a local television reporter, who had been primed for a big confrontation by the antipsychiatry group, called to set up on-camera interviews, the hospital representative (a physician) suggested that the event really wasn't very newsworthy. After all, she offered, it seemed silly to offer publicity to a group that cared so little about patients and their access to good medical care. The protest took place as scheduled, but virtually no one attended. None of the local media gave it prominence; most didn't cover it at all. The hospital and psychiatrists continued to offer ECT without interruption.

No state has actually banned ECT (although Oakland, California, passed a short-lived ordinance against ECT a couple of decades ago). Many states have limited its use, however, often through legislation influenced by social or political factors rather than clinical ones.

Regulation as a professional barrier

State regulations and statutes are sometimes cited as barriers to patient access to ECT. Many states do not mention ECT in their statutes, and those that do focus largely on two things: the consent process and regulations regarding ECT for involuntary or incompetent patients. (Texas is an exception; see next paragraph). Harris (2006) published an excellent review of state laws (including those of the District of Columbia and Puerto Rico) regarding ECT, and noted that APA guidelines have influenced the certification requirements of the Joint Commission on Accreditation of Healthcare Organizations (JCAHO). This, in turn, affects ECT procedures and may help establish a standard of care, but probably does not put up any significant professional barriers.

Texas law stands out from that of other states, creating a situation that probably does prevent at least some psychiatrists and psychiatric hospitals from offering ECT (or offering it to certain clinically eligible patients). Since the early 1990s, Texas has mandated that all nonfederal clinical facilities providing ECT report every treatment to the state's mental health agency. Required data include clinician and hospital identifiers; patient age, sex, ethnicity, diagnosis, and admission/consent status; numbers and types of ECT treatments; symptom severity; symptom response;

payment source; and untoward events occurring within 14 days after treatment (not limited to those that appear to be associated with or caused by the treatment). During a mid-1990s study period, about 6% (117) of Texas psychiatrists performed ECT, at some 50 hospitals. ECT was performed at only one of Texas's 13 state mental hospitals, although a few public-sector patients were treated in private hospitals. Other aspects of the Texas statute make it extremely difficult to perform ECT on involuntary or incompetent patients, and forbids ECT for minors regardless of the circumstances, even though reviews by the state mental health agency consistently support the safety of the treatment and indicate that it is not disproportionately used among poor people, elderly people, women, or minority groups (Reid et al., 1998).

Social and legislative limitations on psychiatrists' ability to secure ECT for their patients often lead to tragedy.

Ms. C., an elderly woman suffering from acute, morbid, depressive psychosis, had been hospitalized for several months. Her psychosis, virtually unresponsive to medications, included almost continuous delusions of being punished and screaming as she believed she was burning in Hell. She often refused to eat and was so self-destructive that her arms were routinely restrained to prevent her from severely scratching her eyes and skin.

Ms. C. had responded well to ECT during a similar episode many years before, and had remained much improved for decades. She was psychotic at that earlier time, but her husband had been able to provide the necessary consent.

Now, once again, ECT could not be given in her psychotic (incompetent) state without a guardian's informed consent. Unfortunately, her husband and only living relative was also incapacitated and unable to accept the guardianship. A call went out to local patient advocates for someone willing to examine her situation and become her guardian for purposes of considering consent on her behalf. Several people responded.

An antipsychiatry group threatened to file allegations of patient abuse against any guardian who would consent to ECT for the patient. The state's federally funded protection and advocacy organization inexplicably refused to intervene on the patient's behalf. Potential guardians, threatened with financial ruin, withdrew. Attending and consulting psychiatrists continued to strongly recommend ECT to alleviate the patient's excruciating symptoms. Doctors and agency administrators unsuccessfully pursued other avenues of permission for treatment. After several more months of unabated symptoms, deterioration, and tube feeding, Ms. C. finally died, exhausted, in the throes of her morbid delusions and hallucinations.

The legislators responsible for clinically restrictive statutes are routinely heavily influenced more by a sensational media, uninformed but vocal zealots, and moneyed antipsychiatry groups than by facts or clinical issues. That inappropriate reliance on unscientific and countertherapeutic influences makes ECT hard to get for ordinary patients and for particular groups of patients (such as those who are psychotically depressed, pseudodemented, and demented), some of whom are the very patients for whom it is most indicated. Anyone can testify at public council or legislative hearings; the council member or legislator may not be able to discern whether or not the testimony is credible (or may not care very much, if the political issue has been billed as "controversial").

Mr. D., an ECT opponent, was well known on the Eastern Seaboard for his sensational, vitriolic comments against the treatment. He told anyone who would listen that ECT had given him a seizure disorder and rendered his life useless, despite observations that he seemed to carry on an active life of antipsychiatry protesting, drove a car, and maintained a valid driver's license. Many, perhaps most or all, of his observed "seizures" occurred at anti-ECT gatherings and city council meetings, notably in the lobby of council chambers where he was protesting.

Malpractice and other liability concerns

One hears anecdotally of psychiatrists' concerns about malpractice liability associated with ECT. Some (not all) malpractice insurance carriers charge an additional premium to psychiatrists who perform ECT. Psychiatric hospitals that need not maintain the general medical environments and staff skills associated with, for example, intravenous medication, anesthesia, cardiopulmonary monitoring, advanced cardiac life support, or even a "crash cart" are often reluctant to move toward the risks of the more "medical" environment associated with an ECT suite.

In more than 30 years of clinical and forensic practice in many states, however, often associated with malpractice allegations or management of practice or facility risk, I have seen almost no lawsuits associated with ECT. It is much more common, in my forensic practice at least, to be referred a case by a plaintiff's or defendant's attorney in which a tragedy allegedly occurred because ECT was *not* adequately considered, or was denied.

A university graduate student about to enter a career in classical music developed morbid depression, sometimes accompanied by paranoid delusions or suicide attempts. He was hospitalized many times during the course of about eight months, in several private and public psychiatric facilities. He received adequate clinical workups for the most part, each of which came to a similar conclusion that he suffered from almost continuous major depressive episodes similar to those reported in a number of his close relatives. Two of those relatives had received ECT in early adulthood many years before, both with good and lasting results.

After unsuccessful trials of different antidepressant and mood-stabilizing medications, his parents raised the subject of ECT with one of his psychiatrists, telling her of the family history of depression and ECT response. The psychiatrist told them that he was "too young" for ECT. Two weeks later, the patient committed suicide.

"Mindset"

"Out of sight, out of mind" seems to explain much of the professional ignoring of (and perhaps ignorance of) ECT. A psychiatry resident can complete training with little or no exposure to the treatment, and often without ever seeing firsthand its positive results. If there is no ECT practitioner in the area, entire communities of psychiatrists may practice for years with only an occasional journal article or Continuing Medical Education (CME) opportunity to bring it into their thoughts. Many psychiatrists, like other physicians, attend CME sessions and read articles that are associated with their practice routines. When ECT is out of a practice community mainstream, it tends to stay there.

Sometimes the avoidance is more direct. A few psychiatrists, and certainly many nonpsychiatric physicians and other clinicians, simply respond to the negative stories they see in the media. "With all this bad publicity," they may say, "there must be something wrong with it."

It is interesting to note that clinicians who do have experience with ECT, whether professional or personal, tend to become lasting supporters of the treatment. I have never talked with a psychiatrist who has performed ECT or observed many ECT patients and come away speaking against it. Even older or retired practitioners, some of whom provided ECT without anesthesia or muscle relaxants and used stimulant doses higher than is now common, speak of its effectiveness and safety. One anecdotal study of a small population of psychiatrists who actually received ECT themselves (or who observed a close family member's treatment) found virtual unanimous acceptance of the treatment and, often, complaints about its now-decreased availability (Reid, 1999).

They know, and most ECT patients know, that the professional barriers to ECT must come down, and the treatment must be taught and used on the basis of its merits, as established in research and practice, not unscientific bias and misunderstanding.

References

Accreditation Council for Graduate Medical Education (ACGME). 2007. ACGME program requirements for graduate medical education in psychiatry, July, 2007. Available at http://www.acgme.org, and present requirements are at http://www.acgme.org/acWebsite/downloads/RRC_progReq/400pr07012007.pdf (accessed September 25, 2008).

American Psychiatric Association Task Force on ECT. 2001. The practice of electroconvulsive therapy: Recommendations for treatment, training, and privileging, 2nd edn. Washington, DC: American Psychiatric Association.

Andrade, C. and Rao, N. S. 1996. Medical students' attitudes toward electroconvulsive therapy: An Indian perspective. Convuls Ther 12(2): 86–90.

Andrews, M. and Hasking, P. 2004. Effect of two educational interventions on knowledge and attitudes towards electroconvulsive therapy. J ECT 20(4): 230–6.

Bertolín-Guillén, J. M., Peiró-Moreno, S., and Hernández-de-Pablo, M. E. 2006. Patterns of electroconvulsive therapy use in Spain. Eur Psychiatry 21(7): 463–70.

Byrne, P., Cassidy, B., and Higgins, P. 2006. Knowledge and attitudes toward electroconvulsive therapy among health care professionals and students. J ECT 22(2): 133–8.

Clothier, J. L., Freeman, T., and Snow, L. 2001. Medical student attitudes and knowledge about ECT. J ECT 17(2): 99–101.

Dolenc, T. J. and Philbrick, K. L. 2007. Achieving competency in electroconvulsive therapy: A model curriculum. Acad Psychiatry 31(1): 65–7.

Gazdag, G., Kocsis-Ficzere, N., and Tolna, J. 2005. Hungarian medical students' knowledge about and attitudes toward electroconvulsive therapy. J ECT 21(2): 96–9.

Harris, V. 2006. Electroconvulsive therapy: Administrative codes, legislation, and professional recommendations. J Am Acad Psychiatry Law 34(3): 406–411.

Hermann, R. C., Ettner, S. L., Dorwart, R. A., et al. 1998. Characteristics of psychiatrists who perform ECT. Am J Psychiatry 155(7): 889–94.

Kramer, B. A. 1999. A teaching guide for electroconvulsive therapy. Compr Psychiatry 40(5): 327–31.

Nelson, A. I. 2005. A national survey of electroconvulsive therapy use in the Russian Federation. J ECT 21(3): 151–7.

Oldewening, K., Lange, R. T., Willan, S., et al. 2007. Effects of an education training program on attitudes to electroconvulsive therapy. J ECT 23(2): 82–8.

Pagnin, D., de Queiroz, V., Pini, S., and Cassano, G. B. 2004. Efficacy of ECT in depression: A meta-analytic review. J ECT 20(1): 13–20.

Reid, W. H. 1999. Electroconvulsive therapy in psychiatrists and their families. J ECT 15(3): 207–12.

Reid, W. H., Keller, S., Leatherman, M., and Mason, M. 1998. ECT in Texas: 19 months of mandatory reporting. J Clin Psychiatry 59(1): 8–13.

Sienaert, P., Filip, B., Willy, M., and Joseph, P. 2005. Electroconvulsive therapy in Belgium: A questionnaire study on the practice of electroconvulsive therapy in Flanders and the Brussels Capital region. J ECT 21(1): 3–6.

Szuba, M. P., Guze, B. H., Liston, E. H., et al. 1992. Psychiatry resident and medical student perspectives on ECT: Influence of exposure and education. Convuls Ther 8(2): 110–17.

UK ECT Review Group. 2003. Efficacy and safety of electroconvulsive therapy in depressive disorders: A systematic review and meta-analysis. Lancet 361(9360): 799–808.

Walter, G., McDonald, A., Rey, J. M., and Rosen, A. 2002. Medical student knowledge and attitudes regarding ECT prior to and after viewing ECT scenes from movies. J ECT 18(1): 43–6.

Warnell, R. L., Duk, A. D., Christison, G. W., and Haviland, M. G. 2005. Teaching electroconvulsive therapy to medical students: Effects of instructional method on knowledge and attitudes. Acad Psychiatry 29(5): 433–6.

Yuzda, E., Parker, K., Parker, V., et al. 2002. Electroconvulsive therapy training in Canada: A call for greater regulation. Can J Psychiatry 47(10): 938–44.

12

Legislation that regulates, limits, or bans electroconvulsive therapy

Alan R. Felthous

Introduction

When properly administered for appropriate indications, electroconvulsive therapy (ECT) is a safe and effective treatment for several severe mental disorders. Nonetheless, ECT is referred to as the "controversial" treatment and is subjected to regulatory legislation and even banning unheard of for other standard treatments. Histories of clinical practice, litigation, cinematic portrayal of ECT, popular and professional literature, and antipsychiatric ideologies that contributed to visceral misperceptions of ECT and the perceived need for increased legal regulation are briefly summarized. The practice of ECT has been affected not only by negative imagery, but also by a passionate anti-ECT movement, the ultimate goal of which is to abolish the use of ECT altogether. After a capsular history of ECT legislation, a more extensive account of the extreme regulatory law in Texas is explained. This is followed by the more moderate and typical approach of Missouri. Rational approaches to ECT legislation would include (a) providing no more statutory regulation than is applied to treatments with comparable risks and benefits and (b) ensuring that any legislation provides adequate informed consent based on fact and reason and protects the patient's autonomy rights as is done for psychotropic medication, while it supports availability of ECT for individuals who would benefit.

Paracelsus said the difference between a medicine and a poison is the dose. ECT, like other modern treatments, is safe and effective when used properly. For specific disorders, the efficacy of ECT is supported by some of the most substantial clinical literature among medical treatments in general (American Psychiatric Association [APA], 2001). Any regulatory law should serve to make effective treatments available to patients in need while protecting individuals from risks associated with improper use. Like the treatments they control, regulatory health laws can achieve useful purposes or create new risks. Health statutes can provide an appropriate balance between availability and access on the one hand and risk control on the other. Given the effectiveness of ECT for specific mental disorders and its relatively low risk of significant side effects, a rational legislative approach would be consistent with the legal regulation of psychotropic medications and of medical or surgical interventions with change in consciousness, namely, general anesthesia.

Unfortunately, the value of ECT has been diminished in popular perception. Because of research on the effectiveness and risks of ECT, improved technology, and clinical practices, public testimonials from persons who have benefited from ECT treatments and greater education of the citizenry about the nature, benefits, and risks of ECT, the treatment's image problem is improving. These beneficiaries include Dick Cavett, TV talk show host; Kitty Dukakis, social worker and spouse of former Massachusetts Governor Michael Dukakis; Patty Duke, star of film, theatre, and television; Vladimir Horowitz, celebrated pianist; Roland Kohloff, first timpanist of the New York Philharmonic; and Leon Rosenberg, M.D., former dean of Yale Medical School (Dukakis and Tye, 2006). Nonetheless, popular and political skepticism is persistent: In Berkeley, California, this persistence was strong enough to have resulted in a ban on ECT treatments altogether (although the ban was invalidated by California courts). As well, outside the United States ECT was banned in Slovenia in 1994 (Smith, 2007, http//www.banshock.org) and in the Swiss Canton of Geneva (Dawson, 2005). In Italy, where ECT originated in 1938, legislative restrictions are so severe that they nearly ban the use of ECT (Dukakis and Tye, 2006).

Public impressions about mental illness, mental health professionals, and psychiatric treatments have traditionally followed superstition and myth rather than knowledge. Public relations efforts by the National Institute of Mental Health (NIMH), the APA, and pharmaceutical firms have lately improved public understanding, tolerance, and appreciation of treatment. However, popular perceptions of ECT, although improved, seem not to have progressed pari passu with the growing appreciation of pharmacotherapy and psychotherapy. The Church of Scientology, with its political action group, Citizens Commission on Human Rights (CCHR), has in recent decades played a leading role in traducing, restricting, and in some cases banning ECT. Their ideology is absolutely opposed to somatic psychiatric treatments in general; but for reasons to be explored, scientologists have targeted with some success ECT in particular. The intransigence of unenlightened views is rooted in the historical evolution of ECT practices and popular perceptions that neglect technological refinements and scientific evidence describing effectiveness and relative safety. Perceptions and regulatory practices of ECT have presumably been influenced by its early, less discriminate, and unmodified use; litigation history; images projected in the media, especially the cinema, but also popular literature; and by antipsychiatric ideology.

Legislation recapitulates litigation

From its inception in the United States in 1940 (Rudorfer et al., 1997, p. 1536) until the 1970s, ECT was used extensively. Over this period, knowledge was gleaned from experience about the treatment's specific therapeutic applications, benefits, and risks. Also during this period, ECT was sometimes notably used excessively or inappropriately. Bromberg reports that one young woman received 200 ECT treatments to correct her homosexual orientation (Bromberg, 1979, p. 372)! Other more systematic examples of excessive or inappropriate ECT use are summarized by Dukakis and Tye (2006, pp. 96–8). Early in this period of heavy ECT administration, refinements in technique for reducing adverse side effects had not yet been developed and uniformly applied.

Without medication to prevent muscle contracture, fractures of bones occurred and sometimes resulted in lawsuits. As early as 1946, a patient sued because, although he suffered severe pain, his hip was not x-rayed until the third day following the ECT treatment (*Quinley v. Cooke*, 1946). Patients were not always informed of the risk of fractures from ECT because such a discussion would upset the patient. This use of the "therapeutic privilege" was said to have been a common practice at the time. A successful defense to malpractice action based on this claim was upheld by the U.S. Court of Appeals for Louisiana (*Lester v. Aetna Casualty Company*, 1957).

The jurisprudence on ECT and informed consent eventually shifted in favor of providing information about the treatment and obtaining written informed consent. In *Mitchell v. Robinson* (1960), the Supreme Court of Missouri upheld a directed verdict in favor of the plaintiff whose mental condition improved from ECT and insulin "subcoma" treatment, but who sustained several vertebral fractures. The high court concluded that clinicians who provide such treatments have a duty to provide their patients with significant information, including consequences of treatment. Because this case was based on failure to obtain written informed consent, expert testimony was not required at trial. Eventually the use of succinylcholine would virtually eliminate the risk of fractures. In another early Missouri case, a patient with paranoid schizophrenia claimed to have sustained total disability related to coma and brain damage from insulin shock therapy (*Aiken v. Clary*, 1965). The Supreme Court of Missouri reaffirmed the necessity of informed consent that included information about such serious side effects. Insulin shock therapy is no longer practiced in the United States, but because both ECT and insulin shock therapy refer to "shock," the two treatments could be confused by persons unfamiliar with the details.

Two legal cases in the 1970s initiated legal regulation that went beyond the requirement for informed consent or prompted corresponding legislation. In

Wyatt v. Hardin (1975), an Alaskan court held that before ECT is administered it must be recommended by two psychiatrists who have ECT experience and by the director of the hospital (Harris, 2006). Moreover, the court ruled some applications of ECT to be forbidden and issued 14 specific restrictions on the uses of ECT (Senter et al., 1984). Thus, without statutory law regulating ECT, the court through this single decision provided the legal regulation of ECT in Alaska (Harris, 2006).

In *Aden v. Younger* (1976), a California court required that three physicians agree that the individual is competent to consent to ECT and that ECT is indicated. The California law specified that written information for consent must include the statement that "there is a difference of opinion within the medical profession on the use of [ECT]" (Harris, 2006, p. 409, citing *Aden v. Younger*). Specific requirements in the California ECT legislation originated from the *Aden v. Younger* court opinion (Harris, 2006).

In 1984, the overregulation of ECT was decried by Winslade and colleagues, who compared federal court orders, state statutes, and other regulatory laws with standards recommended by the APA Task Force on ECT (1978). In recent years, ECT litigation has subsided and most states have remained without ECT statutory regulation (Harris, 2006). Harris attributes government involvement in the regulation of ECT to prior abuse by psychiatrists, patient advocacy groups, and a general trend towards increasing governmental regulation of psychiatric treatment in general (Harris, 2006). Incidentally, physicians have also been criticized in professional negligence litigation for failure to prescribe antidepressant medication or ECT for treatment of serious depression (Kelley, 1996.) Undoubtedly, the media and the U.S. film industry have contributed to a negative public image of ECT that makes it an easy target for regulations.

Cinematic images of ECT

Legislation is the product of politics, and politics, it is said, is driven by perception. Most people are surely more familiar with the movie *One Flew over the Cuckoo's Nest* (Forman, 1975) than with any study of ECT's effectiveness and safety. In this movie, ECT is used not as a treatment of serious mental illness, but as a method to socially control a nonconforming individual on an inpatient service. Alan Stone, a leading psychiatrist, suggested that the fictional book by Ken Kesey (1962) on which the movie is based may not have been far removed from the facts of institutional abuses. Gabbard and Gabbard (1999) described the Golden Age of Psychiatry in the cinema from 1957 to 1963, when psychiatrists were portrayed in film as offering helpful reasoning, and promoting effective adjustment and improved mental health. During this era of favorable cinematic imagery of psychiatry, ECT was presented as therapeutic, but it was also exploited for melodrama.

With the sunset of the Golden Age, films unfavorable to psychiatry became the trend, and ECT was depicted as an instrument of punishment (e.g., *Shock Corridor* [Fuller, 1963]; *Shock Treatment* [Fuller, 1964]; *One Flew over the Cuckoo's Nest* [Forman, 1975]; *The Fifth Floor* [Avedis, 1980]; *Death Wish II* [Winner, 1982]; and *Frances* [Clifford, 1982]) (Gabbard and Gabbard, 1999). Beyond the controlling or punishing motives implicated for persons who administer ECT in film, ECT itself is portrayed anachronistically as inducing a violent convulsion. However inaccurate, exaggerated for dramatic effect, and out of date, the image of a person thrashing about uncontrollably as though being savagely electrocuted is seared permanently in the viewer's affectively charged memory. *A Beautiful Mind,* which won the 2001 Best Picture Oscar (Howard, 2001), was celebrated as refreshingly compassionate toward mentally disordered John Nash and his mental health providers. In the movie, the economics genius and Nobel Laureate was subjected to violent convulsions. As suggested by Dukakis and Tye (2006), most viewers probably mistook his insulin subcoma therapy, which was administered to him in the 1960s and is no longer given, for ECT. For a detailed discussion of ECT in cinema, please see Chapter 10. Here it is important to recognize the contribution of movies in fostering negative popular images of ECT. Opinion of policy makers and of the public may not be explicitly based on the fantasy images created in Hollywood, but such images for many persons constitute an indelible exposure to ECT.

Popular and professional literature on ECT

The incompatibly contrasting images of ECT as both an effective treatment of some of the most severe and disabling mental disorders and as a barbaric practice more punishing than therapeutic were evoked and intensified in the popular press. Jenusky (1992) identified articles in popular magazines as early as 1947 before modified ECT (Not so shocking, 1947) but especially in the 1970s (*New Yorker,* Roueche, 1974; *Newsweek,* Clark and Lubenow, 1975; *Psychology Today,* Friedberg, 1975) and as late as 1980 (*Atlantic Monthly,* Hapgood, 1980) that assailed ECT. Ken Kesey's 1962 fictional book was mentioned earlier and L. Ron Hubbard's writings in the second half of the 20th century will soon be. Writings by John Friedberg, a physician, including his book *Shock Treatment is Not Good for Your Brain* (1976), undoubtedly contributed to negative popular views of ECT.

Sylvia Plath (1971) wrote a book that presumably described her own personal account of recovering from depression after a series of modified ECT treatments but not before experiencing unmodified ECT. Critics of ECT cite her vivid negative impression of experiencing unmodified ECT (e.g., Hapgood, 1980) but without crediting ECT for her recovery. In contrast, articles in popular magazines reported (Electric shock findings, 1949; Meeting on minds, 1949) and rediscovered

(*New York Times* magazine, Scarf, 1979; Comeback for shock therapy?, 1979) the therapeutic value of ECT.

Today the debate continues in popular literature. Individuals and organizations continue to rail against ECT especially on internet Web sites with pithy falsehoods and lurid imagery. Robert F. Morgan's recent book *Electroshock: The Case Against* (2005) perpetuates the effort to discredit ECT treatment. In contrast, Kitty Dukakis' recent autobiographical account *Shock: The Healing Power of Electroconvulsive Therapy* (Dukakis and Tye, 2006) is a compelling testimonial to the value of ECT when other treatments have failed. Larry Tye, her co-author, a newspaper journalist who specializes in medical issues, contributed a balanced and clear discussion of ECT that should be of interest to anyone who wants to learn about this treatment.

Overwhelmingly the scientific and professional literature supports ECT as a safe and effective treatment for certain mental disorders. An exception was an article published in 1977 by John Friedberg in the *American Journal of Psychiatry*. In the article, Friedberg stressed reported adverse effects attributed to ECT. With a survey report he completed on individuals treated with ECT and his popular writings, he promoted impressions that ECT was more harmful than helpful and that there was a difference of opinion on the effectiveness of ECT among physicians.

This brief synopsis illustrates how popular literature may have shaped the common views about ECT. For additional details, see Chapter 10. From popular literature in particular, it is easy to recognize why ECT came to be described as the "controversial treatment."

Anti-ECT ideology and movement

A remarkably politically powerful minority is persons who are not so concerned about the benefits and risks of ECT: They absolutely oppose ECT on religious or ideological grounds. Much more so than for health legislation in general, if ECT is to be made available to those in need, the distorted image of ECT and ECT's religion-based opposition must be taken into account by policy makers committed to the welfare of the citizenry, including citizens afflicted with mental illness.

Lafayette Ronald Hubbard (1911–1986) is regarded by his followers as a spiritual leader; by others as a highly creative, resourceful, and prolific fraud (see http://en.wikipedia.org/wiki/L._Ron_Hubbard). First a science fiction writer, L. Ron Hubbard later developed the spiritual healing technology of "Dianetics" and the religious doctrine of "Scientology." A major aim of the Scientology movement has been to discredit, assail, impede, and ultimately abolish the use of medication and ECT in the treatment of mental disorders.

In 1950, Hubbard published *Dianetics,* which became a best seller. It appeared before the advent of modern psychopharmacotherapy. At that time, ECT was unique in its effectiveness in interrupting profound depression and some cases of what was diagnosed as schizophrenia. However, ECT at that time was unmodified, unrefined, and sometimes used excessively or inappropriately. Dianetics, meaning "through the soul" in Greek, was a system of beliefs and practices intended to bring about "spiritual healing" (Hubbard, 1950, p. 647). Hubbard marketed Dianetics as an alternative to somatic therapies including ECT. Asserting postulates as facts, Hubbard accused psychiatrists of causing painful, but unconscious memories called "engrams" (p. 461), the cause of all psychosomatic disturbances and departures from rational thought (p. 650).

Hubbard gave importance to an electrical field that he assumed envelops and influences the body and is itself influenced by the mind (Hubbard, 1983, p. 58). He asserted that ECT deranges this electrical field, and this leads to poor health and eventually death (p. 59). He claimed that ECT was used for control, not for therapy, thereby turning insanity into a "horror" (p. 59). He described the use of medication, brain surgery, and ECT as "partial euthanasia" (p. 59). Despite the extensive and elaborate theories used to critique ECT and psychopharmacology, Scientology offers no scientific evidence to back its criticisms. Accepting such unsupported claims as factual simply dismisses the usefulness of ECT, without regard for its verifiable – and verified – nature.

In 1969, the Church of Scientology founded the CCHR (so-called "Citizens Committee for Human Rights"). CCHR is sometimes mistaken for a consumer advocacy group, but it has no interest in making evidence-based medical treatment available to mentally ill individuals. Under the guise of campaigning to protect mentally ill individuals from excessive or inappropriate somatic treatment, the CCHR actually advocates separating mentally ill individuals from all medical psychiatric treatments, including medications (see Keller, 2001).

Hubbard (1997) reviles neurosurgery, psychiatry, and ECT, using lurid, evocative imagery. Neurosurgeons use "ice pick[s]" "to rip up and tear up people's brains" (p. 210). They drill holes in people's skulls and slice up their brains. Psychiatrists use "a destructive technology"; "Under a 'drug treatment' engram you often find savage electric shocks of execution strength buried" (p. 210). He explicitly doubts whether one can witness ECT without vomiting. According to Hubbard, such treatments are not only unhelpful, they turn people into "incurable invalids."

Not all critics of ECT are followers of Hubbard and the Church of Scientology, but the shrillest image makers are ideologues who demand the abolition of ECT. Friedberg's concern about possible adverse effects of ECT is not per se unreasonable: Adverse effects of any treatment warrant attention. By referring to the practice of administering ECT as "beating up the insane" and associating ECT with the Nazi program of abusing and killing the mentally ill (1975, p. 20), however, Friedberg reveals a blind aversion that is absolutistic in its opposition to ECT. Similarly, by drawing a comparison between the administration of ECT to a mentally ill individual and "kicking a TV set when the picture begins to fail" (p. 55), Hapgood (1980) illustrates an abolitionist's loathing ideology that opposes ECT without allowance for its substantial therapeutic effectiveness.

Today several antipsychiatry organizations are set on abolishing ECT. The anti-ECT movement began in California and spread to other U.S. states and other countries. Originating in California, the Coalition to Stop Electroshock was chaired by Ted Chabasinski who had received ECT as a child. The Coalition exists on regional, national, and international levels, for example, the Coalition for the Abolition of Electroshock in Texas and the International Coalition for the Abolition of Electroshock. Another "survivor" of ECT, Leonard Roy Frank, claimed to have experienced substantial loss of memory as a result of having received 35 ECT treatments and 50 insulin subcoma treatments while involuntarily hospitalized in the 1960s. In California he brought two anti-ECT groups, the Insane Liberation Front in Oregon and the Mental Patients Liberation Project in New York, together into an antipsychiatric coalition, the Network Against Psychiatric Assault (NAPA) (Dukakis and Tye, 2006), which supports abolition of ECT. Not by accident, anti-ECT activists and image makers stubbornly highlight the outdated term "shock" to exploit its suggestiveness, violent associations, and repulsive double entendres.

Critics of ECT are not without some valid concerns. Achieving specificity of effect, unraveling the mechanisms of action, and reducing the risk of unwanted side effects are concerns for most somatic treatments. Research inquiry to answer these questions and then refine the answers is never-ending. Reasoned criticism is welcome and essential for improvement in therapeutic technologies and practices. The inflammatory rhetoric of ECT abolitionists, however, can leave the medically naïve reader and some policy makers with the false impression that ECT must indeed be controversial, if not condemnable.

A brief legislative history

Utah was the first state to enact ECT legislation beginning in 1967. According to Winslade and colleagues (1984), by 1983, 26 states had some form of statutory ECT regulation and another six had administrative law regulating ECT.

As early as 1976, the State of California enacted ECT regulatory law that stated that a division of opinion existed whether ECT was efficacious, about why and how it works, and about what the risks and side effects were (California Assembly Bill No. 1032, 1976). The APA Task Force on ECT (1978) refuted this assertion, finding "no division of *informed* opinion about the efficacy [of ECT] in appropriately selected cases" (p. 1145, emphasis preserved), and the task force itself explained how risks and side effects can be minimized by proper administration of ECT. This clarification by the APA would not disabuse the Texas legislature 15 years later of the same mistake, or dissuade it from incorporating misinformation about presumed efficacy in the "informed" consent process for ECT.

In contrast to the California law, Massachusetts regulatory legislation in 1973 was favorably appraised by the APA Task Force. The Massachusetts ECT regulation was developed by the staff of the state mental health commissioner (Frankel, 1973). A key requirement of this regulation was periodic reporting of all ECT treatments to the Massachusetts Department of Mental Health. This regulation was reportedly effective in reducing the number of patients who receive more than 35 ECT treatments per year (Grosser et al., 1975). The reporting requirement in Massachusetts was eventually repealed (http://www.maps.org/dissertation/references.pdf). From a current perspective, reporting with possible review can result in more appropriately selective use of ECT, but it can also deter the use of interventional and maintenance ECT. Indeed, between 1974 and 1980, the use of ECT in Massachusetts decreased significantly. Mills and colleagues (1984) attributed this reduction to both advances in psychopharmacotherapy of mental disorders and state regulation. However, from 1975 to 1980, the rate of ECT administration dropped nationwide by 46% (Thompson and Blaine, 1987), presumably largely a result of the negative image created by the media (Kesey's fantasy appeared on the silver screen in 1975) and messages of activists as well as high profile restrictive legislation such as the 1975 California enactment.

Legislation on informed consent for ECT was itself in disarray in the 1970s (see Stone, 1976). An earlier California law provided patients with the right to refuse ECT, but this was a right that could be denied for good cause by the head of the facility (California Welfare and Institutions Code, Section 5326, 1971). In Michigan and New York, permission to administer ECT was required of a "legally responsible person" (Brakel and Rock, 1971). Regulatory law in Kentucky stated that consent was not required for ECT (Brakel and Rock, 1971). The Massachusetts law, in contrast, was the most progressive in requiring written informed consent, a requirement of the Massachusetts Department of Mental Health, not the Commonwealth's legislature (Massachusetts Mental Health Regulation 181, 1973). By the 1990s, informed consent for ECT was the accepted norm (Schwartz and Mack, 2003), and most states with statutory regulation of ECT required consent by the court whenever the patient's competency to give consent came into question (Levine et al., 1991). For a detailed discussion of ECT informed consent, see Chapter 24.

The city of Berkeley, California, passed a referendum that banned ECT (Summary and Analysis, 1982). This ban apparently came from the successful efforts of antipsychiatry groups such as the Coalition to Stop Electroshock and NAPA. When the ban was challenged through litigation, the court held that a municipality does not have jurisdiction over ECT (Freishtat, 1985), and the California Supreme

Court declined to hear the city's appeal. By leaving the lower court's decision in place, the high state court essentially prohibited California cities from enacting laws to ban ECT (Simon, 1990). Nonetheless, the California experience illustrates the possibility of a local pocket of citizenry becoming so persuaded and moved as to attempt to eliminate this useful therapy.

Harris (2006) recently surveyed state laws and administrative codes and determined that most jurisdictions (33, including Washington, DC, and Puerto Rico) do not have state laws or administrative codes that specify the use of ECT. Illinois, Pennsylvania, South Dakota, and Virginia law "requires a court hearing and clear and convincing evidence as the standard of proof and imply substituted judgment" (p. 409) before ECT can be administered involuntarily. Three states – California, New York, and Texas – have statutory requirements that exceed the APA recommendations for ECT. In 1993, Texas replaced California as the state with the most restrictive ECT legislation; thus, here is the evolution of ECT law in this state in point.

The Texas experience

The legislation of ECT in the Lone Star State is unique in several respects. Texas has an unusual method of providing informed consent for medical and surgical procedures in general. Using the state's own structure and procedure for generating new informed consent regulations, the Texas Society of Psychiatric Physicians initiated a successful project that resulted in a progressive, new law for informed consent for ECT. Despite this new informed consent law, which standardized the informed consent procedure and respected the right to self-determination for individual patients, the Texas legislature allowed itself to be moved more by the religious ideology of Scientology than by science, and enacted ECT legislation that further regulated the procedures and created blatant flaws in the informed consent procedure. Because the ideological efforts by Scientologists to limit or ban the use of ECT continue, the Texas experience is especially instructive and timely.

Three years after the Texas Supreme Court's Barclay decision requiring informed consent for antipsychotic medication (*Barclay v. Campbell,* 1986; Felthous, 1987), ECT was proposed as a treatment that should require informed consent (Felthous, 1989). After August 1, 1989, Texas physicians had a statutory duty to obtain written informed consent before administering ECT. Information on ECT modified by sedatives and intravenous muscle relaxants must include the risks of "Memory changes of events prior to, during and immediately following treatment; . . . [f]ractures or dislocations of bones; and . . . [s]ignificant temporary confusion requiring special care" (Texas Revised Civil Statutes Annotated, 1986). (Modification of ECT resulted in fractures occurring only rarely but without entirely eliminating this risk. See Levy, 1988.) With this change in the law, practitioners knew what risks were considered sufficiently material to be shared with patients.

Four years later, in 1993, moved by a lawsuit against the Texas Department of Mental Health and Mental Retardation (TDMHMR) and by scandals of psychiatric abuses in private hospitals (Felthous, 1993), the Texas legislature enacted seven bills to further regulate mental health services. One of these, the ECT bill, also promoted by the Church of Scientology, went far beyond the legally required informed consent already in place. The 73rd Texas Legislature enacted law (Vernon Texas Civil Statutes [VTCS], Chapter 578) that prohibited the use of ECT in individuals younger than 16 years (VTCS, Chapter 578, Section 578.002(a)), mandated quarterly reporting from facilities that provided ECT (VTCS, Chapter 578, 578.007(a) and (b)), and required a misleading, if not misinformative, informed consent procedure (VTCS, Ch. 578, Section 578.003). Compared with more serious procedures such as organ removal or transplantation, life-threatening surgery, and termination of life, the ECT law was overregulative (Scarano et al., 2000a).

Texas ECT regulatory law requires an informed consent that warns simply "that ECT can result in death." This is not the same as informing the patient of the actual statistical risk of death, and that it is about the same as from anesthesia alone. Stating simply that ECT can result in death is unnecessary stigmatizing, as compared with stating the actual numerical fact. Equally misleading is the requirement to inform the patient that "there is a division of opinion as to the efficacy of the procedure" (VTCS, Chapter 578, 578.003).

The Texas law further regulated ECT by requiring that all Texas physicians and hospitals, except U.S. government hospitals, submit information on every ECT treatment administered. This information must be submitted quarterly to the TDMHMR in Austin. Reports must include the "number of fractures, reported memory losses, incidents of apnea, and cardiac arrest without death," as well as "autopsy findings if death followed within 14 days after the date of the administration of the therapy." William Reid, M.D., then medical director of TDMHMR, had the sound judgment to add an inquiry as to whether the treatment was attended with a favorable outcome in the mental disorder (see Chapter 11). Even today, a balanced survey is missing from the statute itself (VTCS, Ch. 578, Section 578.007 (a) and (b)).

Even the most radical ECT statutory regulation in the country did not quiet attempts to ban ECT in Texas altogether. Just two years after this law went into effect, a bill was proposed to ban the use of ECT (Texas House of Representatives Bill 2435). At public legislative hearings, support for this bill was provided by the CCHR/Church of Scientology, the World Association of Electroshock Survivors, Network Against Coercive Psychiatry, DisconnECT News, Advocates for Humanity, and the Texas Association for Women (Editor, *Convulsive Therapy*, 1995). Fortunately, this bill died.

The Texas reporting requirement had a useful outcome. Analyzing the large volume of data collected by virtue of the Texas ECT reporting requirement, several groups of investigators (Reid et al., 1998; Scarano et al., 2000a, 2000b; Shiwach et al., 2001) concluded what was already established from earlier research (e.g., Fink, 1978; Janicak et al., 1985; Sackeim et al., 1991): ECT is a safe and effective treatment.

Fifteen years after the Texas ECT law went into effect and nearly 10 years after the collected data were first analyzed and published, the Texas legislature has yet to make use of the information it created. The flawed law itself remains petrified and unchanged.

The informed consent model

A far more typical legislative approach, illustrated by Missouri ECT regulatory law (Mo. Rev. Stat., Section 630.130) essentially requires informed consent for ECT and court approval if ECT is proposed to be administered against the patient's will.

Toward constructive law making

As a rule, medical treatment decisions and practices are left to the individual practitioners. Regulation to ensure an acceptable level of practice is provided through professional organizations, litigation, and statutory or administrative law. Medical boards endeavor to ensure that physicians are competent to practice medicine and specialty boards, their specialty (such as psychiatry). Professional organizations further provide continuing medical education, practice guidelines, and ethical principles. Within the profession of psychiatry itself, various methods can be used to ensure that practitioners provide safe and effective and ethical treatment, including ECT.

Because ECT is no less safe and no less effective than psychopharmacotherapy, ECT should require legislative regulation that is no more stringent, limiting, or cumbersome than for psychotropic medication or any procedure requiring general anesthesia. Regulatory law can reasonably set parameters for informed consent and involuntary ECT, as is done for psychotropic medication. Risk–benefit analysis of ECT should be based on science, not presupposition and media imagery. Apart from the risks and benefits of ECT itself, policy makers might want to consider litigation trends for further management of risk (See Simon and Sadoff, 1992). The APA Task Force reports on ECT (first and second editions, APA, 1978, 2001), and this comprehensive book can serve as a resource. Noteworthy is that the second

APA ECT Task Force report focuses on clinical and professional recommendations, and the first edition's chapter on "Social, Ethical and Legal Aspects of ECT" was not carried over into the second edition. The introduction to the second edition simply advises practitioners to inform themselves about regulatory law in their jurisdiction of practice.

One legislative approach to ECT is to initiate nothing. After all, most states (33 if the District of Columbia and Puerto Rico are included; Harris, 2006) have no special ECT statutory law. Refraining from proposing legislation, at least in these states, has not resulted in adversive law. Even the no-new-ECT bills approach, nonetheless, should not amount to a totally laissez-faire approach, because the CCHR and others ideologically opposed to ECT could try to introduce their own anti-ECT bill whenever the state legislature is in session. Advocates for making effective and safe treatments available to mentally disordered individuals should have an ongoing, continuously updating strategy for addressing such contingencies, including the most up-to-date information on the nature, indications, clinical standards, efficacy, and risks of ECT.

Proactive initiatives and contingency planning must take into account the possibility of court-generated ECT regulation through lawsuits, however uncommon. As discussed earlier, the *Wyatt v. Hardin* case in Alaska demonstrated that court decisions can be as regulatory as statutory law. *Aden v. Younger* in California illustrated that case law can prompt or inform statutory law, which in turn then mirrors aspects of the court opinion. ECT litigation is much more difficult for the medical and mental health communities to identify and track than is pending legislation.

Proactive ECT regulatory law in Texas did not prevent excessive regulatory law from being enacted. Moreover, the potentially useful information about the effectiveness and safety of ECT registered pursuant to ECT regulatory law itself has so far not led to corrective legislation in the state with the most extreme ECT regulatory law.

After misleading ECT legislation has been enacted, it can remain as though engraved in stone, even when information generated by ECT law itself should correctively inform policy makers. A constructive legislative approach in states with misleading law would be to at least attempt to correct those elements of the law that are especially misleading or misinforming.

Conclusions

In recent decades a strong effort to diminish, restrict, and ban ECT has come from the Church of Scientology and its CCHR, as well as from other ideologically motivated groups such as the Coalition to Abolish Electroshock. It has been allowed some success, however, only because of popular (and therefore political) perceptions shaped by early ECT practices and lawsuits, and by images in the media, in the popular literature, and especially the entertainment media. Through improvements in ECT technique, proper education about the nature of serious depression and psychosis and ECT, and through testimonials from individuals who have benefited from ECT, a more realistic popular understanding of ECT is emerging. Nonetheless, the mental health community must be prepared to respond to litigation claims and legislative initiatives from which misinformed, ideologically driven regulations can appear. When lawmakers concern themselves with patients' autonomy rights, due process, and the availability of safe and effective treatment, rather than with micromanaging treatment based on unscientific ideology, health law legislation will support the availability of safe and effective treatments. Then the patient benefits. Then any absolutist ideology opposed to all somatic therapies has no relevance to judicial and legislative regulation of health care, including ECT and other somatic treatments for individuals with severe mental illness.

References

Aden v. Younger, 129 Cal. Rptr. 535 (Cal. Ct. App., 1976).

Aiken v. Clary, 396 S.W. 2d 668 (Mo., 1965).

American Psychiatric Association (APA). 1978. Electroconvulsive therapy, Task Force Report 14. Washington, DC: APA.

American Psychiatric Association (APA). 2001. The practice of electroconvulsive therapy: Recommendations for treatment, training and privileging, 2nd edn. Washington, DC: APA.

Avedis, H. H. (Director). 1980. The fifth floor [Motion picture]. United States: Hickmar Productions.

Barclay v. Campbell, 704 S.W. 2d 8 (Tex. Sup. Ct., 1986).

Brakel, S. and Rock, R. 1971. The mentally disabled and the law. Chicago: University of Chicago Press.

Bromberg, W. 1979. The uses of psychiatry in the law: Clinical view of forensic psychiatry. Westport, CT: Quorum Books.

California Assembly Bill No. 1032, 1976.

California Welfare and Institutions Code, Section 5326, West Supp., 1971.

Clark, M. and Lubenow, G. 1975. Attack on electroshock. Newsweek (Mr 17) 85: 86.

Clifford, G. (Director). 1982. Frances [Motion picture]. United States. Universal.

Comeback for shock therapy? 1979. Time (N19) 114: 76.

Dawson, J. 2005. Community treatment orders: International comparisons, May 2005. Cited in "ECT is Banned in Swiss Canton." Available at www.ect.org/category/legislation. Accessed September 17, 2008.

Dukakis, K. and Tye, L. 2006. Shock: The healing power of electroconvulsive therapy. New York: Penguin Group.

Editor. 1995. News and notes: Anti-ECT legislation in Texas. Convuls Ther 11(2): 148.

Electric shock findings. 1949. Newsweek (Ja 17) 33: 43.

Felthous, A. R. 1987. Barclay v. Campbell: Informed consent for antipsychotic medication comes to Texas. Newsl Am Acad Psychiatry Law 12(1): 7–9.

Felthous, A. R. 1989. Legislative update. Newsl Am Acad Psychiatry Law 14(2): 51–3.

Felthous, A. R. 1993. Legislative update. Newsl Am Acad Psychiatry Law 18(3): 69–71.

Fink, M. 1978. Efficacy and safety of induced seizures (EST) in man. Compr Psychiatry 19: 1–9.

Forman, M. (Director). 1975. One flew over the cuckoo's nest [Motion picture]. United States: Fantasy Films.

Frankel, F. H.,1973. ECT in Massachusetts: A task force report. Mass Journal Ment Health 3: 3–29.

Freishtat, H. W. 1985. Electroconvulsive therapy: No ban in Berkeley. J Clin Psychopharmacol 5: 52–3.

Friedberg, J. 1975. Electroshock therapy: Let's stop shocking the brain. Psychology Today 9(3): 18, 20–21, 23, 25–26.

Friedberg, J. 1976. Shock treatment is not good for your brain. San Francisco: Glide Publications.

Friedberg, J. 1977. Shock treatment, brain damage, and memory loss: A neurological perspective. Am J Psychiatry 134(9): 1010–14.

Fuller, S. (Director). 1963. Shock corridor [Motion picture]. United States: Leon Fromkess-Sam Firks Productions.

Fuller, S. (Writer, director, and producer). 1964. Shock treatment [Motion picture]. United States: Arcola Pictures.

Gabbard, G. O. and Gabbard, K. 1999. Psychiatry and the cinema, 2nd edn. Washington, DC: American Psychiatric Press.

Grosser, G. H., Pearsall, D. J., Fisher, C. L., et al. 1975. The regulation of ECT in Massachusetts: A follow-up. Mass Journal Ment Health 5: 12–25.

Hapgood, F. 1980. Electroshock: The unkindest therapy of all. Atlantic Monthly 245: 53–6, 58–9.

Harris, V. 2006. Electroconvulsive therapy: Administrative codes, legislation and professional recommendations. J Am Acad Psychiatry Law 34(3): 406–11.

Howard, R. (Director). 2001. A beautiful mind [Motion picture]. United States: Universal Pictures.

Hubbard, L. R. 1950. Dianetics: The modern science of mental health. Los Angeles: Bridge Publications, Inc.: L. Ron Hubbard Library, 1950, 2000, 2002.

Hubbard, L. R. 1983. Scientology: The fundamentals of thought. Los Angeles: Bridge Publications, Inc.: L. Ron Hubbard Library, 1983, 1988, 1991.

Hubbard, L. R. 1997. Scientology: A new slant on life. Los Angeles: Bridge Publications, Inc.

Janicak, P. G., David, J. M., and Gibbons, R. D. 1985. Efficacy of ECT. A meta-analysis. Am J Psychiatry 132: 297–302.

Jenusky, S. M. 1992. Public perceptions of electroconvulsive therapy: A historical review. The Jefferson Journal of Psychiatry 10: 2–11.

Keller, R. 2001. Presenting Rod Keller's alt.religion.scientology week in review 5(40) Jan 21, 2001. Citing article in *Atlantic Monthly*. http://www.xenu.net/archive/WR/wir-40.html.

Kelley, J. L. 1996. Psychiatric malpractice: Stories of patients, psychiatrists and the law. New Brunswick, NJ: Rutgers University Press, pp. 117–133, p. 129. (For sources for Chapter 9, The

Osheroff's Case, Kelley relied on depositions taken in the case, Osheroff v. Chestnut Lodge Hospital, Inc., Claim No. 82-262, Health Claims Arbitration Office, State of Maryland.)

Kesey, K. 1962. One flew over the cuckoo's nest. New York: Viking Press.

L. Ron Hubbard. http://en.wikipedia.org/wiki/L._Ron_Hubbard, accessed December 22, 2007.

Lester v. Aetna Casualty Company, 240 F. 2d 676, Cir., 5th Dist. (La., 1957).

Levine, S. B., Blank, K., Schwartz, H. I., and Rait, D. S. 1991. Informed consent in the electroconvulsive treatment of geriatric patients. Bull Am Acad Psychiatry Law 19: 395–403.

Levy, S. 1988. Letter to the Editor. "Cuff" monitoring, osteoporosis and fracture. Convuls Ther 4(3): 248–9.

Massachusetts Mental Health Regulation 181, effective May 1, 1973.

Meeting on minds. 1949. *Newsweek* (Je 6): 47–9.

Mills, M. J., Pearsall, D. T., Yesavage, J. A., and Salzman, C. 1984. Electroconvulsive therapy in Massachusetts. Am J Psychiatry 141(4): 534–8.

Missouri Revised Statute, Section 630.130.

Mitchell v. Robinson, 334 S.W. 2d 11 (Mo., 1960).

Morgan, R. F. 2005. Electroshock: The case against. Morgan Foundation Publisher: International Published Innovation.

Not so shocking. September 8, 1947. *Time*. Available at: http://www.time.com/time/magazine/article/0,9171,804181,00.thml?iid=digg_share, accessed December 26, 2008.

Plath, S. 1971. The bell jar. New York: Harper & Row.

Quinley v. Cooke, 192 S.W. 2d 992 (Tenn., 1946).

Reid, W. H., Keller, S., Leatherman, M., and Mason, M. 1998. ECT in Texas: 19 months of mandatory reporting. J Clin Psychiatry 59(1): 8–13.

Roueche, B. 1974. Annals of medicine: Empty as Eve. *New Yorker* (89)50: 84.

Rudorfer, M. V., Henry, M. E., and Sackeim, H. A. 1997. Electroconvulsive therapy. In Psychiatry (eds. Tasman, A., Kay, J., and Liberman, J. A.). Vol. 2. Philadelphia: W. B. Saunders Company, pp. 1535–1556, 1536.

Sackeim, H. A., Prudic, J., and Devanand, D. P. 1991. Stimulus intensity, seizure threshold and seizure duration: Impact on the efficacy and safety of electroconvulsive therapy. Psychiatr Clin North Am 14: 803–43.

Scarano, V. R., Felthous, A. R., and Early, T. S. 2000a. The state of electroconvulsive therapy in Texas, Part 1. Reported data on 41,660 ECT treatments in 5971 patients. J Forensic Sci 45(6): 1197–202.

Scarano, V. R. Felthous, A. R., and Early T. S. 2000b. The state of electroconvulsive therapy in Texas, Part 2: Contact with physicians, hospitals, medical liability insurance companies, and manufactures of stimulus generating equipment. J Forensic Sci 45(6): 1203–6.

Scarf, M. 1979. Shocking the depressed back to life. New York Times Magazine (June 17): 32–4, 38, 42.

Schwartz, H. I. and Mack, D. M. 2003. Informed consent and competency. In Principles and practice of forensic psychiatry, 2nd edn. (ed. Rosner, R.). London: Arnold, pp. 97–106.

Senter, N. W., Winslade, W. J., Liston, E. H., et al. 1984. Electroconvulsive therapy: The evolution of legal regulation. Am J Soc Psychiatry 4: 11–15.

Shiwach, R. S., Reid, W. H., and Carmody, T. J. 2001. An analysis of reported deaths following electroconvulsive therapy in Texas, 1993–1998. Psychiatr Serv 52(8): 1095–7.

Simon, R. I. 1990. Somatic therapies and the law. In Review of clinical psychiatry and the law (ed. Simon, R. I.). Vol. 1. Washington, DC: American Psychiatric Press, pp. 3–79.

Simon, R. I. and Sadoff, R. L. 1992. Psychiatric malpractice: Cases and comments for clinicians. Washington, DC: American Psychiatric Press.

Smith, W. 2007. First in world: Shock free zone announced: Republic of Slovenia. http://www.banshock.org. Accessed December 15, 2007, and September 17, 2008.

Stone, A. A. 1976. Mental health and law: A system in transition. New York: Aronson.

Summary and analysis. 1982. Mental Disability Law Reporter 6: 366.

Texas House of Representatives Bill 2435.

Texas Revised Civil Statutes Annotated, Article 4590; 6.07 (b) (Vernon Supp., 1986).

Thompson, J. W. and Blaine, J. D. 1987. The use of ECT in the United States in 1975 and 1980. Am J Psychiatry 144(5): 557–62.

Vernon Texas Civil Statutes. Title 7. Mental Health and Mental Retardation. Chapter 578. Electroconvulsive and other therapies.

Vernon Texas Civil Statutes. Title 7. Mental Health and Mental Retardation. Chapter 578. Electroconvulsive and other therapies. Section 578.002(a).

Vernon Texas Civil Statutes. Title 7. Mental Health and Mental Retardation. Chapter 578. Electroconvulsive and other therapies. Section 578.003.

Vernon Texas Civil Statutes. Title 7. Mental Health and Mental Retardation. Chapter 578. Electroconvulsive and other therapies. Section 578.007(a) and (b).

Winner, M. (Director). 1982. Death wish II [Motion picture]. United States: Cannon Films.

Winslade, W. J., Liston, E. H., Ross, J. W., and Weber, K. D. 1984. Medical, judicial and statutory regulation of ECT in the United States. Am J Psychiatry 141: 1349–5.

Wyatt v. Hardin. U.S. Dist. (M.D. Ala., 1975).

Part III

International perspectives

Electroconvulsive therapy availability in the United States

Michelle Magid and Barbara M. Rohland

Introduction

Electroconvulsive therapy (ECT) was first administered in Rome by Ugo Cerletti and Lucio Bini in 1938 (Cerletti, 1950). Dr. Renato Almansi, an associate of Dr. Cerletti in Rome, brought a treatment apparatus from Italy to the United States, where it was used by Dr. David Impastato, an American psychiatrist, at Columbus Hospital in New York City in 1940 to perform ECT treatment (Impastato, 1960). Lebensohn (1999) describes the historical context of the introduction of ECT to American psychiatry. The ambivalence that the public and the psychiatric community have toward ECT has many explanations (see Chapters 9–12), and these presumably contribute to the regional variation in ECT use.

During the past 60 years, ECT trends in the United States have fluctuated. Thompson et al. (1994) analyzed nationally representative data from the National Institute of Mental Health (NIMH) to evaluate trends in the use of ECT in psychiatric hospitals in the United States in 1975, 1980, and 1985. In 1975, the NIMH reported that 58,667 patients received ECT treatments. Despite a growing population, this number decreased to 31,514 in 1980, and remained unchanged (when accounting for population growth) in 1986 at 36,558 patients. ECT was used primarily in private hospitals, rather than public general, state, or county mental hospitals. In 1986, more than 90% of patients who received ECT were White, and 84% carried the diagnosis of a mood disorder. Age was found to be more important than gender in predicting ECT use, but more than 70% of the ECT patients in the 1986 sample were female. Patients older than 65 years, primarily insured by Medicare, received ECT in greater proportion than the number of patients hospitalized.

Despite growing evidence of the safety and efficacy of ECT (e.g., Chapters 6, 7, 9, 11, 12, 19, 20, 22–28, 31), there are large variations in the use of ECT in the United States. ECT availability increases with higher population density and closer proximity to an academic medical center, and varies with geographic region (higher in the Northeast and Midwest than the West or South). Availability is greater in private and nonprofit hospitals than in state hospitals and is increasing in outpatient settings. Patients older than 65 treated under Medicare are more likely to receive ECT than younger, uninsured, or non-Medicare insured patients. Here we review the details of these patterns.

Sources of variation

In a study by Hermann et al. (1995), wide variation in ECT use was observed, suggesting that ECT is among the highest variation procedures in medicine. Recognizing the inverse relationship between variability and quality, the U.S. Agency for Health Care Policy and Research (now reorganized as the Agency for Healthcare Research and Quality) has encouraged medical specialties such as the American Psychiatric Association (APA) to develop guidelines to reduce variation in its practices, including ECT. However, research studies to determine factors associated with variation in the utilization of ECT in this country are limited.

In their study, Hermann et al. (1995) measured variation in ECT utilization rates across nonrural areas of the United States using data from the APA 1988–1989 Professional Activities Survey. This was a survey of 17,729 psychiatrists practicing in 317 metropolitan statistical areas across the United States. In the 202 metropolitan statistical areas in which ECT was reported, annual ECT use varied from 0.4 to 81.2 patients per 10,0000 population. The estimated rate of national ECT utilization was 4.9 patients per 10,000. Sources of variation that they examined included health care system characteristics, demographic factors, and state regulations affecting the initiation and delivery of ECT treatment. The strongest predictors of variation in ECT were the number of psychiatrists, the number of primary care physicians, the number of private hospital beds per capita, and the stringency of state regulations.

Small-area analysis

Our understanding and approach to the identification of determinants of small-area variation have been informed by health service researchers such as Wennberg and Gittelsohn (1973). In a population-based analysis of health service delivery, epidemiologic factors, such as characteristics of the health system, may explain variation in the delivery of procedures and treatments beyond that associated with the medical condition itself. Approximately 90% of ECT patients receive it for the treatment of depression, consistent with APA guidelines (APA, 2000). Regarding beneficiaries of a large New England insurance company in 1994–1995, 86.5% of ECT courses were performed on patients with a diagnosis within evidence-based indications, and one half of the 13.5% courses of ECT outside the indications were on patients with depressive disorders (Hermann et al., 1999). In this study, patients who received ECT for diagnoses outside evidence-based indications were more likely to be treated by psychiatrists who graduated between 1940 and 1980 than by those who graduated after 1981.

The incidence of depression has little regional variation and does not explain the variation in the rates or availability of treatment. Among the five sites of the Epidemiologic Catchment Area (ECA) Study, the one-year prevalence of depression was remarkably consistent and ranged from 1.7% to 3.4% (Robins and Regier, 1991). Moreover, little variation is explained by psychiatrists using ECT for disorders other than major depression.

State and regional variation

In the 1995 study by Hermann et al., several ECT regions of high utilization were identified within the United States. Specifically, high ECT use occurred in the northeastern region of the United States, and low ECT use occurred in the western region. Olfson et al. (1998), in a study looking at the use of ECT for inpatient treatment of recurrent major depression, also noted geographic variation in ECT use. Patients with depression in midwestern states (i.e., Minnesota, Iowa, Missouri, North Dakota, South Dakota, Nebraska, and Kansas) were four times more likely to receive ECT than were patients with similar illness characteristics in the mountain states (i.e., Montana, Idaho, Wyoming, Colorado, New Mexico, Arizona, Utah, and Nevada). Patients in the Northeast (particularly the New England states) and the Midwest were twice as likely to receive ECT as were their counterparts in western states. A study of Medicare patients (Rosenbach et al., 1997) showed similar geographic distribution; ECT use was the highest in the Northeast, the lowest in the West.

A strong relationship between ECT use and the presence of an academic medical center has also been described (Hermann et al., 1995). Almost one half (43.6%) of the metropolitan areas in which ECT was performed had one or more academic centers. The highest rates of ECT utilization were in small metropolitan areas with prominent academic medical centers, for example, Rochester, Minnesota (Mayo Clinic); Charlottesville, Virginia (University of Virginia); Iowa City, Iowa (University of Iowa); Ann Arbor, Michigan (University of Michigan); and Raleigh-Durham, North Carolina (Duke University/University of North Carolina).

Service system variation

The strongest determinants of ECT use in a metropolitan area are the number of psychiatrists and primary care physicians per capita (Hermann et al., 1995). ECT use is also related to the number of private hospital beds per capita. A paucity of ECT use in rural areas was noted both in a study looking at ECT use in patients with depression (Olfson et al., 1998) and in a study looking at the use of ECT in North Carolina, a predominantly rural state (Creed et al., 1995).

Service site: Public versus private hospital

ECT utilization varies with whether the hospital is public or private. Several studies have documented that ECT is more commonly used in private hospitals than in public hospitals (Bailine and Rau, 1981; Kramer, 1990, 1999; Mills et al., 1984; Olfson et al., 1998; Thompson and Blaine, 1987; Thompson et al., 1994) and that more than 90% of inpatient ECT occurs in private hospitals (Kramer, 1990, 1999; Olfson et al., 1998). It is not clear if state-funded academic medical centers are classified as public or private, but in most studies public hospitals are defined as state, county, district, Veterans Administration (VA), or forensic hospitals. ECT was once commonly and indeed primarily performed in state hospitals, but ECT availability in state hospitals is now extremely variable from state to state, and sometimes from one state hospital to another within the same state. In addition to economic factors, state-run facilities can have more extensive administrative steps than private hospitals have in authorizing or providing ECT, especially if the patient is involuntary or has a guardian (Grosser et al., 1975; Kramer, 1985; Mills et al., 1984). In 1987, only 19% of state hospitals in the southern United States offered ECT. This is a 40% decrease from 10 years earlier (McCall, 1989). Mandatory ECT reporting in Texas revealed that ECT was offered on-site at only 1 (7%) of its 13 state-run mental institutions (Reid et al., 1998). In California, fewer than 6% of ECT recipients received this treatment at a state hospital. Between 1975 and 1980, Thompson et al. reported a 74% decrease in the number of state hospital patients receiving ECT (Thompson and Blaine, 1987; Thompson et al., 1994); this corresponds to 1.2% of all state inpatients receiving ECT in 1975, but only 0.3% in 1980. A 10-year review of patients receiving ECT in a state hospital in Pennsylvania revealed that only 21 patients were treated with ECT during that entire time period, representing 0.4% of all admissions there (Sylvester et al., 2000). In short, during the past few decades, state hospitals have gone from having the highest to the lowest ECT availability, and state hospital patients make up the hospitalized seriously ill psychiatric group least likely to receive ECT.

Service site: Inpatient versus outpatient

Except for its early introduction in this country (when ECT was sometime administered in patients' homes with a portable unit or in private doctors' offices) (Lebensohn, 1999), ECT has been almost exclusively considered and performed as an inpatient procedure, largely because the administration and risks of anesthesia. In 1993, approximately 10% of all general hospital adult inpatients admitted for recurrent major depression received ECT treatments (Olfson et al., 1998). Because of advances in anesthesiology and cardiac care, ECT has become safer and more tolerable (see Chapters 25 and 26). In addition, third party payors have associated the length and subsequent costs of hospital stays with inpatient ECT treatment and have created financial incentives to provide outpatient options for ECT treatment. Olfson et al. (1998) and others have presented data suggesting that prompt administration of ECT is associated with shorter and less costly hospital stays, and that higher treatment costs and longer stays associated with ECT delivery are a consequence of delay in beginning ECT. Rosenbach et al. (1997) reported that the proportion of ECT patients who were outpatients has more than doubled, from 7% to 16% in recent years. In this study, the proportion of Medicare reimbursement for ECT for outpatient versus inpatient expenditures was shown to vary by region, with a low of 9.8% in the West, and 19.1% in the North Central region.

Demographic variation: Age, gender, race/ethnicity, and socioeconomic factors

The "typical" ECT patient in the United States is an elderly White woman with insurance (often Medicare) who is admitted to a private hospital. Hence, the demographic factors that are associated with variation in the use of ECT include age, gender, race/ethnicity, and socioeconomic factors, particularly insurance or third party coverage.

Age

Age is the most powerful predictor of ECT use in the United States (Olfson et al., 1998). Major depressive disorder is prevalent in the elderly population, and many persons who receive ECT for the treatment of their depression are older than 65 years, partly because older depressed patients respond favorably to ECT and are more accepting of the risks associated with it (Kahn et al., 1957; O'Connor et al., 2001). It is estimated that ECT use increased by 30% in the geriatric population between 1987 and 1992. This percentage is equivalent to a total increase from 12,000 to 15,560 geriatric patients receiving ECT annually (Rosenbach et al., 1997). Conversely, ECT is seldom used in children and teenagers. Fewer than 1% of ECT patients are younger than 18 years (Kramer, 1999; Olfson et al., 1998).

Gender

The lifetime risk for major depressive disorder in the United States is 10% to 25% in females and 5% to 12% in males (APA, 2000). One study indicated that males and females were equally likely to receive ECT when factors such as age and diagnosis were controlled (Thompson and Blaine, 1987). However, most studies indicate that females are twice as likely as males to receive ECT (Babigian and Guttmacher, 1984; Grosser et al., 1975; Kramer, 1985; Mills et al., 1984; Reid et al., 1998; Rosenbach et al., 1997; Scarano et al., 2000; Sylvester et al., 2000), and this closely correlates to gender prevalence rates of major depressive disorder.

Race/Ethnicity

Several studies have shown that more than 80% (in most studies, closer to 90%) of U.S. patients receiving ECT are White (Breakey and Dunn, 2004; Kramer, 1999; Olfson et al., 1998; Reid et al., 1998; Scarano et al., 2000; Sylvester et al., 2000). ECT is less likely to be used for Hispanics and African Americans than for Whites. Texas, for example, reported that 87.3% of patients receiving ECT were White, with the remainder being 8.5% Hispanics, 3.3% African Americans, and 0.7% Asians (Scarano et al., 2000). In California, even fewer minority patients make up the population of patients receiving ECT (Kramer, 1999). Given that the U.S. percentages of Caucasian, Hispanic, African American, and Asian populations are 66.9%, 14.4%, 12.8%, and 4.3%, respectively, these data provide strong evidence that minority groups are less likely to receive ECT if one assumes that their risk for a disorder with an evidence-based indication for ECT is at least equal. This disparity in access to ECT may be caused by minorities having less access to physicians, private hospitals, and ECT from economic factors, less likelihood of geographic proximity, attitudes of psychiatrists toward minority group patients (i.e., are less likely to see minority patients or less likely to recommend ECT treatment to minority patients), or misdiagnosis of minority patients. Conversely, patients belonging to a minority group may be less likely to accept ECT, even when it is recommended, because of historical, cultural, or health education factors and may be less likely to receive it even when it is indicated.

Socioeconomic factors/insurance

Socioeconomic factors are related to variation in ECT utilization across patient groups. Patients who are affluent are more likely to be treated with ECT regardless of diagnosis (Babigian and Guttmacher, 1984; Kramer, 1985; Olfson et al., 1998), suggesting that affluence may place patients at risk for overutilization. This trend is a reversal from the 1950s, when impoverished patients were more likely to receive ECT (Kahn et al., 1957). Patients with insurance receive ECT at a much higher rate than that of their uninsured counterparts. More than half of patients receiving ECT are insured by Medicare. This is not surprising because Medicare insures the geriatric population, and geriatric patients, when depressed, are more likely to receive ECT. Patients with private insurance account for 25% to 40% of ECT patients, and fewer than 10% of ECT patients are insured by Medicaid or are self-pay (Breakey and Dunn, 2004; Olfson et al., 1998).

State regulations (sociopolitical factors)

Political and legislative factors affecting the availability of ECT in the United States and its regions are addressed in Chapters 11 and 12. States with more ECT restrictions and regulations tend to have lower rates of ECT use. California and New York have populations with similar demographic characteristics such as socioeconomic status, percentage of White population, and proportion of elderly persons (U.S. Census Bureau Web site). However, total ECT use in New York is much greater than in California, although California has twice as many residents as New York has. California requires extensive record keeping and complicated consent forms, along with competency evaluations by a second physician for voluntary ECT patients. In addition, ECT treatments in California are time limited and are restricted for minors (Hermann et al., 1995). Despite the increasing population in California, ECT use continues to decline and is considered underutilized relative to the use of ECT that would be expected because of the size of its population and its population demographics. The use of ECT in California has been reported by Kramer for the time periods 1977 through 1983 (Kramer, 1985) and 1984 through 1994 (Kramer, 1999).

The future of ECT

A notable challenge in ensuring appropriate patient access to ECT is identifying when ECT is overutilized, underutilized, and appropriately utilized. Additional research is needed to describe and compare short- and long-term treatment outcome in selected population groups. We know that utilization patterns of ECT in the United States have changed dramatically since its introduction to the United States in 1940. During the past 60 years, ECT has gone from an informally effective somatic treatment largely used in state hospitals for the poor to a treatment with proven efficacy and effectiveness predominantly available to those of relative affluence, particularly for the treatment of depression in elderly persons.

Although preliminary studies have demonstrated some regional, socioeconomic, and demographic factors related to its utilization, there are concerns about regional variations in diagnosis, patient selection for ECT, and the ECT procedure itself; together these represent variations in ECT clinical outcome. The variation in ECT use also suggests that psychiatrists do not have a consistently high level of educated awareness about ECT and unhindered accessibility to ECT, despite the development of APA guidelines and task force findings strongly supporting its use in the

treatment of mood disorders. Wennberg et al. (1982) speculated that high variation in the use of a specific procedure (like ECT) can result from lack of consensus
among clinicians about the clarity of diagnosis, the procedure's efficacy (when
compared with alternative treatments), and the timing of the procedure among
a sequence of alternatives. Among psychiatrists (including those who make decisions about medical necessity for third party payors), judgment about when ECT is
needed surely varies widely. There is a clear difference between the recommended
use of ECT in this book (see Chapter 22) and the place accorded ECT in the "Texas
Algorithm" for treating major depression in state hospital patients in Texas.

Although substantial gains have been achieved in the administration, understanding, and use of ECT, additional study is needed about ECT underutilization
and its consequences. Perhaps the greatest advances in ECT-related treatment yet
to be made are service oriented and await a more consistent level of educated
awareness by psychiatrists about ECT.

Acknowledgments

The authors would like to give special thanks to Brent Turnipseed, MD, for his
assistance in data gathering and Jason Reichenberg, MD, for his assistance in
editing.

References

American Psychiatric Association (APA). 2000. Diagnostic and statistical manual of mental
disorders, 4th edn. Washington, DC: APA.

Babigian, H. M. and Guttmacher, L. B. 1984. Epidemiologic considerations in electroconvulsive
therapy. Arch Gen Psychiatry 41: 246–53.

Bailine, S. H. and Rau, J. H. 1981. The decision to use ECT: A retrospective study. Compr
Psychiatry 22: 274–81.

Breakey, W. R. and Dunn, G. J. 2004. Racial disparity in the use of ECT for affective disorders.
Am J Psychiatry 161: 1635–41.

Cerletti, U. 1950. Old and new information about electroshock. Am J Psychiatry 107: 87–94.

Creed, P., Froimson, L., and Mathew, L. 1995. Survey of the practice of electroconvulsive therapy
in North Carolina. Convuls Ther 11: 182–7.

Grosser, G., Pearsall, D., and Fisher, C. 1975. The regulation of electroconvulsive therapy treatment in Massachusetts: A follow-up. Mass Ment Health J 5: 12–25.

Hermann, R., Dorwart, R., Hoover, C., and Brody, J. 1995. Variation in ECT use in the United
States. Am J Psychiatry 152: 869–75.

Hermann, R. C., Ettner, S. L., Dorwart, R. A., et al. 1999. Diagnoses of patients treated with ECT:
A comparison of evidence-based standards with reported use. Psychiatr Serv 50: 1059–65.

Impastato, D. J. 1960. The story of the first electro shock treatment. Am J Psychiatry 116: 1113–14.

Kahn, R., Pollack, M., and Fink, M. 1957. Social factors in selection of therapy in a voluntary mental hospital. J Hillside Hosp 6: 216–28.

Kramer, B. 1985. Use of ECT in California, 1977–1983. Am J Psychiatry 142: 1190–2.

Kramer, B. 1990. ECT use in the public sector: California. Psychiatr Q 61: 97–103.

Kramer, B. 1999. Use of ECT in California, revisited: 1984–1994. J ECT 15: 245–51.

Lebensohn, Z. M. 1999. The history of electroconvulsive therapy in the United States and its place in American psychiatry: A personal memoir. Compr Psychiatry 40: 173–81.

McCall, W. V. 1989. Physical treatments in psychiatry: Current and historical use in the southern United States. South Med J 82: 345–51.

Mills, M. J., Pearsall, D. T., Yesavage, J. A., and Salzman, C. 1984. Electroconvulsive therapy in Massachusetts. Am J Psychiatry 141: 534–8.

O'Connor, M., Knapp, R., Husain, M., et al. 2001. The influence of age on the response of major depression to electroconvulsive therapy: A C.O.R.E. report. Am J Geriatr Psychiatry 9: 382–390.

Olfson, M., Marcus, S., Sackeim, H., et al. 1998. Use of ECT for the inpatient treatment of recurrent major depression. Am J Psychiatry 155: 22–9.

Reid, W., Keller, S., Leatherman, M., and Mason, M. 1998. ECT in Texas: 19 months of mandatory reporting. J Clin Psychiatry 59: 8–13.

Robins, L. and Regier, D. (eds.). 1991. Psychiatric disorders in America. New York: Free Press.

Rosenbach, M., Hermann, R., and Dorwart, R. 1997. Use of electroconvulsive therapy in the Medicare population between 1987 and 1992. Psychiatr Serv 48: 1537–42.

Scarano, V., Felthous, A., and Early, T. 2000. The state of electroconvulsive therapy in Texas. Part I: Reported data on 41,660 ECT treatments in 5971 patients. J Forensic Sci 45: 1197–202.

Sylvester, A., Mulsant, B., Chengappa, K., et al. 2000. Use of electroconvulsive therapy in a state hospital: A 10-year review. J Clin Psychiatry 61: 534–9; quiz 540.

Thompson, J. and Blaine, J. 1987. Use of ECT in the United States in 1975 and 1980. Am J Psychiatry 144: 557–62.

Thompson, J., Weiner, R., and Myers, C. 1994. Use of ECT in the United States in 1975, 1980, and 1986. Am J Psychiatry 151: 1657–61. (A p. 1613).

U.S. Census Bureau Web site. Retrieved December 28, 2007, from http://quickfacts.census.gov/qfd/

Wennberg, J. and Gittelsohn, A. 1973. Small area variations in health care delivery. Science 182: 1102–8.

Wennberg, J. E., Barnes, B. A., and Zubkoff, M. 1982. Professional uncertainty and the problem of supplier-induced demand. Soc Sci Med 16: 811–24.

14

Electroconvulsive therapy in Scandinavia and the United Kingdom

Susan Mary Benbow and Tom G. Bolwig

This chapter examines the history and present state of electroconvulsive therapy (ECT) practice in Scandinavia and the United Kingdom, considers recent changes, and looks to the future of treatment provision in these regions.

The practice of ECT in Scandinavia, past and present

ECT is given in all Nordic countries, but more so in Denmark and Sweden than in Norway, Finland, and Iceland. The two latter countries are not strictly within geographical Scandinavia.

The first reported sporadic use of ECT in Norway, as well as in Sweden and Denmark, was about 1940, but it was not in regular use in university clinics (in Sweden and Denmark) until the late 1940s. With the introduction of anesthesia, muscle relaxation, and artificial ventilation by Holmberg and Thesleff (1952) in Sweden, ECT gradually became an accepted therapeutic modality, particularly in Denmark. The indications were mainly melancholic or psychotic depression. Catatonic states and various forms of delirium were also considered appropriate for ECT treatment by the majority of clinicians. Based on anecdotal reports, practice in Sweden was similar to that in Denmark, whereas ECT acceptance in Norway was negligible outside a few institutions.

These differences in ECT practice within Scandinavia may be viewed alongside the far more enthusiastic adoption of various psychotherapeutic approaches (psychoanalysis/dynamics, therapeutic community) in Norway than in Denmark and Sweden. The latter countries generally took a more Continental approach to diagnosis and classification, and they incorporated a tradition of research.

In their report on ECT in Oslo from 1988 through 2002, Moksnes and colleagues (2006) refer to a previous report from 1968 through 1978 (Volden and Gøtestam, 1982). This earlier report noted that the number of ECT courses within Norway was substantially lower than in the other Scandinavian countries. In 1978, ECT was given to 2.8% of psychiatric inpatients in Norway, 4.1% in Sweden, and 10.1%

in Denmark. With such limited use in Norway, teaching, training, and research efforts concerning ECT were rare.

After 1979, when the Italian-born Swedish psychiatrist Giacomo d'Elia became a professor at Bergen University, there was renewed interest in ECT in Norway. Research programs were established, training became mandatory, and gradually the respectability of ECT in Norwegian psychiatry seems to have become comparable to that in Sweden and Denmark (Moksnes et al., 2006).

The use of ECT in Scandinavia has not been investigated systematically. However, the preceding impressions are based on longitudinal observation of published studies conducted in the Scandinavian countries. The first Scandinavian nation-wide survey of ECT was the Danish study by Heshe and Röder (1976), who reported that ECT was given to more than 10% of inpatients in Denmark during the early 1970s for the indications mentioned above, and they confirmed its high degree of safety. At the same time, Frederiksen and D'Elia (1979) published Swedish data showing that about 4% of inpatients were treated with ECT, mainly for affective disorders and confusional states.

The rate of Swedish usage has been largely unchanged in the ensuing years. However, the Danish situation has changed considerably since the Heshe and Röder report. Denmark became the most "ECT-positive" Scandinavian nation for several years (Andersson and Bolwig, 2002). The latest national survey in Denmark found that 5% of all patients hospitalized for psychiatric illness are treated with ECT. Still, there was a fivefold variation between different hospitals, ascribed to different treatment traditions. Altogether, among inpatients with a diagnosis of major depression, 18% were treated with ECT. The survey found a 17% decrease in the number of ECT sessions and a decrease in the number of patients of 27% from 1979 to 1999, suggesting that treatment courses were longer in 1999.

The most recent data examining the use of ECT within Scandinavia are those of Moksnes et al. (2006), dealing specifically with the University of Oslo area, and those of Andersson and Bolwig (2002), covering Denmark (including Greenland). These data suggest that the frequency of ECT use is fairly similar throughout Scandinavia, at least in academic hospitals.

As in many other countries, ECT in Scandinavia has been demonized by certain political and ideological factions, and in the 1970s and 1980s ECT was used to exemplify a so-called authoritarian malevolence of psychiatry. Despite the demonization, there never was a powerful anti-ECT lobby in Scandinavia. However surprising that may seem, it is most probably the reason why there was never the same suspicion or mistrust of psychiatry in the public arena and, more important, in the general population, as has been observed in most countries of the Western world.

The fact that the public via the media has been aware that ECT is the subject of lively research activity, and the fact that research-active psychiatrists have stood up for ECT in public debates may well have played a role in the relatively high level of acceptance of ECT in the Scandinavian countries.

A Scandinavian research tradition

From the start of the 1960s a highly influential Swedish group of researchers headed by Jan-Otto Ottosson in Gothenburg conducted a series of studies on both clinical and pathophysiological issues that became central in Scandinavian and international ECT concepts (Ottosson, 1960). Working together with the American psychiatrist Max Fink, Ottosson proposed a theory of ECT action (Fink and Ottosson 1980). The role of the seizure, mechanisms of post-ECT memory impairment, electrode placement (D'Elia, 1970), and the implication of brain monoamines (Modigh, 1976) represent distinguished Swedish research traditions in the area of ECT.

In Denmark, ECT research has likewise focused on both clinical (Strömgren, 1976) and pathophysiological (Bolwig et al., 1977) studies. Since the early 1970s, a search to understand the working mechanism behind ECT has continued, especially at the University Department of Psychiatry in Copenhagen. During the last decade it has continued in close collaboration with Swedish and international university research units. This collaboration led to the first demonstration of hippocampal neurogenesis (Madsen et al., 2000). A recent hypothesis associating the hippocampus with the mechanism of ECT in melancholia was proposed by Bolwig and Madsen (2007).

Norway has reported some ECT research. Notable are studies at the University of Bergen where Bergsholm investigated a variety of physiological factors influenced by anesthesia and electrode placement (Bergsholm, 1995).

Research is mentioned only to illustrate that ECT has remained a generally accepted treatment choice in the Scandinavian countries, even throughout the difficult antipsychiatry period.

Standards and practice of ECT: The United Kingdom context before the National Institute for Clinical Excellence

Shorter and Healy's recent book (2007) notes that ECT was readily accepted into the United Kingdom following its inception in 1938 and comments that well-known leading psychiatrists such as Michael Shepherd were "great fans" of the treatment. However, they take the view that later, from about the 1960s, ECT became more heavily stigmatized in the United Kingdom than in the United States. In 1977 the Royal College of Psychiatrists (1977) published a memorandum on ECT and decided to survey the use of ECT in England. Later, the survey was extended to

Scotland, Wales, the Channel Islands, and the Isle of Man. A postal questionnaire was sent to all members of the Royal College of Psychiatrists to establish how they prescribed and used ECT, and a second questionnaire was sent to all clinics administering ECT. A three-month prospective study aimed to collect information on all people given ECT during a three-month period, and a short survey was sent to more than 600 family doctors to investigate their patients' experience of ECT. The findings were published as a report in 1981 (Pippard and Ellam, 1981). Standards in 30% of clinics were described as "not satisfactory" and 27% had "serious deficiencies." At that time consultants were rarely involved in the work of the ECT clinic. About half of physicians training to become consultant psychiatrists ("junior doctors") received "minimal training," and in 90% of the clinics treatment was left to junior doctors. The report noted obsolete machinery, unsuitable premises, low standards of care, and lack of policies to guide practice. In relation to the national statistics on ECT usage in 1979, the Yorkshire Region administered three times as much ECT as the Oxford Region, and some hospitals gave 17 times as much ECT as others. This report heralded the onset of official concern about the quality of ECT practice in the United Kingdom.

In 1989 the Royal College of Psychiatrists published its first *ECT Handbook* (Freeman, 1989). This was followed by a second audit (Pippard, 1992), which compared practice in two English regions with the standards set in the 1989 *Handbook*. Despite some areas of improvement, many clinics failed to meet the 1989 standards. There was particular concern about the training of junior doctors and the use of outdated machines.

The second *ECT Handbook* was published in 1995 (Royal College of Psychiatrists Special Committee on ECT, 1995). It was criticized for not recommending electroencephalographic (EEG) monitoring of seizures and routine determination of seizure threshold in the United Kingdom, but at that time very few ECT clinics in the United Kingdom had instruments capable of performing these tasks.

A third audit was subsequently carried out and reported by Duffett and Lelliott (1998). They found that only one third of the clinics they visited met College standards. Only 16% of consultant psychiatrists responsible for ECT attended their ECT clinic weekly, and only 6% had time for ECT in their job plan. Only one third of clinics had policies to guide junior doctors in administration of ECT. Duffett and Lelliott noted that ECT facilities were at that time inspected when the College visited to accredit psychiatric training schemes, but asked, "What sanctions should replace exhortation and education?" They mentioned two possible options: special training and accreditation of psychiatrists (along the lines of the American Psychiatric Association [APA] system) or accreditation of the ECT clinics themselves.

The Final Report of the Scottish ECT Audit Network was published in 2000 (Freeman et al., 2000). It reported a national audit of all ECT centers in Scotland.

This report found that ECT was mainly given to white adult inpatients with a diagnosis of depressive illness. The female-to-male ratio was approximately 2:1, and 76% of patients were informal (voluntary). Of all patients receiving ECT, 81.8% gave informed consent, and there was documented definite clinical improvement in 71.2% with a diagnosis of depressive illness and in 65% with other (psychotic) illnesses. The audit had been well received, and the methodology was becoming incorporated into routine clinical practice. Facilities and equipment at ECT centers were up to date and of a generally high standard, and the overall standard of ECT provision across the country was high. Areas highlighted for further improvement were the ongoing supervision of trainee doctors, dedicated time for ECT coordinators, and standards in the clinical workplace.

The National Institute for Clinical Excellence and ECT in the United Kingdom

The National Institute for Clinical Excellence (NICE) in 2003 published a health technology appraisal (HTA) on the use of ECT (NICE, 2003). It states, "it is recommended that ECT is used only to achieve rapid and short-term improvement of severe symptoms after an adequate trial of other treatment options has proven ineffective or when the condition is considered to be potentially life-threatening in individuals with severe depressive illness, catatonia, a prolonged or severe manic episode." The Special ECT Committee of the Royal College of Psychiatrists appealed against the draft guidance on the grounds that it was "perverse," arguing that the evidence for the efficacy of ECT relates to the treatment of moderate depressive illness (rather than severe), that patients should be able to choose to have ECT if they so wish, and that there is evidence to support the use of continuation and maintenance treatment. The appeal was unsuccessful, and the guidance went ahead unchanged. The appraisal concluded that ECT is likely to be cost-effective for appropriate patient groups, but took "special note" of the evidence from users' experiences of adverse effects. Outside observers regarded the outcome as heavily influenced by the anti-ECT lobby, which tipped the balance toward the side effects of ECT and away from the evidence of efficacy, and noted that, of the 24 people listed as Appraisal Committee members, none was a psychiatrist.

There are two other important factors to take into account when contemplating the effect of NICE's ECT guidance. First, what is specifically meant by "severe" depressive illness (in the United Kingdom)? Second, inside all NICE's guidance (and the ECT HTA is no different) is an important disclaimer, which reads as follows: "Health professionals are expected to take (this guidance) fully into account when exercising their clinical judgement. This guidance does not, however, override the individual responsibility of health professionals to make appropriate decisions in the circumstances of the individual patient." The impact of NICE's technology appraisal on clinical practice in the use of ECT in the United Kingdom is unclear.

Post-NICE developments in the United Kingdom

The same year that the NICE HTA was published, two other influential articles appeared in the United Kingdom medical press. The UK ECT Review Group (2003) published the findings of their systematic review and meta-analysis of the efficacy and safety of ECT in depressive disorders, and concluded that ECT is an effective short-term treatment for depression, probably more effective than drug treatment. They found that "bilateral ECT is moderately more effective than unilateral ECT, and high dose ECT is more effective than low dose." Rose et al. (2003) published their analysis of patient perspectives of ECT. They found 26 studies by clinicians and 9 studies by or with patients. One third of patients reported persistent memory loss, and they noted that patient-led studies reported lower benefit than did studies led by professionals. Curiously, there appears to be an idea that patient researchers are free of the biases that supposedly influence professionals.

The ECT Accreditation Service (ECTAS) was also launched in 2003. The Service is a joint initiative involving three Royal Colleges: the Colleges of Psychiatrists, Anaesthetists, and Nursing. They set three types of standards:

- Type 1: essential to safety and must be met
- Type 2: good quality clinic
- Type 3: excellent clinic

Accreditation involves an audit of health records; examination of ECT documentation; observation of ECT; and inspection of facilities, equipment, staffing, and questionnaire information from staff and service users. After the accreditation procedures are completed, a report is considered by the accreditation advisory committee, and, if ratified by the College, the clinic is accredited. It then undertakes an annual self-review and is fully reviewed every three years.

The first ECTAS report (ECTAS, 2005) covered the period from October 2003 to October 2005 and found that about 40% of the total eligible clinics joined over that period. Approximately half of those that joined were accredited, and a small number were "deferred," most commonly for reasons of poor documentation. Others were still undertaking self-review at the time of the report. Numbers had increased by the time of the second ECTAS report, and some clinics were entering their second review cycle. ECTAS reported evidence of improvements in ECT practice, investment in new equipment, the introduction of new policies and procedures, some streamlining of clinic provision, and changes to clinic staffing. The system of accreditation has been credited with leading to these improvements.

The updated *ECT Handbook* published in 2005 (Royal College of Psychiatrists Special Committee on ECT, 2005) required EEG monitoring (a minimum of one channel from each side of the head) to be available in all ECT clinics from January 1, 2006, and consolidated the move to ECT practice more closely aligned with that in the United States.

The second report produced by ECTAS (2007) covers a two-year period between 2005 and 2007. It notes two phenomena that may relate to the combined impact of NICE's guidance and the introduction of an accreditation system. First, rates of ECT in England, Wales, and Ireland are decreasing. It is estimated that the number of patients and treatment applications there has halved since 1999. Second, there is evidence that the total number of clinics providing an ECT service has decreased. Concern is expressed that this might exacerbate the decrease in ECT usage and ultimately lead to patients being denied access to treatment. One important question raised is whether, in some areas of the United Kingdom or the Republic of Ireland, ECT is already being underused.

Training in ECT in Scandinavia

ECT occupies the same place in specialist training as do psychotherapy and psychopharmacology in the three Scandinavian countries. In Denmark, an annual specialist training course is held for psychiatrists in charge of their local ECT unit.

Training in ECT in the United Kingdom

Training in the administration of ECT cannot be separated from practice, and the audits referred to earlier highlighted major shortcomings in the training of the junior doctors who were administering ECT and in the supervision practices of the consultant psychiatrists who might have been reasonably expected to provide training/supervision in the clinic. When one author (SMB) started training in psychiatry in 1978, it was normal practice for a newly appointed doctor to be shown how to "press the button" by a doctor who had administered treatment previously. It was certainly not normal for consultant psychiatrists to visit ECT clinics! Even in the late 1990s, supervision of treatment and training of junior doctors remained an issue, with few consultant psychiatrists spending time in the clinic supervising the administration of ECT. Thankfully, practice has changed considerably since then.

The ECTAS standards published in 2006 (Cresswell et al., 2006) require clinics to have a named consultant psychiatrist who has dedicated time included in the job plan. This psychiatrist takes responsibility for developing treatment protocols, training and supervising clinic staff, liaising with and advising other professionals, developing audit and quality assurance, and undertaking continuing professional development. The standard for ECT administration is that ECT is administered by "a small cohort of experienced psychiatrists who regularly attend" the clinic (a type 2 standard). There are also type 1 standards that apply to the training of doctors, requiring that only "psychiatrists with formal training" administer treatment and that administering psychiatrists receive instruction covering the theoretical basis of effective treatment, local protocols, and clinic layout. They should observe the administration of ECT prior to administering it for the first time (type 1 standard). In addition, they should be directly supervised by the ECT consultant or an "appropriately trained deputy" for at least three sessions before administering treatment on their own, and be supervised directly (or through examination of treatment charts) at least once weekly while administering ECT (type 2 standard). The implementation of these standards represents a considerable shift in practice, and, by the time that the sixth ECTAS newsletter (Hood, 2007) was written, there were 93 member clinics, which is probably just less than 50% of the total number of eligible clinics (based on 2005 numbers).

Recently, the Royal College of Psychiatrists ECT Committee produced some draft competencies for doctors involved in ECT. These are currently being piloted.

The future of ECT in Scandinavia and the United Kingdom

ECT has continued to have a role, particularly in the treatment of severe depressive illness, in Scandinavia and the United Kingdom. Practice in the United Kingdom has made considerable progress since the advent of ECTAS, and it is likely that this will continue with further updating into the immediate future. Unilateral ECT may well become more commonly used in the United Kingdom now that treatment is more consistently supervised and monitored, perhaps more in line with clinical practice in Scandinavia. Training in the United Kingdom has developed rapidly over recent years, and there is interest across both geographical regions in further developing the training and updating of the professionals involved in the ECT clinic, alongside ways of maintaining high clinical standards. The formation of the European Forum for ECT (for further information, see www.theeffect.eu) also offers the opportunity for sharing experience and learning from one another across Europe as a whole.

References

Andersson, J. E. and Bolwig, T. G. 2002. Electroconvulsive therapy in Denmark 1999. A nation-wide questionnaire study. Ugeskr Laeger 164(26): 3449–52.

Bergsholm, P. 1995. Electroconvulsive therapy. Issues related to narcosis, physiology, radiological anatomy, electrode placement, endocrinology. Ph.D. Dissertation, University of Bergen.

Bolwig, T. G., Hertz, M. M., Paulson, O. B., et al. 1977. The permeability of the blood-brain barrier during electrically induced seizures in man. Eur J Clin Invest 7: 87–93.

Bolwig, T. G. and Madsen, T. M. 2007. Electroconvulsive therapy in melancholia: The role of hippocampal neurogenesis. Acta Psychiatr Scand Suppl 433: 130–5.

Cresswell, J., Rayner, L., Hood, C., and O'Sullivan, J. (eds.) 2006. The ECT Accreditation Service. Standards for the administration of ECT. Available at: http://www.rcpsych.ac.uk/ PDF/The%20ECTAS%20Standards%20Dec%2006.pdf.

D'Elia, G. 1970. Unilateral electroconvulsive therapy. Acta Psychiatr Scand Suppl (215): 1–98.

Duffett, R. and Lelliott, P. 1998. Auditing electroconvulsive therapy. The third cycle. Br J Psychiatry 172: 401–5.

The ECT Accreditation Service (ECTAS) 2005. First national report. October 2003 – October 2005 (eds. Cresswell, J., Fortune, Z., and Lelliott, P.). Download at http://www.rcpsych.ac.uk/ PDF/ECTAS%201st%20National%20Report.pdf, accessed September 26, 2008.

The ECT Accreditation Service (ECTAS). 2007. Second national report (eds. Cresswell, J., Hood, C., and Lelliott, P.). Download at http://www.rcpsych.ac.uk/PDF/Ectas%20Report%202.pdf, accessed September 26, 2008.

Fink, M. and Ottosson, J.-O. 1980. A theory of convulsive therapy in endogenous depression. Significance of hypothalamic functions. Psychiatry Res 2: 49–61.

Frederiksen, S. O. and D'Elia, G. 1979. Electroconvulsive therapy in Sweden. Br J Psychiatry 134: 583–7.

Freeman, C. P. L. 1989. The practical administration of electroconvulsive therapy. ECT Sub-committee of the Royal College of Psychiatrists. London: Gaskell.

Freeman, C. P. L., Hendry, J., and Fergusson, G. 2000. National audit of electroconvulsive therapy (ECT) in Scotland. Final Report. Available at http://www.sean.org.uk/AuditReport/ HomePage, accessed November 30, 2007.

Heshe, J. and Röder, E. 1976. Electroconvulsive therapy in Denmark. Br J Psychiatry 128: 241–5.

Holmberg, G. and Thesleff, S. 1952. Succinyl-choline-iodide as a muscular relaxant in electroshock therapy. Am J Psychiatry 108(11): 842–6.

Hood, C. (ed.) 2007. ECTAS Newsletter Issue 6, July 2007. Download at http://www.rcpsych. ac.uk/pdf/ECTAS%20July%202007.pdf, accessed September 26, 2008.

Madsen, T. M. M., Treschow, A., Bengzon, J., et al. 2000. Increased neurogenesis in a model of electroconvulsive therapy. Biol Psychiatry 47: 1043–9.

Modigh, K. 1976. Long-term effects of electroconvulsive shock therapy on synthesis, turnover and uptake of brain monoamines. Psychopharmacology 49: 179–85.

Moksnes, K. M., Vatnaland, T., Eri, B., and Torvik, N. H. 2006. Electroconvulsive therapy in the Ullevaal region of Oslo 1988–2002. Tidsskr Nor Laegeforen 26(13): 1750–3.

National Institute for Clinical Excellence (NICE). 2003. Guidance on the use of electroconvulsive therapy. Technology Appraisal 59. London: NICE. Download at http://www.nice. org.uk/guidance/index.jsp?action=download&o=32597, accessed September 26, 2008.

Ottosson, J.-O. 1960. Experimental studies of the mode of action of electroconvulsive therapy. Acta Psychiatr Neurol Scand Suppl (145): 1–131.

Pippard, J. 1992. Audit of electroconvulsive treatment in two National Health Service regions. Br J Psychiatry 160: 621–37.

Pippard, J. and Ellam, L. 1981. Electroconvulsive therapy in Great Britain, 1980. A report to the Royal College of Psychiatrists. London: Gaskell.

Rose, D., Fleischmann, P., Wykes, T., et al. 2003. Patients' perspectives on electroconvulsive therapy: Systematic review. Br Med J 326: 1363–4.

Royal College of Psychiatrists. 1977. Memorandum on the use of electroconvulsive therapy. Br J Psychiatry 131: 261–72.

Royal College of Psychiatrists Special Committee on ECT. 1995. ECT Handbook. The Second Report of the Royal College of Psychiatrists Special Committee on ECT. Council Report CR39. London: Royal College of Psychiatrists.

Royal College of Psychiatrists Special Committee on ECT. 2005. The ECT Handbook. Council Report CR128, 2nd edn. (ed. Scott, A .I. F.). London: Royal College of Psychiatrists.

Shorter, E. and Healy, D. 2007. Shock therapy. A history of electroconvulsive treatment in mental illness. Piscataway, NJ: Rutgers University Press, Chapter 10, pp. 219–52.

Strömgren, L. S. 1976. Unilateral and bilateral ECT. Depression and memory. Dissertation, University of Århus.

UK ECT Review Group. 2003. Efficacy and safety of electroconvulsive therapy in depressive disorders: A systematic review and meta-analysis. Lancet 361(9360): 799–808.

Volden, O. and Götestam, K. G. 1982. The use of electroconvulsive treatment in Norway during 1968–79. Tidsskr Nor Laegeforen 102(7): 411–2.

15

Electroconvulsive therapy in continental Western Europe: A literature review

Pascal Sienaert and Walter W. van den Broek

Introduction

Both convulsive therapy and electroconvulsive therapy (ECT) are European achievements. At the Budapest-Lipotmezö State Hospital (Hungary), on January 23, 1934, Ladislas Meduna decided to produce "epileptic attacks" by means of an intramuscular injection of camphor in oil to treat a man in catatonic stupor (Fink, 1984, 2001). Although within Hungary Meduna's work was criticized, psychiatrists from all over Europe visited him and adopted his treatment at a number of centers in Europe (Fink, 1984). In April 1938, at the Clinic for Mental and Nervous Diseases in Rome, Cerletti and Bini went ahead with the first ECT treatment in humans (Accornero, 1988; Kalinowsky, 1986; Shorter and Healy, 2007). By 1940, at least 32 treatment units had been established in Italy (Shorter and Healy, 2007). Outside Italy, Switzerland was the first country in which ECT visibly flourished for the international community. From there, ECT spread to the rest of continental Western Europe, in large part thanks to the efforts of Lothar Kalinowski (Shorter and Healy, 2007). In both the United Kingdom and Scandinavia, ECT has been used frequently throughout its history, whereas in other European countries the use of ECT has been highly variable.

Few data on the use of ECT in other European countries are available, however. Official central data collection is lacking in most countries, and published data are provided in different formats, making it difficult to compare practice between countries. Data have been published on the use and practice of ECT in Belgium, France, Germany, The Netherlands, and Spain.

Belgium

A nationwide survey among all Belgian psychiatric services providing ECT revealed that from 2003 through 2004 ECT was performed in 32 psychiatric services (21.5% of all psychiatric services) (Sienaert et al., 2005a, 2005b, 2006b). ECT is available

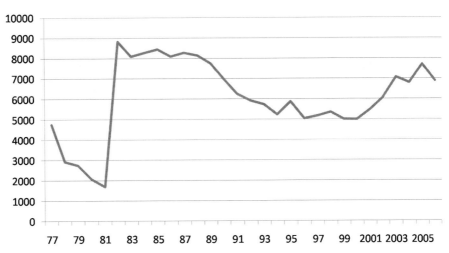

Figure 15.1   Data on use of electroconvulsive therapy in Belgium from 1977 through 2006.

in 13.6% of psychiatric hospitals and 32.8% of general hospitals with a psychiatric department, but two thirds of these ECT facilities treat fewer than two patients per month. ECT is probably still regarded as a last resort for patients severely resistant to medication. Moreover, ECT is used primarily for depressive disorders; fewer than 10% of patients receive ECT for a psychotic disorder. In all hospitals modified ECT is used, and propofol is the most commonly used hypnotic (74% of hospitals). Surprisingly, as late as 2003, 34% of departments still used sine wave devices. In 65.6% of the hospitals, bitemporal electrode placement is used for all patients, and in 37% a combination of bitemporal electrode placement and a fixed, high-stimulus dose is used. Continuation ECT is underused: Only two hospitals use it frequently (>30 sessions per month), whereas about half of the hospitals never use this treatment modality.

According to the National Sickness and Invalidity Insurance Institute (D. Van Gucht, November 13, 2007, personal communication), the annual rate of ECT use in Belgium is increasing (Figure 15.1). In 2000, the ECT rate was 4.8 per 10,000 inhabitants. By 2006, it had increased to 6.6 per 10,000 inhabitants. This small increase is largely due to the establishment of a large university-based ECT department. It was criticized in the lay press, and questions were raised in Parliament regarding the use of informed consent (Sienaert et al., 2005a). Nevertheless, the survey introduced the revival of ECT in Belgium. A collaborative Workgroup on ECT (WEV) was founded in 2004 as part of the Flemish Association of Psychiatry and the Belgian College of Neuropsychopharmacology and Biological Psychiatry. In 2006, Sienaert and colleagues published national guidelines for ECT in practice (Dhossche, 2007; Sienaert et al., 2006a). Finally, it was in Belgium that a European

Forum for Electroconvulsive Therapy (EFFECT) was founded in February 2006 at the ECT Department of the University Psychiatric Center-Catholic University Leuven (Bolwig et al., 2006).

France

According to a survey in 1981 in the French region of Aquitaine, ECT was never used in 15 of the 26 public psychiatric services. In nine facilities, two courses per year were performed on average. Reasons for not using ECT included the absence of indications for its use, fear of legal problems, and public opinion (Bourgeois et al., 1981). In private hospitals ECT was used more frequently. About 10 years later, a survey of 770 psychiatrists (with 400 respondents) showed a more favorable attitude toward ECT (Auquier et al., 1994). A minority (16%) of respondents stated that they would never use ECT because of ethical considerations. Only 22% of respondents used ECT. A large subgroup (58%) stated that they were aware of the beneficial effects of ECT, were willing to use it in severe cases, but did not have access to this treatment (Auquier et al., 1994). In a later survey into the practice of ECT (1996–1997) in all French psychiatric public hospitals (response rate 47%, $n = 382$), 195 psychiatrists (51%) reported using ECT (Benadhira and Teles, 2001). Medication-resistant depression seemed to be the main indication for ECT (63%).

More than half of the psychiatrists practicing ECT did not know what anesthetic hypnotic was used in their service; those who did know used propofol most frequently (65%). A sine wave device was used in 44% of services. Unilateral electrode placement was used in 18% of services. About 40% of services stated that they used continuation ECT as a method of relapse prevention. Although it cannot be concluded from these data in the surveys, some authors suggest that the number of hospitals providing ECT is decreasing. This suggestion was attributed partly to higher standards (e.g., for anesthesia) stipulated in a French government paper of 1996 and in the national guidelines for ECT published in 1997 (Agence Nationale d'Accréditation et d'Évaluation en Santé [ANAES], 1997). Several services stopped ECT practice and referred patients to accredited specialized hospitals (Benadhira and Teles, 2001).

Germany

The first ECT survey in Germany was published in 1981 (Reimer and Lorenzen, 1981). A questionnaire was sent to 295 psychiatric services in Western Germany and West Berlin, and 227 (77.2%) replied. ECT was used in 98 (42%) of the psychiatric services. Deliberately limited use of ECT was confirmed in another survey among 76 state mental hospitals, 84 psychiatric departments of general hospitals, and

28 university hospitals (Lauter and Sauer, 1987); the response rate was 80%. The number of ECT courses was lowest in state mental hospitals (2.04/1,000 beds) and highest in university hospitals (41.3/1,000 beds). About half of the departments used bilateral ECT. Depressive disorders were the main indication. The overall use of ECT in Germany in 1985 was 0.08 per 10,000 inhabitants, one third the rate in Switzerland and about 1/60 the rate in the United Kingdom.

ECT use in Germany is increasing, however. In 1994, the number of patients treated with ECT was 1,050, twice the number treated in 1985 (Muller et al., 1998). This increase is partly because of the reunification of West and East Germany. It was estimated that between 0.015 and 0.036 treatments per 1,000 inhabitants were performed in Eastern Germany. Between 1992 and 1994, Eastern Germany contributed almost one third of all patients treated with ECT (Muller and Geretsegger, 2004). According to the University of Munich, the renaissance of ECT in Germany is still ongoing; from 1995 through 2002, the number of treatments in that hospital more than doubled (Baghai et al., 2005). However, it is unknown if these numbers reflect an increase in the use of ECT in the rest of the country. A renewed interest in ECT is also reflected in the publication of national guidelines for ECT in 2004 and of a multi-authored textbook (Baghai et al., 2004).

The Netherlands

After World War II, ECT was administered in The Netherlands on a large scale. By the end of the 1960s, ECT use started to decline because of the use of psychopharmacological drugs and public assertions of ECT as oppressive. In 1976, the antipsychiatry group, National Anti-Shock Action, requested a complete abolishment of ECT, inspired by the successful actions of the anti-ECT movement in California (Verwey and Sienaert, 2005; Vijselaar, 2007). National Anti-Shock Action published a "black list" of psychiatrists and hospitals using ECT, demonstrated outside psychiatric hospitals, and gained considerable media support. By 1979 only 46 patients were treated with ECT, and only 4% of Dutch psychiatrists used ECT (Oei et al., 1985). In 1984, the Department of Public Health issued a statement that ECT is a viable treatment in patients with severe melancholic depression and could be performed in a limited number of hospitals. Patients had to give informed consent and a second opinion was obligatory. From 1985 onward, ECT treatments were to be registered with the Inspectorate of Mental Health. Since then, there has been a steady increase in the annual number of patients treated with ECT (Figure 15.2).

In 1992, the Dutch Association for Psychiatry issued a more liberal report with recommendations for the practice of ECT, including mania and schizophrenia as possible indications. In 1993, a joint task force from the Dutch Association for

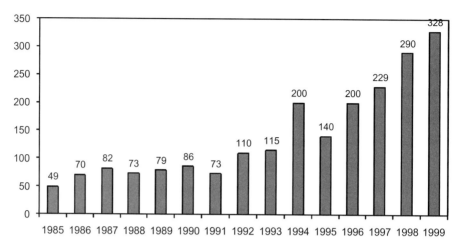

Figure 15.2 Numbers of patients in The Netherlands treated with electroconvulsive therapy per year (from Verwey & Sienaert, 2005).

Psychiatry and the Inspectorate of Mental Health recommended the establishment of an ECT evaluation committee, and a nationwide registration of ECT treatments started in 1996. The committee evaluated the indications and application of ECT. Meanwhile, a Dutch ECT Society (WEN) was organized in 1995. The success of this working group made the ECT evaluation committee superfluous. In 1999, the ECT evaluation committee produced its last report. In that year, 328 patients were treated with ECT at 20 sites, in a population of 15 million people. The average age was 60 years, and 84% of the patients were treated as inpatients. In about 60% of the cases, the indication was treatment-resistant depression; waiting time was on average 44 days.

In 2000, a guideline for ECT (approved by the Dutch Association for Psychiatry) was developed (van den Broek et al., 2000), to be updated in 2008. In 2005, van den Broek and colleagues published the Dutch Handbook on ECT (Dhossche, 2005; van den Broek et al., 2005), reflecting the renaissance of ECT in The Netherlands (Fink, 2006).

Portugal

No data have been published on the use and practice of ECT in Portugal. In February 2008, a well-attended national conference on ECT was held at the Electricity Museum in Lisbon. It was shown that, in Portugal, in the past few years, a total of six ECT units became active, three of which are situated in the Lisbon area (Lisbon, Amadora). These units performed a total of 500 to 1,200 treatment sessions in 2007, which corresponds to an ECT rate of 0.5 to 1.2 per 10,000 inhabitants. At least one new unit (Azores) will start activities in 2008. As in other European countries, the main indication for ECT is medication-resistant depression; the bitemporal electrode position is used most frequently, as is the hypnotic propofol.

Spain

Only two publications on the practice of ECT in Spain could be found (Bernardo et al., 1996; Bertolin-Guillen et al., 2006). Bernardo et al. (1996) described the pattern of ECT use in Barcelona in 1993. In 12 of the 20 hospitals surveyed, ECT was provided. Technical application was highly variable, but most hospitals used bilateral sine wave ECT, without monitoring seizure duration or electroencephalogram (EEG). Thiopental was the anesthetic most frequently used, and pharmacological agents were used simultaneously with ECT (Bernardo et al., 1996). In a recent survey of all psychiatric units in Spain ($n = 233$), it was shown that 108 psychiatric units (46.4%) provided ECT to a median of 15 patients per unit in 2001 (Bertolin-Guillen et al., 2006). Of these units, 66% used a brief-pulse device, and 15% still used sine wave devices. In 87% of the units, bilateral ECT was prescribed almost exclusively, on a three-times-per-week schedule. Seizure duration was measured in 76% of the units, and EEG monitoring was performed in 61%. General anesthesia was used in 95% of units, with propofol being the hypnotic most often used (34%). Surprisingly, three units (2.8%) did not administer muscle relaxants in 50% to 75% of patients, and five units (4.6%) used no muscle relaxants at all. About 50% of the units practiced outpatient ECT, whereas continuation ECT was only occasionally used. The attitude of the responding psychiatrists to ECT was generally favorable. The reason most mentioned for not administering or prescribing ECT (25% of psychiatric units, $n = 59$) was the lack of equipment – although this can hardly be seen as a reason for not referring patients to a hospital that does provide ECT. In a previous survey, 100% of psychiatrists working in a hospital where ECT was offered had a favorable attitude, whereas in hospitals that did not offer ECT only 36% of psychiatrists expressed a favorable attitude (Bertolin-Guillen et al., 2001). A similar pattern was seen in a survey with a sample of 47 Spanish anesthetists; 78% of the anesthetists had no objection to performing ECT anesthesia, whereas 13% refused application of the treatment (Bernardo et al., 1993).

There is great variability in the use of ECT across Spain, with a higher use in the northern "autonomous communities" (Catalonia, Navarre, Murcia) and a very low use in the south (Extremadura, Cantabria, and Ceuta-Melilla). The estimated annual ECT rate, measured in patients per 10,000 inhabitants, is 0.61.

Discussion

Data on the use and the practice of ECT in continental Western Europe are scarce. To our knowledge, there are no published reports on ECT in Italy, Portugal, Austria, and Switzerland. The available data suggest that ECT practice could be improved. For example, in some countries ECT is still administered without general anesthesia for a small number of patients (e.g., 0.6% of patients in Spain) or without muscle relaxants (e.g., 2.3% of patients in Spain) (Bertolin-Guillen et al., 2006). Some psychiatric hospitals find it difficult to recruit anesthetists for ECT, and often anesthetists have no experience with ECT (Bourgeois et al., 1981; Sienaert et al., 2005a). At least recently some hospitals continued to use sine-wave devices (Benadhira and Teles, 2001; Bertolin-Guillen et al., 2006; Sienaert et al., 2006b). In most countries, bitemporal ECT is the technique of first choice, whereas unilateral and bifrontal ECT are used infrequently. The main indication for ECT in Western Europe (as in the United States) is medication-resistant depression, whereas in the Central and Eastern European regions schizophrenia remains the main indication (Baudis, 1992; Gazdag et al., 2004). It appears that ECT training for psychiatric residents and psychiatrists is rarely provided in Europe. In only some countries, experienced ECT practitioners primarily give training. Most European national psychiatric associations have formulated no specific ECT standards or requirements.

Although ECT is available in all Western European countries (in specialized psychiatric facilities and in psychiatric departments of general hospitals), there are large national and regional differences. The large national and regional differences appear to be analogous to surveys reporting differences in the practice of ECT among countries, regions, and hospitals (Hermann et al., 1995; Westphal and Rush, 2000).

In some countries the ECT rate is low and, at least in some countries, the availability of ECT is problematic. In Italy, for example, ECT may be administered only as an emergency procedure in government hospitals in life-threatening situations, and only after other treatments have failed (Abrams, 2000). Low rates of use are probably largely from nonmedical concerns such as a negative public image (Hoffmann-Richter et al., 1998), obstructive legal regulations, and lack of knowledge and education about ECT. These variations contribute to controversies about equal access to medical care for all citizens wherever they may live (Benadhira and Teles, 2001).

Nevertheless, the available data seem to indicate an increasing acceptance of ECT throughout Europe. A growing scientific interest in ECT is reflected in the increasing number of scientific publications in most Western European countries in the last decade (Figure 15.3). On February 4, 2006, as a notable sign of the renaissance of ECT in Europe, at the University Psychiatric Center-Catholic University Leuven (Belgium), the EFFECT organization was founded on the initiative of Pascal Sienaert (Belgium), King Han Kho (The Netherlands), and Björn Wahlund (Sweden). This forum aimed to unite European practitioners and researchers on ECT, to ensure and promote access to safe and effective ECT for patients throughout

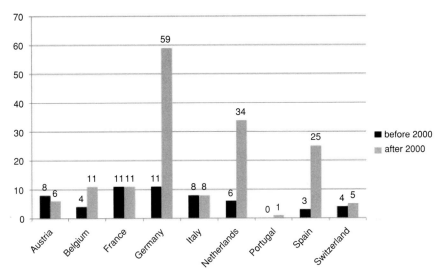

Figure 15.3 Publication activity in Western European countries (Medline search: "Electroconvulsive Therapy [Mesh] AND country [affiliation]").

Europe, to work toward a high standard of ECT practice across all countries in Europe, and to develop guidelines relating to ECT practice (Bolwig et al., 2006). In its wake, an Italian association for ECT (the *Associazone Italiana per la terapia elettroconvulsivante*) was established under the leadership of Athanasios Koukopoulos (A. Koukopoulos, 2005, personal communication). In February 2008, in Lisbon, a Portuguese national conference on ECT was organized. As part of this conference, a Portuguese association for ECT (the *Sociedade Portuguesa de Electroconvulsivoterapia*) was established, with António Gamito as president.

References

Abrams, R. 2000. Use of ECT in Italy. Am J Psychiatry 157: 840.

Accornero, F. 1988. An eyewitness account of the discovery of electroshock. Convuls Ther 4: 40–9.

Agence Nationale d'Accréditation et d'Évaluation en Santé (ANAES). 1997. Indications et modalités de l'electroconvulsivitherapie: Recommendations professionelles. Paris: ANAES.

Auquier, P., Hodgkinson, M., Thirion, X., and Tramoni, A. V. 1994. Attitude of psychiatrists to electrotherapy. Encephale 20: 713–7.

Baghai, T. C., Frey, R., Kasper, S., and Moller, H. J. 2004. Elektrokonvulsionstherapie: Klinische und wissenschaftliche Aspekte. Vienna: Springer-Verlag.

Baghai, T. C., Marcuse, A., Moller, H. J., and Rupprecht, R. 2005. Electroconvulsive therapy at the Department of Psychiatry and Psychotherapy, University of Munich. Development during the years 1995–2002. Nervenarzt 76: 597–612.

Baudis, P. 1992. Electroconvulsive therapy in the Czech Republic 1981–1989. Cesk Psychiatr 88: 41–7.

Benadhira, R. and Teles, A. 2001. Current status of electroconvulsive therapy in adult psychiatric care in France. Encephale 27: 129–36.

Bernardo M, Arrufat F, Pintor L, Catarineu S, Buisan E, Ballus C. 1996. Patterns of the use of electroconvulsive therapy in Barcelona. Med Clin (Barc) 106: 201–4.

Bernardo, M., Catarineu, S., Minarro, A., et al. 1993. Actitudes de los médicos anestesiologos ante la terapia electroconvulsiva. Rev Psiquiatria Fac Med Barna 20: 108–12.

Bertolin-Guillen, J. M., Peiro, M. S., Hernandez De Pablo, M. E., and Saez, A. C. 2001. Variability in attitudes and used conditions of electroconvulsive therapy. Results of a preliminary study. Actas Esp Psiquiatr 29: 390–5.

Bertolin-Guillen, J. M., Peiro-Moreno, S., and Hernandez-de-Pablo, M. E. 2006. Patterns of electroconvulsive therapy use in Spain. Eur Psychiatry 21: 463–70.

Bolwig, T., Wahlund, B., Kho, K. H., and Sienaert, P. 2006. A European foundation for electroconvulsive therapy. J ECT 22: 91.

Bourgeois, M., Palem, R., Tignol, J., et al. 1981. Current status of electroconvulsive therapy (ECT). I. Numerical aspects, indications, efficacy, media, prejudices and ideologies. Ann Med Psychol (Paris) 139: 1122–35.

Dhossche, D. 2005. Handboek elektroconvulsietherapie. J ECT 21: 256–7.

Dhossche, D. 2007. Elektroconvulsietherapie: Aanbevelingen voor de praktijk. J ECT 23: 296.

Fink, M. 1984. Meduna and the origins of convulsive therapy. Am J Psychiatry 141: 1034–41.

Fink, M. 2001. Convulsive therapy: A review of the first 55 years. J Affect Disord 63: 1–15.

Fink, M. 2006. The renaissance of ECT. In Elektroconvulsietherapie: Aanbevelingen voor de praktijk (eds. Sienaert, P., De Fruyt, J., and Dierick, M.). Gent: Academia Press.

Gazdag, G., Kocsis, N., and Lipcsey, A. 2004. Rates of electroconvulsive therapy use in Hungary in 2002. J ECT 20: 42–4.

Hermann, R. C., Dorwart, R. A., Hoover, C. W., and Brody, J. 1995. Variation in ECT use in the United States. Am J Psychiatry 152: 869–75.

Hoffmann-Richter, U., Alder, B., and Finzen, A. 1998. Electroconvulsive therapy and defibrillation in the paper. An analysis of the media. Nervenarzt 69: 622–8.

Kalinowsky, L. B. 1986. History of convulsive therapy. Ann NY Acad Sci 462: 1–4.

Lauter, H. and Sauer, H. 1987. Electroconvulsive therapy: A German perspective. Convuls Ther 3: 204–9.

Muller, N. and Geretsegger, C. 2004. Die Anwendung der Elektronvulsionstherapie in deutschsprachigen Landern. In Elektrokonvulsionstherapie: Klinische und wissenschaftliche Aspekte (eds. Baghai, T. C., Frey, R., Kasper, S., and Moller, H. J.). Vienna: Springer-Verlag.

Muller, U., Klimke, A., Janner, M., and Gaebel, W. 1998. Electroconvulsive therapy in psychiatric clinics in Germany in 1995. Nervenarzt 69: 15–26.

Oei, T. I., Koopmans, A., and Kalenda, Z. 1985. Recent developments in ECT in Holland. J Clin Psychopharmacol 5: 311.

Reimer, F. and Lorenzen, D. 1981. Use of electroconvulsive therapy in psychiatric treatment centres in West Germany. Nervenarzt 52: 554–6.

Shorter, E. and Healy, D. 2007. Shock therapy: A history of electroconvulsive treatment in mental illness. Piscataway, NJ: Rutgers University Press.

Sienaert, P., Bouckaert, F., Milo, W., and Peuskens, J. 2005a. De praktijk van elektroconvulsietherapie in Vlaanderen en het Brussels Hoofdstedelijk Gewest. Resultaten van een enquêteonderzoek. Tijdschr v Psychiatr 47: 279–89.

Sienaert, P., De Fruyt, J., and Dierick, M. 2006a. Elektroconvulsietherapie: Aanbevelingen voor de praktijk. Gent: Academia Press.

Sienaert, P., Dierick, M., Degraeve, G., and Peuskens, J. 2006b. Electroconvulsive therapy in Belgium: A nationwide survey on the practice of electroconvulsive therapy. J Affect Disord 90: 67–71.

Sienaert, P., Filip, B., Willy, M., and Joseph, P. 2005b. Electroconvulsive therapy in Belgium: A questionnaire study on the practice of electroconvulsive therapy in Flanders and the Brussels Capital region. J ECT 21: 3–6.

van den Broek, W., Huyser, J., Koster, A. M., et al. 2000. Richtlijn elektroconvulsietherapie. Amsterdam: Boom.

van den Broek, W., Leentjens, A. F. G., van Vliet, I. M., and Verwey, B. 2005. Handboek elektroconvulsietherapie. Assen: Van Gorcum b.v.

Verwey, B. and Sienaert, P. 2005. Geschiedenis van ECT. In Handboek electroconvulsietherapie (ed. van den Broek, W.). Assen: Van Gorcum b.v.

Vijselaar, J. 2007. Psyche en elektriciteit. Universiteit Utrecht, Faculteit Geesteswetenschappen.

Westphal, J. R. and Rush, J. 2000. A statewide survey of ECT policies and procedures. J ECT 16: 279–86.

16

Electroconvulsive therapy in Asia

Sidney S. Chang

Introduction

Electroconvulsive therapy (ECT) utilization has varied widely among countries and changed periodically since ECT was introduced in 1938. In Western countries, ECT use has varied not only among countries but within the same country (Glen and Scott, 1999; Hermann et al., 1995). Similar variation and evolution in ECT use occur in Asian countries. ECT in Japan was first reported in 1939, and modified ECT in Japan was first noted in 1958 (Motohashi et al., 2004). During the 1960s, ECT use in Japan decreased by 50% and has continued to decrease for more than 30 years (Chanpattana et al., 2005a). The general impression has been that ECT usage in Asian countries is much lower than in Western countries, data are limited, and ECT practice remains largely undocumented in this region. Recently there has been a revival of interest in ECT in Asia, with more publications about ECT usage.

Here the history of ECT and then ECT usage based on surveys are reviewed. ECT indications in Asia, age and gender distributions, and technical aspects of the ECT procedure such as electrode placements, devices, and ECT anesthesia are also reviewed.

ECT rates

From a centralized database of ECT treatment in Hong Kong, annual rates of ECT use from 1997 to 2002 varied from 2.7 to 3.4 patients treated per 100,000 population and from 1.34 to 1.88 patients treated per 100 patients discharged (Chung, 2003). This rate is much lower than the rates of 8 to 49 patients per 100,000 population in the United States (Kramer, 1999; Thompson et al., 1994); in Victoria, Australia (Wood and Burgess, 2003); and in the United Kingdom (Department of Health, England, 2002; Duffett et al., 1999; Glen and Scott, 1999; Hermann et al., 1995) (see Figure 16.1). Similarly, in terms of ECT use per 100 patients discharged, Hong Kong's use was lower, with rates of 1.34% to 1.64%, compared with 0.4% to 1.7% in state hospitals in the United States (Sylvester et al., 2000) and 0.8% to 15% among consultant teams in Edinburgh (Glen and Scott, 2000).

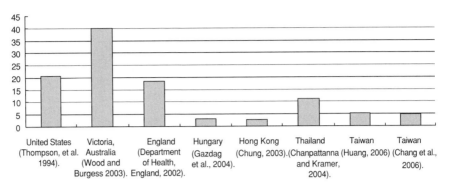

Figure 16.1 Electroconvulsive therapy (ECT) rates of some Asian and Western countries (ECT/100,000 population).

In Taiwan, the government provides comprehensive health insurance covering 96% of the population. The medical claims database reveals an ECT use rate per 100,000 adult population in Taiwan during 1997 through 2001 of 5.2% to 6.0% per year, and a rate per 100 inpatients of 3.6% to 2.2% (Huang, 2006). Another report using this database found an ECT rate per 100 patients discharged of 1.97% and a rate of 4.7 per 100,000 population per year in 2001 (Chang et al., 2006). These results are similar. Even though the ECT rate is higher in Taiwan than Hong Kong, it is still much lower than in Western countries. Whereas the population ECT rate remained stable from 1997 to 2001, the rate per 100 inpatients declined significantly from 3.6% to 2.2% ($p = .004$). The number of psychiatric inpatient beds increased markedly, but total ECT usage remained unchanged (Huang, 2006).

In Thailand, a mail survey during the period from September 2001 through August 2002 revealed that ECT was available in 26 institutes (64%) and the usage rate was 11.5 per 100,000 population per year (Chanpattana and Kramer, 2004). The authors believed that the results generally represented ECT practice because only two institutions that performed ECT did not respond to the survey; overall 53 of 67 institutes replied. The ECT usage rate of 11.5 per 100,000 population per year in Thailand is the highest known among Asian countries. The authors believed that a shortage of psychiatrists and mental health facilities and the unavailability of newer medications such as second generation antipsychotic drugs might be the explanation.

ECT was introduced to Japan in 1939 and was widely used until the 1960s. Its use then decreased by 50% and continued to decrease during the next 30 years. Japan has the highest number of physicians and psychiatrists in Asia, and has adequate medical resources. Motohashi et al. (2004) conducted a mail survey to 123 national and university hospitals with psychiatric beds. The study period was from 1997 through 1999, and the reply rate was 71% (86/123). ECT was performed in 56 hospitals (65%), but the number of patients receiving ECT per year varied widely, from 0.5 to 120 per year. However, there are more than 1,600 hospitals with psychiatric beds in Japan. The author concluded that ECT is underdeveloped in Japan and ECT practice should be improved and made more accessible.

A second ECT survey in Japan was taken during the period from September 1, 2001, through August 31, 2003, with a 29-item questionnaire sent to 271 institutions (Chanpattana et al., 2005a). A total of 100 institutes replied (40% rate). ECT was available in 83 institutes (83%). The results confirmed the previous report that ECT usage is low in Japan, but has increased slightly since 1999. Low ECT usage was attributed to opinion in the absence of experience.

Mental illness carries a huge stigma in Pakistan. ECT there carries many misconceptions, and there is great resistance by patients and their families to accepting it. A 13-year naturalistic review of ECT usage in a university hospital in Karachi, Pakistan, was reported by Naqvi and Khan (2005). During this period of 4,013 inpatients, 136 (3.38%) received ECT. This rate is high relative to Asian standards, and not typical of Pakistan as a whole.

ECT is more actively used in India. A total of 13.4% of psychiatrists in India used ECT during the six months preceding a survey in 1991 (Agarwal et al., 1992, 1993). A more recent survey found that 66 institutions (of 74 replying) made ECT available (Chanpattana et al., 2005b).

In a survey of ECT in the Asian Pacific region, Little (2003) found the percentage of inpatients receiving ECT varied from less than 1% to 9%, except in Nepal, where it was 25.6%. No ECT was given in Cambodia. The only detail available about ECT in Malaysia, the Philippines, and China is that it is used. In Asia, cultural attitudes toward ECT and mental illness are negative, except in the Philippines.

In an earlier mail survey, Kramer and Pi (1990) reported low ECT usage in Asia and that many psychiatrists had lost interest in ECT. In China, ECT was available but seldom used. During the period of the cultural revolution, ECT was officially pronounced as cruel and was severely criticized. In Korea, ECT use was essentially nonexistent, and most psychiatrists had no awareness of it.

Although data describing ECT usage in many Asian countries are rare, ECT appears to be widely used but at rates lower than in Western countries. As shown in Figure 16.1, rates in the United States, Australia, and England are 20 to 40 per 100,000 population per year (Department of Mental Health, England, 2002; Thompson et al., 1994; Wood and Burgess, 2003) and 5 to 10 per 100,000 population in Hong Kong, Taiwan, and Thailand (Chang et al., 2006; Chanpattana and Kramer, 2004; Chung, 2003; Huang, 2006). Shortages of psychiatrists and low budgets probably account for some of the ECT underuse. Misunderstandings about ECT by both the public and mental health professionals are probably a stronger influence against ECT. Recent reports of increasing ECT use in Asia seem to signal renewed

Table 16.1 Psychiatric diagnosis of patients receiving electroconvulsive therapy

Country	Mood disorders (%)	Schizophrenia (%)	Other (%)
United States (Thompson et al., 1994)	84	6	9
Victoria, Australia (Wood and Burgess, 2003)	83	16	1
England (Department of Health, 2002)	81	6	12
Hong Kong (Chung, 2003)	68	31	1
Thailand (Chanpattana and Kramer, 2004)	16	74	10
Taiwan (Huang, 2006)	25	70	4
Japan (Chanpattana et al., 2005a)	42	56	2
Pakistan (Naqvi and Khan, 2005)	79	16	5

interest in ECT. Patient and public education remains an important measure to take to counter the stigmatization of mental illness and its treatment in Asia.

Indications for ECT

Characteristic of ECT usage in Asia is that it used in more patients diagnosed with schizophrenia than with mood disorders (Kramer and Pi, 1990; Little, 2003). As illustrated in Table 16.1, in the United States, Australia, and England more than 80% of ECT patients had a diagnosis of mood disorder. In Taiwan and Thailand, more than 80% of ECT recipients had a schizophrenia diagnosis. Hong Kong and Japan fell in between. In India, ECT was used equally for schizophrenia and major depression (Agarwal et al., 1992, 1993).

In Hong Kong, ECT usage was lower than in Western countries, and mood disorders were the primary target. Differences in expression and lower prevalence of depressive illness in Chinese people might partially account for the rarity of ECT use in Hong Kong (Chung, 2003). Chinese patients might have a similar clinical response to ECT whether the diagnosis is schizophrenia or depression (Chung, 2003). Relatively high usage of ECT in patients with schizophrenia is probably associated with widespread belief that ECT produces more rapid response than drugs in this patient group (Chanpattana et al., 2005b).

Another reason for ECT use for schizophrenia in Asia is the high cost of second generation antipsychotic drugs. Although a course of six ECTs costs about US$130

Table 16.2 Age classification of patients receiving electroconvulsive therapy

Country	Younger than 65 years (%)	65 years old or older (%)
United States (Thompson et al., 1994)	66	34
Victoria, Australia (Wood and Burgess, 2003)	67	33
England (Department of Health, 2002)	54	46
Hong Kong (Chung, 2003)	85	15
Thailand (Chanpattana and Kramer, 2004)	97	3
Taiwan (Huang, 2006)	96	4
Japan (Chanpattana et al., 2005a)	61	39
Pakistan (Naqvi and Khan, 2005) (cutoff age = 61 years)	91	9

in developing countries (Naqvi and Khan, 2005), this is substantially less than the cost of second generation antipsychotic drugs.

Traditions in clinical orientation might contribute to ECT usage for schizophrenia in Taiwan and Japan. Psychiatry practices in both countries have been connected with German psychiatric teachings emphasizing ECT usage in schizophrenia. This situation appears similar to the situation of Hungary, which was strongly influenced by German psychiatry and where a high proportion of ECT patients have the diagnosis of schizophrenia (Gazdag et al., 2004). The historically strong influence of Japanese psychiatry on practice in Taiwan may explain the high proportion of ECT patients with schizophrenia in Taiwan.

Age classification of patients receiving ECT

A larger percentage of ECT patients are elderly in Western countries than in Asia (Table 16.2). In the United States (Thompson et al., 1994), England (Department of Health, England, 2002), and Australia (Wood and Burgess, 2003), more than one third of ECT patients are older than 65 years. In Taiwan, Hong Kong, Thailand, and Pakistan, elderly persons account for less than 15% of ECT patients. Japan is the exception to this trend; there 39% of ECT patients are older than 65 years. This finding might partially result from the longer life expectancy in Japan and the higher proportion of elderly citizens in Japan.

Perhaps underrecognition and undertreatment of depressive disorders in elderly patients in Hong Kong explain the low usage of ECT (Chung, 2003). Another reason for underuse of ECT in elderly patients is shortage of medical resources, anesthesiologists, or recovery facilities.

Table 16.3 Sex distribution of patients receiving electroconvulsive therapy

Country	Male (%)
United States (Thompson et al., 1994)	29
Victoria, Australia (Wood and Burgess, 2003)	37
England (Department of Health, 2002)	29
Hong Kong (Chung, 2003)	32
Thailand (Chanpattana and Kramer, 2004)	72
Taiwan (Huang, 2006)	41
Japan (Chanpattana et al., 2005a)	46
Pakistan (Naqvi and Khan, 2005)	44

Sex distribution of patients receiving ECT

Most reports from Asian countries show greater usage of ECT in women than men (Table 16.3). This sex distribution is the same as in Western countries. Thailand is the exception, apparently because they have more psychiatric beds for men than for women and relatively high ECT use in schizophrenia ECT is used more in men than women in Thailand (Chanpattana and Kramer, 2004). Similarly, in other countries in which most ECT patients had mood disorders, the proportion of female patients receiving ECT is higher (Tables 16.2 and 16.3).

Technical aspects of ECT

In Asian countries, bitemporal ECT is the most commonly used electrode placement. In Thailand (Chanpattanna, 2004), Taiwan (Chang et al., 2006), Pakistan (Naqvi and Khan, 2005), and India (Agarwal et al., 1992, 1993), bitemporal ECT is used almost exclusively. In Japan, unilateral ECT is used in some academic institutes, but bitemporal ECT generally predominates (Chanpattana et al., 2005a; Motohashi et al., 2004). In Hong Kong, unilateral ECT was used in 22% of ECT patients during a five-year study period, and its use gradually increased (Chung, 2003).

ECT modified with muscle relaxants is not common in Asia. In Thailand, unmodified ECT was used in 94.2% of ECT treatments (Chanpattana and Kramer, 2004) and in Taiwan about 85% (Chang et al., 2006). In Japan, 61% of 60 institutes used unmodified ECT exclusively, and another 32% used modified ECT most of the time (Chanpattana et al., 2005b). A university hospital in Karachi routinely used modified ECT (Naqvi and Khan, 2005). In comparison, modified ECT is routine in Western countries. The reason for unmodified ECT in Asia is a shortage of medical resources and anesthesiologists. This is not the case in Japan; the use in Japan of unmodified ECT has been attributed to stigmatization of psychiatric illness and treatment hindering adoption of modern ECT practices (Chanpattana et al., 2005b). Many Asian psychiatrists recognize the benefits of modified ECT and promote its use. One group in India seeks to ban ECT without anesthesia (Mudur, 2002). In Japan, individual psychiatrists (but no group) have urged uniform use of modified ECT (Motohashi et al., 2004).

Modern brief-pulse devices such as MECTA and Thymatron instruments are used in many Asian countries, but so are sine wave devices. In India, sine wave ECT devices were more common, although the last data are outdated (Agarwal et al., 1992, 1993). In Thailand, 12 of 26 institutes used MECTA or Thymatron instruments (Chanpattana and Kramer, 2004). In Japan, brief-pulse ECT devices were not approved at the time of the survey from 1997 through 1999 (Motohashi et al., 2004). A second survey five years later showed increased use of brief-pulse ECT, but still 46 respondents used sine wave, 16 used brief-pulse, and 5 used both types (Chanpattana et al., 2005b). In Taiwan, most hospitals use brief-pulse devices, but some public mental hospitals still use sine wave devices (Chang et al., 2006). The use of brief-pulse ECT has increased recently. For example, more than 200 brief-pulse instruments are in use in Japan, a considerable number are in China, a dozen are in Malaysia, and there are several in Vietnam (Somatics Company, March, 2008, personal communication).

The number of sessions in an ECT course in Asia is between 5 and 10 treatments, as in Western countries. Reports of ECT outcome in Asia are also similar, indicating high efficacy and tolerability, and only very rarely mortality. Outpatient and maintenance ECTs are rare in Asia.

Regulation of ECT and training of ECT professionals in Asia

In Asian countries, regulation of ECT is left to the health professions, and legislators have not enacted laws involving ECT (Chanpattana et al., 2005b). In addition, laws have not been enacted about ECT administration to patients declared incompetent. For example, when a patient is unable to make an informed decision about ECT treatment in Hong Kong, a second senior psychiatrist's written opinion and consent from a relative are sufficient (Chung, 2003). This is similar to the author's experience in Taiwan.

There is no specific credentialing or training requirement for ECT privileges in Asia, even in Japan (Chanpattana et al., 2005b). ECT policy and procedure statements were written in 16 of the 46 hospitals surveyed in Japan (Motohashi et al., 2004). Thailand has no formal training program or supervision standards for ECT, and instruction in the ECT procedure for a psychiatry resident is usually by the preceding resident assigned to ECT or by a senior resident (Chanpattana and Kramer, 2004). In Pakistan, anecdotal evidence is noted of ECT usage without clear clinical indications or informed consent (Naqvi and Khan, 2005). After a 20-year-old survey in a state mental hospital in Singapore, it was concluded that ECT was given primarily according to impressionistic managerial decisions rather than criterion-based diagnosis, and informed consent was virtually unknown (Chee, 1992). Fortunately, Singapore has changed markedly since that time, with large improvements in individual patient rights. Although no later survey was published, it is reasonable to expect that practices there are modernized. Generally, ECT regulation and supervision are less restrictive in Asia than in the West. There are efforts in Japan to ensure quality in ECT practice (Kurita, 2007).

No report from an Asian country indicated that ECT training is required during psychiatry residency. Of course, systematic ECT training is important for the professional development and advancement of ECT practice in Asia.

Summary

ECT practice is alive in Asia, particularly in Japan, Taiwan, Hong Kong, Thailand, Pakistan, and India. ECT use is reported in Singapore, Malaysia, China, and the Philippines, but is probably underutilized. In Cambodia and South Korea, it is essentially nonexistent. ECT is generally used there in 1% to 9% of inpatients, and more frequently in Nepal. Public perceptions of psychiatric illness and ECT are more as stigmatization than illness, except in the Philippines.

ECT usage rates are much lower in Asia than in Western countries, approximately 5 to 10 per 100,000 persons per year compared with 20 to 40 per 100,000 persons, respectively. Shortages of psychiatrists, anesthesia personnel, and funding presumably account for some of the lower ECT usage. Stigmatization associated with psychiatric illness and treatment is probably also responsible. Public education in Asia about psychiatric illness is similarly behind that of Western countries.

In Asia, bitemporal ECT is typical, unmodified ECT is common, ECT usage for patients with schizophrenia is more prevalent than for those with mood disorders, the ECT patient population is relatively young, and sine wave ECT devices are widely used. Some of these practices are not consistent with modern expectations, and efforts are growing in Japan and India to routinely use anesthesia with ECT. Japan and China are widely replacing sine wave devices with brief-pulse instruments.

More professional publications about ECT from Asia have been appearing. Publications from Japan recently reached 50 per year, an increase from an average of

13 per year from 1983 through 2005 (Kurita, 2007). Between these modernizations and the growing number of publications, it is clear that ECT clinical activity and interest are advancing in Asia, but required ECT education during psychiatry residency is needed.

References

Agarwal, A. K., Andrade, C., and Reddy, M. V. 1992. The practice of ECT in India. I. Indian J Psychiatry 34: 28–97.

Agarwal, A. K., Andrade, C., and Reddy, M. V. 1993. The practice of ECT in India. II. Indian J Psychiatry 35: 81–6.

Chang, S., Chang, I.-S., and Lin, K.-M. 2006. Electroconvulsive therapy (ECT) usage in Taiwan. Annual Meeting of Taiwanese Society of Psychiatry (Symposium #20).

Chanpattana, W., Kojima. K., Kramer, B. A., et al. 2005a. ECT practice in Japan. J ECT 21: 139–44.

Chanpattana, W. and Kramer, B. A. 2004. Electroconvulsive therapy practice in Thailand. J ECT 20: 94–8.

Chanpattana, W., Kunigiri, G., Kramer, B. A., et al. 2005b. Survey of the practice of electroconvulsive therapy in teaching hospitals in India. J ECT 21: 100–4.

Chee, K. T. 1992. Medico-legal implications of electroconvulsive therapy – a Singapore viewpoint. Singapore Med J 33: 271–2.

Chung, K. F. 2003. Electroconvulsive therapy in Hong Kong: Rates of use, indications, and outcome. J ECT 19: 98–102.

Department of Health, England. Electroconvulsive therapy survey covering period of January 2002 to March 2002. Available at http://www.markwalton.net/statistic.asp, accessed May, 2005, and at http://www.dh.gov.uk/en/Publicationsandstatistics/Statistics/StatisticalWork Areas/Statisticalhealthcare/DH_4000216, accessed September 24, 2008.

Duffett, R., Siegert, D. R., and Lelliott, P. 1999. Electroconvulsive therapy in Wales. Psychiatr Bull R Coll Psychiatr 23: 597–601.

Gazdag, G., Kocsis, N., and Lipcsey, A. 2004. Rates of electroconvulsive therapy use in Hungary in 2002. J ECT 20: 42–4.

Glen, T. and Scott, A. I. F. 1999. Rates of electroconvulsive therapy use in Edinburgh (1992–1997). J Affect Dis 54: 81–5.

Glen, T. and Scott, A.I. F. 2000. Variation in rates of electroconvulsive therapy use among consultant teams in Edinburgh (1993–1996). J Affect Dis 58: 75–8.

Hermann, R. C., Dorwatt, R. A., Hoover, C. W., et al. 1995. Variation in ECT use in the United States. Am J Psychiatry 152: 869–75.

Huang, L. Y. 2006. Electroconvulsive therapy in Taiwan: Findings from analysis of the national health insurance database. Annual Meeting of Taiwanese Society of Psychiatry (Oral Presentation #26).

Kramer, B. A. 1999. Use of ECT in California, revisited: 1984–1994. J ECT 15: 245–51.

Kramer, B. A. and Pi, E.- H. 1990. A survey of ECT use in Asia. Convuls Ther 6: 26–31.

Kurita, S. 2007. Future direction of the guideline for electroconvulsive therapy (ECT). Seishin Shinkeigaku Zasshi 109: 348–53 (in Japanese).

Little, J. D. 2003. ECT in the Asia Pacific region: What do we know? J ECT 19: 93–7.

Motohashi, N., Awata, S., and Higuchi, T. 2004. A questionnaire survey of ECT practice in university hospitals and national hospitals in Japan. J ECT 20: 21–3.

Mudur, G. 2002. Indian groups seek ban on use of electroconvulsive therapy without anesthesia. Brit Med J 324: 806.

Naqvi. H. and Khan, M. M. 2005. Use of electroconvulsive therapy at a university hospital in Karachi, Pakistan: A 13-year naturalistic review. J ECT 21: 158–61.

Sylvester, A. P., Mulsant, B. H., Roy Chengappa, K. N., et al. 2000. Use of electroconvulsive therapy in a state hospital: A 10-year review. J Clin Psychiatry 61: 534–9.

Thompson, J. W., Weiner, R. D., and Meyers, C. P. 1994. Use of ECT in the United States in 1975, 1980 and 1986. Am J Psychiatry 151: 1157–61.

Wood, D. A. and Burgess, P. M. 2003. Epidemiological analysis of electroconvulsive therapy in Victoria, Australia. Aust N Z J Psychiatry 37: 307–11.

17

History of electroconvulsive therapy in the Russian Federation

Alexander I. Nelson and Nataliya Giagou

Introduction

To those who are familiar with the current situation in the Russian Federation, it will come as a surprise that the USSR was one of the first countries that began using electroconvulsive therapy (ECT). In the 1930s, "Meduna's method" of chemical convulsive therapy (with the help of camphor or pentylenetetrazol) was already well known and officially recognized (Goldenberg, 1938; Guidelines on convulsive therapy, 1940; Sereisky and Rotshtein, 1940; Shapiro, 1940; Zhivotovsky, 1941). In the first year after its invention (1939), ECT was introduced in Professor Sereisky's clinic in Moscow and Professor Frumkin's clinic in Kiev (Frumkin et al., 1950; Rodzevskaya, 1951).

ECT in the 1940s and 1950s: The bloom and the freeze

The precipitous development of this method in the USSR in the 1940s was particularly striking, considering that the atmosphere of mass repressions at the end of the 1930s was not conducive to new treatment methods. Moreover, World War II, which began three years after the invention of ECT, was expected to hinder new developments in psychiatry. However, Soviet scientists and clinicians immediately appreciated the enormous therapeutic potential of ECT, and their enthusiasm overcame these obstacles.

Still, in 1941 the influential book *The Convulsive Therapy of Schizophrenia* by G. A. Rotshtein (Rotshtein, 1941) did not mention ECT, focusing entirely on chemically induced seizures and "Meduna's method." In 1942, the first Russian experiences with ECT were described in print, and the advantages of ECT over chemical convulsive therapy were emphasized (Sereisky and Rotshtein, 1942). Six years later, G. A. Rotshtein wrote about the experience "of longstanding use of electroconvulsive therapy in psychiatric clinics and hospitals of the Soviet Union" (Rotshtein, 1948).

Indeed, Soviet psychiatric practice promptly accepted ECT. By 1948, 5.3% of hospitalized mentally ill patients were treated with ECT (Banschikov and Rapoport, 1952). Professor A. I. Molokhov from Kishinev wrote that ECT "is becoming the main instrument of medical treatment of schizophrenia" (Molokhov, 1948). In 1949, among "the active methods" of treatment of psychosis, ECT was second to insulin shock therapy. The report data indicated that by 1950 ECT was used in many psychiatric hospitals in the USSR. By 1951, tens of thousands of patients had been treated with ECT in the USSR.

It seems that all the prerequisites needed for vigorous study and development of ECT in the Soviet Union were then present, but they did not occur because of the scientific atmosphere in the USSR during those years. The political regime at that time raged against intellectuals, including those in medicine and science, regardless of talent. Many intellectual physicians and scientists lost their jobs, were reduced in rank, or were stripped of all credentials. Even extreme adverse actions were common, including exile, concentration camp, or execution.

Psychiatry, among other branches of medicine, was not able to avoid the dreadful millstones of Stalin's regime. Medical administrators who were followers of the Communist Party separated all psychiatrists by their loyalty to the principles of Pavlov. They decreed that Pavlov had "the only correct socialistic theory of behavioral medicine." All whose work suggested any doubt in conformity to Pavlov's concepts were "extirpated" as "socially extraneous elements" infected with bourgeois ideology. In accordance with political traditions of the time, Soviet medical leaders declared nonconforming methods and trends in medicine as "fascist," "barbarian," "not corresponding with socialistic ideology," and so forth. The authoritarian condemnations, presented as scientific articles in central journals, often included political testimonials at the end of the text: "To Stalin the Great, the leader of our triumphs at the war front, at the peace front, and at the science front; long live the luminary of science!" (Gilyarovsky, 1951).

The activities that promoted the isolationism of Soviet psychiatry were propagated under the banner of "the fight against cosmopolitanism." It became dangerous to have any knowledge of foreign literature and experience. It was particularly risky to quote or try to adopt it. Here is an eloquent excerpt from a Soviet psychiatric journal published during that time, which accompanied savage punishment of the scientists from the Serbsky Institute:

"The regulations of the Central Committee of the Communist Party of the Soviet Union urged Soviet intellectuals, including scientists, to firmly adhere to the position of Bolshevik Party's spirit." "The authors . . . excessively used multiple citations of foreign authors. Such citations most of the time are absolutely unnecessary and sometimes simply distort the true status of the matter. They confuse the reader and cause damage to the priority of Russian science." "The transfer into the Russian psychiatric literature . . . of foreign terms is absolutely unjustified." (Kalashnik, 1950).

The supreme party and government administrators did not have any bona fide evidence against the use of particular treatment methods in any area of medicine. A posture of "pursuit of the enemy" and "fight for purity" was propagated from the top. Uneasiness and fear for one's own work and life dictated specific modes of behavior within the scientific environment. If they did not demonstrate vigilance and did not denounce anybody, they themselves could be denounced. In the science of that time, as always, many people were compelled in their behavior by envy, ambition, and vanity. Some scientists had fully mastered the science of self-affirmation at the cost of the destruction of their colleagues, compensating for their own lack of talent and productivity. In the scientific environment of those times, proximity to the administrators conveyed more empowerment than scientific prestige and achievements did.

ECT became a target for malicious attacks on Soviet psychiatry because it came from abroad. The method of ECT was somewhat unusual, both nonpharmaceutical and effective. It came from Italy, a country that was an enemy during World War II as a member of the fascist coalition. ECT was actively developing in Western countries, considered political opponents. The method seemingly embodied internal inconsistencies: High efficacy was combined with the appearance of physical roughness, medical complications, inability to prevent relapses, and the suggestion of psychosurgery. More difficult was that ECT did not blend with Pavlov's theory, and it was difficult to ascribe Soviet ownership of concepts. Finally, many of the most active researchers and advocates of ECT appeared to be Jewish, and anti-Semitism was strong. All these things made ECT a natural object for "eradication" both by morally unscrupulous persons and by those who did not like ECT because of personal or ideological considerations.

Although some renowned Soviet psychiatrists at that time vigorously rejected ECT, others enthusiastically advocated it. In 1949 at Plenum II of the Soviet Scientific Society of Neurologists and Psychiatrists, the members discussed ECT with favorable or at least neutral impressions (Likhterman and Likhterman, 2000). However, the environment surrounding ECT gradually became more tense. In 1950, the frequency of ECT use in psychiatric hospitals started decreasing (Banschikov and Rapoport, 1952). The hospitals where ECT had not been introduced continued to refrain from it.

In 1950, at the Kharkov Medical Institute, A. I. Ploticher presented a brilliant dissertation about ECT (Ploticher, 1950). His dissertation was remarkably inclusive, with a logical theoretical basis, scrupulous research about the presentation of seizures, and elegantly organized discussions of experiments. It described the development and use of an original ECT device of his design. Ploticher reported different methods of conducting individual treatments and courses of ECT, including using anesthesia. He elucidated a method of stimulus dosing based on physiology.

He reported on his studies of ECT effectiveness in 500 patients with a variety of disorders and syndromes, analyzing subtle psychopathological and physiological changes, methods of prophylaxis, management of complications, and anticipation of relapses. It was so far ahead of its time that it could now be mistaken for a contemporary work. Unfortunately, it was not published, and few people are familiar with it. We hope it will eventually be published and recognized.

During the following two years, the Higher Certification Board considered approval of Ploticher's dissertation. On May 16, 1952, the Academic Council of the Department of Clinical Medicine of the Academy of Medical Sciences of the USSR held a session dedicated to "the discussion of the expediency and possibility of ECT use in the treatment of psychiatric disorders." This was an awkward political event to dispose of ECT. Ploticher was compelled to contritely announce that he had "revised indications and counterindications for ECT," but his dissertation was just the same suppressed. The report of this session appeared in the journal *Zhurnal Nevrol Psikhiatr Im S S Korsakova* (About use of electroshock for treatment of psychical diseases, 1952). The pronouncement was that ECT may be used "only as a method of final resort, after other methods have not been successful, mainly in involutional melancholia and some forms of schizophrenia. The use of ECT is absolutely inadmissible in reactive depressions, neuroses, and as a method of rapid relief of agitation in children. The course of ECT may not be long and intensive. Its use is permissible only within a hospital." The content of this resolution did not stop ECT, but its tone and implications did. It was perceived as prohibition.

In 1952, the Academy of Medical Sciences of the USSR and the USSR Academy of Sciences held a series of sessions dedicated to "the problems of Pavlov's physiological teaching" and "the distribution of scientific and teaching personnel in the system of Public Health of the USSR." The resolutions of these scientific meetings were perceived as a call for the evaluation of all the current work in neurology and psychiatry on ideological adherence to Pavlov's teaching and elimination of all "ideologically unfaithful" scientists. This was terrorism in the halls of medicine, and it changed the views of Soviet psychiatrists on ECT. There were many political publications in the medical literature claiming harm from ECT. New publications stated that markedly lower percentages of patients were responding to ECT treatment (Dain, 1958).

The central psychiatric press newsletter printed that "it is necessary to put an end to such broad indications to ECT" (Banschikov and Rapoport, 1952). Professor O. V. Kerbikov lectured in 1952 and 1953 that "the indications to this grave method of therapy are drastically limited" (Kerbikov, 1955). Such statements were clearly understood as prohibition.

In this environment ECT was impossible, as ECT device production stopped after it barely started. It was dangerous for individual physicians; they could lose their medical licenses or their freedom. Stopping ECT was rationalized by unrealistically high expectations of cure with the new breed of psychotropic medications such as chlorpromazine, imipramine, lithium, and iproniazid.

Oddly, in the heat of battle against ECT, chemical convulsive therapy remained uncontroversial. Its greater discomforts and risks did not matter. The issue was "electric shock." Indeed, a 1952 dissertation on chemical convulsive therapy with an ammonium preparation in treating epilepsy and schizophrenia was approved promptly (Borzunova, 1952).

However, the discussion about ECT continued. A conference of the Moscow Society of Neurologists and Psychiatrists focusing on ECT took place in 1952, and leading specialists participated. Alongside flat authoritarian calls to prohibit ECT were sensible arguments describing its helpfulness to patients. The conclusion of the conference was that, despite many drawbacks, practicing physicians should not reject ECT. The Academy of Medical Sciences of the USSR delivered a special decision that the use of ECT was allowed but only as a final resort after other methods had proven ineffective. Although a funeral for ECT did not occur, an underlying spirit of ominous malevolence by medical administrators was clear and painfully felt, and the method fell into nearly total disuse in the USSR for several years.

Close to the end of the 1950s, written mention of ECT was tolerated in textbooks in a neutral tone, with mention of its therapeutic affinity for catatonic schizophrenia, and including photos of an ECT treatment (Kerbikov et al., 1958). In 1957, the main psychiatric journal printed this text about ECT: "Not even one article about ECT has been published in our journals within the past two years. In many provincial psychiatric hospitals this method has been abandoned entirely. Beyond doubt, this situation does not promote the effective treatment of mentally ill patients" (Lebedev, 1957).

ECT in the 1960s and 1970s

In the 1960s, the ECT situation started to improve. The texts of articles about ECT during that time seem to suggest that official antipathy to ECT was diminishing. Some reports described substantial ECT research efforts. The principal Soviet book on insulin shock therapy (Lichko, 1962) included several courageous recommendations for combination with ECT, brave even from our present perspective. Research directed to identify hormonal predictors of ECT effectiveness was conducted at the Department of Psychiatry at Leningrad's State Institute for the Advanced Training of Physicians (Timofeeva, 1962). At the end of the 1960s, ECT was mentioned straightforwardly in the standard psychiatry textbook for medical students (Banschikov and Nevzorova, 1969).

In 1970, the Department of Psychiatry of the First Moscow Institute of Medicine published an article indirectly advocating ECT treatment because of its high efficacy

(Nevzorova and Romanovsky, 1970). However, the official administrators were in no hurry to approve it. At the Sixth World Congress on Psychiatry (Honolulu, HI, 1977) the Soviet delegation was put on the spot with accusations about inappropriate and political use of psychiatric knowledge. Their reply claimed "particular humanism" in Soviet psychiatry by stating that ". . . The Ministry of Public Health of the USSR introduced new amendments to its instructions about the use of ECT. The indications for its use are strictly limited. At the present time ECT is used extremely rarely in our country" (Babayan, 1978). These statements about ECT were of little import, and the USSR was expelled from the World Psychiatric Organization for misuse of psychiatry.

At the end of the 1970s, the political climate in the USSR had warmed a little to new ideas, and the first dissertation on ECT after a 23-year hiatus was presented (Nikolaenko, 1978). The first brief instructive guide to ECT use, 10-pages long, was published at that time (Health Ministry of the USSR, 1979).

From the 1980s through the end of the 20th century

Ten more years passed before a Russian-made brief-pulse ECT device became available (the Elikon-01; 1987) and for the Health Ministry to provide another ECT manual, this one 34-pages long (Health Ministry of the USSR, 1989). The end of the 1980s might be considered the rebirth of ECT in Soviet psychiatry. Two dissertations about ECT were defended during that decade (Moschevitin, 1989; Rakhmazova, 1985). However, even in that period of time modified ECT was used only rarely, and notations in publications indicated that many hospitals continued to use antiquated ECT devices.

In the 1990s, ECT development continued as slowly as in the 1980s. An unofficial ECT teaching center appeared in Naro-Fominsk near Moscow, but it had a national scope. Psychiatrists training there spread knowledge of modern ECT methods into many psychiatric hospitals around the Russian Federation. The obstacles they faced in providing ECT (primarily indifference and procrastination by local medical facility administrators) were more passive than in previous decades. ECT methods found growing use in neurology, led by the Department of Neurology of the Moscow State University of Stomatology. A dissertation on the use of ECT in addiction psychiatry was presented after extensive clinical study (Ostankov, 2002).

Present ECT use in the Russian Federation

In the 21st century, ECT use in Russia is increasing. According to a national survey (Nelson, 2005), ECT is used regularly in some states and geographic areas, comparably with Europe and the United States. However, most physicians, scientists, and health care administrators lack substantial knowledge of modern ECT. Even the doctors who actively use ECT in their everyday practice are not usually aware of basic concepts such as seizure threshold and rational stimulus dosing. Many have never evaluated the therapeutic quality of ECT seizures. Confusion is widespread about contraindications to ECT and pre-ECT evaluation. Such basic deficiencies in ECT knowledge result from inadequate training and unfamiliarity with the ECT literature. Moreover, no particular credentials or privileging process is needed to administer ECT in Russia.

Unmodified ECT is still more common than ECT with anesthesia in the Russian Federation. This is not unusual in third world countries. However, there are no reliable data about the comparative rates of complications for modified and un-modified ECT as practiced in Russia. Regrettably, modern ECT devices are not available in Russia; the devices in use were manufactured several decades ago.

In the Russian Federation, ECT is sometimes used for several conditions for which it is not used elsewhere. These include treatment of acute opiate and alcohol withdrawal syndromes, including delirium tremens. These are acute syndromes that are usually readily observable by the physician, and the effect of ECT on them is similarly observable. ECT is sometimes used for maintenance of alcohol abstinence in patients who have alcohol dependence. It is hypothesized that ECT suppresses pathologic cravings and helps to mitigate the mood disturbances that provoke drinking. Another unusual use of ECT is in trigeminal neuralgia status, a seriously painful condition. These uses of ECT are accepted as ordinary and not considered experimental.

It finally seems sure to say that, as of the 21st century, ECT is safe to discuss and use without political reprisals, and indeed that in Russia ECT is received more favorably than in many other countries. We are grateful that historically no significant antipsychiatry or anti-ECT organization has appeared in the Russian Federation. Russian psychiatry is open to the use of active and efficient methods of biological therapy. This is a tradition founded by one of the most outstanding scholars of Russian psychiatry and neurology, S. S. Korsakov, and continued by the schools of the brilliant Russian psychiatrists M. Y. Sereysky and G. Y. Avrutsky. Moreover, ECT has shown dramatic observable clinical benefits in addiction psychiatry, long one of the most vigorous and influential fields of Russian medicine. These positive factors open doors for interest in ECT and its propagation.

The current situation with ECT in the Russian Federation is reassuring. Still, psychiatrists in other countries have accumulated ECT experience over more than 60 years, whereas Russian psychiatrists must proceed from the circumstances of no hospital tradition and little experience. In most Russian psychiatric institutions, ECT is being introduced as if new, with corresponding administrative, methodical, and attitudinal hindrances.

Editor's note

The anti-ECT activities described in this chapter have counterparts in the United States and Europe, as reported in Chapters 10–15 here. –CMS.

References

About use of electroshock for treatment of psychical diseases. 1952. [In Russian.] Zh Nevrol Psikhiatr Im S S Korsakova 52(8): 71–3.

Babayan, E. A. 1978. Legal aspects of psychiatry in legislation of the USSR [in Russian]. Zh Nevrol Psikhiatr Im S S Korsakova 78(4): 598–603.

Banschikov, V. M. and Nevzorova, T. A. 1969. Psychiatry [in Russian]. Moscow: Meditsina, 344 pp.

Banschikov, V. M. and Rapoport, A. M. 1952. Electroconvulsive therapy in psycho-neurological hospitals of the USSR [in Russian]. Zh Nevrol Psikhiatr Im S S Korsakova 52(3): 67–81.

Borzunova, A. S. 1952. About pathogenesis of epilepsy and schizophrenia in connection with their treatment with convulsive remedies [in Russian]. Abstract of Ph.D. Dissertation, Ufa, Psychiatric Clynic of Bashkir Medical Institute, 16 pp.

Dain, E. G. 1958. Distant results of electroconvulsive therapy of schizophrenia [in Russian]. In Proceedings of Chernovitskaya regional psycho-neurological hospital, Vol. 1. Chernovitsy, pp. 233–53.

Device for electroconvulsive therapy "Elikon-01." 1987. [In Russian.] Zh Nevrol Psikhiatr Im S S Korsakova 87(11):4 (cover).

Frumkin, Ya. P., Slivko, I. M., and Mizrukhin, I. A. 1950. Prolonged intermittent sleep (electro-comatose therapy, electro-narcoshock) in treatment and research of schizophrenia and so-called functional psychical pathology [in Russian]. In Proceedings of the 3rd All-Union Congress of Neuropathologists and Psychiatrists, Moscow, pp. 362–6.

Gilyarovsky, V. A. 1951. Evolution of ideas of I. P. Pavlov in psychiatry [in Russian]. Nevropatologiia i Psikhiatriia 20(1): 17–8.

Goldenberg, M. A. 1938. Psychopathology of symptomatic (camphor) epilepsy in connection with treatment of schizophrenia with Meduna's method [in Russian]. Sovetskaia Psykhonevrologiia 4: 11–24.

Guidelines on convulsive therapy. 1940. [In Russian.] Nevropatologiia i Psikhiatriia 9(3–4): 109–16.

Health Ministry of the USSR. 1979. Guidelines on use of electroconvulsive therapy No 21-59/PS59-1/ET [in Russian]. Moscow: Health Ministry of the USSR.

Health Ministry of the USSR. 1989. Use of electroconvulsive therapy in psychiatric practice. Methodical recommendations [in Russian]. Moscow: Administration of Special Medical Aid, Moscow Scientific-Research Institute of Health Ministry of the USSR, 34 pp.

Kalashnik, Ya. M. 1950. Critical remarks on some scientific works of Serbsky Institute of forensic psychiatry [in Russian]. Nevropatologiia i Psikhiatriia 19(3): 74–5.

Kerbikov, O. V. 1955. Lectures on psychiatry [in Russian]. Moscow: Medgiz, 240 pp.

Kerbikov, O. V., Ozeretsky, N. I., Popov, E. A., and Snezhnevsky, A. V. 1958. Handbook of psychiatry [in Russian]. Moscow: Medgiz, 368 pp.

Lebedev, V. A. 1957. Use of home preparation dithylin for facilitation of electroconvulsive therapy and prophylaxis of its complications [in Russian]. Zh Nevrol Psikhiatr Im S S Korsakova 57(12): 1487–93.

Lichko, A. E. 1962. Insulin comas [in Russian]. Moscow-Leningrad: Publishing House of the Academy of Sciences of the USSR.

Likhterman, L. and Likhterman, B. 2000. How they prohibited psychosurgery in the USSR [in Russian]. Meditsinskaia Gazeta 87: 12–3.

Molokhov, A. I. 1948. About indications for electroconvulsive therapy of schizophrenia [in Russian]. Nevropatologiia i Psikhiatriia 17(2): 38–41.

Moschevitin, S. Yu. 1989. Place of electroconvulsive therapy in modern treatment of endogenous psychoses [in Russian]. Zh Nevrol Psikhiatr Im S S Korsakova 89(3): 145–53.

Nelson, A. I. 2005. A national survey of ECT use in the Russian Federation. J ECT 21(3): 151–7.

Nevzorova, T. A. and Romanovsky, A. I. 1970. About electroconvulsive method of treatment of psychoses [in Russian]. In Problems of theoretical and clinical medicine. Zaporozhje, pp. 342–3.

Nikolaenko, N. N. 1978. Clinical and electrophysiological study of unilateral electroconvulsive seizures [in Russian]. Abstract of Ph.D. Dissertation, Leningrad, The Bekhterev Leningrad Scientific-Research Psycho-Neurological Institute, 19 pp.

Ostankov, S. B. 2002. Electroconvulsive therapy of opioid dependence [in Russian]. Abstract of Ph.D. Dissertation, Tomsk, Scientifical-Resesrch Institute of Psychical Health of Scientific Center Of Siberian Department of the Russian Academy of Medical Sciences, 26 pp.

Ploticher, A. I. 1950. Theory and practice of treatment of psychoses with electrical shock [in Russian]. Abstract of Ph.D. Dissertation, Kharkov, Ukrainian Psycho-Neurological Institute, 23 pp.

Rakhmazova, L. D., 1985. Place of ECT in the entire rehabilitation of schizophrenic patients with lingering course of disease. Abstract of Ph.D. dissertation. Tomsk: Tomsk Medical Institute, 21 pp.

Rodzevskaya, T. F. 1951. Our experience of electroconvulsive therapy of schizophrenia (preliminary report) [in Russian]. In Proceedings of Khabarovsk Medical Institute, collection 11. Khabarovsk, pp. 116–20.

Rotshtein, G. A. 1941. Convulsive therapy of schizophrenia [in Russian]. Moscow.

Rotshtein, G. A. 1948. Guidelines on electroconvulsive therapy of psychical diseases [in Russian]. In Therapy of psychical diseases (ed. Sereisky, M. Ya.). Moscow: Moskovsky Bolshevik, pp. 230–54.

Sereisky, M. Ya. and Rotshtein, G. A. 1940. About provoking epileptic seizures with intravenous infusion of camphor [in Russian]. Klin Med 18(5): 141–5.

Sereisky, M. Ya. and Rotshtein, G. A. 1942. Electroshock in treatment of psychical diseases [in Russian]. Nevropatologiia i Psikhiatriia XI(6): 57–65.

Shapiro, M. L. 1940. Follow-up periods of patients treated with Meduna's camphor method [in Russian]. In Proceedings of the first Moscow psychiatric hospital, Issue 3. Moscow, pp. 80–90.

Timofeeva, A. N. 1962. About correlation of effectiveness of electroconvulsive therapy and reactivity of cortex of suprarenal glands [in Russian]. In Psychiatric clinic and problems of supreme nervous activity. SM Kirov State Lenin's Order Institute of doctors' qualifying, Collection of works of psychiatry department (ed. Sluchevsky, I. F.). Issue 4(25). Leningrad, pp. 272–7.

Zhivotovsky, S. D. 1941. Camphor therapy of schizophrenia, from materials of Astrakhan State Medical Institute in 1939–1940 [in Russian]. In Collection of scientific works of Psychiatric Clinic of the Astrakhan first clinical hospital, Issue 1. Astrakhan, pp. 161–8.

18

Electroconvulsive therapy in Latin America

Moacyr Alexandro Rosa and Marina Odebrecht Rosa

Introduction

Latin America usually includes Mexico, South America, and most countries of Central America. It is a huge territory and includes countries with widely varying environments, from the tiny Caribbean Islands, some with a population of a few thousand people, to Brazil with almost 190 million people. It incorporates diverse ethnicities, including European, Native American, and African origins. It has varying languages, with Spanish the most common but Dutch in the Caribbean, French in Guyana, English in Belize (formerly British Honduras), and Portuguese in Brazil, with many regional dialects of each. Paradoxically, contrasts within the countries of Latin America are what makes them similar: differing life conditions and opportunities between "haves and have nots" and between powerful and disempowered, rural and urban, and migrant and fixed populations. Another common influence is runaway urbanization, with newly arrived migrant populations crowded into dense slums on the rims of great cities, and development of these cities independently from the rest of the country. In the background of most Latin American countries is a small, highly educated intellectual elite (Brody, 1966).

After its creation, electroconvulsive therapy (ECT) reached virtually every country in Latin America. Especially in its unmodified form (sine wave devices, without anesthesia or muscle relaxation), it represented a safe, inexpensive, and clearly effective treatment that developing countries could benefit from. Indiscriminate use and delay in the use of the modified (anesthetized) technique has contributed to a negative public opinion and, added to the influence of antipsychiatric movement ideologies, has been responsible for some decline in ECT use. Consequent to the influence of North American psychiatry, ECT is experiencing a renaissance in South and Central America, although perhaps too slowly to meet the clinical needs in these countries.

Overview

The population of Central and South America totals 513 million people, 60% of whom (almost 346 million) live in South America (with Brazil, Argentina, and Colombia the most populated), and 20% (almost 99 million) in Mexico. Guatemala has the largest population in Central America (11 million), and the populations of Cuba (11 million) and the Dominican Republic and Haiti (8 million each) surpass those of the rest of the Caribbean countries. Spanish is the official language in 17 countries of the region; Portuguese is spoken in Brazil (which is responsible for almost 30% of Latin America's total population); and French, English, Flemish, and a variety of dialects are spoken in the other 13 countries, particularly the Caribbean countries (Alarcón, 2003).

Despite efforts of professional medical associations, sparseness of information is another similar feature among Latin American countries. Few papers can be found providing data about mental health in general or ECT use in particular. According to the Pan American Health Organization (PAHO; 2005), 114 million people in the Americas suffered some type of mental disorder in 1990, and this is projected to increase to 176 million by the year 2010.

Mental health in Latin America

It is estimated that 64.5% of Latin American countries have specific mental health policies, 80.6% have plans and programs, 67.9% have specific mental health legislation, and 87.1% provide disability benefits for psychiatric patients. What is not well documented is whether such instruments are effectively implemented and utilized (Alarcón, 2003).

Epidemiological studies show a consistent prevalence of 18% to 25% of mental disorders in communities, and up to 27% to 48% in clinical settings (Almeida Filho and Canino, 1995). Depression and anxiety in all their clinical variants, plus somatoform and alcohol and drug abuse disorders (the latter, more than 20% of the estimated prevalence), in addition to the so-called "major" psychiatric disorders, are the most frequent risks. Estimate rates of the prevalence of mental disorders are as follows: Unipolar depression represents 35.7% among psychiatric entities, alcoholism 18.2%, schizophrenia 7.8%, bipolar affective disorder 6.6%, and substance abuse 5.6%.

Mental health resources in Latin America are scarce. The estimated figures of 1.6 psychiatrists, 2.7 psychiatric nurses, 2.8 psychologists, and 1.9 social workers per 100,000 are much lower than those of Europe and the United State (Saraceno and Saxena, 2002). The concentration of these professionals in metropolitan areas leaves unattended at least 45% of the total population in need. In contrast, patients are seen first by nonprofessionals, second by nonpsychiatric professionals, and last by mental health professionals. Insurance coverage is minimal, and mental health professionals in these countries are among the lowest paid of those in all countries. Their training takes place in insufficient facilities with limited teaching staffs, scarce equipment, and loose monitoring by academic centers or governmental agencies. Countering the suggestion of improvement through some growth in absolute numbers of resident trainees in psychiatry, the risk of emigration by present and future trainees is high.

In Latin America, there are approximately 3.3 psychiatric beds per 10,000 inhabitants; 47.6% of these are in psychiatric hospitals, 16.8% are in general hospitals, and 35.6% are in other community settings. In contrast, 86.7% of Latin American countries have policies related to supply and provision of psychotropic agents, but more than one third experience significant problems in the actual implementation of such policies.

Regarding research in mental health, Latin America has made some progress, but it is not comparable with that in the United States or Europe. Brazil, Argentina, Mexico, and Chile are ahead in resources and productivity, but Mexican authors publish more consistently, despite a proportionately lower budget than the other three countries (US$20 per capita in Mexico vs. US$60 in Brazil; in the United States, the figure is US$827 per capita) (Mari, 2001). Eight countries have institutes intended for mental health research, but only the one in Mexico works consistently toward this goal. The others may have the infrastructure but lack policies, rules, operational systems, and qualified personnel. The absence of solid financial support by the government is probably at the root of this disappointment.

In clear contrast to this, Latin American psychiatry has produced significant research contributions, particularly in epidemiology, clinical studies, cultural issues, and psychopharmacology. There is an intense debate on the fate of basic research in the subcontinent, with slight dominance of persons who advocate a social and clinical orientation closely related to the plight of the impoverished majorities (Alarcón, 1993).

The use of ECT

The information here is based mainly on one relatively comprehensive report on ECT in Latin America and the Caribbean (Levav and González Uzcátegui, 1998). These investigators contacted directors of the mental health divisions or departments of the Ministries of Health through the representative offices of the PAHO/World Health Organization. Where Ministries lacked such a division or department (as in many Caribbean countries), the survey was directed to the officials responsible for mental health programs or the directors of the national public psychiatric hospital. Seventeen of 19 countries contacted in Latin America

(89%) answered most of the survey, and the other two provided some responses. Unfortunately, the report does not identify how individual countries participated in the survey, so the results provide a nonspecific panoramic view.

Rate of use

ECT is used in all Latin America countries that answered the questionnaire. Relative to the countries or territories in the English- or Dutch-speaking Caribbean, 13 of 17 (76%) responded to the survey, including those with the largest populations; only four reported the use of ECT. In Latin America as well as the Caribbean, use varies from country to country and even within individual countries. As a rule, public institutions use ECT more frequently than do private ones. Brazil is an exception. After a decree of the Federal Medical Council (2002) prohibiting ECT without general anesthesia and muscle relaxation, virtually no public institution provides ECT. With few exceptions, only public institutions linked in some way with medical universities offer this kind of treatment for the most poor and needy. Otherwise, ECT is an expensive and hard-to-find treatment. In addition, devices made in Brazil use sine wave stimuli, and costly electrical testing within Brazil is required for foreign-made instruments. A trend away from using ECT was reported in eight Latin American countries and in the two most populous ECT-using countries in the English-speaking Caribbean.

ECT technique

Written technical standards exist in the four Caribbean countries that use ECT, but in only 10 of the 19 Latin American countries. Two additional countries reported in the cited study that they have developed standards and were seeking approval from national authorities and professional associations.

Only 26% of countries in Latin America reported that anesthesia is given with ECT in all institutions, as did three of four Caribbean countries. In some Latin American countries, the use of anesthesia is more frequent in the private sector than in the public sector. Muscle relaxants are given in all institutions in 32% of Latin American countries, and in some institutions in another 36%. As with anesthesia, administration of muscle relaxants tends to be more routinely used in the private than the public sector.

Informed consent

The safeguarding of patients' rights in psychiatric institutions varies from country to country. The greatest gap is found within countries between the public and the private sectors. In private health care, there is a greater degree of awareness about patients' rights than in public institutions (Levav and González Uzcátegui, 2000).

In only 37% of Latin American countries do all institutions obtain informed consent for ECT from the patient or authorized individual. In 26% of the countries, informed consent is obtained sometimes, and in another 26% never. Informed consent is routinely obtained in the four Caribbean countries that administer ECT.

Especially in Central America, mental health is an area where patients' rights are not respected (Levav and González Uzcátegui, 2000). Therapeutic interventions are provided after obtaining written consent on admission. However, the wording is so general that it allows the treating institution to conduct any intervention without further justification or permission. In practice, no patient is permitted to refuse treatment. If a patient's family requests early discharge, permission is granted provided there is no danger to the individual or to others. Specific consent to administer ECT is seldom requested, but informed consent is most often obtained in the private sector.

ECT training

No official information is available about specific training in ECT practice. Psychiatry residency training programs usually make reference to ECT within general teaching about "biological treatments" and include some conceptual information about "indications" and "side effects." No training or knowledge updating is required for ECT practitioners and they usually start providing ECT after observing a senior physician give the treatment and simply copy what they observed.

History and use of ECT in specific countries

It is believed that, after ECT reached the United States in 1940, the first Latin American countries to use ECT were Argentina, Chile, and Cuba. Published materials are scarce, and references are mainly personal communications. In the following subsections, the history and current use of ECT in some countries of Latin America are considered, based on published information.

Argentina

The first information about ECT use in Argentina came from Osvaldo Loudet, who observed some treatments in Rome in 1938. The initial use of ECT in Argentina is in dispute and has been claimed by both Orlando y Fontanarrosa and Cesar Castedo (Villanueva, 1985). The work of J. Thenon on unilateral ECT in 1956 highlighted its potential to preserve cognitive functions (Thenon, 1956).

Chile

In the early 1940s, ECT was already used in the Psychiatric Hospital of Santiago. However, no specific information about dates or names is available. No data about its current use could be found. The work of Trucco et al. (1983) suggested a relatively high rate of ECT use (22% of inpatients, ranging from 13.5% in the Psychiatric Hospital to 26% in private clinics), an almost exclusive use of bilateral electrode placement, and a low rate of use of anesthesia and muscle relaxation (7.5%). More than 20 years have passed since these data were published. Recently, modern brief-pulse ECT instruments were widely adopted in Chile and several are in use in Peru, Colombia, and Venezuela (personal communication, Somatics Co.).

Cuba

According to Diaz and Agramonte (1987), ECT reached La Habana in 1942, just four years after Cerletti's first treatment. An Offner device was used. No official information about these first treatments is available. Although not the first, Rafael J. Larragoiti Alonso was the greatest early exponent of ECT in Cuba. Because of World War II, he was not able to buy a commercial device so he built one himself for use with his patients. In October 1944, he had treated 150 patients in more than 1,000 sessions. A few months after treating his first patients, he began to administer atropine to patients, and was cited by Kalinowsky and Hoch (1961) as one of the first to use it. In addition, Larragoiti studied electrocardiographic changes during treatments, started building brief-pulse devices, and introduced ECT with general anesthesia and muscle relaxation in Cuba (Larragoiti et al., 1956).

Mexico

Samuel Ramirez Moreno performed the first ECT treatment with a Rahm device on March 17, 1941, to treat a patient with schizophrenia in Mexico. He had extensive previous experience in using pentylenetetrazol. His assistant, Mauricio Rubio y Yarza, published the first complete monograph on ECT in Mexico ("Los electro-choques en el tratamiento de la esquizofrenia"; "Electroshock in the treatment of schizophrenia") in 1942. Dr. Ramirez Moreno promoted the use of ECT in patients older than 50 years (which had been considered too risky at that time) and also in patients younger than 12 years, based on his direct professional experience. He used a basic concept of seizure threshold, suggesting that ECT start with a low current for a short period of time and that the stimulus be repeated if a seizure is not induced. He also suggested a maximum of two stimulations per day. He used curare in his first treatments, but abandoned it because of toxicity.

In the 1950s ECT was overused in Mexico, as in the rest of the world. In the Manicomio de La Castaneda, 2,756 treatments were reported in 1950, 5,838 in 1952, and 8,380 in 1954. Likewise ECT use declined with the advent of psychotropic drugs in the 1960s and returned again in the 1980s. Current data suggest that ECT use is mainly bitemporal, with fixed high charge and only rare use of general anesthesia (Colin Piana and Ruiz Lopez, 1997).

Uruguay

There is some detailed information on ECT practice in Uruguay (Casarotti et al., 2004; Lyford Pike et al., 1995). Convulsive therapy has continued since its introduction. There is a report by the Psychiatric Society of 1939 of a special session in honor of and with the presence of Ladislas Meduna, who presented two lectures about the use of pentylenetetrazol (Meduna, 1939; Meduna and Rohny, 1939). An early report about "shock" therapy (Bruno, 1941) was published and included descriptions of the first electroconvulsive treatments.

In the 1960s, ECT was used indiscriminately in Uruguay. With the introduction of psychotropic medications, a small decrease in use was observed between 1970 and 1990. A notable survey on Uruguayan psychiatrists' opinions about ECT (di Segni and Cusmanich, 1993) reported that 82.3% used ECT, 91.2% considered it appropriate for melancholia, and 62% stated that there were no human rights issues involving ECT.

An ECT revival occurred in Uruguay and, after 1994, a commission standardized the use of ECT based on the American Psychiatric Association's recommendations. It is estimated that 12,000 to 12,500 treatments in the capital (Montevideo) and 1,000 to 2,000 treatments in the country's other regions are given per year – a rate of 70 to 75 per 10,000 inhabitants in the capital and 12 to 15 per 10,000 elsewhere. This is a high rate.

Brazil

ECT in Brazil started just a few years after its invention (Rosa, 2007). It was introduced by Antonio Carlos Pacheco e Silva. In 1941, soon after he came back from the American Psychiatric Association Annual Meeting held in Richmond, Virginia, he brought the first ECT devices (one Offner and one Rahm) to Brazil from the United States, as well as knowledge of its use. He first carried out experiments with animals before starting to use them to treat patients.

The first ECT sessions in Brazil were performed in July 1941 in three different hospitals, including the Psychiatric Clinic of the University of São Paulo. He described his first results as follows: "We have treated so far 21 patients with electroshock, with a total of 139 treatments. Sixteen were schizophrenic and 5 melancholic. Of the 16 schizophrenic, 5 reached total remission, 3 a partial remission, 4 had amelioration of symptoms and are still on treatment; the rest of them, chronic schizophrenics, continue stationary. Among the melancholic, 2 had total remission, being discharged from hospital; 1 has just started treatment, but has already signs of improvement; one had an improvement after the first 3 treatments, followed by recurrence to the previous state" (Rosa, 2007). The success of these results encouraged ECT use in Brazil, and it soon completely displaced pentylenetetrazol therapy.

Since then, ECT has been consistently used in Brazil (Rigonatti et al., 2004). In the 1970s, anesthesia was introduced routinely in the Institute of Psychiatry of the University of São Paulo and several other academic centers. In other regions of the country, anesthesia and muscle relaxation was routinely used only after it was mandated by the 2002 resolution of the Federal Medical Council. Currently, public psychiatric services seldom offer ECT, except those linked with a school of medicine. Private clinics are the best choice for patients in need, although they are few and the treatment is relatively expensive. Devices used are mainly brief-pulse machines imported from the United States, although in many places sine wave devices produced in Brazil are still used because they are less expensive.

Conclusion

ECT is an important tool in treating psychiatric disorders in Latin America. Unfortunately, as with health care generally, Central and South America lack prepared ECT practitioners, and the technique used is not always modern. Medical associations and schools should present ECT knowledge at the same level of expertise as in psychopharmacology, psychopathology, and psychotherapy, and specific training in concepts and procedures should be made available to psychiatrists interested in ECT. Substantial efforts are needed to inform patients and families about the nature of depressive illnesses and the risks and benefits of ECT. The virtues and ethics of informed consent need greater appreciation by clinicians, health care administrators, and patients in these countries.

References

Alarcón, R. D. 1993. Perspectivas de la investigación psiquiátrica en América Latina. Acta Psiq Psicol Am Latina 39: 19–31.

Alarcón, R. D. 2003. Mental health and mental health care in Latin America. World Psychiatry 2(1): 54–6.

Almeida Filho, N. and Canino, G. 1995. Epidemiología psiquiátrica. In Enciclopedia Iberoamericana de psiquiatría. Vol. 2. (eds. Vidal, G., Alarcón, R. D., and Lolas, F.). Buenos Aires: Editorial Médica Panamericana, pp. 487–501.

Brody, E. B. 1966. On the psychiatry of Latin America. Am J Psychiatry, 123: 475–7.

Bruno, A. U. 1941. Resultados obtenidos en clínica psiquiátrica con el empleo de los métodos modernos de shockterapia en cuatro años de experiencia personal. Rev Psiquiatr Urug 6(35): 33–8.

Casarotti, H., Otegui, J., Savi, G., et al. 2004. Electroconvulsoterapia: Fundamentos y pautas de utilización. Rev Psiquiatr Urug 68(1): 7–41.

Colin Piana, R. and Ruiz Lopez, I. 1997. Inicios de la terapia electroconvulsiva en Mexico. Arch Neurociencias 2(1): 25–8.

Diaz, E. G. and Agramonte, E. A. G. 1987. La azarosa historia de la terapia electroconvulsivante (II Parte). Rev Hosp Psiquiatr La Habana 28(2): 227–39.

di Segni, M. And Cusmanich, S. 1993. Electroshock: Studio de los reparos de los psiquiatras para su uso. Rev Psiquiatr Urug, 57(326): 19–30.

Kalinowsky, L. B. and Hoch, P. H. 1961. Somatic treatment in psychiatry. New York: Grune and Stratton.

Larragoiti, R. J., Valenzuela, E. V., and Machado, R. 1956. Fundamentos y tecnicas de la electro-convulsoterapia modificada. Arch Soc Estud Clin Hab 49: 261–72.

Levav, I. and González Uzcátegui, R. 1998. The use of electroconvulsive therapy in Latin America and the Caribbean. Rev Panam Salud Publica/Pan Am J Public Health 3(2): 121–3.

Levav, I. and González Uzcátegui, R. 2000. Rights of persons with mental illness in Central America. Acta Psychiatr Scand 101: 83–6.

Lyford Pike, A., Otegui, J., Savi, G., and Fernández, M. 1995. ECT: Changing in Uruguay [letter]. Convuls Ther 11: 58–60.

Mari, J. J. 2001. Mental health research in Latin America. Presented at the Conference on Mental Health in the Americas: Partnering for Progress; Washington, DC. November 5th and 6th.

Meduna, L. 1939. La técnica actual de la Cardiazolterapia. Rev Psiquiatr Urug 4(22): 27–34.

Meduna, L. and Rohny, B. 1939. Estudio comparativo del tratamiento con insulina y cardiazol. Rev Psiquiatr Urug 4(22): 9–24.

Pan American Health Organization (PAHO). 2005. World Mental Health Day 2005 focuses on life span. http://www.paho.org/English/DD/PIN/pr051006.htm.

Rigonatti, S. P., Rosa, M. A., and Rosa, M. O. (Eds.) 2004. Electroconvulsoterapia. São Paulo, Brazil: Lemos Editorial.

Rosa, M. A. 2007. Pacheco e Silva and the origins of electroconvulsive therapy in Brazil. J ECT 23(4): 224–8.

Saraceno, B. and Saxena, S. 2002. Mental health resources in the world: Results from Project ATLAS of the WHO. World Psychiatry 1: 40–4.

Thenon, J. 1956. Electrochoque monolateral. Acta Neuropsiquiatrica Argentina 2: 292–6.

Trucco, M., Larach, V., and Duran, E. 1983. Terapia electro-convulsiva: Su utilizacion en establec-imientos psiquiatricos de Santiago. Rev Chil Neuropsiquiat 21: 283–9.

Villanueva, M. A. 1985. Historia y actualidad de la terapia electroconvulsive en la psiquiatria Argentina. Quiron 16(1): 33–7.

Part IV

Administrative perspectives

Electroconvulsive therapy hospital policy and quality assurance

Barry Alan Kramer

Introduction

In the not too distant past, medical progress notes consisted of a few cryptic words followed by an illegible signature. Policies and procedures consisted of either one or two paragraphs or were kept in your head. For better or worse, it is not likely that those days will ever return. Medical practice has become too complex to assume that what must be done is self-evident. How we practice medicine is governed by a complex array of rules and regulations dictated by a diverse group of institutions. Each state has a set of laws and regulations governing medical practice generally and sometimes electroconvulsive therapy (ECT) specifically. These laws may be changed and reinterpreted periodically. The Joint Commission has an extensive set of often-revised requirements governing health care, including some specifically for ECT. The Centers for Medicare & Medicaid Services have their own requirements. Regulations from the U.S. Food and Drug Administration (FDA) and the Emergency Medical Treatment and Active Labor Act (EMTALA) may affect hospital policies regarding ECT.

Hospitals and other health care settings are expected to develop policies and procedures to demonstrate compliance with the regulations from these highly visible agencies and delivery of good medical care. This is not a task for one person alone but for administrative and clinical personnel to collaborate on. These hospital policies and procedures should be available for outside regulatory reviewers to read, consider if regulations are being followed, and envision how patient care is delivered in the particular setting. Likewise, the policies and procedures should be available for physicians to read and apply in their clinical work. This means that the policies and procedures should be easily understood and followed by clinical staff, so they can identify their roles and responsibilities. Although they are often written to comply with complex regulatory and legal language, straightforward unambiguous statements will help medical personnel (who have not attended law school) easily interpret and follow them. Policies should be dated so that, as they are changed with changes in regulations, the current version is clearly identified. It is usually helpful to identify the immediate past version that is superseded.

Most of this chapter is a model for policies and procedures. It is meant to be used as a guide, with its contents adjusted to your particular setting rather than copied verbatim. It is presented as "hospital" policies and procedures because most ECT in the United States is given in a hospital setting – be it inpatient or outpatient. It is *not* the policies and procedures of any specific hospital. These policies are compliant with the laws of California but not specifically with the laws of other states. It is wise to obtain a copy of *all* the laws and regulations in your state prior to writing any new policies. It is possible to write one global set of policies and procedures document to cover everything. As regulation has expanded over the years, writing multiple documents attending to each specific area is another approach. Although this writing of multiple documents results in some duplication, it can make specific information easier to find. This approach is used here.

General policies for ECT are listed first. These policies include a statement that they are in compliance with the applicable regulatory agencies. It sets out the policies for providing ECT legally in California: what ECT is, issues with informed consent and the consent form, patients unwilling or unable to give informed consent, rules for treating minors, required review committees, and required reporting to the state. This section is the largest section of policies and the one that most differs under different governments – although the general issues covered should be routinely included. For example, the state of California stipulates the contents of the informed consent form, so that substitution is not permitted. The state specifies the maximum length of time the consent is valid. It requires another psychiatrist to verify the patient's capacity to consent. It defines "Excessive Use of Convulsive Treatment" and what legally constitutes a treatment. Although the reader can debate the value of each of these items, California law allows no flexibility, so these regulations are followed exactly. Some states and countries are just as inflexible, and others are not. This section is followed by general guidelines for ECT, including patient selection, medical workup, preparation of the ECT suite, requirements for who can give ECT (although requirements for obtaining and maintaining ECT privileges are included in a previous chapter), and general nursing requirements.

A separate policy for nursing responsibilities specifies step-by-step expectations for the nursing staff. This policy includes information on preparing the room and equipment, medical record responsibilities, preparing the patient, interacting with the psychiatrist and anesthesiologist, the role in the actual treatment, and room cleanup.

The next sections include special situations. There is a policy for treating patients who are inpatients at other facilities that do not provide ECT. Given the irregular availability of ECT in many areas, this is a way to improve access. There is a section for treating patients with developmental disabilities, because California imposes additional legal and procedural rules for these patients. Although intended to protect these individuals from exposure to reckless handling, in my experience it has resulted in depriving many of them from access to needed care.

Last, a brief section deals with the scope of the ECT service, including location, hours of operation, role in the hospital or departmental organization, and staffing. This document, the "Scope of the ECT Service" section, should be most useful in larger hospitals and probably less useful in smaller settings. It can easily be incorporated in the general policies for ECT. Chapter 21 of this book contains suggested forms, so these are not included here. Chapter 20 discusses practical aspects of many of these policies and procedures.

General policies for ECT

I. Purpose

To provide guidelines in the application, administration, and documentation of electroconvulsive therapy (ECT) and in the care of the patient post-ECT in order to ensure a safe and responsible implementation.

II. Policy

To ensure that ECT will be administered in compliance with the Welfare and Institutions Code (WIC), Sections 5326.15–5326.95, and California Code of Regulations (CCR), Title 9, Sections 835–849, and will be safely and responsibly implemented.

III. Definition

"Convulsive treatment" is the planned induction of a seizure through electrical or chemical means for therapeutic purposes. [*Defined by State of California*]

IV. Procedure

A. Legal requirements for informed consent

ECT will be administered in conformance with the applicable provisions of the Welfare and Institutions Code (WIC) and California Code of Regulations (CCR), as follows:

1. Written informed consent means that a person knowingly and intelligently, without duress or coercion, clearly and explicitly manifests consent to the proposed therapy to the treating physician and in writing on the standard consent form.
2. A person shall be deemed to have the capacity to consent or to refuse to consent if it is determined that such person has actually understood and can

knowingly and intelligently act upon the information specified in Paragraph 8. Understanding of the potential benefits and risks of the proposed treatment is the primary factor in determining such capability to consent or to refuse treatment. A person shall not be deemed to lack capacity to consent or refuse consent solely by virtue of any psychiatric or medical diagnosis.

3. The patient shall be deemed incapable of giving written informed consent if such a person cannot understand, or knowingly and intelligently act upon, the information as specified in WIC Section 5326.6 (c).

4. Consent shall be for a specified maximum number of treatments, not to exceed twelve (12) over thirty (30) days, and shall be revocable by the patient at any time before or between treatments. Such withdrawal of consent may be either oral or written and shall be given effect immediately.

5. No convulsive treatment shall be performed if the patient, whether admitted to the facility as a voluntary or involuntary patient, is deemed to be able to give informed consent and refuses to do so.

6. The physician may urge the proposed treatment as the best one, but may not use, in an effort to gain consent, any reward or threat, expressed or implied, nor any other form of inducement or coercion, including, but not limited to, placing the patient in a more restricted setting, transfer of the patient to another facility, or loss of the patient's hospital privileges. No one shall be denied any benefits for refusing treatment.

7. If a patient is deemed by the physician to have the capacity to give informed consent, but refuses to do so, the physician shall indicate in the clinical record that the treatment was refused despite the physician's advice, and that the physician has explained to the patient the patient's responsibility for any untoward consequence of the refusal.

8. The attending physician must give to the patient and a responsible relative if the patient designates one and the patient's guardian or conservator, if there is one, a clear and explicit oral explanation of specifics:

   a). The reason for treatment, i.e., the nature and seriousness of the patient's illness, disorder, or defect.

   b). The nature of the procedures to be used in the proposed treatment, including its probable frequency and duration.

   c). The probable degree and duration (temporary or permanent) of improvement or remission, expected with and without such treatment.

   d). The nature, degree, duration, and the probability of the side effects and significant risks, commonly known by the medical profession, of such treatment, including its adjuvants, especially noting the degree and the duration of memory loss (including its irreversibility) and how and to what extent they may be controlled, if at all.

e). That there exists a division of opinion as to the efficacy of the proposed treatment, why and how it works, and its commonly known risks and side effects.

f). The reasonable alternative treatments, and why the physician is recommending this particular treatment.

g). That the patient has the right to accept or refuse the proposed treatment, and that if the patient consents, the patient has the right to revoke his/her consent for any reason, at any time prior to or between treatments.

9. The standard State Department of Mental Health consent form is to be used. This form sets forth clearly, and in detail, the matters listed above, along with further information with respect to each item as deemed generally appropriate to all patients. The treatment physician must utilize the standard form and, in writing, supplement it with those details that pertain to the particular patient being treated.

10. The treating physician shall explain to the patient orally, clearly, and in detail all of the above information. The patient must be allowed at least 24 hours in which to consider the information provided prior to actually signing the consent form.

11. The consent form must be dated, timed, and witnessed. The witness must be someone other than the treating or attending physician who explains the procedure. The consent must include the maximum number of treatments to be administered, not to exceed twelve (12) over a thirty (30) day period and the consent is in effect for a maximum of thirty (30) days from the date of first treatment.

12. The treating physician must enter into the medical record the date and time on which the required information was discussed with the patient, which must be at least 24 hours prior to the date on which the patient signs the consent form. The consent form shall be available to the person, and to his/her attorney, guardian, or conservator, and, if the patient consents, to a responsible relative of the patient's choosing. The fact of the execution of the written consent form shall also be entered in the treatment record. The patient may withdraw consent at any time.

13. If this information has been discussed with the patient in the attending or treating physician's office prior to admission, this must be documented in the Medical Record, along with the date(s) and time(s) of discussion.

14. The treating or attending physician shall give a responsible relative of the patient's choosing and the patient's guardian or conservator, if there is one, the oral explanation as outlined under the Voluntary Informed Consent. Responsible relative is defined as the spouse, parent, adult child, or adult brother or sister of the patient.

15. Should the patient desire not to inform a relative, this requirement is dispensed with, and the patient's request for notification or non-notification will be documented in the patient's Medical Record. The treating or attending physician must enter into the Medical Record that the required oral explanation was given to the relative and the guardian or conservator, if there is one. If the patient names a relative who is unavailable, the attempt made to locate the relative, or any other reason the relative may be unavailable for the oral explanation must be entered into the record. The physician's notification and attempts at notification shall be documented in the patient's Medical Record.

B. Convulsive treatment procedures for voluntary patients

Convulsive treatment may be administered to VOLUNTARY patients only if:

1. The treating physician or attending physician enters adequate documentation in the patient's treatment record of the reasons for the procedure, that all reasonable treatment modalities have been carefully considered, and that the treatment is definitely indicated and is the least drastic alternative available for this patient at this time. Such statement in the treatment record shall be signed by the attending or treating physician.

2. All other treatment modalities need not to be tried prior to convulsive treatment, but they must be considered. Treatment modalities are to be construed to mean general categories such as chemotherapy, psychotherapy, etc., but not all specific subcategories of each general category.

3. All requirements for informed consent contained in Section A above have been met and written consent obtained from the patient.

4. A board-certified or board-eligible psychiatrist or neurologist other than the patient's attending or treating physician has examined the patient and verifies that the patient has the capacity to give and has given written informed consent. Such verification shall be documented in the patient's treatment record and signed by the physician either in the Progress Note or on the "Informed Consent Consultation for Convulsive Therapy" form.

5. A responsible relative (if the patient designates one) and the patient's guardian or conservator, if there is one, have been given the oral explanation (as outlined under Section A) by the treating or attending physician. Responsible relative is defined as the spouse, parent, adult child, or adult brother or sister of the patient. The patient may request that no relative be notified, and this request will be documented in the patient's Medical Record.

6. The treating or attending physician must enter into the Medical Record that the required oral explanation was given to the relative or the guardian or conservator, if there is one. If the patient does not desire to inform a relative, this fact must be

entered into the record. If the named relative is unavailable, attempts to locate him/her should be documented in the patient's Medical Record.

7. If the required verification of the capacity to give written informed consent is not met or if it is determined that the patient does not have the capacity to give informed consent, then WIC 5326.7, section f. must be followed (see IV.C.9 & 10 of this policy, below).

C. Convulsive treatment procedures for involuntary patients (including anyone under Lanterman-Petris-Short (L-P-S) guardianship or conservatorship)

1. Convulsive treatment may be administered to an involuntary patient, including anyone on a 72-hour hold, 14-day hold certification, second 14-day hold and 30 day hold certification, 180-day post certification, or under L-P-S guardianship or conservatorship, only if all of the following provisions have been met.

2. The attending or treating physician enters adequate documentation in the patient's treatment record of the reasons for the procedure, that all reasonable treatment modalities have been carefully considered, and that the treatment is definitely indicated and is the least drastic alternative available for the patient at the time. Such statement in the treatment record shall be signed by the attending or treating physician.

3. All other treatment modalities need not be tried prior to convulsive treatment, but they must be considered. Treatment modalities are to be construed to mean general categories such as chemotherapy, psychotherapy, etc., but not all specific subcategories of each general category.

4. A review of the patient's treatment record is conducted by a committee of two physicians, at least one of whom shall have personally examined the patient. Both physicians must be either board-certified or board-eligible psychiatrists or neurologists. One physician may be appointed by the facility responsible for the ECT. The other physician shall be taken from a list approved by the county mental health director. Both of the physicians must agree with the treating physician's determinations as noted in Section I, item 2 Section IV, C. 2. above. Such agreement shall be documented in the patient's treatment record and signed by both physicians.

5. The treating or attending physician shall give a responsible relative of the patient's choosing and the patient's guardian or conservator, if there is one, the oral explanation as outlined under the Voluntary Informed Consent. Responsible relative is defined as the spouse, parent, adult child, or adult brother or sister of the patient.

6. Should the patient desire not to inform a relative, this requirement is dispensed with, and the patient's request for notification or non-notification will be documented in the patient's Medical Record. The treating or attending physician

must enter into the Medical Record that the required oral explanation was given to the relative and the guardian or conservator, if there is one. If the patient names a relative who is unavailable, the attempt made to locate the relative, or any other reason the relative may be unavailable for the oral explanation must be entered into the record. The physician's notification and attempts at notification shall be documented in the patient's Medical Record.

7. The patient gives informed consent as outlined above under Section A, "Legal Requirements for Informed Consent."

8. The patient's attorney, or, if none, a public defender appointed by the Superior Court, agrees as to the patient's capacity or incapacity to give written informed consent and that the patient who has capacity has given written informed consent. If the attorney agrees that the patient can give informed consent, this must be documented in the Medical Record by the attorney.

9. If either the attending physician or the attorney believes that the patient does not have the capacity to give a written informed consent, then a petition shall be filed in the Superior Court to determine that patient's capacity to give written informed consent. The court shall hold an evidentiary hearing after giving appropriate notice to the patient, and within three judicial days after the petition is filed. At such hearing, the patient shall be present and represented by legal counsel.

10. If the Court determines that the patient does not have the capacity to give written informed consent, then treatment may be performed upon gaining the written informed consent from the responsible relative or the guardian or the conservator of the patient.

11. At any time during the course of treatment of a person who has been deemed incompetent, that person shall have the right to claim regained competency. Should the person do so, the person's competency must be reevaluated accordingly.

D. ECT procedures for minors

1. Under no circumstances shall convulsive treatment be performed on a minor under 12 years of age.

2. Persons 16 and 17 years of age shall personally exercise their rights with regard to ECT. They are thus subject to the provisions mentioned above under Section A "Legal Requirements for Informed Consent," if voluntary, and may grant or withhold consent for convulsive treatment to the same extent as adults who are voluntary patients.

3. For adolescents ages 12–15, in addition:

   a) It is an emergency situation and convulsive treatment is deemed a life-saving treatment.

b) This fact and the need for and appropriateness of the treatment are unanimously certified by a review board of the three board-certified or board-eligible child psychiatrists appointed by the local mental health director. ECT is otherwise performed in full compliance with regulations promulgated by the Director of the State Department of Mental Health.

c) If substitute consent is authorized by the court, the custodial parent(s), or individual or agency with legal custody, shall be considered the guardian for purposes of granting or withholding substituted consent.

d) ECT is thoroughly documented and reported immediately to the Director of Mental Health. The state DMH will provide the required form for reporting convulsive treatment given to minors 12–15 years of age, exclusively. This form must be submitted immediately after the first treatment.

E. Review and post-treatment audit committee

1. Any facility in which convulsive treatment is performed, whether on a voluntary or an involuntary patient, shall designate a qualified committee of at least three psychiatrists or neurologists knowledgeable about the treatment and its effect to verify the appropriateness and need for such treatment.

2. This committee shall review all convulsive treatments given in that facility on a quarterly basis.

3. If treatments are initiated in a facility, and then continued outside that facility, the physician who continues treatments shall report the total number to the facility, and any such treatments shall be reviewed by the facility's review committee.

4. Records of these committees will be subject to availability in the same manner as are the records of other committees and to such other hospital utilization and audit committees and to such other regulations as are promulgated by the State Director of Mental Health.

5. Persons serving on such review committees will enjoy the same immunities as other persons serving on utilization, peer review, and audit committees of health care facilities.

6. Persons who serve on review committees shall not otherwise be personally involved in the treatment of the patient whose case they are reviewing. This restriction applies to pre-treatment review committees and post-treatment audit committees.

7. When more than one seizure is induced in a single treatment session, each seizure shall be considered a separate treatment for record keeping and reporting purposes.

8. The local mental health director shall establish a post-audit review committee for convulsive treatments administered anywhere other than in any facility as defined in the Health and Safety Code in which psychiatric evaluation or

treatment is offered. The post-treatment review committee will have the responsibility to review all convulsive treatments given anywhere other than in a health facility. There must be at least a quarterly review.

F. Excessive use of convulsive treatment

1. Convulsive treatment shall be considered excessive if more than 15 treatments are given to a patient within a 30-day period, or a total of more than 30 treatments are given to a patient within a one-year period.
2. If, in the judgment of the attending physician, more than the above limits are indicated, prior approval for continued ECT therapy must first be obtained from the review committee of the facility or, if ECT is not administered under the auspices of a facility, by the County.
3. Requests for approval shall include documentation of the diagnosis, the clinical findings leading to the recommendation for the additional treatments, the consideration of other reasonable treatment modalities, and the opinion that additional treatments pose less risk than other potentially effective alternatives available for the particular patient at the present time. A maximum number of additional treatments shall be specified.
4. The review committee shall act upon any such request within seven days of its receipt and shall document the maximum number of additional treatments approved. All applicable informed consent procedures shall also be followed.

G. Reports on convulsive treatment

1. Any doctor or facility which administers convulsive treatments or which considers such treatment methods a part of their program shall submit a monthly report to the local mental health director, who shall transmit the data to the State Director of Mental Health. These reports shall be made regardless of whether or not any of these treatment methods were used during the month. Likewise, any physician who considers any of these methods a service that he/she provides, and whose use of the above-mentioned treatment methods is not included in any facility's report, must submit a monthly report to the local mental health director even if such treatments were not administered during that particular time.
2. The reports shall indicate:
   a) Voluntary patients who gave informed consent.
   b) Voluntary patients deemed incapable of giving informed consent.
   c) Involuntary patients (including patients under L-P-S guardianship or conservatorship) who gave informed consent.
   d) Involuntary patients (including patients under L-P-S guardianship or conservatorship) deemed incapable of giving informed consent.

e) Age, sex, and the race of the patients undergoing convulsive treatment.

f) The major source of payment for the treatment by type: private, public (including, but not limited to Medicare and Medicaid), third-party payor or other funding source which is specified.

g) Number of treatments administered. When more than one seizure is induced in a single treatment session, each seizure shall be considered a separate treatment for record-keeping and reporting purposes.

h) Complications that arise during the course of administering convulsive treatment including the following: cardiac arrests regardless of outcome i.e., fatal or nonfatal; fractures, with medical diagnosis of the fracture accompanying the report; apnea, persisting 20 minutes or longer after initiation of treatment; memory loss extending for more than 3 months after treatment has stopped; deaths – all deaths during or within the first 24 hours after the convulsive treatment must be reported to the coroner as well as deaths subsequent to the treatment but attributable to the treatment. If an autopsy is performed by the coroner, a report of the findings should accompany this report. If no autopsy is performed, the reason for noncompliance must be stated. Requirements of Section 5328 of the Welfare and Institutions Code on confidentiality must nevertheless be observed.

3. Monthly reports shall be made on a form which shall be issued by the State Department of Mental Health which shall include all necessary instructions and definitions. (Form not included)

4. A facility, clinic, or physician who fails to submit required reports by the 15th of the month following completion of the month shall be notified by the local mental health director of the legal obligation to submit these reports. Failure to comply within 15 days after such notification shall be reported to the Director of the State Department of Mental Health, who may take any or all of the action specified in Section 5326.9 of the Welfare and Institutions Code.

5. The local mental health director shall transmit copies of all quarterly reports received to the Patients' Rights Office, State Department of Mental Health, by the last day of the month following the end of the quarter.

6. In keeping with the privacy and confidentiality policies of the Hospital, persons having access to protected health information will only access the minimum necessary information to carry out their job duties. Persons carrying out external regulatory reporting activities must only release the minimum information necessary to accomplish the purpose of the report as determined by the requestor. Persons releasing protected health information for other purposes must follow established release of information policies.

H. Violation penalties

1. Alleged or suspected violation of the laws governing the denial of rights (all rights, not just the rights involving convulsive treatment) shall be reported to the Director of the State Department of Mental Health, who shall investigate and report each such allegation or suspected violation and the results of the investigation to the Board of Medical Quality Assurance. The board will impose the necessary penalty, if any.

2. Intentional violation of the above provisions regarding convulsive treatment shall be subject to a civil penalty of not more than $5,000 for each violation as the result of an action brought by the Attorney General. This penalty is in addition to, not in substitution for, any other remedies which an individual may have under the law. Also, intentional violation is grounds for revocation of the physician's license.

3. Either the local director of mental health or the State Director of Mental Health, upon issuing a notice of violation, may take any or all of the following actions:

    a. Assign a specified time period during which the violation shall be corrected.

    b. Referral to the Medical Board of California or other professional licensing agency. Such board shall investigate further, if warranted, and shall subject the individual practitioner to any penalty the board finds necessary and is authorized to impose; revoke a facility's designation and authorization to evaluate and treat persons detained involuntarily; refer any violation of law to a local district attorney of the State Attorney General for prosecution in any court with jurisdiction.

I. General guidelines for electroconvulsive therapy

1. ECT patients must have a history and physical evaluation completed within 7 days prior to the first or initial ECT treatment in a series of ECT treatments, and at least annually thereafter. When a series of ECT treatments is given, changes in physical health status of the patient will be assessed and documented in the patient's medical record by the RN, Psychiatrist, and Anesthesiologist prior to each subsequent ECT treatment within the series of treatments. This includes changes in the History and Physical examination.

2. There is no "routine" lab workup for ECT. A CBC, chemistry panel, urinalysis, chest X-ray and EKG should be obtained and repeated whenever clinically indicated.

3. Given that ECT is a brief, repetitive procedure that may have the patient transfer from Inpatient and Outpatient status over time, the workup in one section

shall be valid for subsequent sections unless specifically prohibited by WIC or CCR.

4. Patients will be kept NPO after midnight the day prior to treatment.

5. ECT will be performed in the designated ECT Suite. If the ECT psychiatrist, anesthesiologist and internist determine that a different location is clinically indicated for a specific patient, this can be arranged.

6. ECT may be administered only by a board-eligible or board-certified psychiatrist who has been certified for this privilege. The electrotherapist shall demonstrate familiarity with current American Psychiatric Association (APA) guidelines.

7. The Department of Anesthesiology will supervise all anesthesia procedures and administration of anesthetic agents. [This is only one of several possible scenarios for the administration of anesthesia for ECT. In some settings, anesthesia would be administered by a nurse anesthetist. In other settings, the psychiatrist may administer the anesthesia in addition to the ECT. These scenarios would determine how the wording in this section (7) and the next section (8) are changed.]

8. The choice of specific medications and doses to be used during the pre-anesthesia, intra-anesthesia, and post-anesthesia periods will be determined by collaboration between the ECT psychiatrist and anesthesiologist.

9. All patients should have EKG monitoring and baseline vital signs taken prior to treatment.

10. All patients should have EKG, vital signs, and pulse oximetry monitoring during the treatment until awake.

11. EKG, vital signs, and pulse oximetry will continue to be monitored at least every 15 minutes until stable post-ECT.

J. Care of the patient receiving ECT: See "nursing responsibilities"

K. Outpatient ECT

1. Outpatient ECT is available to patients if the treating psychiatrist assesses that it is both psychiatrically and medically safe and appropriate for the patient.

2. Patients treated on an outpatient basis need someone to bring them to and from each ECT. A responsible adult must be available to be with them for at least 24 hours after each treatment. If the availability cannot be verified, the treatment will be cancelled.

3. The patient cannot drive or work during the acute phase of the outpatient ECT. For outpatient maintenance ECT, the restriction on driving and working shall be determined on an individual basis, but will be for at least 24 hours.

4. Patients receiving ECT on an outpatient basis must be registered through Outpatient Registration on or before the first ECT treatment and will check in with ECT Department prior to each outpatient treatment.

5. The Medical Record of an outpatient receiving ECT will include all of the documentation required for a hospitalized patient who is receiving ECT.

6. The ECT consent that is on the Medical Record must be the original consent signed by the patient unless the original consent is on the Hospital Inpatient Medical Record.

7. If the patient is receiving a series of ECT treatments, the medical record will be secured per the Medical Records Department Policy.

8. Once the patient has met criteria for discharge as indicated in the hospital's standardized post-sedation/anesthesia discharge criteria, they may be discharged to the care of a responsible adult.

9. The patient and the person responsible for transporting the patient will be given written ("Outpatient Electroconvulsive Therapy (ECT) Instructions") and verbal instructions regarding post-treatment care, information about next treatment date and time and pre-ECT instructions, if indicated.

10. Outpatients who are inpatients at other facilities will be discharged to responsible staff from that facility and transported back to their facility by means established by contract or letter of agreement with that facility and in full compliance with Hospital policy. Please see "Treating Patients who are Inpatients Elsewhere."

11. The patient will be transported by wheelchair to the pick-up area.

L. ECT forms

The following list of forms is to be used to ensure compliance with the Welfare and Institutions Code (WIC) and California Code of Regulations (CCR) – [Not included here].

ECT nursing responsibilities

I. Purpose

To outline nursing staff responsibilities for the administration of Electroconvulsive Therapy (ECT). This policy will be used in conjunction with the "General Policies for Electroconvulsive Therapy."

II. Policy

To ensure that ECT will be administered in compliance with the Welfare and Institutions Code (WIC), Sections 5326.15–5326.95, and California Code of

Regulations (CCR), Title 9, Sections 835–849, and will be safely and responsibly implemented.

III. Procedures

A. Pre-ECT patient preparation

The Charge Nurse/designee will assure that the following are completed:

1. The patient will be kept NPO from midnight the night before each treatment unless physician orders specify otherwise.
2. The nursing staff will arrange to have breakfast for inpatients held until after the ECT treatment.
3. For all outpatients receiving ECT, the ECT RN will:
    a) Contact the patient by phone, prior to the first treatment. A Patient Profile and Assessment must be completed prior to the first treatment.
    b) On the morning of ECT treatment, the RN/designee will: greet the patient and the responsible accompanying adult; escort the patient to the pre-treatment area in the ECT suite; escort the accompanying adult to ECT Suite waiting area; take the patient's vital signs; assist the patient into a patient gown; complete the pre-ECT checklist; assess and document the patient's status including any change from initial assessment, brief mental status, any evidence (or lack of) of suicidality, and any significant change in the patient's functional ability. The blood pressure, temperature, pulse, and respiration of the patient will be taken and recorded prior to the ECT treatment.
    c) The patient will be encouraged to void prior to the ECT treatment.
    d) Dentures, bridges, artificial limbs, hearing aids, eyeglasses or contacts, or other prostheses will be removed and their disposition documented. If the patient requests to keep the above until they arrive in treatment area, this must be documented in the medical record, and the ECT nurse informed.
    e) List all allergies or "no known allergies" on the Medicine Administration Record.
    f) Check that the patient is wearing an I.D. bracelet.
    g) Have patient change into hospital gown. If the patient requests to wear personal clothes to the treatment area, they will be permitted.

B. Inpatient transportation

The Charge Nurse/designee will ensure that:

1. Patient is transported to the ECT Treatment Area by unit staff at least 15 minutes prior to scheduled treatment time.

2. The Patient Care Record, addressograph plate, and at least three face sheets are to be taken with the patient to the treatment area.

C. Treatment room preparation

The RN/designee will:

1. Prepare the stretcher with a clean sheet and a bath towel at the head.
2. Check the Emergency Cart. A complete inventory of the Cart is to be completed every Monday (or first treatment day of the week if not Monday) and whenever the Cart is used. Daily checks of the top of the Cart, emergency supplies and equipment, expiration dates, and integrity of the lock are to be done on each treatment day.
3. Assure that all monitoring equipment, including cardiac monitor, pulse oximeter, and sphygmomanometer, is available and functional.
4. Open ECT cart and set up equipment:
   a). Stimulus electrodes, recording electrodes, Thymopads™, handheld paddles, and electrode gel.
   b). ECT paper in the machine (extra paper is in the cart).
   c). Bite Blocks (all sizes). A sterile bite block or disposable bite block is used for each treatment. After each treatment, the rubber bite blocks are given to the anesthesia technician for sterilization per hospital policy.
   d). Alcohol sponges – at least four per scheduled patient.
   e). Washcloths – at least two per scheduled patient.
5. Attach oxygen mask to wall outlet and check that it is working (for post-treatment if needed).
6. Set up Yankhauer suction and tubing, turn it on, and assure that it is functional.
7. Arrange anesthesia tubing and mask and attach to anesthesia machine.
8. Arrange the following forms on top of the chart: Last anesthesiology record from previous treatment, if applicable, for the anesthesiologist to review; New anesthesia record; Copy of the face sheet; Anesthesia medication record; Anesthesiology Post-Operative Order Sheet.
9. Assist the patient to change into a gown, if not already in a gown.
10. Assure that all consults and consents are complete and on the patient's chart.
11. Assure that the number of treatments and the timeframe covered by the consent has not been exceeded.
12. Start IV of 0.9% sodium chloride at a TKO rate, unless ordered otherwise. The ECT nurse or anesthesiologist will do this.
13. Assure that the Emergency Cart, its keys, and diazepam (10 mg. IV) are available in the Treatment Room.
14. Assure that the intubation equipment is available in the Treatment Room.

D. Nursing staff assistance during the ECT treatment

1. Staffing is based on identified volume and acuity of patients determined by patient needs. Core staffing is determined by analysis of annualized data from the patient classification system. The registered nurse to patient ratio is based on patient care needs and number of patients on the unit.

2. Nurses are educated to care for the patient population primarily consisting of adult and geriatric psychiatry patients receiving ECT. All staff who assist with ECT must successfully complete ECT orientation and cross training.

3. The patient will not be left alone at any time.

4. The nursing staff will ascertain that the routine preparation of the patient has been completed.

5. The medical record of the patient will be checked to ensure that it contains: A Consent Form which indicates the number of treatments and is properly signed and dated by the patient or parent or legal guardian; A completed ECT checklist for subsequent treatments verifying limits of consent (for time and number of ECT) has not been exceeded; The time of administration and the dosage of any medication given after the preceding midnight.

6. The patient will be assisted onto the gurney in a supine position with side rails up.

7. All patients will have EKG monitoring, pulse oximeter, and baseline vital signs taken prior to the treatment.

8. The mouth of the patient will be checked for any foreign objects (toothpicks, gum, etc.) that will be removed.

9. Body jewelry and piercings in the patient's mouth or face will be removed unless permitted by the anesthesiologist and psychiatrist.

10. The patient will be connected to the vital signs monitoring device.

11. Treatment will be administered by the psychiatrist with the anesthesiologist administering medication/anesthesia.

12. The ECT nurse will assist with the procedure.

13. All patients will have EKG monitoring and pulse oximeter during the treatment until awake.

14. The nursing staff will be available at the side of the gurney to protect and support the extremities as needed.

15. The anesthesiologist will monitor the respirations and the patient's blood pressure and pulse; the blood pressure, pulse, and SAO_2 will be automatically monitored.

16. The anesthesiologist will determine when to transfer the patient to the recovery area by completing the "Anesthesiology Post-Operative Orders Form" and will advise the nurse responsible for post-anesthesia care of any specific problems presented by the patient's condition.

17. The nurse assisting with ECT will record: The patient's vital signs pre- and post-ECT indicating the times the vital signs were taken; and the behavioral observation of the patient's condition pre-ECT, during recovery, and post-ECT, including physiological or psychological events.
18. The nurse will enter patient's name and date of treatment in the ECT log.

E. ECT recovery procedure

The RN is responsible to assure that:

1. A nursing staff member will remain with the patient at all times from the administration of the anesthesia until the patient meets criteria for discharge.
2. The nursing staff will be responsible for maintaining an adequate and clear airway. If the patient is snoring, the airway may be obstructed.
3. The nursing staff will protect the patient from harm: Side rails will be up at all times; If the patient is thrashing, pillows or other safety interventions will be used to cushion the extremities; the nursing staff will be aware that some patients have a startled response upon awakening, and may become agitated for a short period of time. When this occurs, the patient will be oriented, i.e., by being told where they are and that the treatment is completed.
4. The patient's vital signs (blood pressure, pulse, and respiration) will be taken immediately upon recovery and at least every 15 minutes until the vital signs are stable and the patient is alert.
5. The anesthesiologist or psychiatrist in charge will decide when to allow the patient to leave the recovery area based on the Aldrete Scoring System in the Clinical Procedures Manual and return to his/her own room. When possible, the patient will be allowed to sleep until he/she awakens spontaneously.
6. Prior to transferring the patient from the recovery area, the RN who assisted in the treatment will:
   a). Evaluate the patient using the Aldrete Scoring system to determine when the patient may be transferred out of the treatment area.
   b). Assess the patient for orientation.
   c). Record the presence or absence of anesthesia-related complications.
   d). Record observations concerning the patient's emotional and mental condition and behavior.
   e). Document this information.
7. Assess and document the patient's condition on the flow sheet, and discontinue the IV unless contraindicated by physician order.
8. All patients will be escorted from the recovery area by the nursing staff. Inpatients will be transported back to the unit, accompanied by an RN, post-treatment.

9. Unit nursing staff will be notified by the RN that the patient is returning to the unit by wheelchair and will be responsible for the patient's care at that time.

10. The RN escorting the patient back to the unit will provide the RN responsible for the care of the patient with a report to include patient response to treatment, vital signs, and post-anesthesia precautions.

11. The unit staff will complete following when the patient returns:

   a). The patient's vital signs (blood pressure, pulse, and respirations) will be taken and recorded on return to the unit as indicated. If either the systolic or diastolic blood pressure registers either higher or lower than the last post-treatment reading, contact the physician with the results and monitor vital signs at least every 30 minutes or more as indicated until stable.

   b). The patient will be assessed post-ECT for the following, and the nurse will document: ambulation ability; level of orientation; food and fluid intake; and effects of/response to treatment.

   c). Patient may eat or drink as tolerated when returned to the unit, unless contraindicated by physician order.

12. The patient will be restricted to the unit until orientation to the surroundings has been re-established.

13. No unsupervised activity is to be performed by the patient for at least two (2) hours following the ECT procedure unless the staff is certain that the patient can manage it.

14. Verbal and written post-ECT care instructions will be given to responsible person(s) escorting all outpatients and will include but is not limited to post-treatment instructions, emergency contact information, next treatment date and time, and pre-treatment instructions.

15. Outpatients will be escorted by the RN/designee via wheelchair to the Discharge Area, to transportation with responsible adult as arranged.

F. General post-ECT duties

The RN/designee will:

1. Bill for ECT treatment and supplies via the computer.
2. Schedule the next ECT treatment with scheduling personnel.
3. Prepare staff nursing schedule for ECT.
4. Fax the supply requisition to Central Issue for supplies.
5. Put equipment away and tidy up as necessary.
6. Send all equipment, mouth props, and face masks to Central Sterile Supply Department for resterilization and return to unit.

7. Clean head straps with soap and water.
8. Clean electrodes with alcohol wipes only.
9. Place clean linens on the stretcher.
10. Turn off the oxygen and any equipment.
11. Assure that all medications in the treatment area are secured.
12. Assure that the ECT suite is secured.

Treating patients who are inpatients elsewhere

I. Purpose

To outline guidelines for administration and documentation of Electroconvulsive Therapy and the care of the patient who is currently an inpatient at another acute care facility. This policy will be used in conjunction with the "General Policies for Electroconvulsive Therapy" and "Nursing Responsibilities" and will meet all guidelines as established by the Hospital Transfer Center.

II. Policy

A). All guidelines established by the Hospital Transfer Center will be implemented and followed in the care of the patient transferred from another acute health-care facility for the purpose of receiving ECT treatments. ECT will be administered in compliance with the Welfare and Institutions Code (WIC), Sections 5326.15–5326.95, and California Code of Regulations (CCR), Title 9, Sections 835–849, and will be safely and responsibly implemented.

B). In keeping with the privacy and confidentiality policies of the Hospital, persons having access to protected health information will only access the minimum necessary information to carry out their job duties. Persons carrying out external regulatory reporting activities must only release the minimum information necessary to accomplish the purpose of the report as determined by the requestor. Persons releasing protected health information for other purposes must follow established release of information policies that are maintained by the Health Information Department.

III. Procedure

A. Pre-treatment

1. The patient must meet all legal requirements for informed consent, history and physical evaluation, pre-operative testing as indicated per "General Policies for ECT."
2. Prior to the first treatment, the ECT Psychiatrist will instruct the Attending Physician at the sending facility regarding the need to keep the patient NPO

after midnight the night before each treatment and the time that the patient needs to arrive at ECT Suite on the morning of the treatment.

3. Prior to transport of the patient to ECT Suite, and in order for the ECT Suite to accept the patient for ECT treatment, the attending physician at the sending facility evaluates the patient and documents in the Medical Record that "the patient is stable for transfer."

4. The sending facility is responsible for transporting the patient with appropriate staff accompaniment and the patient's Medical Record to the ECT Suite.

5. The patient registers as a Hospital outpatient through the Admitting Office the morning of the first treatment at the scheduled hour. The registration must be renewed periodically as per hospital policy. The patient and accompanying staff proceed to the Visitors Waiting Area adjacent to the ECT Suite and notify the ECT nurse of his or her arrival.

6. The ECT RN/designee greets the patient and accompanying staff and brings them to the ECT Suite.

7. The ECT RN completes the pre-ECT treatment procedure per "ECT Nursing Responsibilities".

8. The ECT RN enters the following information into the Transfer Log: the patient's name, date and time of the patient's arrival; Medical Record number of the referring facility; diagnosis; referring physician and facility; Hospital accepting physician; reason for transfer; if the patient is accepted for ECT treatment; and if consent for treatment is obtained.

B. Treatment

1. Prior to the treatment being administered, the treating physician and the anesthesiologist evaluate the patient and document that he or she is stable for treatment and that the patient consents to the treatment.

2. The treatment is administered per policy and is documented in the patient's Hospital Outpatient Medical Record by the treating physician and the anesthesiologist.

C. Post-treatment/recovery

1. The patient is monitored and care provided and documented per policy.

2. When the patient meets Post-Sedation/Anesthesia Discharge Criteria, the patient may be discharged if the patient is assessed by the treating physician to be stable for transport/transfer back to the sending facility.

3. The treating physician assesses the patient and documents in the hospital Outpatient Medical Record that "the patient is stable for transport/transfer to the sending facility with staff accompaniment."

4. The ECT RN notifies the sending facility that the patient is stable for transport, confirms that the patient can return, and documents this notification in the Hospital Medical Record including the name of the RN at the sending facility accepting the return of the patient.

5. The ECT RN/designee prepares a copy of the treatment records for the sending facility which includes treatment number and detail; time of treatment; medications administered; and patient's response to treatment. These records are given to the staff from the sending facility to be included in the Medical Record of the sending facility.

6. The patient and the accompanying staff are given written post-procedure instructions, the telephone number of the person(s) to contact if any problems arise, the date and time of their next scheduled ECT treatment, and other information as per written "Outpatient Electroconvulsive Therapy (ECT) Instructions." The accompanying staff signs as the "Responsible Adult" receiving the instructions. The original is kept in the Hospital Medical Record and the copy is given to the patient and accompanying staff.

7. The ECT RN enters the date and time of the patient's discharge and enters the patient's condition at time of discharge, and the name of the accepting physician in the Transfer Log. The ECT RN/designee will submit the hospital Transfer Log to the Hospital Transfer Center weekly.

8. The patient and the accompanying staff are then transported back to the sending facility by transportation as arranged by both hospitals and within the guidelines of the Transfer Center as an approved method of patient transportation.

D. Medical emergencies

1. If the patient is assessed to need emergency treatment, the hospital physician will arrange for the patient to be seen and evaluated in the Hospital Emergency Department as clinically indicated.

2. The patient will be treated at Hospital as indicated by the patient's clinical condition until stable for transport/transfer to an appropriate treatment facility as indicated.

3. The Hospital attending physician will communicate with the attending physician at the sending facility regarding the patient's status initially and ongoing during the course of clinical emergency treatment. The physicians will assist in deciding the patient's final disposition once the patient is stabilized.

4. All care provided will be documented in the patient's Medical Record.

ECT for regional center patients

(In California these are patients with developmental disabilities)

I. Purpose

To develop a policy for ECT treatment of Regional Center Patients that complies with Title 17, Division 2, Chapter 1, Subchapter 8, Section 5080 (J) and Article 4, Section 50830–50835 of California Code of Regulations.

II. Policy

A. Regional Center patients shall not receive ECT unless the use of ECT has been developed into a program that is fully described in a proposed treatment plan that has been approved by the ECT Review Committee approved by the Regional Center.

B. In keeping with the privacy and confidentiality policies of the Hospital, persons having access to protected health information will only access the minimum necessary information to carry out their job duties. Persons carrying out external regulatory reporting activities must only release the minimum information necessary to accomplish the purpose of the report as determined by the requestor. Persons releasing protected health information for other purposes must follow established release of information policies that are maintained by the Health Information Department.

III. Procedure

A. All proposals to use ECT shall be developed into a program that is fully described in a treatment plan. The proposed treatment plan shall include at a minimum:

1. A description of:
   a. The reasons for proposing the use of ECT, which shall include:
      (1) A list of the behaviors, symptoms, and diagnoses leading to the decision to propose the use of ECT.
      (2) The results of other, less restrictive alternative treatments used to modify these behaviors or alleviate the described symptoms.
   b. The anticipated benefits to the client of using ECT, with a statement of the probable consequences of denying the use of ECT.
   c. The number and frequency of proposed treatments.
   d. The methods to be used to determine and document the results of the treatments.
   e. Consent that shall be subject to all requirements for voluntary patients.
   f. The proposed treatment plan shall be submitted in writing to the ECT Review Committee approved by the Regional Center.

B. The ECT Review Committee for Regional Center patients shall be established and shall consist of at least four persons, including:

1. Two board-certified psychiatrists or neurologists, licensed in California with experience in electroconvulsive treatment; one of whom shall be appointed by the facility and one of whom shall be appointed by the local mental health director. Neither of these physicians shall be the client's treating physician.

2. A representative from the Department of Development Services appointed by the Director of the Regional Center who will function as a Clients Rights Advocate;

3. A representative from the Regional Center in which client resides, appointed by the Chairperson on the Area Board (an Area Board Representative).

C. The following criteria are required, at a minimum, for approval of ECT:

1. The ECT Review Committee shall consider for approval or denial only those proposed treatment plans which have met the requirements specified in Item A above.

2. Approval is predicated on the unanimous agreement of the ECT Review Committee with the treating physician's determinations.

3. If the ECT Review Committee approves the proposed treatment plan, their approval shall be limited to 30 days, commencing with the first ECT. Further, the approval of the ECT Review Committee shall be nullified if the treatment plan is not followed exactly as written when approved.

4. Approval of the proposed plan by the Regional Center ECT Review Committee shall not supersede or replace the review requirements necessary under "General Policies for ECT, Section IV." The review of a proposal to use ECT with a person with both developmental disabilities and a mental illness that might justify the use of ECT shall be completed separately and independently by both the Regional Center ECT Review Committee pursuant to these regulations and the reviewing entity required by General Policies for ECT."

D. Procedures for Review of Proposed ECT:

1. The Regional Center ECT Review Committee shall complete its review of all treatment plans submitted pursuant to Section 50831 within 30 calendar days of receipt of the plans. The chairperson of the ECT Review Committee shall telephone the requesting physician and relay the committee's approval or denial of the proposed treatment plan on the day the review is completed.

2. Written notice of the approval or denial shall: Be mailed within five working days of the telephone notice pursuant to paragraph III-D-1; include express findings of conformity or nonconformity to the criteria in Section 50833 with statements of reasons for each finding; be documented in the client's treatment record; be signed by all members of the ECT Review Committee; and be permanently attached to the treatment plan as proposed.

3. ECT can commence when the mailed notice or faxed copy is received.

IV. Reporting requirements

The physician conducting the ECT shall submit a narrative progress report within 30 days of completion of the treatment to the Regional Center ECT Review Committee. The report shall include, but not be limited to, the number of treatments given and the benefits derived. A copy will be a part of patient's medical record.

V. Patients residing in "Family Home" situations cannot be referred directly to ECT. They must first be on L-P-S conservatorship and then referred through the above procedure.

Scope of service: electroconvulsive therapy (ECT)

Location and hours of operation

Electroconvulsive Therapy (ECT) is located at _____.

The normal service hours are Monday, Wednesday, and Friday from 7:00 AM to 12:00 PM, but the hours and days are flexible.

Scope of services provided

ECT provides treatment for adult patients (18 years and over) either on an inpatient or outpatient basis. The treatment is provided based on the patient's individual needs and focuses on maximizing the patient's health care status.

Staffing plan

Staffing is based on identified volume and acuity of patients determined by patient needs. Nurses are educated to care for the patient population primarily consisting of adult and geriatric psychiatry patients receiving ECT. Core staffing is determined by analysis of annualized data from the patient classification system. The registered nurse to patient ratio is based on patient care needs and number of patients on the unit.

Departmental performance improvement

The Department has one Performance Improvement Committee. The committee is co-chaired by psychiatrists, and comprises physicians, nurses, clinical staff, and administration. The Performance Improvement Committee monitors a variety of activities such as ECT, seclusion/restraint use, falls, patient/physician/staff satisfaction, adverse events, and documentation. ECT performance improvement indicators include those required by law and those specific to trends that develop. An ECT Committee meets quarterly and reports to the Performance Improvement Committee.

Additionally, the Department nursing staff has specific indicators that are monitored and reported to the Performance Improvement Committee and Nursing Council. The Nursing Council is chaired by the Chief Nursing Officer. The Nursing Council monitors outcomes for the following: Patient satisfaction with discharge education and compassion and caring by nurses; physician and staff satisfaction; restraint use; patient falls; dermal ulcers; conscious sedation; patient education; and prevention of delays.

Quality assurance monitors

Quality assurance is an approach to ensure that you are doing the best job possible. Retrospective results of predetermined issues are compared against benchmark measures. When the benchmarks are not attained, the ECT unit should try to determine why they were not attained and set a plan for improvement. The goal of any Quality Assurance Program is to improve patient care, patient safety, and patient satisfaction. It should also lead to improvement in the mechanisms for the delivery of care. Although this may lead to a more cost-effective way to deliver care, quality and patient satisfaction should never be sacrificed for cost. Quality assurance measures should change as the maturity of the program changes. Initially, it is important to assess the integrity of the program itself. Are the charting requirements of the hospital being followed? Are history and physical examinations, laboratory tests, and EKGs being completed in a timely manner? Are nursing intake assessments completed in a timely manner? Although the goal should be 100%, the ECT unit should perform at least as well as the other parts of the hospital. Are all of the legal requirements being met? Is the consent process being appropriately handled? The goal for these should be 100%. In the state of California, these are required measures that must be reported to the state quarterly. Less than 100% compliance could result in sanctions from the state. What percentage of patients is achieving response and what percentage remission – broken down by diagnosis? These should be consistent with national norms. Patient satisfaction monitors could also be measured. What is the waiting time? How do patients and their families view the program? Can they suggest areas of improvement? Do they feel included in the treatment decisions? Do they feel that their concerns are listened to? Can they reach the doctor or nurse easily after treatment if there is a question or problem? Changes in functioning can be measured. Are there differences in quality of life and disability measures before and after ECT? Side effects such as post-discharge headache, falls, medical complications, and hospital re-admission for outpatients are all valuable monitors after the basic monitors have been consistently performing well. Quality assurance measures that are dropped because of consistent good performance should still be periodically revisited to ensure that levels are maintained.

Having a quality assurance system in place and monitoring and improving care also is necessary for the hospital to comply with regulatory requirements of the Joint Commission, Centers for Medicare and Medicaid Services, and various state agencies. Increasingly, accreditation and review agencies have been asking us to show them our quality assurance work since their prior reviews.

References

American Psychiatric Association (APA). 2001. The practice of electroconvulsive therapy: Recommendations for treatment, training and privileging. Washington, DC: APA.

(As laws and regulations are frequently being updated, I believe that the Web sites with the most up-to-date regulations are more appropriate than the specific volume used for these procedures).

California Code of Regulations (CCR), Title 9 can be found at http://www.oal.ca.gov/index.html

California Code of Regulations (CCR), Title 17 can be found at http://www.oal.ca.gov/index.html

Up-to-date manuals for the Centers for Medicare and Medicaid Services can be found at http://www.cms.hhs.gov/

Up-to-date manuals for EMTALA regulations can be found at: http://www.emtala.com/

Up-to-date manuals for The Joint Commission regulations can be found at http://www.jcrinc.com/Welfare and Institutions Code (WIC) for California can be found at http://www.leginfo.ca.gov/cgi-bin/calawquery?codesection=wic&codebody=&hits=20

20

Staff management and physical layout for electroconvulsive therapy

Jerry Lewis

General concerns

The physical layout of the electroconvulsive therapy (ECT) suite and the allocation of staff can influence ECT outcome, patient comfort, and staff satisfaction. Most of the information here is directed to those providers who plan to deliver 5 to 30 ECT treatments on a given day, but some should apply to any ECT setup.

The art of ECT evolves with the clinical science, aiming toward improved efficiency and patient comfort. Delivering ECT in a dedicated area helps to preserve privacy and confidentiality. The ECT procedure room must be large enough to accommodate the personnel, devices for ECT and defibrillation, anesthesia equipment including oxygen and suction, and monitoring equipment needed to observe patients while anesthetized.

ECT is not appropriate for a surgical operating room. There it is an unpleasant and cumbersome process requiring both the patient and treatment team to change into surgical clothing, which is quite unnecessary for ECT. Operating rooms are not readily accessible and slow down patient flow. Ideal is a dedicated ECT suite located near a psychiatry unit or in a separate area of an outpatient surgical facility. If outpatient ECT is provided, having the suite directly accessible to the public is generally helpful and efficient as outpatients can present directly to the suite without needing to be accompanied by a transport aide. Patient privacy should be emphasized by each clinician involved. Performing ECT in an area that can be observed (even heard) by other patients violates privacy, even if the area is curtained off.

In the following sections, discussion centers on the type of area needed, designs for treating a large number of patients, and how intravenous (IV) access, subdermal ports, recovery area, and other factors may influence patient flow and safety. Types of personnel and their training are described.

This writer has 20 years of experience in psychiatric practice in a small hospital where three to five ECT treatments per treatment day were administered. For the subsequent seven years, I worked in a large university hospital setting with 15 to

20 ECT treatments on each treatment day. My work has included directing ECT services, redesigning the ECT suite, and visiting other hospitals to assess their ECT operations. This article is a result of this experience.

Equipment necessary for ECT

A. Suction and oxygen are needed in both the treatment area and recovery room. An anesthesia machine is preferred, and equipment for emergency intubation should be available. Disposable breathing masks and circuits and devices (commonly called bite blocks or mouth protectors) to protect the teeth during treatment are needed as well. Airways, both nasal and oral, are helpful and an ambu bag is needed.

B. An electrocardiogram (ECG) monitor, pulse oximeter, and automatic blood pressure monitor should be present in the treatment area. A nerve stimulator is also helpful.

C. A fully stocked medication and equipment cabinet and crash cart should be in the treatment area. These should be inventoried on a regular basis for expiration dates and adequacy of the equipment.

D. The ECT machine with all necessary leads and equipment should be located near the treatment bed. The machine instruction manual and accompanying informational tables should be within easy reach.

E. A spare ECT machine and monitoring equipment should be stored on site in case the original machine or monitoring equipment malfunctions. This is typically an administrative requirement.

The small hospital and small-volume operations

ECT can be done effectively in small hospitals and can be a great service to many people. In many rural areas, inpatient units have closed during the past few years, and some patients drive several hundred miles to receive outpatient ECT at large hospitals. A local hospital could provide this service and save patients both time and travel expense. The negative aspects of the small hospital setup are the lack of privacy and the time limitation (having to be finished before the operating room schedule starts).

In a small hospital, the usual practice is to do the ECT early in the morning before the operating room schedule starts. When ECT was first started in the small hospital where I practiced, they scheduled the procedure in turn with other surgical procedures. It became clear that making ECT patients wait unit late afternoon to have the procedure was not practical. An agreement was made with the surgeons that the ECT treatments would be done first thing in the morning and would be completed by a particular time.

Usually, in a small hospital, the anesthesia team will want to do the ECT in an area very close to the operating room where the anesthesia equipment is located. This area might be in a room in or close to the recovery area. If, on average, fewer than five treatments per day are done, considerations of efficiency and economy allow no convincing alternative. However, it is extremely important to provide privacy for the patient. Ethically, other patients should not be able to see or even hear the procedure. Hanging curtains around the bed is not acceptable because it does not mute the noise that sometimes accompanies the treatment. A waiting area adjacent to the actual treatment room may be helpful in facilitating patients arriving close together or from different parts of the hospital.

A recovery room area is needed to take the patient for first-stage recovery. In a small hospital, this usually is the same room used for patients recovering from general surgical procedures. Inpatients can then be taken back to their rooms for second-stage recovery. If outpatient ECT is given, another part of the hospital could be used for second-stage recovery, or patients could stay longer in the general recovery room area.

At least three people are needed in the actual treatment room. These include an anesthesiologist or registered nurse anesthetist, an ECT nurse, and the psychiatrist. Their job functions are described in detail later, but in brief the anesthetist is responsible for managing the airway, the psychiatrist is responsible for determining treatment parameters and managing the therapeutic efficacy of the seizure, and the ECT nurse is responsible for coordinating and monitoring patient care and patient flow. The anesthetist, in conjunction with the psychiatrist, will decide which anesthetic medications are to be used and help decide if the general medical condition of the patient allows the treatment to proceed (see Chapter 19).

High-volume operations

Special consideration needs to be given to the personnel and physical layout needed if a moderate to large volume of patients (6 to 30) is going to be treated in one day. The issues that usually slow down the progression of treatments are IV access problems and recovery room complications. Having to cancel planned patient treatments, especially patients in the middle of an ECT course, because of problems that delay the ECT schedule so that all treatments are not completed, can lengthen inpatient stay. Missed treatments in the early part of a series can result in relapse of the patient or slow down a patient's improvement. Deliberate efforts are needed to run an efficient and smooth schedule and make contingency plans to deal with problems as they occur. These issues can affect the design of the ECT suite and personnel requirements.

IV access

Good and dependable IV access is critical to success of the procedures. IV access is needed to administer most of the agents, especially the anesthetic agents, and provide access for emergency medications if complications should develop. Difficulties in obtaining IV access can greatly slow down the schedule, for example, with patients who are obese, dehydrated, or have no visible veins. Sometimes an hour or more can be spent trying to start an IV on a patient. Of course, this delay can destroy a schedule, and it is very uncomfortable for the patient. Some patients complain more about the IV than about ECT itself. Several ways of dealing with the problem of the difficult IV have been developed.

First, patients can indeed be allowed to drink small amounts of clear fluids from midnight until 5 A.M. the morning before treatment to prevent dehydration and allow veins to be more accessible. Still, the responsible anesthesiologist has the authority to veto this.

The waiting area or receiving room adjacent to the actual treatment room can be designed to have two to three patients at a time. The personnel staffing this room are assigned the task of starting IVs while the treatment team is giving ECT. This assignment accomplishes two things. If starting one patient's IV is difficult, and the next patient has easy access, then the second patient can bypass the obstruction, keeping delays in the schedule to a minimum. Personnel as available can then work on accessing the difficult vein. Additionally, the personnel starting IVs, if assigned that duty on a regular basis, become very proficient; their proficiency is a real benefit to economy, efficiency, and morale. At University of Iowa Hospitals and Clinics (UIHC), this person is usually a nurse. Another major institution assigns their senior respiratory therapists this task.

Another technique that can be used is to administer the inhaled anesthetic sevoflurane to the patient before the IV is started. Sevoflurane causes the veins to dilate and spares the patient awareness of ECT preparation. However, it can raise the seizure threshold (Carllarge et al., 2003) and thereby reduce the effectiveness of the ECT seizure.

If a patient has difficult IV access and will require continuation or maintenance ECT, a subdermal port should be considered. At UIHC a significant number of patients receiving outpatient ECT have subdermal ports. The nurses undergo special training to learn to access this port, which is usually placed in the thoracic area. A special needle accesses the port after the skin area above the port has been sterilized. Figure 20.1 shows a picture of ports before insertion, and Figure 20.2 is a diagram of a port in place having been accessed by a needle.

A vascular surgeon places the port, which is the same as those used for chemotherapy, in a 30-minute procedure in a vascular laboratory at the UIHC cancer center. Subdermal ports have had very few complications. Infection is the most common

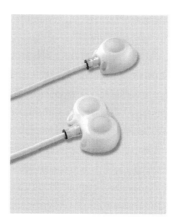

Figure 20.1 Ports before insertion.

complication but is unusual. In one case, the patient picking at the incision caused an infection. The port is flushed with heparin after each treatment and should be flushed once a month if not used during that month. After ECT is discontinued, the port should be surgically removed if it is expected that there will be no further ECTs in the foreseeable future.

A percutaneous IV central catheter (PICC) line can be used for inpatients with very difficult IV access who are going to receive only an index series or a very limited number of ECTs. Again, special care and monitoring of PICC lines are necessary, and complications such as infection can occur.

In summation, if a patient's veins are very difficult to access (requiring more than 20 minutes or four or more punctures at each session), a subdermal port or PICC line should be strongly considered. If an IV line cannot be inserted within

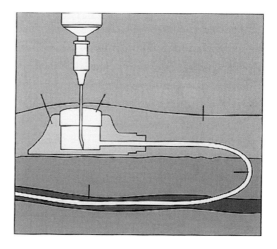

Figure 20.2 Port in place.

20 minutes, that patient's treatment should probably be postponed to another day and either a subdermal port or PICC line placed for further treatments.

Outpatient considerations

Outpatients receiving ECT have special considerations. Optimally the patient presents to the waiting area adjacent to the treatment room from the street. The patient is checked in and examined by the personnel, and an IV is started. However, if the treatment area and waiting room are deep within an area not accessible to the general public or the street, as at UIHC, the patient has to be transported from the check-in area to the treatment area by a transport aide.

Patients receiving outpatient ECT are not required to change into a hospital gown if the ECT is not done in an operating room. They are advised to wear loose clothing and to bring an extra change of clothes in case of incontinence. One extra step (changing into a gown) is avoided, and patients in general prefer wearing their street clothes. If a patient is regularly incontinent, changing into a gown may be advisable.

After the ECT and first-stage recovery are accomplished, the outpatient may be transported to another area for second-stage recovery if there are only two or three beds in the immediate recovery area. Inpatients are transported back to their room for second-stage recovery. Outpatients must be discharged from second-stage recovery to a responsible adult. Occasionally a patient will say that he or she is able to drive or get home by bus alone. Nevertheless, if a patient does not have a responsible adult to take custody on discharge, the ECT should not be given until such arrangements are made. If it is discovered after the ECT is done that no one is present to take charge of the patient, the patient should be admitted overnight (or until a relative can arrive). It is required by policy at UIHC that an adult stay with the patient for the whole day and, if the patient is receiving three ECT treatments a week, the patient have constant supervision every day of the week. This requirement is in place because patients on the day of ECT can be confused and forgetful and may get lost or make dangerous errors in judgment. The more frequently ECT is administered, the greater the maximum cognitive side effects; generally three-times-per-week ECT is the maximum (Shapira et al., 1998).

Treatment room considerations

The treatment room itself is probably the most easily managed part of the treatment. The personnel duties described for the low-volume operation in the treatment room hold true in the large-volume operation. However, with large volume there may be more than one nurse to deal with the paperwork, two or three persons on the anesthesia team to help deal with IV problems, and sometimes several people on the psychiatric team. In a university setting, residents, medical students, or student nurses may assist any of the teams.

Having medications and anesthetic agents drawn up and ready to administer to each patient, even before the schedule begins, can be very helpful. A nurse can do this before the day starts. The anesthetist and the psychiatrist generally work together to determine the agents and changes in agents to be given to the patient. They also work together to decide whether a patient has developed a condition that would contraindicate the treatment.

In all operations, but especially the high-volume operation, a procedure should be developed to verify the patient's identity and treatment parameters. This procedure is called a "Time Out" at UIHC. The psychiatrist calls "time out," and the patient's name, birth date, and hospital number are read out loud, then the patient is asked if he or she is the person named. The settings of the ECT machine are often verified as well. When the person is determined to be the correct patient, then the treatment proceeds.

In setting up the treatment room, the equipment should be organized so that the personnel can access what they need without interfering with others. The organization will often be dependent on the personnel habits and needs of individual practitioners.

Recovery room issues

After the ECT seizure the patient begins recovery in the treatment room. The anesthetist determines that the patient is breathing adequately and that vitals are stable before the patient is moved to first-stage recovery. After the patient's vitals have been stable for about 15 or 20 minutes in first-stage recovery, and he has recovered enough to speak and knows his whereabouts, he is transferred back to his inpatient room for full recovery or to outpatient recovery. If there are enough beds in the recovery area, the outpatients can be recovered fully in the immediate or first-stage recovery area.

Problems arising in the recovery room can slow down the schedule, especially if there are not enough recovery room nurses or recovery room beds. With one nurse and two recovery room beds, ECT patient flow will probably be three or four patients an hour as long as things go well. However, if any difficulties such as postictal delirium, prolonged sedation, or other medical problems develop, a patient may occupy a bed for a prolonged period. Unless more beds and nurses are available, the whole schedule will be delayed. The optimal solution is to have at least three recovery room beds and two nurses for first-stage recovery and five or six beds in the recovery area if outpatients are going to remain until recovery is complete. There should probably be at least one nurse for every two patients in the recovery area, and more if complications develop. Of course funds, budget, and space can limit the fulfilment of these recommendations.

Personnel attitude is important. The recovery room area is where psychiatry may interface with the general hospital. Here the ECT team may encounter attitudes about psychiatry and ECT based on old beliefs, myths, and obsolete concepts left over from old training and ideas promulgated by uninformed training and pop culture such as *One Flew over the Cuckoo's Nest*. Special education of the personnel may be needed. Staff unwilling to accept ECT as a beneficial treatment may have to be culled from the area. Unfortunately, it is also important to notice personnel who discriminate against or make fun of patients with mental illnesses; either retrain them or have them work elsewhere. Personnel working in the recovery area should have been trained in restraining without injury patients who become agitated because of postictal excitement or delirium.

The design of the ECT suite

Based on considerations described for the pretreatment room, the treatment area, and the recovery area, the ECT suite generally consists of three major rooms (Figure 20.3).

The room patients enter is the pretreatment room, as in Figure 20.1. Here, the IV person or nurse checks in the patient. Pretreatment personnel ensure that all paperwork is in order, including a current consent. The patient is screened for any conditions that might affect the treatment that day, and if no problems are noted, the IV is started or the venous port accessed. There should be at least two or three beds in the pretreatment room so that if there are problems in starting an IV, or if other issues develop that require more time, the next patient can be prepared and taken to the treatment room while the first patient's issues are resolved. After the IV is started, the nurse can administer some of the medications such as glycopyrrolate while waiting for access to the treatment room.

Next, the patient is taken to the treatment room where the ECT nurse, psychiatrist, and anesthetist are waiting (Figure 20.3). After monitoring leads are applied and time out is called, the anesthetic agent is administered. The muscle relaxant is administered, and, after muscle relaxation occurs, the actual treatment stimulus is given. After the seizure, when the patient is stable as described earlier, the patient is taken to the recovery room to undergo first-stage recovery. If there are as many beds as depicted in Figure 20.3, outpatients can recover fully in the suite.

Bottlenecks will occur if there is only one bed in the pretreatment area or if there are no IV personnel. If there are only one or two beds in recovery, the whole process can be backed up.

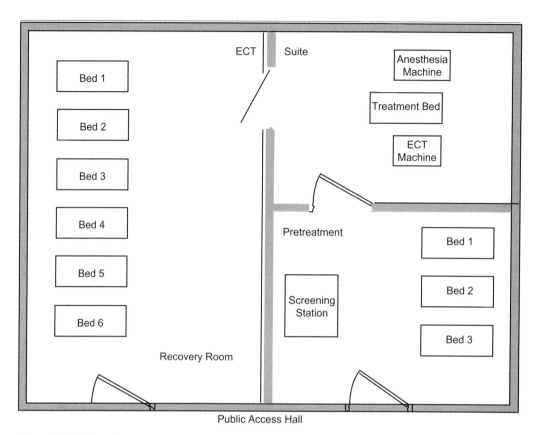

Figure 20.3 ECT suite.

Personnel summary

IV personnel or pretreatment room personnel

The staff in this room most likely will have nursing training, but people with other types of background can be utilized. In some facilities respiratory therapists are used in this capacity. Training and proficiency in starting IVs is required as well as knowledge of accessing subdermal ports if those devices are being used. Being able to do a brief screening physical is helpful. In addition to accessing the veins, this same person can attach monitoring leads and administer some of the pretreatment medications.

ECT nurse

The role of the ECT nurse may vary from place to place, but coordination is the key word to describe the function of this nurse. The nurse makes sure the patient has had preanesthetic and other needed evaluations. This person sets up the schedule or order of patients for the day, taking into account the patients' needs such as being diabetic. The psychiatrist calls the nurse to place a patient on the schedule. The nurse draws up the medications for the patients after consulting with the psychiatrist and anesthetist, preferably before the day begins, and ensures that the paper work is completed and the consent has been signed.

During the actual procedure, the nurse helps monitor vital signs and assists in applying the electrodes for the ECT. She sees that the cuff is applied to a limb to monitor the ECT. In most facilities, a cuff is applied to the right ankle to prevent the entry and effect of succinylcholine on the foot, to monitor the duration of the motor convulsion.

A nursing background is a requirement for this position because of the medical issues. Being trained and up to date in basic life support resuscitation is required.

Psychiatrist

As a physician responsible for the procedure, the psychiatrist decides if a patient is to have the procedure and what the contraindications are, if any. In conjunction with the anesthetist, he selects the anesthetic agents, other medications, and their doses to be given during the procedure.

During the actual procedure the psychiatrist supervises the process, being sure that electrodes are applied correctly and determining when the patient is actually prepared for stimulation. He may assist in administering the medications, select the settings (the electrical dosing) of the ECT machine, and determine if the patient has had a therapeutic seizure. From the patient's response, the psychiatrist may change the actual charge administered to the patient via the ECT machine. The psychiatrist should be available during the patient's recovery period to provide emergency care if needed.

The psychiatrist's training involves completion of a psychiatry residency and board certification in psychiatry. He or she should have training in ECT, either in residency or from a course that involves hands-on training, and he or she should show evidence of updating this training every two or three years. The hospital in which the ECT treatments are done should actively consider credentials for ECT and dispense privileges to physicians to perform it. It should have an ECT Policy and keep it up to date (see Chapter 19).

Anesthetist

The anesthetist's primary concern is airway management. Because of the muscle paralysis caused by the succinylcholine or like agent given during the procedure, the patient will be unable to breathe for several minutes, and the anesthetist will provide active ventilatory support. The majority of the time this can be managed by an ambu bag, but rarely intubation may be needed. The anesthetist is responsible for the medication given during the procedure but should proactively consult with the psychiatrist because it can affect psychiatric outcome. In some localities an anesthetist administers the agents, but in other hospitals the psychiatrist does this. In some hospitals, the anesthetist is responsible for starting the IVs. The anesthetist should be consulted ahead of time for special problems such as heart disease, lung disease, and other special conditions that may cause risk during the treatment.

The anesthetist can be either a board-certified physician in anesthesia or a certified nurse anesthetist operating under the supervision of an anesthesiologist. It is best if the anesthetist has experience in providing anesthesia for ECT so that he or she is familiar with the special issues that occur during the procedure.

The relationship between the anesthetist and psychiatrist is very important. In smaller facilities where there are only one or two anesthetists or psychiatrists, good professional relationships (in which each knows the other's skills, preferences, and idiosyncrasies) are easy to develop. Such relationships can be helpful in providing good continuity of care. However, in large settings where there may be 20 or more anesthetists and even more psychiatrists, these kinds of relationships may be hard to develop, especially if the ECT service rotates among different practitioners on each treatment day.

For example, anesthetists at the UIHC disagreed as to whether anesthesia should be given to patients on monoamine oxidise inhibitors (MAOIs). Often an index series would start with an anesthetist who agreed to give anesthesia to such a person, but on the third or fourth treatment another anesthetist would be assigned who would refuse to treat the patient on MAOI. The patient might miss one or two treatments, causing regression.

The anesthesia department solved this problem by appointing one of their members to be an ECT liaison, who established policy that all the anesthetists would follow. An even better solution would be to have only two or three anesthetists in the department do ECT. A more systematic solution is to have a standing written ECT procedure statement approved by the hospital chairmen of both Psychiatry and Anesthesiology, in addition to an ECT policy statement. (For details on ECT anesthesia, see Chapter 26.)

Recovery room nurse

The recovery room nurse is responsible for monitoring the patient during the recovery process and notifying the psychiatrist or anesthetist if any problems develop. He or she provides support and care while the patient is recovering and monitor the patient to be sure that no problems develop. The recovery room nurse administers any medications necessary, monitors vital signs, and provides emotional support as needed. In some cases, patient restraint may be needed if agitation develops. The recovery room nurse should notify the psychiatrist of any problems so that they may be avoided during the next treatment if possible.

The recovery room nurse should have nursing training and experience in recovering ECT patients and familiarity with the special problems associated with ECT. It is best if an identified and limited group of nurses provides ECT recovery at the facility to help to develop familiarity not only with ECT but with each patient's particular problems with recovery.

Miscellany

An ECT team can treat four patients an hour. This rate requires optimal IV access and at least three recovery room beds. It should be added that some of the nursing staff are more comfortable with three patients an hour because they feel that some of the safety concerns are neglected at a faster rate. Some practitioners allude to doing six ECT treatments an hour. The skill and personality of the treatment providers and condition of the patients affect the rate. Treating young, physically robust patients is typically faster than managing fragile elderly or obese patients with several medical problems.

Maintaining consistent personnel in the ECT treatment service is distinctly helpful in providing continuity of care. Knowing that a particular patient has an airway problem or that in the past he or she has had the syndrome of postictal excitement allows for preparation and treatment of that problem. In turn, this saves time and stress on both the staff and the patient.

References

Carllarge, C., Crowe, R., Gergis, S., et al. 2003. The comparative effects of sevoflurane and methohexital for electroconvulsive therapy. J ECT 19(4): 221–5.

Shapira, B., Tubi, N., Prexler, H., et al. 1998. Cost and benefit in the choice of ECT schedule: Twice versus three times weekly ECT. Br J Psychiatry 172: 44–8.

21

Electroconvulsive therapy forms

Jerry Lewis

This chapter includes sample forms to facilitate documenting the details of the electroconvulsive therapy (ECT) procedure. These forms may be copied or adapted as needed. Most of these forms correspond to discussions presented in this book, for example, informed consent (Figure 21.1), (Chapter 24), pre-ECT medical evaluations (Chapter 25), and ambulatory ECT (Chapter 34).

Standing orders lists

Standing orders lists (Figures 21.2 and 21.3) may facilitate compliance by physicians and nurses with hospital medical procedures and policies, which in turn will help compliance with other governing and inspecting agencies. Examples included are standing orders lists for inpatients, ambulatory patients, and patients with diabetes coming to ECT. Use of standing orders lists is generally not compulsory.

The progress note

The progress note template (Figure 21.4) includes a place to record each stimulus given, including subthreshold stimuli. Periodically a cognitive function rating, such as from the Folstein Mini-Mental State Exam (MMSE) or the modified mental status exam might be written in the progress note. A structured depression scale such as the Beck Depression Inventory can be given to the patient at intervals (e.g., weekly) to help document treatment progress.

Nursing record and procedure verification

This form (Figures 21.5 and 21.6) corresponds to the nurse's detailed record. An important aspect of this form is the second section of the form, the "time out" section. This is used to verify the correct patient, the chart, and the procedure details. Time out is completed while the patient is fully conscious and can verify the details. On the fourth section of this form the recovery room nurse records vital signs and other recovery details. Typically, three sets of vital signs, taken ten minutes apart, are required before discharge from the recovery area.

**G-4₁ CONSENT TO ELECTROCONVULSIVE
THERAPY (ECT) RECORD**
(See reverse for Anesthesia/Sedation Consent)
Monitored Telephone Consent recorded electronically via IPR

Dotted lines are to be completed by patient or representative.

• File with corresponding Nursing ECT Record (G-4₂) and ECT Therapy Record (G-4) •
• File most recent set ON BOTTOM •

DATE

HOSP.#

NAME

BIRTH DATE

ADDRESS

IF NOT IMPRINTED, PLEASE PRINT DATE, HOSP. #, NAME AND LOCATION

1. I hereby authorize Doctors _____, and such other associates
_____(Attending and Resident Physicians)_____

(Residents, Medical students, other medical personnel may perform important parts of the procedure and/or administer anesthesia and will only perform tasks within their scope of practice that the hospital has granted privileges) as may be selected by the attending doctor to perform upon _____
_____(Myself or Name of Patient)

the following procedure: electroconvulsive therapy at a frequency and number the doctor deems advisable.

2. I understand that this treatment consists of passing an electric current to the patientís temples. The patient is given anesthesia prior to treatment, and the electric current is administered while the patient is anesthetized. Convulsive muscular contractions occur for 30 to 60 seconds, after which the patient gradually regains consciousness. Electrode placement can be either bilateral or unilateral. The doctors have explained the advantages and disadvantages of both placements with me.

   I understand that after the treatment the patient may experience confusion, headache, nausea and muscle soreness. These effects are temporary.

   An initial series of ECT consists of between 6-12 ECT in some situations even more, This consent is applicable to the whole series. If this series is a continuation/maintainnce ECT, then consent needs to be obtained every 6 months.

   Shortly after the series of ECT, the patient may experience difficulties remembering events that happened before and during ECT. This spottiness in memory for past events may extend back to several months before the ECT, and in rare instances, to one or two years. Many of these memories will return during the first several months following the ECT course. However, the patient may be left with some permanent gaps in memory, particularly for events that occurred close in time to the ECT course. In addition, for a short period following ECT, the patient may experience difficulty in learning and remembering new information. This difficulty in forming new memories should be temporary and will most likely subside within several weeks following the ECT course.

   The risk of relapse of illness after ECT is completed is high, especially if further treatment is not sought. The patient should plan with his physician how to prevent relapse of illness.

   Because of the possible problems with confusion and memory, it is important that the patient not make any important personal or business decisions during or immediately following the ECT course. For the same reason the patient should avoid any activities on the day of treatment where mental alertness is required for the safety of the patient or others (e.g., driving a motor vehicle).

   I understand that this consent is voluntary and that I may have the right to withdraw my consent at any time before or during the treatment course.

   The nature of the my condition, the nature and purpose of the procedure, anticipated benefits, possible alternative methods of treatment, the risks involved and the possible consequences and complications have been explained to me. Complications include but are not restricted to the slight possabliity of accidental death, cardiac arrtyhmias, stroke and other central nervous conitions.

3. In the event that developments indicate that further operations / procedures may be necessary, I authorize the physicians to use their own judgment and do as they deem advisable during operation / procedure for the patientís best interests. Note any exceptions here, (if no exceptions, write or circle NONE):_ _ _ _ _ _ _ _ _ _ _ _ _ _ _ _ _
_ _

4. Should I (the patient) have an Advance Directive / Do Not Resuscitate (DNR) order, please be aware that it may be temporarily suspended during this procedure. I will discuss any questions with my physician.

Figure 21.1 Electroconvulsive therapy consent and anesthesia consent form.

G-4₁ Consent to ECT (Cont'd)   Pt. Name: _____

Hosp. #:_____

5. I am aware that the practice of dentistry, medicine, and surgery is not an exact science and acknowledge that no guarantees have been made to me by anyone concerning the results of the aforementioned operation / procedure.

Signature: _____ Date _____
                    (Patient or person authorized to consent for patient)

I declare that I have personally explained to _____ the nature of the patient's
                                              (Patient or Representative)

condition, the procedures to be undertaken, the risks involved and the alternatives on _____ at _____ a.m./p.m.
                                                                          (Date)   (Time)

_____   _____   _____
(Signature of Physician/dentist/PA/ARNP)   (Printed name of Physician/Dentist/PA/ARNP)   (CLP #)

CONSENT FOR SEDATION AND/OR ANESTHESIA

Information has been offered about the selection of anesthesia or sedation, and monitoring, for this procedure; the choices depend on the procedure, your physical condition and your preferences. A responsible practitioner has explained an initial plan, and the relative risks and benefits of any alternatives. Conditions may change unexpectedly, therefore it is possible that without further discussion the initial plan may have to be changed accordingly, and other practitioners may become involved in your care. You may decline anesthesia or sedation, but this might make the procedure uncomfortable, less safe, or impossible.

Most people receive anesthesia or sedation without any problem. Minor complications and side effects do occur and may include, but are not limited to: sore throat, damage to teeth and mouth, scratches on the eyes, nausea, vomiting, headache, wrong site of injection, pain, bleeding, bruises, localized swelling and redness, muscle aches, and unwanted recall of noise or conversations.

Serious complications may include, but are not limited to: allergic reaction, loss of air-way (inability to breathe), brain damage, coma, paralysis, seizure, confusion, memory-loss, need for prolonged mechanical breathing, pneumonia, nerve damage, difficulty with swallowing and speech, blindness, heart attack, damage to other organs, infection, and unintended awareness. Some of these complications can result in permanent disability or death.

Other hazards or risks discussed:_____

Further comments:_____

Initial plan includes:_____

I agree to the plan for anesthesia or sedation, and to any unforeseen intervention necessary for my welfare:

_____ Date _____
(Signature of patient or person authorized to consent for patient)   (Date)

_____   _____   _____   _____
(Signature of Responsible Practitioner)   (CLP#)   (Date)   (Time)

Figure 21.1 (*cont.*)

A-1a DOCTORS' ORDERS

Remove TOP carbon copy to send to Pharmacy
• File most recent sheet of this number on bottom •

Affix date and signature to each set of orders.
Write orders to change or discontinue a current order on next blank line.
Medication orders must include the four character (alpha-numeric) prescriber's code.

IF NOT IMPRINTED, PLEASE PRINT DATE, HOSP. #. NAME AND LOCATION

DRUG ALLERGIES RECORDED ELECTRONICALLY

DATE / TIME	DRUG OR I.V. SOLUTION	DOSE	ROUTE	INTERVAL / REMARKS
	INPATIENT ECT ORDERS			
	Patient weight _____ Kg			
	1. Glycopyrrolate	0.2 mg	IV	q Monday, Wednesday, Friday
	2. Methohexital	___mg	IV	q Monday, Wednesday, Friday
	3. Succinylcholine	___mg	IV	q Monday, Wednesday, Friday
	4. Esmolol	___mg	IV	PRN HTN or tachycardia
	5. Labetalol	___mg	IV	PRN HTN or tachycardia
	6. Lorazepam	___mg	IV	PRN prolonged seizure/agitation
	7. Caffeine and Sodium Benzoate	___gm	IV	PRN failure to seize
	8. Acetaminophen	650 mg	PO	q 4 hr PRN after ECT HA/body aches (max. x 2 doses)
	9. Ibuprofen	400-600 mg	PO	q 6 hr PRN after ECT HA/body aches (max. x 2 doses)
	10. Lidocaine 1% injection	___ml	subq	PRN for IV starts
	STANDARD ORDER FOR DIABETIC PATIENT RECEIVING ECT			
	1. Hold all oral diabetic agents or all morning insulin orders before ECT, except insulin glargine (Lantus).			
	2. Insulin glargine (Lantus) is to be given at the usual time already ordered for this patient.			
	3. After ECT and patient returned to unit, usual morning diabetic agents or insulin medications are to be given with patient's breakfast.			
				64503/5-07

DATE / TIME	DIAGNOSTIC, THERAPEUTIC AND DIETARY ORDERS:
	INPATIENT ECT ORDERS

PERMANENT MEDICAL RECORD DOCUMENT

Figure 21.2 Standing orders for inpatient ECT including diabetic management.

A-1a DOCTORS' ORDERS

Remove TOP carbon copy to send to Pharmacy
• File most recent sheet of this number on bottom •

Affix date and signature to each set of orders.
Write orders to change or discontinue a current order on next blank line.
Medication orders must include the four character (alpha-numeric) prescriber's code.

DRUG ALLERGIES, TO BE COMPLETED BY PRACTITIONER ONLY
☐ No Known Allergies
☐ Specify

IF NOT IMPRINTED, PLEASE PRINT DATE, HOSP. #. NAME AND LOCATION

DATE / TIME	DRUG OR I.V. SOLUTION	DOSE	ROUTE	INTERVAL / REMARKS
	OUTPATIENT ECT ORDERS			
	Patient weight _____ Kg			
	1. Glycopyrrolate	0.2 mg	IV	Once
	2. Methohexital	___ mg	IV	Once
	3. Succinylcholine	___ mg	IV	Once
	4. Esmolol	___ mg	IV	PRN HTN or tachycardia
	5. Labetalol	___ mg	IV	PRN HTN or tachycardia
	6. Lorazepam	___ mg	IV	PRN prolonged seizure/agitation
	7. Acetaminophen	650 mg	PO	q 4 hr PRN after ECT HA/body aches (max. x 2 doses)
	8. Ibuprofen	400-600 mg	PO	q 6 hr PRN after ECT HA/body aches (max. x 2 doses)
	9. Lidocaine 0.1% injection	___ ml	subq	PRN for IV starts

DATE / TIME **DIAGNOSTIC, THERAPEUTIC AND DIETARY ORDERS:**

OUTPATIENT ECT ORDERS

Date: Time:

Discharge from first stage recovery when:

1. Vital signs are stable and have returned
   to their pretreatment range.
2. Patient conscious, verbally responsive
   and able to follow commands.

Signature:

Date: Time:

Admit to Unit:

Occupancy Category: Recovery

Staff Attending Physician Name:

Diet:

Discharge from second stage recovery after
one hour and meets the following criteria:

1. Vital signs remain stable within
   pretreatment range.
2. Returned to pretreatment ambulation
   and orientation level.
3. Post ECT side effects and discomforts
   manageable with minimal support and
   improving with time.
4. Accompanied by responsible adult.

A
1a
B CLM. NOTES
C LABORATORY
D X-RAY EXAM
E CONSULTATION
F SPEC. EXAM
G THERAPY
H PATHOLOGY
I PT. QUES.

PERMANENT MEDICAL RECORD DOCUMENT

Figure 21.3 Standing orders for ambulatory ECT.

G-4 ELECTROCONVULSIVE THERAPY (ECT) RECORD

DATE

HOSP. #

NAME

BIRTH DATE

ADDRESS

• File with corresponding Nursing ECT Record (G-4$_2$) and Consent for ECT (G-4$_1$) •

• File most recent set ON BOTTOM •

IF NOT IMPRINTED, PLEASE PRINT DATE, HOSP. #. NAME AND LOCATION

Age _____   Weight _____

Special Instructions:

The following have been obtained prior to beginning treatments:

_____ consent   _____ urine

_____ physician examination   _____ EKG

_____ blood work   _____ chest X-ray

Signature of Physician _____   Date _____

TREATMENT RESULTS			
DYNAMIC IMPEDANCE	OHMS	_____	
AVERAGE VOLTAGE	VOLTS	_____	
DYNAMIC ENERGY	JOULES	_____	
PULSE WIDTH	M SEC	_____	
FREQUENCY	HERTZ	_____	
DURATION	SECONDS	_____	
CURRENT	AMPS	_____	

Treatment number/date:

Electrode Placement:

Seizure duration:

Location of seizure:

Notes:

Medications:

Resident signature:

Date:

I was present for the entire ECT procedure

Staff signature:

Charge (mC)

Date:

TREATMENT RESULTS			
DYNAMIC IMPEDANCE	OHMS	_____	
AVERAGE VOLTAGE	VOLTS	_____	
DYNAMIC ENERGY	JOULES	_____	
PULSE WIDTH	M SEC	_____	
FREQUENCY	HERTZ	_____	
DURATION	SECONDS	_____	
CURRENT	AMPS	_____	

Treatment number/date:

Electrode Placement:

Seizure duration:

Location of seizure:

Notes:

Medications:

Resident signature:

Date:

I was present for the entire ECT procedure

Staff signature:

Charge (mC)

Date:

G-4

H   PATHOLOGY

I   PT. QUES

Figure 21.4 Detailed ECT progress note record.

<table>
<tr><td colspan="2">

G-4$_2$ NURSING ELECTROCONVULSIVE THERAPY (ECT) RECORD AND PROCEDURE VERIFICATION

• File with corresponding ECT Record (G-4) and Consent for ECT (G-4$_1$) •

• File most recent set ON BOTTOM •
</td><td>

DATE

HOSP. #

NAME

BIRTH DATE

ADDRESS

IF NOT IMPRINTED, PLEASE PRINT DATE, HOSP. # NAME AND LOCATION
</td></tr>
</table>

PRE-ECT	Date:	Time:	ID bracelet:	Void: Yes No	NPO: Yes No

Belongings w/patient: Dentures   Vitals: time

Glasses/contacts/none   T

Jewelry/other: P

Code Status: Isolation: BP

Pre-medications:

Blood Glucose: Time tested:

Oriented to: person   place   date: Additional Assessment:

RN Signature:

To ECT suite per: W/C   cart   ambulatory   Escort Signature:

Patient received in ECT suite   RN Signature:

TIME OUT/ANTIBIOTIC VERIFICATION

Immediately prior to the start of the operation/procedure an active "time out" was performed by all members of the team. The patient was identified using two patient identifiers, the correct side and site were identified (if applicable), the operation/procedure was agreed upon, the correct patient position was identified (if applicable) and the availability of correct implants and any special equipment or special requirements was confirmed (if applicable).

For electroconvulsive therapy procedures, one signature is required below.

(Signature of Responsible Practitioner/Assistant)   (Title)   (Date)

ECT TREATMENT #:   Time: Legal Status: Vitals:

Date of last COC appt.:   P

Pt. verbalizes agreement to ECT: BP

Pt. physically cooperative to ECT: SaO$_2$

Pts report of side effects or discomforts after last treatment

Additional assessment:

Physicians:

Vitals: P   BP   SaO$_2$

To Recovery Room per cart   Pt. position: Time: RN Signature:

Figure 21.5 Nursing ECT record including verification of procedure.

G-4$_2$ Nursing ECT Record (Cont'd)   Pt. Name:_____

                                            Hosp. #:_____

DATE	RECOVERY ROOM				Side rails up (circle) yes no Wheels locked (circle) yes no
	TIME				TIME NURSING COMMENTS
Vital Signs:	BP				
	HR				
	rr				
	SaO$_2$				
Skin:	Dusky				
	Warm				
	Cool				
	Dry				
	Moist				
Respirations:	Deep				
	Shallow				
	Irregular				
	Regular				
Pulse:	Regular				
	Irregular				
	Strong				
	Weak				
Level of Consciousness	Unresponsive				
	Responsive				
	Alert				
Oriented to:	Person				
	Place				
	Date				
Pain, if yes, describe	Yes				
	No				

(EKG Strip)

Bed in lowest position (circle):   yes   no   Transfer assessment:

Personal belongings with patient:

RN Signature from ECT Suite:

Returning patient to unit per: W/C   cart   Escort Signature:

Figure 21.6 Nursing ECT record continued.

	B-19b₁ CLINICAL NOTES	DATE

B-19b₁ CLINICAL NOTES

PATIENT INFORMATION/INSTRUCTIONS

ADULT PSYCHIATRY OUTPATIENT ECT
INFORMATION SUMMARY

• File most recent sheet of this number ON BOTTOM •

DATE
HOSP. #
NAME
BIRTH DATE
ADDRESS

IF NOT IMPRINTED, PLEASE PRINT DATE, HOSP. #. NAME AND LOCATION

DATE

Section A:
Pre-ECT
Screening

Contact Physician _____ Phone No. _____ (8 am-5 pm)
Hospital Operator _____ Ask for psychiatrist on call. (After hours)
SHORT PSYCH EVAL & NOTE!

Brief Physical Exam:

M.D. Signature _____ Date

Section B:
ECT
Treatment

ECT # _____ Time: _____ Comments:

Medications Given During ECT: Robinul ____ mg Etomidate ____ mg Succinylcholine ____ mg
Esmolol ____ mg Labetalol ____ mg Caffeine ____ mg Other _____

M.D. Signature _____ Date

Section C:
ECT
Recovery

BP _____ P _____ R _____
Circle Appropriate Response:
<u>Gait</u>: Steady   Needs Assistance
<u>Oriented to</u>:   Person   Place   Date
<u>Comfort</u>:   Denies Discomfort   Reports HA   Reports Body ache

Medications given during ECT Recovery:

Medication	Dose	Time Given	RN Initials

Comments:

Section D:
Instructions

HOME CARE INSTRUCTIONS AND RETURN APPOINTMENT:
Return to ECT Department for next ECT on _____ Time: _____ AM
Do not eat or drink after midnight on _____ . Medications to be taken before each
ECT with a small sip of water: _____

Please call _____ if unable to keep your appointment.

Temporary "side effects" following ECT include: confusion, muscle soreness, headache, nausea, forgetfulness, dizziness. Tylenol and rest will generally relieve these discomforts. Contact UIHC if any of these symptoms become severe or are persisent, <u>PATIENT SHOULD STAY IN THE COMPANY OF A RESPONSIBLE ADULT FOR THE ENTIRE DAY. DO NOT DRIVE A MOTOR VEHICLE OR OPERATE MACHINERY FOR 24 HOURS.</u>

Signature of relative or responsible adult _____ Date

Side tabs: B-19b | C LABORATORY | D X-RAY EXAM | E CONSULTATION | F SPEC. EXAM | G THERAPY | H PATHOLOGY | I PT. QUES.

58817/7-06

Figure 21.7 Physicians ambulatory ECT record given to patient (copy kept).

A-1c₁ NURSES' DETAILED NOTES

OUTPATIENT POST ECT NURSING NOTES

DATE

HOSP. #

NAME

BIRTH DATE

ADDRESS

• File most recent sheet of this number ON BOTTOM •

IF NOT IMPRINTED, PLEASE PRINT DATE, HOSP. # NAME. AND LOCATION

A -1c₁

DATE TIME	NURSING COMMENTS
	INITIAL ASSESSMENT: BP P R
	Level of Consciousness: Alert Drowsy
	Oriented to: Person Place Date
	Pain/Discomfort: Absent Present (if present describe):
	Gait: Steady Needs assistance (if needs assistance describe):
	Safety/Comfort Interventions:
	Disposition of Patient Belongings:
	Additional RN Assessment:
	RN Signature:
	ASSESSMENT: BP P R
	Level of Consciousness: Alert Drowsy
	Oriented to: Person Place Date
	Pain/Discomfort: Absent Present (if present describe):
	Safety/Comfort Interventions:
	Additional RN Assessment:
	RN Signature:

B CLIN. NOTES
C LABORATORY
D X-RAY EXAM
E CONSULTATION
F SPEC. EXAM
G THERAPY
H PATHOLOGY
I PT. QUES.

Figure 21.8 Nurses ambulatory recovery record.

A-1c₁ NURSES' ASSESSMENT (Cont.)   Name: _____ **Hosp. No.**_____

DATE TIME	NURSING COMMENTS
	ASSESSMENT: BP P R
	Level of Consciousness: Alert Drowsy
	Oriented to: Person Place Date
	Pain/Discomfort: Absent Present (if present describe):
	Safety/Comfort Interventions:
	Additional RN Assessment:
	RN Signature:
	RELEASE ASSESSMENT: BP P R
	Level of Consciousness: Alert Drowsy
	Level of Orientation: Person Place Date
	Pain/Discomfort: Absent Present (if present describe):
	Gait: Steady Needs assistance (if needs assistance describe):
	Patient Behaviors
	Short Term Memory:
	Discharge order written: Yes
	Belongings returned to patient: Yes
	Home Care Instructions (B-19b1) given: Yes
	Person patient released with:
	Additional RN Assessment:
	RN Signature:

Figure 21.9 Nurses ambulatory recovery record continued.

Ambulatory forms

Ambulatory patients receive written instructions for their next treatment, and an example of this is included (Figure 21.7). On this ambulatory record the physician documents a brief history and physical and mental status exam in section A. This is followed by medications given during the procedure and recovery notes. In section D, the physician provides instructions to the patient, including date and time for the next treatment. The patient receives a copy of this form so that if the patient sees a physician in the interim he or she can share these details with that physician. A separate form is for post-ECT nursing recovery details (Figures 21.8, 21.9).

Part V

The clinical manual

Patient selection and electroconvulsive therapy indications

Conrad M. Swartz

Introduction

My colleague Everett Simmons accurately identified patients for electroconvulsive therapy (ECT) from across the room, before talking with them. He enthusiastically delivered his impressions to me. He did not give ECT himself, referring cases to me, and I found his referrals always merited. Dr. Simmons's love was psychodynamics, but he claimed that I taught him how to select patients for ECT by observing them. This claim was made within a year of my joining Dr. Simmons on the faculty. My teaching was not deliberate, but Dr. Simmons was a fast learner. As he was 60 years old, his long previous experience of not selecting patients for ECT is apparently common for psychiatrists. This chapter addresses what Dr. Simmons learned about selecting depressed patients for ECT.

Unfortunately, the diagnostic criteria of major depression obstruct selectivity in using ECT because the criteria do not have clear boundaries. Rather, they allow major depression to be stretched and wrapped onto any unhappy patient at the vagaries of the doctor, patient, or other stakeholder. Verifiable observable evidence is not required for diagnosing major depression according to *The Diagnostic and Statistical Manual of Mental Disorders* (DSM). More peculiarly, it is not sufficient. DSM is the standard for diagnosis because of consensus and politics, but patient selection for ECT needs more specificity than the DSM embodies.

Before addressing the specifics, we should consider general philosophy. ECT is a biological treatment, and separate from psychological therapies. Psychotherapies treat psychological but not biological disturbances, conditions that are subjective and not observable by others. In contrast, ECT treats only illness that is observable. ECT should not be used in conditions that are entirely subjective. One cause for confusion between biological and psychological conditions is that biological interventions can diminish psychological symptoms, for example, tranquilizers can lessen worrying. These are nonspecific effects and do not comprise treatment, although they can be mistaken for it. ECT too has nonspecific effects, and using it for these effects does not incorporate treating according to diagnosis. Understanding ECT patient selection and outcome depends on identifying both its specific and nonspecific effects.

Supplementing this philosophy of diagnosis is that medical conditions and drug effects can mimic any psychiatric disorder. Simply, exposure to antipsychotic drugs, benzodiazepines, alcohol, or drugs of abuse prior to hospitalization necessitates a substantial drug-free observation period before diagnosis and ECT. For example, olanzapine produced the appearance and symptoms of melancholia, with (Nelson and Swartz, 2000) or without (Swartz, 2002a) concurrent fluoxetine; merely withholding olanzapine produced remission. As another example, I gave a couple of ECT treatments to a patient who appeared to have a mixed manic-depressive state before he confessed to deception, that he drank very heavily and did not want to be seen as "just another alcoholic." The duration of the drug-free period that is needed can be 3 to 14 days, depending on the drug.

The depression that ECT does not treat

Everyone knows that ECT treats major depression. However, a course of ECT does not treat all types of major depression, such as atypical depression (i.e., with atypical features). This was once known as "neurotic depression." Peculiarly, atypical depression is the most common subtype of major depression. It is not clearly distinguishable from anxiety disorders that make patients unhappy (Parker et al., 2002), and anxiety disorders are the most common psychiatric conditions. Anxiety disorders and atypical depression have the same basic psychopathology, with only vague differences in phrasing (Swartz, 2003). This common pathology includes being easily upset by small things (excessive mood reactivity and rejection sensitivity), restlessness (agitation), muscle tension (leaden feelings), and rejection hypersensitivity (social phobia). While subjective unhappiness is an explicit aspect of atypical depression, it is a common consequence of most anxiety disorders; the difference is impalpable. Anxiety disorders and atypical depression have the same treatments, primarily selective serotonin reuptake inhibitors (SSRIs) and psychotherapy, sometimes with tranquilizers, sympatholytics, or sedating anticonvulsants added. The longitudinal time courses are similarly chronic with varying severity, so it is no surprise that they are reported as usually comorbid.

An acute course of ECT does not reliably and stably treat either anxiety disorders or atypical depression. I say this in the face of a recent report (unjustifiably) claiming that bitemporal ECT treats atypical depression (Husain et al., 2008). That study compared atypical depression with nonatypical major depression, but not placebo. However, atypical depression responds well to placebo and psychological therapy (Jarrett et al., 2000), so treatment studies of atypical depression need a placebo control for validity, here sham ECT. Their comparison with nonatypical major depression does not control for placebo effect and so does not support the claims. That study is simply an open uncontrolled trial of treating an entirely subjective and unobservable condition. Moreover, diagnosis in that study was peculiar because 14% of the patients with atypical depression were said to have psychotic features. Patients with anxiety disorders or atypical depression do not have psychotic symptoms; rather they have dissociative symptoms. These dissociations are pseudopsychotic (Swartz and Shorter, 2007). This report also did not mention examining or accounting for anxiety disorders in their patients, a notable omission in any study of patients said to have atypical depression.

Another major problem with that study is that anxiety disorders respond to ECT temporarily but not stably. Husain et al. (2008) did not examine for a stable response to ECT; the response was rated only within 24 to 48 hours of the final ECT treatment. Relapse occurring after that was not reported. This 24–48-hour rating is not sufficient for judging the outcome of treating atypical depression. These patients have problematic mood reactivity. In the hospital 24 to 48 hours after the last ECT treatment they are still recovering from the ECT procedure. The placebo effect includes the suggestion of cure by a treatment (ECT) well known as beneficial for depression that is "no fault" of the patient. To judge bona fide response to treatment, patients with atypical depression must be examined while residing at home, not in hospital, and after three weeks or more and while exposed to the same stimuli for rejection sensitivity and mood reactivity that precipitated hospitalization.

Clear evidence that anxiety disorders show a strong but only brief response to ECT comes from studies of treating obsessive-compulsive disorder (OCD). In treating nine patients with chronic OCD, Khanna et al. (1988) reported that ECT response was distinct but lasted only about a month. Complementing this, Maletzky et al. (1994) gave ECT to 32 patients with refractory OCD, 19 of whom did not have concurrent major depression. Maintenance ECT for a year produced sustained improvement and worked as well in patients without major depression as in those with it. Taking these two studies together implies that an acute course of ECT has only short-term benefits in anxiety disorders (including atypical depression), but not persistent effects as it does in melancholic, catatonic, psychotic, or manic episodes.

There are simple explanations for patients with anxiety disorder (or atypical depression) responding temporarily to the nonspecific effects of ECT, especially the bitemporal placement used by Husain et al. (2008). Anxiety disorders and atypical depression have two basic groups of symptoms, psychological anxiety symptoms and somatic tension. Psychological anxiety symptoms include dissatisfaction, worry, obsessions, and recurrent unpleasant memories; they are decreased by serotonin-enhancing drugs such as SSRIs. Somatic tension is decreased by central sympatholytic action, particularly treatments that decrease central nervous system (CNS) β-adrenergic-1 receptors, because of high epinephrine neurotransmitter activity in the reticular activating system cells that mediate sympathetic elevation of heart rate and adrenal medullary release of catecholamines (Jansen et al., 1995). The temporary cognitive side effects of bitemporal ECT interrupt psychological anxiety symptoms. The somatic tension (described later in this chapter) is mitigated by the sympatholytic effects of ECT. ECT markedly decreases both β-adrenergic receptor sensitivity and the number of β-receptors (Nimgaonkar et al., 1985). In this way it should diminish CNS epinephrine and norepinephrine neurotransmitter activity, sympathetic nervous system activity and excitability, and thereby somatic tension. The progressive decrease in resting blood pressure along a course of ECT presumably has a sympatholytic basis (Swartz and Inglis, 1990). These sympatholytic effects should wear off within a month.

In my clinical practice, of patients referred for ECT by nonfaculty colleagues, a third were not suitable. Their unhappiness was part of an anxiety disorder (with concurrent or equivalent atypical depression). Unfortunately, it is not well known how to obtain stable remission from marked anxiety disorders. At the same time, few psychiatrists are experienced with ECT, so the many psychiatrists unfamiliar with ECT can suppose it treats the unhappiness of anxiety disorders. Several high-profile doctors promote antipsychotics off label for anxiety disorders, but this mismatch is analogous to attacking a mosquito with a brick, and causes collateral damage.

Of course, patients with an anxiety disorder are dysphoric from it, that is, anxiety disorders worsen mood. So do most psychiatric disorders. Sleep is broken, patients do not feel well, demoralization can set in (and be called anhedonia or apathy), energy is low (sometimes leading to overeating), composure is unstable (with rejection hypersensitivity and mood hyperreactivity), concentration is distracted, and irritable bowels and dyspepsia are common (with disturbed eating and appetite). Probably because of intense dissatisfaction and impressions of victimization, typical patients with anxiety insist that they are depressed. These symptoms are common and often sufficient to permit diagnosing DSM major depression. Yet, DSM gives no guidance about forbearing a major depression diagnosis the criteria of which are met and diagnosing solely anxiety disorder, albeit a dysphoric one. It is up to the psychiatrist to judge.

This judgment should involve the patient's appearance, not just subjective symptoms. However, visibly disturbed behavior is not enough. The noticeable signs of anxiety disorder can accompany virtually any other psychiatric condition, because they represent somatic tension anxiety. The point is that the presence of visible somatic tension anxiety does not by itself indicate major depression. Somatic anxiety corresponds to activation of the sympathetic nervous system, including agitated movements, agitated speech, need to ventilate, restlessness, unstable composure, irritability, jumpiness, grating voice, loudness, muscle tension or tightness, and repetitiveness. Impulsive, destructive, or suicidal behavior or violent threats can occur from the discomfort of somatic tension anxiety. Although these signs beg urgent relief, and patients with melancholia can show any of them, they are not specific to any psychiatric condition and they do not by themselves suggest using ECT. Conversely, with patients who do have a suitable ECT-treatable condition, these signs suggest an urgent need for ECT.

Half or more of patients with DSM major depression have a diagnosable DSM anxiety disorder (Zimmerman et al., 2002), even elderly patients (Beekman et al., 2000). This number is too high to be mere coincidence. Depressive symptoms can be epiphenomena of anxiety disorders, and vice versa. DSM does not recognize the difference between an artifactual depression that depends on anxiety disorder and a distinct major depression that does not. Nevertheless, *we* must.

Beyond mathematical coincidence is the harsh reality that the personally threatening experiences of a severe psychiatric illness such as melancholia or acute psychosis generate anxiety disorders such as post-traumatic stress disorder (PTSD). These threats include stigmatization, career interruption, financial stress, inpatient hospitalization, violent or suicidal acts by the patient, and thought disorder, even if temporary. They also include witnessing or being involved in menacing experiences on psychiatric wards, which are unfortunately commonplace (Frueh et al., 2005). A November 2006 inspection documented numerous threatening events in state hospitals, including patient-to-patient assaults, self-injurious behavior, improper use of restraints, and multiple serious overdose errors by nurses (Cole, 2008). Resulting PTSD symptoms are routinely mistaken for resistant symptoms of depression. PTSD is more likely to occur with repeated exposure to threatening stresses. Indeed, anxiety disorders were present cross-sectionally in 47% of patients with recent psychosis (Ciapparelli et al., 2007). This is a straightforward and not disproven explanation for the apparent growing resistance to treatment of patients who have multiple episodes of depression or bipolar disorder.

Of course it is not feasible to examine for anxiety disorders while the patient is ill with melancholia, catatonia, or acute psychosis, because these conditions interfere. They can obscure anxiety disorder symptoms or they can generate anxiety themselves. Only after the ECT course can a diagnostic evaluation for anxiety disorder be completed. However, I have not seen a published research study that did this. Diagnostic evaluation for anxiety disorders after the ECT course is important because depression rating scales will score continuing depression after ECT in patients with an anxiety disorder or atypical depression, regardless of depression response to ECT. Depression rating scales including global scales, Hamilton Rating

Scale for Depression, and Montgomery-Åsberg Depression Rating Scale were never intended to help distinguish between anxiety disorders and major depression, only to rate severity in patients with depression alone.

Unfortunately, ECT circumstances are yet more complex, because ECT temporarily mitigates symptoms of anxiety disorders. Although anxiety disorder symptoms can be present immediately after a course of ECT, their return is typically about three to four weeks after the last ECT treatment and up to six weeks after ECT. So, apparent relapse within the first month of ECT can represent returning symptoms of an anxiety disorder rather than a bona fide relapse of depression. The doctor must determine if observable depressive signs that were present before ECT have returned – indicating relapse – or if there is a different reason for the patient to claim low mood.

This is a long section because undertreated anxiety and personality disorders are pervasive problems in all psychiatric populations, including ECT patients. Probably because remission from anxiety disorders is not commonly obtained, comorbid anxiety disorders are underdiagnosed. It is striking that former ECT patients who seek public attention to their dissatisfaction typically display prominent anxiety symptoms. They are apparently suffering, indeed, from largely untreated anxiety disorders.

ECT preventing anxiety disorders

Clinicians might be able to prevent anxiety disorders such as PTSD from developing in conjunction with exposure to threatening stress by decreasing patients' exposure to the psychiatric episodes they experience (Swartz, 2002b). ECT accomplishes this by stopping the patients' experience with threatening thoughts and behaviors that are part of their episodes of psychiatric illness. As an example, when given to suicidal patients, ECT promptly stops suicidal thoughts and behaviors (Kellner et al., 2005). When given promptly, ECT shortens hospital stay, decreasing exposure to threats in the hospital (Markowitz et al., 1987).

Accordingly, patients who are at risk of developing an anxiety disorder should be considered for ECT early in their course. Specifically, these patients are those with previous exposure to life-threatening situations, anxiety disorders in the family, past anxiety episodes, or whose present episode is clearly threatening to them. Unfortunately, meeting DSM major depression criteria can often result from merely having an anxiety disorder. Although hypomania can similarly be an artifact of anxiety, manic episode is too severe and specific for such confusion. The high concurrence of anxiety disorders with bipolar I disorder points to the threatening experiences of bipolar I causing anxiety. Although genetic explanations have been hypothesized, direct causation is simpler and logical. So, bipolar I patients are at high risk for anxiety disorders, and should be considered for ECT sooner rather than later.

However, the life experiences of patients with bipolar disorder resemble those of patients with acute or episodic psychosis, catatonia, or melancholia. This is clearly so with suicidality, destructive or humiliating thoughts, loss of personal honor or dignity, self-stigmatizing behavior, or substantial restrictions on personal autonomy. These are the circumstances in which ECT should be kept in mind as high priority, if medication is not likely to rapidly restore the patient's mental health and abilities to manage his own affairs.

DSM versus observable melancholia

Many more patients fulfill DSM criteria for "with melancholic features" than have observable (classic) melancholia. In the latter, the patient appears sickly or slowed, in an observable vegetative state different from usual (Hamilton, 1989). Peculiarly – and at odds with classic melancholia – DSM melancholia is diagnosable from unverifiable patient complaints alone, for example, feeling deprived of pleasure, sad or apathetic mood, feeling worse in the morning, unverified early morning awakenings, eating less, or guilty thoughts. Unfortunately, DSM melancholia symptoms are not associated with good outcome in response to treatment, but features of classic melancholia are (Nelson and Charney, 1981). Only 57% of patients with DSM melancholia show observable psychomotor disturbance (Parker et al., 1995). Its commonly unobservable nature presumably explains why the assessment of DSM melancholia was found to be unreliable (Chelminski et al., 2000). Unreliability means that we cannot clinically apply the results of treatment studies of patients with DSM melancholia unless these patients were described further, objectively and reliably. Here we focus on the subset of DSM melancholia that is verifiably observable.

ECT as first choice treatment

Although a large fraction of ECT patients have melancholia, for most patients with melancholia ECT is usually not the first treatment given because melancholia can respond to antimelancholic medications, especially in mild cases but even in severe or psychotic melancholia. Antimelancholics are tricyclics, bupropion, venlafaxine, and MAOIs. In contrast, SSRIs such as paroxetine and citalopram are markedly inferior to these drugs in treating classic melancholic depression (Nobler and Roose, 1998; Roose et al., 1994). Simply, there is no overlap between SSRIs and either ECT or antimelancholics; they treat different kinds of depression. Numerous conversations I have had with pharmaceutical industry personnel indicated they were opposed to narrowing the indicated use of their antidepressant drugs to a sub-group of major depression; they wanted to preserve their privilege to promote it for any depression. This opinion translates into powerful politics opposing recognition of diagnosis-related limitations on "antidepressant" drug indications.

ECT does become the first treatment of choice when there a clear urgency or a history of resistance to medications. Urgency might come from psychopathology such as suicidality or destructive behavior. It might be associated with medical factors such as dehydration, inanition, or weakness, perhaps doubly complicated by consequent respiratory problems or arrhythmias, or urgency might derive from personal circumstances that demand a prompt and reliable remission. This range of urgencies can point to ECT for patients with any acute episode of functional psychosis (e.g., psychotic depression, psychotic mania) or bipolar disorder.

Suicidality in an endogenous mood disorder deserves special attention. Suicide eventually occurs in the 25% of bipolar patients and the 17% of unipolar depressives who claim suicidality. Rapid benefit from ECT decreases the period of risk for suicide (Kellner et al., 2005). Suicide despite ECT still can result from untreated underlying anxiety disorder or weak ECT treatments. After discharge, suicide risk also depends on prophylactic medication, substance abuse, or relapse.

ECT can be preferred by patients who value its reliability and dislike the prospect that medication is more likely to fail than succeed in treating melancholia of at least moderate severity. Patient preference (but not physician preference) is a reasonable justification for ECT in hospitalized patients with suitable conditions. Hospitalized patients appreciate the high likelihood of discharge within three weeks with ECT versus the uncertainty when medication is prescribed, along with the two thirds likelihood of medication failure. Moreover, costs are on average lower when ECT is started promptly, because hospitalization is shorter (Markowitz et al., 1987).

ECT can be a first choice in depressed elderly patients who are unable to tolerate antimelancholic drugs. This path to ECT was common when tricyclics were the only available antimelancholics, because of their orthostatic and anticholinergic effects. Risk from adding a modern antimelancholic medication can still be a problem in patients who have multiple medical problems or take multiple medications.

ECT is also the first treatment of choice in conditions that are not reliably brought to a stable and complete remission by medications. Prominent, common, and underdiagnosed examples of these conditions are acute illnesses with catatonic features, for which the ECT response rate is near 100% (Hatta et al., 2007; Chapter 7 of this volume). Unfortunately, catatonia is not reliably and persistently mitigated by any medication. No longitudinal study has shown lorazepam or another benzodiazepine to provide a stable remission from catatonia. Rather, studies have reported only briefly observed mitigation of catatonic signs, analogous to the effect of a test dose of Tensilon (edrophonium) in diagnosing myasthenia gravis.

Lorazepam-induced improvements can be abrupt and marked, even astonishing. They can also be weak or negligible (Hatta et al., 2007). In the hope of avoiding ECT, patients' families will contend that lorazepam has brought full remission. None of this drama heralds the stable remission we are obliged to seek. Accordingly, rational practice regarding catatonia is to use lorazepam only as a temporary diagnostic and management aid and treat with ECT.

The ability of antidepressant drugs to bring patients to a stable and complete remission has similarly been overrated; indeed, it is systematically misrepresented in the medical literature (Turner et al., 2008). Meta-analysis reveals that only half of U.S. Food and Drug Administration (FDA)-registered antidepressant trials had positive results, as compared with 94% of the subset of these studies that were published in the medical literature. This meta-analysis tallied 74 total registered studies. Of the 38 positive studies, 37 were published. Of the 36 negative studies, only 3 were published as negative, but 11 were misrepresented as positive. The recent (and huge) Sequenced Treatment Alternatives to Relieve Depression (STAR*D) study of treating nonpsychotic major depression found an overall 27% remission rate (Lesser et al., 2007); this result is disappointing and hardly reliable.

Even acutely, antipsychotic drugs do not reliably mitigate catatonia. Acute response to risperidone was 26%, to intravenous haloperidol 16%, and to chlor- promazine 68% (Hatta et al., 2007). This study too included no follow-up, so that discharging these patients on antipsychotic drugs is not justified by medical study.

Depending on co-occurring symptoms, acute catatonia can be part of major depression, manic episode, mixed manic-depressive state, schizophreniform ill- ness, brief psychosis, or atypical psychosis, in DSM terminology. In some coun- tries, the latter three or four conditions can be called cycloid psychosis, oneiroid state, or periodic catatonia. In these cases, the presence of catatonic features pri- marily indicates the treatment of choice as ECT, although the primary diagnosis is initially peripheral and sometimes quite obscured by catatonia. Catatonia often fades quickly after a few ECT sessions, leaving symptoms of melancholia, mania, or psychosis to dominate the psychopathology and then fade with further ECT treatments.

Catatonia is obvious when the patient spontaneously displays dramatic signs such as grimacing, posturing, or severe echolalia or echopraxia; however, these occur in only a small minority of patients with acute catatonia. Perhaps the most noticeable sign in the majority of patients with acute catatonia is an affect of puzzlement, confusion, or extreme vacancy. The archetype is staring silently with a deeply furrowed brow, perhaps at other people, or perhaps at nothing. Although we depend on mutism, immobility, and staring to qualify these patients for "catatonic features," these signs are often incomplete. Using just a few words can distract the examiner from pervasive albeit partial mutism. Diagnosing acute catatonia with high sensitivity is important because uninterrupted (or antipsychotic drug-treated) catatonia can become chronic and then be called schizophrenia.

A further extreme is lethal catatonia, which includes fever, weakness with prostration, autonomic instability with tachycardia or fluctuating heart rate, diaphoresis, obtundation, and perhaps muscle enzyme elevations. It can be fatal within five days if ECT is not given. Giving an antipsychotic drug to patients in acute catatonia risks abrupt exacerbation into lethal catatonia. Lethal catatonia is easily confused with neuroleptic malignant syndrome. Lorazepam can rapidly mitigate only the former; benztropine, bromocriptine, and dantrolene treat only the latter. Even "nonlethal" catatonia can be fatal or debilitating, by causing pulmonary embolus, skeletal muscle injury with myoglobinemia and consequent acute tubular necrosis and renal failure, exhaustion and arrhythmia, dehydration and other electrolyte imbalance, self-injury, or muscle contracture.

Besides catatonia, another condition for which medications have not proven reliable is mixed manic-depressive episode. Its DSM classification is based on bureaucratic details; these collect dysphoric manic episodes and agitated melancholia together with bona fide mixed states. This is a classification but not a diagnosis. Fortunately, ECT works on the lot, except in patients who show only epiphenomena of PTSD or borderline personality disorder. The goal here is to identify mixed states because of expected medication resistance, and to consider nonmixed states (such as irritable mania or euphoric mania) first for medications. In bona fide mixed states, the patient shows sickly melancholia together with specific signs of mania that are not merely agitation or its variations; one such sign is flight of ideas with press of speech. Sometimes the interaction of melancholia with mania prevents meeting criteria for either major depression or manic episode, and DSM fails us here.

Using ECT in first-episode psychosis is another opportunity to prevent chronic psychosis and long-term antipsychotic drug use. This topic is detailed in the chapter comparing medications with ECT (Chapter 23), but in summary there are both neurobiologic and political reasons. Giving antipsychotic drugs for a year or so (four months in the elderly population) can induce tardive psychosis in patients who were never psychotic before (Lu et al., 2002; Swartz, 2004). Symptoms of tardive psychosis are indistinguishable from those of schizophrenia. Moreover, antipsychotic usage promotes diagnosing schizoaffective disorder or schizophrenia; the politics of these diagnoses increases physician liability – at least for conflict with colleagues – associated with discontinuing antipsychotic drugs. ECT sidesteps these problems, at least in patients whose first episode has not yet become resistant to ECT because of duration alone.

My impression is that ECT can restore patients to the best condition they have shown in the previous two to three years, regardless of the details of functional psychopathology. Still, patients vary widely, and exceptions can occur. Illustrating that chronicity can override the details of psychopathology, a 65-year-old man I treated with 40 years of hospitalized continuous untreated but otherwise typical motor-retarded melancholia showed only one- to two-week remissions from repeated courses of bitemporal ECT. Although his psychopathology was typical for patients who remit with ECT, the long duration apparently had a greater effect than ECT could correct. Illustrating that acuteness can override psychopathology, a 17-year-old girl I treated with ECT achieved stable remission from symptoms typical for hebephrenic (disorganized) schizophrenia, without antipsychotic drugs. These symptoms included "witzelsucht" (silly shallow laughter for no reason), unrelated and flat affect, and Schneiderian delusions. The onset had been distinct and two months prior to ECT. Her mother was enthusiastic about avoiding a diagnosis of schizophrenia, and she identified ECT as less threatening to her daughter's well-being. Although this psychopathology was not typical for patients who remit with ECT, the brevity of illness presumably allowed ECT to work.

Experience has suggested that I should avoid allowing skeptical expectations alone to disqualify ECT in treating psychosis. To illustrate, a 35-year-old man paid no attention to me during my examination, calmly mumbling incoherently while looking around the ceiling, with an unrelated flat affect. Veterans Administration (VA) hospital records revealed he was admitted depressed 16 years prior and was never discharged. Notes for recent years detailed only caretaking, without details of psychopathology. After two ECT treatments he showed typical euphoric mania, and after two to three more ECT treatments he achieved full remission, which proved stable.

ECT or antipsychotics as first choice

In treating psychotic depression, antipsychotic drugs are often tried, with or without antidepressants. Antipsychotic dosage must be maintained above the equivalent of 400 mg/d chlorpromazine to effectively diminish symptoms (Nelson et al., 1986), although in practice this is rarely done (Mulsant et al., 1997). Nevertheless, decreasing symptoms by antipsychotic tranquilization is hardly preferable to specific treatment. The adverse psychological, psychiatric, and medical effects of antipsychotics on patients who do not have schizophrenia are profound (see Chapter 23).

Even when rated merely by symptom severity, ECT is clearly superior to the combination of antidepressants and neuroleptics in treating psychotic depression (Parker et al., 1992; Perry et al., 1982). If it were possible to rate the frequency of return to the patient's premorbid persona, the advantage of ECT would surely be manyfold. Of course, even in patients who will receive ECT, antipsychotics can be useful in the short term for rapid suppression of problematic agitation, somatic tension, or violent behavior.

Antidepressant-resistant depression

Antimelancholic medication alone brings remission in about one third of patients with severe melancholic depression, including psychotic depression (Swartz and Shorter, 2007). A larger fraction of patients with milder melancholia should remit with antimelancholic medications alone. If there is no urgency, it is usually reasonable to try such a medication. Absence of any improvement after five to seven days suggests that it is time to start ECT because the time course of remission shows improvement gradually and substantially within that five to seven days. Because medication failure selects for ECT it is noteworthy that SSRIs are inferior in treating melancholia (Roose et al., 1994), and an antimelancholic should be used instead.

Patients with depression treated before the advent of pharmaceutical antidepressants and ECT generally used to recover spontaneously, except those with psychotic depression, who tended to suffer chronically (Kantor and Glassman, 1977). About 25% of patients with major depression presenting at mixed secondary–tertiary care facilities have psychotic depression (Parker et al., 1991). The incidence is much smaller in pure secondary care, of course.

Response to antidepressant medication is much lower if delusions are present in melancholia (Avery and Lubrano, 1979; Brown et al., 1982; Davidson et al., 1978; Glassman et al., 1975; Kantor and Glassman, 1977; Minter and Mandel, 1979; Nelson and Charney, 1981), likewise if cognitive impairment is present in melancholia (Aronson et al., 1988; La Rue et al., 1986). ECT is markedly superior to antidepressants in treating psychotic depression and also works well on medication nonresponders (Avery and Lubrano, 1979; Glassman et al., 1975; Lykouras et al., 1986a, 1986b; Parker et al., 1992). ECT efficacy exceeds that of combining phenelzine and amitriptyline (Davidson et al., 1978). Likewise, it exceeds that of antidepressants in corticosteroid-induced depression (Brown et al., 1982; Lewis and Smith, 1983).

Delusions in melancholia are themselves distressing, and the usual delusional themes have a narrow range (Parker et al., 1991). Guilt and paranoia are common; for example, the patient believes he is unwanted by his family, has committed an evil act or sin and deserves punishment, or is condemned to hell. Although delusions can be rigid and organized into a system, they differ from paranoid schizophrenia by the emotional concern and affect the patient displays about them. Not only can delusions indicate likely resistance to medications, their content can identify risks for suicide or assault. Other melancholic delusions can include poverty, nihilism (i.e., he doesn't exist, he is now in hell), worthlessness, or sickness.

Sickness can include delusions of being full of waste, poisoned, having organ dysfunction (especially stomach or intestines), or parasitosis. Sensory distortions or hallucinations can accompany these delusions. Middle-aged or elderly patients with psychotic melancholia often have constipation or other gastrointestinal complaints (Parker et al., 1991).

Psychotic melancholia is one of several common types of psychotic depression, most of which are treatable with ECT, but for some types ECT is not suitable (Swartz and Shorter, 2007). Some other types of psychotic depression are bipolar mixed depression, deteriorative psychotic depression, catatonic psychotic depression, psychotic-equivalent demented depression, tardive psychotic depression, drug-induced psychotic depression, and coarse brain disease psychotic depression. ECT should help patients with these types of depression but should be only a last resort in tardive and coarse brain disease psychotic depressions.

Several reports from Columbia University claim that medication-resistant major depression responds poorly to ECT (Prudic et al., 1990, 1996). Indeed, the outcome of their studies was markedly worse than expected. Response – which is a substantially lower outcome than remission – was obtained in only 35% to 65% of their patients with an average ECT course of 10 treatments, a long course. Their claim of medication resistance predisposing to poor ECT outcome contrasts markedly with other studies – some quite large – reporting that medication-resistant patients respond very well to ECT (e.g., Pluijms et al., 2002). In the DeCarolis study (Avery and Lubrano, 1979) 85% of 110 patients who failed to respond to one month of imipramine achieved remission with 8 to 10 ECT treatments. The "endogenous depression" that these patients had presumably corresponds to melancholia or simultaneous melancholia and catatonia. The inability of an acute course of ECT to treat comorbid anxiety disorders such as PTSD may explain the poor results at Columbia.

The Columbia study patients had long suffered with psychiatric conditions with averages of 15 to 20 years since illness onset. Still, the reports do not state that anxiety disorders were accounted for, disqualified, or even examined for. The simple explanation for the bad outcome is that the Columbia patients had comorbid dysphoric anxiety disorders that increased depression rating scores. Hints that this was so include the regular use of lorazepam in 84% (67/80) of their ECT study patients and the fact that higher depression scores at the end of the ECT course were strongly associated with more frequent relapse (Sackeim et al., 2000). Anxiety disorders are present in at least half of patients with DSM major depression (Zimmerman et al., 2002), and long-suffering patients should have a still higher incidence. Indeed, having concurrent anxiety symptoms predicts worse long-term outcome to antidepressant medication (Andreescu et al., 2007), and anxiety is so common in this group that the converse is surely true, that worse long-term outcome to antidepressant medications corresponds to comorbid anxiety disorder. We must assume that anxiety disorders affected the results, and specifically that anxiety increased depression rating scores after ECT, falsely indicating ECT nonresponse. We must also expect that anxiety increased depression rating scores before ECT, incorrectly indicating depression severity higher than from major depression alone and perhaps provoking ECT use itself.

Results of other studies from the same Columbia group suggest a large effect of anxiety disorders. Specifically, one month after ECT there was an abrupt increase in relapse (Prudic et al., 2005). Studies of treating OCD with ECT suggest that this is the expected timing for relapse after ECT in anxiety disorders, as noted earlier in this chapter.

Antimanic medication–resistant manic episode

Despite the drama and satisfaction of treating patients in an acute manic episode with lithium, valproic acid, or carbamazepine, only about half achieve remission with these medications alone. Still, each remission is a blessing, because the alternative to remission is impairment, severe life disruption, and high service usage. Medication-resistant acute manic episodes respond well to ECT, and ECT has several profound advantages over antipsychotic drugs. Of course, even with ECT, antipsychotic drugs are often needed temporarily. The basic issue is whether the patient will be discharged on antipsychotic drugs and thereby exposed to their long-term adverse effects and impairments. When bipolar patients are discharged on antipsychotic drugs it is rare for these drugs to be discontinued (Sernyak et al., 1994).

Antimanic medication–resistant patients face two very different paths, of long-term ECT or long-term antipsychotics. The comparative consequences are detailed in Chapter 23. The differences are so profound that the doctor should occasionally prod patients and their families to reevaluate their plan. In summation, patients on long-term ECT will be more normal in personality but more likely to be rehospitalized, whereas patients on antipsychotics will be more passive and simplistic and probably develop medical and neurological disorders from the medication.

Several bipolar patients I have seen developed temporary resistance to ECT. They were managed by alternating several months of antipsychotic drugs with an acute course of ECT followed by maintenance ECT. Eventually maintenance ECT would not suffice and they would return to antipsychotics for several months.

Medication-resistant acute psychosis

This description typically reflects an urgency in the patient's presentation, as described earlier for ECT as first choice, and that this urgency has continued despite antipsychotic tranquilizers. ECT should calm the urgency and then remove the psychosis.

Acute psychosis could mean that the patient has a mood disorder with psychotic features, in which the psychosis is so forceful and resistant that the mood disorder is obscured. The severity of drama, agitation, disorganization, hallucinations, or delusions in a psychosis does not disqualify a mood disorder; neither does the content of these phenomena. The psychosis of a mood disorder is not a separate entity, and the patient does not have both a mood disorder and a psychosis. Rather, the psychosis is a symptom of the mood disorder, and fully treating the mood disorder produces remission of both psychosis and mood symptoms. Sometimes ECT will diminish psychotic symptoms faster than mood symptoms, and the mood disorder will become more noticeable partway through the course.

In treating medication-resistant acute psychosis with ECT, the key to expecting improvement is acuteness. The clearer and more focused the onset, the stronger we should expect that ECT will quickly succeed. Because acute usually means less than six months, all acute functional psychosis should respond to ECT (until proven otherwise).

Schizoaffective illness is a common diagnosis. Yet, the reliability of this diagnosis has always been low (Maj et al., 2000), probably because of variability in detecting and interpreting the symptoms and signs of depression and mania when psychosis is present. This means that there is no reliability in distinguishing between schizoaffective disorder and mood disorder with psychotic or catatonic features. It is well worth noting that new-onset psychosis is significantly more likely to be psychotic depression than schizophrenia (Crebbin et al., 2008). There is a basic issue of professional ethics here. It harms patients to forecast chronic psychosis when there is no compelling evidence of chronicity (this means diagnosing schizophrenia or schizoaffective disorder when alternative diagnoses of better prognosis and different treatment are possible, such as a mood disorder with psychotic features – for example, psychotic depression – or catatonic features/catatonic depression). Operationally this means that if antimelancholic or antimanic medications do not succeed by themselves during the first two years of psychotic illness, ECT should be considered.

Medication-resistant intermediate-duration psychosis versus schizophrenia

Coursewise, between acute (six months) and chronic (two years) is intermediate duration. Although the prognosis might be intermediate, it is not patient centered to pronounce a psychiatric illness irreversible after six months and plan to continue antipsychotic tranquilizers permanently. This forecast of irreversibility flatly conflicts with the course of untreated melancholic depression, lasting about a year and not becoming chronic. Yet, a six-month course suffices to diagnose DSM schizophrenia. DSM allows schizophrenia to be diagnosed even more loosely: A one-month course suffices if it just follows or precedes nonspecific symptoms such as apathy for five months, symptoms so-called prodromal or residual. This one-month minimum obviously is a diagnostic shortcut, it has never been justified by evidence, and it disempowers patients from control over their lives as it empowers persons who aim to supervise them.

In this context ECT can empower patients, destigmatize them, and divert them into remission instead of into long-term antipsychotic tranquilization with psychopathology indistinguishable from that of patients with schizophrenia. Accordingly, I consider ECT if the patient functioned well premorbidly. The decision to give ECT for intermediate-duration patients often turns into the question of who will advocate for it. The decision to try ECT often follows the personal preferences of the patient and his or her family, in view of the patient's individual circumstances. Patients who have no emergencies and whose family members are not dissatisfied will probably prefer to continue with their present treatment, whatever it is. Conversely, ECT should be appreciated by patients who repeatedly or urgently need psychiatric services or whose family members crave better quality of recovery.

If the psychosis began in association with abuse of psychotogenic or stimulant drugs, a coarse brain disease, or traumatic brain injury, the prognosis for remission with ECT is probably lower, but not zero. Remission is less likely if the patient recently abused drugs or alcohol, because these neurotoxic agents contribute to psychosis, depression, anxiety, physical illness, and noncompliance. With continuing drug abuse, the prognosis is for further emergencies and hospitalizations, regardless of ECT. So, until a patient shows clear-cut mania or catatonia after five to seven days of drug abstinence, melancholia after two weeks, or psychosis after three weeks, I do not consider him or her a candidate for ECT.

Medication-resistant chronic psychosis or schizophrenia

Futility is abundant when trying to distinguish between a bipolar disorder long managed with antipsychotic drugs and schizophrenia on the basis of pre-ECT psychopathology and history. What counts more than diagnosis in considering the patient for ECT is uncontrolled psychotic behavior or recent exacerbations of psychotic symptoms that resist medication changes. The former might be seen in a long-institutionalized patient who is frequently placed in restraints, holds no coherent conversation, or does not maintain basic hygiene, despite medication efforts. Drug-resistant exacerbation of psychosis might be seen in an outpatient who has long kept a job or maintained a role in a protected environment, but several months prior became too distracted by paranoia or hallucinations to continue.

These patients are good candidates for ECT, but it is typically necessary to continue antipsychotic medication during and after the ECT course. In a few severe chronic patients, long-term management was with clozapine and either maintenance ECT or periodically repeated courses of ECT.

ECT as prerequisite for other procedures

A trial of ECT is typically a prerequisite for several surgically invasive psychiatric treatments, for example, psychosurgery, focused ablation via intersecting gamma-rays (e.g., gamma-knife, cyberknife), deep brain stimulation, and vagus nerve stimulation. Psychosurgery and intersecting gamma-rays involve destruction of brain tissue. Deep brain stimulation begins with electrode implantation in the brain, has some morbidity, and might have irreversible effects (Gimsa et al., 2006). Vagus nerve stimulation involves permanent implantation of an electrode around the vagus nerve in the neck.

Patients receiving ECT as a prerequisite will not necessarily match ECT patient selection considerations, as noted earlier in this chapter. Primarily, many of these patients have a treatment-resistant anxiety disorder, such as OCD. Accordingly, we must here consider specific drug treatment of anxiety disorders or atypical depression. Detailed discussion of evaluating and treating anxiety disorders is outside the purview of this book. Still, there are noteworthy aspects of anxiety disorders that are candidates for ECT as a prerequisite. These anxiety disorders typically include uncontrolled somatic tension anxiety symptoms, associated with arousal of the catecholaminergic sympathetic nervous system. Somatic tension symptoms are not reliably treated by SSRIs, bupropion, or buspirone, as these drugs are not sympatholytic. The usefulness of serotonergic drugs in mitigating psychological anxiety symptoms such as dissatisfaction, worrying, and recurring unpleasant memories still leaves somatic tension anxiety untreated. Continuing distress from untreated symptoms raises questions about "last resort" and the invasive treatments noted earlier in this chapter. Nevertheless, the vast majority of these patients respond quickly – and observably – to medications that smoothly and persistently reduce CNS β-adrenergic activity, specifically betaxolol (Swartz, 1998) and/or topiramate. These methods are detailed elsewhere (Swartz and Shorter, 2007), and if ECT is a prerequisite, so should these methods be.

Medication-resistant agitated dementia

The medical literature contains nothing but a few case reports about ECT mitigating the agitation of dementia. This tiny literature can rationalize such use only occasionally and as a last resort. Because no medications have received an FDA indication for agitated dementia – and antipsychotics are officially discouraged – the meaning of medication resistance here is unclear. To illustrate, my experience is that pindolol, quetiapine, and topiramate are useful separately or together, but because they have not been impartially tested I cannot dispute overlooking them. Conversely, because there are no indicated drugs for this condition, prescribing these drugs can be reasonable. Nevertheless, the standard of practice for treating agitation in dementia is to administer unproven drug treatments and turn to ECT only rarely.

Closing

These perspectives focus more on verifiable observation of the patient and smaller details than DSM does, and they are more specific. This is similarly true compared to the American Psychiatric Association (APA) Task Force Report on ECT (APA, 2001). The latter did not limit the use of ECT within the group of patients who can be diagnosed with major depression, nor did it limit the use of this diagnosis. Limiting administrative obstructions to clinical practice is what a Task Force Report should do. Administrative reports identify what should not be done. In comparison, this book and particularly this chapter aim to describe what we should prefer to do.

In practice, diagnosis is the main determinant of ECT efficacy, although outcome can be subverted by grossly deficient ECT method. The ECT method should not be grossly deficient if a distinct tonic phase of convulsion occurs (per Ottosson, 1960), especially with any form of bilateral ECT, and the course length includes at least seven such ECT treatments. This expectation should be consistently met by the vast majority of ECT practice. Claims that deficient ECT method is the main cause of weak ECT outcome are unproven because the investigators overlooked the effects of untreated – and common – comorbid anxiety disorders and atypical depression (Prudic et al., 2005). The weak outcomes reported should not occur with due attention to these disorders that ECT does not treat.

References

American Psychiatric Association. 2001. The practice of ECT: Recommendations for treatment, training, and privileging, 2nd edn. Washington DC: American Psychiatric Press.

Andreescu, C., Lenze, E. J., Dew, M. A., et al. 2007. Effect of comorbid anxiety on treatment response and relapse risk in late-life depression: Controlled study. Br J Psychiatry 190: 344–9.

Aronson, T. A., Shukla, S., Hoff, A., and Cook, B. 1988. Proposed delusional depression subtypes: Preliminary evidence from a retrospective study of phenomenology and treatment course. J Affect Disord 14: 69–74.

Avery, D. and Lubrano, A. 1979. Depression treated with imipramine and ECT: The DeCarolis study reconsidered. Am J Psychiatry 136: 559–62.

Beekman, A. T., de Beurs, E., van Balkom, A. J., et al. 2000. Anxiety and depression in later life: Co-occurrence and communality of risk factors. Am J Psychiatry 157: 89–95.

Brown, R. P., Frances, A., Kocsis, J. H., and Mann, J. J. 1982. Psychotic vs. nonpsychotic depression: Comparison of treatment response. J Nerv Ment Dis 170: 635–7.

Chelminski, I., Zimmerman, M., and Mattia, J. I. 2000. Diagnosing melancholia. J Clin Psychiatry 61: 874–5.

Ciapparelli, A., Paggini, R., Marazziti, D., et al. 2007. Comorbidity with axis I anxiety disorders in remitted psychotic patients 1 year after hospitalization. CNS Spectr 12: 913–19.

Cole, M. 2008, January 17. Feds slam state hospital safety. *The Oregonian* (Portland newspaper) p. 1.

Crebbin, K., Mitford, E., Paxton, R., and Turkington, D. 2008. First-episode psychosis: An epidemiological survey comparing psychotic depression with schizophrenia. J Affect Disord 105: 117–24.

Davidson, J., McLeod, M., Law-Yone, B., and Linnoila, M. 1978. A comparison of electroconvulsive therapy and combined phenelzine-amitriptyline in refractory depression. Arch Gen Psychiatry 35: 639–42.

Frueh, B. C., Knapp, R. G., Cusack, K. J., et al. 2005. Patients' reports of traumatic or harmful experience within the psychiatric setting. Psychiatr Serv 56: 1123–33.

Gimsa, U., Schreiber, U., Habel, B., et al. 2006. Matching geometry and stimulation parameters of electrodes for deep brain stimulation experiments – numerical considerations. J Neurosci Meth 150: 212–27.

Glassman, A. H., Kantor, S. J., and Shostak, M. 1975. Depression, delusions, and drug response. Am J Psychiatry 132: 716–19.

Hamilton, M. 1989. Frequency of symptoms in melancholia (depressive illness). Br J Psychiatry 154: 201–6.

Hatta, K., Miyakawa, K., Ota, T., et al. 2007. Maximal response to electroconvulsive therapy for the treatment of catatonic symptoms. J ECT 23: 233–5.

Husain, M. M., McClintock, S. M., Rush, A. J., et al. 2008. The efficacy of acute electroconvulsive therapy in atypical depression. J Clin Psychiatry 69: 406–11.

Jansen, A. S. P., Nguyen, X. V., Karpitskiy, V., et al. 1995. Central command neurons of the sympathetic nervous system: Basis of the fight-or-flight response. Science 270: 644–6.

Jarrett, R. B., Schaffer, M., McIntire, D., et al. 2000. Treatment of atypical depression with cognitive therapy or phenelzine: A double-blind, placebo-controlled trial. Arch Gen Psychiatry 56: 431–7.

Kantor, S. J. and Glassman, A. H. 1977. Delusional depressions: Natural history and response to treatment. Br J Psychiatry 131: 351–60.

Kellner, C. H., Fink, M., Knapp, R., et al. 2005. Relief of expressed suicidal intent by ECT: A consortium for research in ECT study. Am J Psychiatry 162: 977–82.

Khanna, S., Gangadhar, B. N., Sinha, V., et al. 1988. ECT in obsessive-compulsive disorder. Convuls Ther 4: 314–20.

La Rue, A., Spar, J., and Hill, C. D. 1986. Cognitive impairment in late-life depression: Clinical correlates and treatment implications. J Affect Disord 11: 179–84.

Lesser, I., Castro, D., Gaynes, B., et al. 2007. Ethnicity/race and outcome in the treatment of depression: Results from STAR*D. Med Care 45: 1043–51.

Lewis, D. A. and Smith, R. E. 1983. Steroid-induced psychiatric syndromes. A report of 14 cases and a review of the literature. J Affect Disord 5: 319–32.

Lu, M. L., Pan, J. J., Teng, H. W., et al. 2002. Metoclopramide-induced supersensitivity psychosis. Ann Pharmacother 36(9): 1387–90.

Lykouras, E., Malliaras, D., Christodoulou, G. N., et al. 1986a. Delusional depression: Phenomenology and response to treatment. Psychopathology 19: 157–64.

Lykouras, E., Malliaras, D., Christodoulou, G. N., et al. 1986b. Delusional depression: Phenomenology and response to treatment. A prospective study. Acta Psychiatr Scand 73: 324–9.

Maj, M., Pirozzi, R., Formicola, A. M., et al. 2000. Reliability and validity of the DSM-IV diagnostic category of schizoaffective disorder: Preliminary data. J Affect Disord 57: 95–8.

Maletzky, B., McFarland, B., and Burt, A. 1994. Refractory obsessive compulsive disorder and ECT. Convuls Ther 10: 34–42.

Markowitz, J., Brown, R., Sweeney, J., and Mann, J. J. 1987. Reduced length and cost of hospital stay for major depression in patients treated with ECT. Am J Psychiatry 144: 1025–9.

Minter, R. E. and Mandel, M. R. 1979. The treatment of psychotic major depressive disorder with drugs and electroconvulsive therapy. J Nerv Ment Dis 167: 726–33.

Mulsant, B. H., Haskett, R. F., Prudic, J., et al. 1997. Low use of neuroleptic drugs in the treatment of psychotic major depression. Am J Psychiatry 154: 559–61.

Nelson, J. C. and Charney, D. S. 1981. The symptoms of major depressive illness. Am J Psychiatry 138: 1–13.

Nelson, J. C., Price, L. H., and Jatlow, P. I. 1986. Neuroleptic dose and desipramine concentrations during combined treatment of unipolar delusional depression. Am J Psychiatry 143: 1151–4.

Nelson, L. A. and Swartz, C. M. 2000. Melancholic symptoms from concurrent olanzapine and fluoxetine. Ann Clin Psychiatry 12: 167–70.

Nimgaonkar, V. L., Goodwin, G. M., Davies, C. L., and Green, A. R. 1985. Down-regulation of beta-adrenoceptors in rat cortex by repeated administration of desipramine, electroconvulsive shock and clenbuterol requires 5-HT neurones but not 5-HT. Neuropharmacology 24: 279–83.

Nobler, M. S. and Roose, S. P. 1998. Differential response to antidepressants in melancholic and severe depression. Psychiatr Ann 28: 84–8.

Ottosson, J. O. 1960. Effect of lidocaine on the seizure discharge in electroconvulsive therapy. Acta Psychiatr Scand Suppl 35(145): 7–32.

Parker, G., Hadzi-Pavlovic, D., Austin, M. P., et al. 1995. Is psychomotor disturbance necessary and sufficient to the definition of melancholia? Psychol Med 25: 813–23.

Parker, G., Hadzi-Pavlovic, D., Hickie, I., et al. 1991. Psychotic depression: A review and clinical experience. Aust N Z J Psychiatry 25: 169–80.

Parker, G., Roy, K., Hadzi-Pavlovic, D., and Pedic, F. 1992. Psychotic (delusional) depression: A meta-analysis of physical treatments. J Affect Disord 24: 17–24.

Parker, G., Roy, K., Mitchell, P., et al. 2002. Atypical depression: A reappraisal. Am J Psychiatry 159: 1470–9.

Perry, P. J., Morgan, D. E., Smith, R. E., and Tsuang, M. T. 1982. Treatment of unipolar depression accompanied by delusions. ECT versus tricyclic antidepressant – antipsychotic combinations. J Affect Disord 4: 195–200.

Pluijms, E. M., Birkenhager, T. K., Huijbrechts, I. P., and Moleman, P. 2002. Influence of resistance to antidepressant pharmacotherapy on short-term response to electroconvulsive therapy. J Affect Disord 69: 93–9.

Prudic, J., Haskett, R. F., Mulsant, B., et al. 1996. Resistance to antidepressant medications and short-term clinical response to ECT. Am J Psychiatry 153: 985–92.

Prudic, J., Olfson, M., Marcus, S. C., et al. 2005. Effectiveness of ECT in community settings. Biol Psychiatry 55: 301–12.

Prudic, J., Sackeim, H., and Devanand, D. 1990. Medication resistance and clinical response to electroconvulsive therapy. Psychiatry Res 31: 287–96.

Roose, S. P., Glassman, A. H., Attia, E., and Woodring, S. 1994. Comparative efficacy of selective serotonin reuptake inhibitors and tricyclics in the treatment of melancholia. Am J Psychiatry 151: 1735–9.

Sackeim, H. A., Prudic, J., Devanand, D. P., et al. 2000. A prospective, randomized, double-blind comparison of bilateral and right unilateral electroconvulsive therapy at different stimulus intensities. Arch Gen Psychiatry 57: 425–34.

Sernyak, M. J., Griffin, R. A., Johnson, R. M., et al. 1994. Neuroleptic exposure following inpatient treatment of acute mania with lithium and neuroleptic. Am J Psychiatry 151: 133–5.

Swartz, C. M. 1998. Betaxolol in anxiety disorders. Ann Clin Psychiatry 10: 9–14.

Swartz, C. M. 2002a. Olanzapine-induced depression. J Pharm Technol 18: 321–3.

Swartz, C. M. 2002b, September 19. PTSD from psychiatric illness. Psychiatric Times 9: 18–20.

Swartz, C. M. 2003, April 20. Evidence versus subjectivity in major depression. Psychiatric Times 4: 30–2.

Swartz, C. M. 2004, October 21. Antipsychotic psychosis. Psychiatric Times 11: 17–20.

Swartz, C. M. and Inglis, A. E. 1990. Blood pressure fall with ECT response in males: Evidence for depression-induced hypertension. J Clin Psychiatry 51: 414–16.

Swartz, C. M. and Shorter E. 2007. Psychotic depression. New York: Cambridge University Press.

Turner, E. H., Matthews, A. M., Linardatos, E., et al. 2008. Selective publication of antidepressant trials and its influence on apparent efficacy. N Engl J Med 358: 252–60.

Zimmerman, M., Chelminski, I., and McDermut, W. 2002. Major depressive disorder and axis I diagnostic comorbidity. J Clin Psychiatry 63: 187–93.

23

Electroconvulsive therapy or antipsychotic drugs (or benzodiazepines for catatonia)

Conrad M. Swartz

Introduction

Whether from obstruction or proclivity, many psychiatrists who treat acutely ill patients do not arrange electroconvulsive therapy (ECT) for their patients. As several writers describe in this volume (e.g., Dr. Reid, Dr. Rohland), ECT is not reasonably accessible – or flatly unavailable – in many areas of the United States and elsewhere. There is no mystery in how to manage patients without giving ECT for the acute and episodic conditions for which ECT is indicated. It is by giving antipsychotic drugs, benzodiazepines, or both. These conditions include psychotic depression and other major depressions resistant to antidepressants, acute psychotic episode, acute catatonic episode, mixed manic-depressive state, and manic episode resistant to specific antimania medication (e.g., lithium, valproate, carbamazepine). The basic question about this substitution is: For these patients, how do these drugs compare with ECT in psychiatric side effects, medical risks, and benefits?

In the medical order of things, adverse effects precede benefits, as "Above all do no harm" is an overarching tenet. Accordingly, first we compare antipsychotic drugs with ECT on adverse effects and risks, and then on benefits.

Comparing antipsychotics with ECT for patients with schizophrenia is a matter outside our focus. Still, it is important to note that, for new onsets, psychotic depression by itself is more common than schizophrenia (Crebbin et al., 2008). Add to psychotic depression the other ECT indications noted earlier, and the importance of the comparison between ECT and antipsychotics is clear. Also outside the focus here is comparing ECT with antidepressant drugs; this is dealt with in Chapter 22.

"When everybody knows that something is so, it means that nobody knows nuthin'."
—Andrew S. Grove, Intel co-founder, Fortune magazine interview, 2005.

Experts in any field have difficulty imagining – or tolerating – the idea that what they have long known is not so. This was true in the times of Plato, Copernicus, Darwin, and Lysenko, and surely continues today. In treating patients with psychosis, psychiatrists usually operate as has been routine for more than 50 years. They give an antipsychotic drug. Acceptance of the "antipsychotic" name for this class of drugs both recognizes and urges this tradition. It reflects the widespread belief that antipsychotics are intrinsically and specifically antipsychotic.

Of course they are not. Most antipsychotic prescription is off label because these drugs have powerful psychotropic actions on people who are not psychotic. There is hardly an Axis I condition in the *The Diagnostic and Statistical Manual of Mental Disorders* (DSM) for which antipsychotic drugs have not been advocated in a peer-reviewed journal article, along with hordes of industry-sponsored publications. Lately some pharmaceutical firms have obtained U.S. Food and Drug Administration (FDA) permission to market antipsychotic drugs to patients with nonpsychotic major depression. This is merely rephrasing of an old tale. The neuroleptics perphenazine (in Triavil®) and thioridazine (Mellaril®) were widely used for neuroses, including "neurotic depression." That diagnosis is superseded by major depression with atypical features, minor depression, dysthymic disorder, or an anxiety disorder.

As another example of traditional antipsychotic use outside psychosis, chlorpromazine was the longstanding benchmark for antimanic action. It was lithium's virtue to match chlorpromazine's scores when rating scales were used on patients with acute mania. Despite the similar scores, there is a world of difference between these two drugs in the quality of clinical improvement.

Simply put, patients whose rating scores fell to normal range with lithium returned to normal personae, including their normal qualities of behavior and judgment. Patients whose rating scores fell similarly with chlorpromazine did not appear normal, did not resume their pre-illness behavior, and showed oversimplistic judgment. Our psychiatric rating scales aim to rate the gross behavioral disruptions generated by illnesses such as mania and melancholia and reflect a need for hospitalization and supervision. They are not even designed to be sensitive to the impairments produced by antipsychotic drugs, such as changes in personality, creativity, judgment, individuality, and appreciation of complexity. Of course, each of these is a substance of the quality of life and contributes fundamentally to its meaning. We professionals hold each of these dear and close, and we know that we could not do our jobs well without them. The contrast between lithium and chlorpromazine is the same as the contrast between ECT and antipsychotic drugs, and it is what this chapter is about.

Just as antipsychotics mitigate numerous nonpsychotic conditions, response to antipsychotics demonstrates nothing about diagnosis or disease. The responding disorder might be entirely psychological, because antipsychotics and other tranquilizers bluntly decrease psychological concerns. Antipsychotics do not precisely excise psychosis and bring patients to full remission. Rather, substantial psychopathology persists, and we are usually unsure how much of the negative symptoms results from the antipsychotic drug and how much comes from the illness. In contrast, full remission is an ordinary occurrence with ECT.

Fundamental psychiatric and psychological issues are overlooked in publications that advocate antipsychotic drugs for patients who have depression or another condition that is not schizophrenia. One issue is adverse mental side effects. I ask the physician reader to now pause and identify the adverse mental side effects of antipsychotic drugs as taught in psychiatry residency, medical school, continuing medical education (CME) conferences, textbooks, and review articles. These effects are in addition to adverse neurological effects such as movement disorders and akathisia, and in addition to medical problems such as weight gain, diabetes, strokes, and myocardial infarction.

The only commonly taught adverse mental effects of antipsychotics are somnolence and tiredness. Of course, some antipsychotics are not sedating but still would have robust mental effects on normal volunteers. Surely these adverse mental consequences must be understood and appreciated by doctor and patient before any bona fide informed consent can occur. Basic medical ethics demand this understanding even if written consent is not required, such as is always done before ECT in the United States.

In addition to mental effects, the adverse medical effects of antipsychotic drugs are profound. They markedly decrease life span. Recent data show that patients with schizophrenia who take antipsychotic drugs show markedly increased mortality. Similar life-span-shortening effects should occur with patients who take antipsychotic drugs for any reason, because the effects derive from the medication. Indeed, patients with bipolar disorder or schizophrenia showed high similar prevalences of smoking, obesity, diabetes, and cardiovascular risk factors (Birkenaes et al., 2007). Likewise, patients with unipolar depression, bipolar disorder, schizoaffective disorder, and schizophrenia had similar overall excess mortality rates, and patients with schizophrenia showed fewer deaths from unnatural causes, for example, suicide (Laursen et al., 2007). In Sweden, a 10-year study of 255 patients and 1,275 population controls found a mortality rate in patients with schizophrenia of 23% but an age- and sex-matched rate in controls of 11.2% (Fors et al., 2007), with significant excess rates of occurrence in patients for both cardiovascular disease and unnatural causes. A meta-analysis similarly found the overall ratio of mortality rates between patients and controls to be 2.5, with ratios for suicide of 12.9, infection 4.3, neurological disease 4.2, genitourinary disease 3.7, respiratory disease 3.2, endocrine disease 2.7, and digestive disease 2.4 (Saha et al., 2007). The survival gap between controls and patients with schizophrenia and schizoaffective disorder was reported as increasing during the past 30 years (Capasso et al., 2008).

These higher mortality rates mean shorter life spans. A study of 20,018 psychiatric patients of state hospitals in Ohio – a huge number – found their life span 32 years shorter, on average (Miller et al., 2006). Because they were patients in state hospital in times of tight budgets, it is reasonable to expect that the vast majority received antipsychotic drugs. This medication-induced life shortening contrasts with the massive efforts and expense that people commonly invest to extend their lives in the face of heart disease, cancer, and renal failure, even by a few months. The medications Vioxx and Celebrex were withdrawn for much less.

In contrast, as a brief time-limited treatment, ECT should not generate chronic medical conditions. Beyond this, ECT is associated with longer life span. Patients who received ECT for depression were more likely to be alive at 5- to 12-year follow-ups than were those who received only antidepressant medications (Philibert et al., 1995). This finding complements those of a previous study that patients who received either ECT or adequate tricyclic antidepressant dosage survived longer than those who did not (Avery and Winokur, 1976). Similarly, patients who received ECT showed a lower death rate than patients who did not, although there was a slightly higher suicide rate during the first week after hospital discharge (Munk-Olsen et al., 2007). Forty percent of patients who did not receive ECT for psychotic depression at Yale University Hospital died within 15 years (Vythilingam et al., 2003). This high rate is obviously excessive. Ninety percent of those deaths were from medical causes. Similarly, after hospital discharge, patients who received ECT died less frequently than other psychiatric patients did from lung diseases, including pneumonia (Joseph et al., 1996).

Mental side effects: Hypofrontality

In serious psychiatric illnesses such as mania, melancholia, and schizophrenia, the prefrontal regions of the brain do not function normally (Cohen et al., 1989). Antipsychotic drugs suppress neural activity in the prefrontal lobes or disconnect them from the rest of the brain (Cohen et al., 1997; Potkin et al., 1994). This effect decreases the influence of the prefrontal regions on the rest of the brain. It presumably explains how these drugs diminish the severity of psychiatric illnesses, and why they affect the psychopathology of many different psychiatric conditions. In normal humans, the prefrontal region comprises almost half the brain cortex. It is centrally involved in novel problem solving, recognition and management of complexity in human relationships, salience, initiative, delayed reward motivation, and multitasking. These prefrontal lobe functions represent the differences in psychological performance between humans and animals and also between mature and childlike behaviors. Correlating with this, in animals and human children the prefrontal region is relatively smaller than in human adults.

Three syndromes of prefrontal dysfunction ("hypofrontality") have been described, although they have some overlaps and similarities. The "apathetic syndrome" is associated with mesial prefrontal dysfunction. The "orbitofrontal syndrome," named for the orbital frontal region, consists primarily of disregard of social complexity such as disinhibited behavior, rudeness, and childlike behavior. The "dysexecutive syndrome" is associated with impairment of the dorsolateral prefrontal cortex (DLPFC), particularly on the left. The "executive" cognitive functions of problem solving, planning, novel thought, and organization and management of complexity are associated with the DLPFC. These three syndromes were identified from the study of brain injuries. The notorious case of Phineas Gage (Bigelow, 1850) is primarily orbitofrontal syndrome.

Antipsychotic drugs can induce any of these syndromes, as can Parkinson's disease (Bassett, 2005). The symptoms of Parkinson's disease express the loss of dopaminergic brain cells in the deep brain region called the pars compacta of the substantia nigra. The functioning of dopaminergic brain cells is similarly deficient in Parkinson's disease and with exposure to dopamine-blocking antipsychotic drugs. Further similarity occurs in the shared physical signs of muscle rigidity, tremor, tendency to fall, and akinesia. Deficient functioning of the dopaminergic cells in the striatum diminishes connections between the prefrontal lobes and the rest of the brain.

There is extensive overlap between these frontal syndromes and the negative symptoms associated with schizophrenia. That is, the same negative symptoms can be induced by psychiatric illness and by the medications given to manage it. Typical negative symptoms include poverty of expressed thought, simplistic speech, monotone voice, blunted or flattened affect with limited range of emotional expression, social deficits, poor rapport, lack of friends, low motivation, passive unproductive behavior, sloppy grooming, observably deficient hygiene, disinterest in hobbies and world events, vague or absent life goals and meaningfulness, and slowed movements. This list is illustrative rather than complete. Antipsychotic drugs can generate any of these symptoms in people who never experienced them before. Overall, antipsychotic drugs make minds dull and simple, whereas ECT does not do this and does not impair learning.

Behavioral and mental changes vary somewhat among antipsychotic drugs, apparently because specific neurotransmitter effects do. Dopamine blockers such as haloperidol, risperidone, and perphenazine decrease the quantity of physical movement and speech as they lessen complexity and amount of thought. Some second generation antipsychotics such as olanzapine, clozapine, and quetiapine decrease thought complexity more than they diminish motor activity and speech. This difference might make the thought simplicity that they cause easier to notice. Disinhibition from decreased orbitofrontal function and diminished executive cognitive functions presumably contribute to the problematic weight gain patients experience with olanzapine, clozapine, and quetiapine. In addition to these effects, olanzapine and clozapine suppress the medial prefrontal cortex, producing somnolence, apathy, asthenia (physical weakness), and abulia (loss of willpower) (Nelson and Swartz, 2000).

Olanzapine-induced apathy and abulia have been mistaken for the anhedonia, anergy, indecisiveness, poverty of expressed thought, and motor retardation of melancholia (Swartz, 2002). Other antipsychotic drugs generate akathisia, provoking patients to pace or show other signs of agitation and thereby appear worse psychiatrically. Elderly patients are at particularly high risk for rigidity, akinesia, and other parkinsonian symptoms from antipsychotics, which can be mistaken for melancholia because of motor slowing and impoverishment of thought and speech. Of course these side effects can lead to incorrect ratings of depression when using the Hamilton Rating Scale for Depression (HRSD), Montgomery-Åsberg Depression Rating Scale (MADRS), and global scales typically involved in studies of depression treatment.

Somnolence from antipsychotics is an adverse experience in itself, but also more than that. Somnolence is a significant cause of unintentional injury, with excess rates of 61% and 25% for quetiapine and olanzapine, respectively (Said et al., 2008).

Although ECT can cause orbitofrontal syndrome and dysexecutive syndrome, they fade within one to five weeks after the last ECT treatment. Such cognitive side effects are more pronounced when ECT is given more frequently, particularly with two or more treatments under the same anesthesia (Roemer et al., 1990). Orbitofrontal syndrome resembles hypomania, with disinhibition, intrusiveness, hypersexuality, silliness, distractibility, and immodesty. Although there is no hyperactivity, insomnia, flight of ideas, or psychosis, orbitofrontal syndrome probably accounts for most cases of supposed ECT-induced hypomania. Frank disorientation or delirium can result from ECT but is also temporary; these problems can also result from antipsychotic drugs (Swartz, 2001).

Mental side effects: Tardive

The mental effects noted earlier begin promptly, within a few days of drug initiation. Another set of adverse mental effects accompanies long-term use of antidopaminergic drugs. As the acute side effects resemble Parkinson's disease, the chronic side effects resemble Huntington's chorea. In addition to the well-known tardive movement disorders are several tardive behavioral disorders, including psychosis, depression, obsessions and compulsions, vomiting, and hiccupping (Stueber and Swartz, 2006; Swartz, 1995, 2004b).

Tardive psychosis was originally called dopamine supersensitivity psychosis (Chouinard et al., 1986; Weinberger et al., 1981). In the conceptual explanation for it, both deficiency and excess of dopamine generate neurological and psychiatric symptoms, of somewhat opposite nature. Acutely, antipsychotic drugs block dopamine, but eventually homeostatic processes generate resistance to this blockade. Indeed, long-term use of various different types of medications produces effects opposite those produced by short-term use. For example, antiarrhythmic drugs, antibiotics, and benzodiazepines eventually promote arrhythmias, superinfections, and rebound anxiety, respectively. In analogy, the possible tardive behavioral effects of antipsychotic drugs include actions opposing their acute effects of suppressing psychosis, depression, obsessions, and compulsions; nausea and vomiting; and hiccups. Besides dopamine supersensitivity and excess, cholinergic deterioration (Miller and Chouinard, 1993), gamma-aminobutyric acid (GABA-)ergic insensitivity, and glutamatergic excess (Gunne and Andren, 1993) might contribute to tardive phenomena.

Just as with tardive dyskinesia, these other tardive phenomena begin to develop after about two years of drug exposure in adults but as soon as three months in elderly patients (Lu et al., 2002). Rapid onset in older patients who never previously experienced psychotic symptoms draws a clear line between these symptoms and exposure to dopamine-blocking drugs. Relevant to our immediate interest, young adults with nonpsychotic bipolar disorder who were prospectively followed showed first onset of mood-incongruent delusions while taking dopamine-blocking antipsychotic drugs for three years (Downs et al., 1993). This psychosis occurred despite their continuing to receive these drugs. Tardive obsessive-compulsive disorder (OCD) presumably explains the frequent onset of compulsions after several years of taking antipsychotic drugs. Most worrisome is that tardive psychosis presumably resembles tardive dyskinesia in being usually irreversible and then functionally indistinguishable from schizophrenia. In other words, patients who have what should be an acute or episodic mood disorder or psychosis become at risk for chronic psychosis if maintained on an antipsychotic drug long term. Methods to obtain remission from this "antipsychotic psychosis" have not been established, and only a few cases of remission without antipsychotic drug continuation have been reported (Swartz, 1995).

Presumably reflecting the permanence of tardive psychosis, longitudinal studies of patients receiving antipsychotic drugs for schizophrenia show virtually 100% stability of their diagnosis. This rate is higher than for any other serious psychiatric condition. It is higher than is credible. It is far higher than expected for a diagnosis that should be made on the basis of exclusion (Carpenter and Buchanan, 1994). Moreover, patients maintained on antipsychotic drugs for other conditions (e.g., delusional disorder, schizoaffective disorder, psychosis not otherwise specified) were usually rediagnosed as having schizophrenia (Whitty et al., 2005). The simple and logical explanation for the virtually perfect diagnostic stability of schizophrenia – and for diagnosing it in other patients taking antipsychotics – is that the syndrome of schizophrenia can result from taking these drugs. Schizophrenia symptoms can result from the schizophrenialike side effects of antipsychotic drugs, for example, flattening of affect, impaired problem solving, and poor grooming and rapport. Schizophrenia symptoms can also result from tardive psychosis. Diagnosing schizophrenia can also result from the behavior of diagnosticians, that is, the well-worn path of continuing to prescribe antipsychotic drugs is associated with diagnosing schizophrenia.

The situation of tardive psychosis and dyskinesia resembles giving alcohol to an alcoholic shaking from early withdrawal. It calms the symptoms, but it was the underlying cause. Continuation progressively makes the symptoms worse. Decreasing or stopping acutely makes symptoms temporarily worse. There are irreversible changes to the brain, including the frontal lobes, and these changes persist even after stopping intake permanently. For alcoholism, completely stopping alcohol intake is generally desirable. The most desirable path is to avoid persistent substantial use of alcohol. It is only a small extrapolation to say that persistent substantial use of antidopaminergic drugs is similarly unhealthy and is plainly the *very last resort* in psychiatry. The apparent irreversibility of tardive phenomena resembles lobotomy. In comparison with antipsychotic drugs, ECT has only temporary risks, toxicity, adverse effects, and no known persisting substantial adverse effects except for minor retrograde memory issues that are intertwined with memory interference from illness, medication, and the personally threatening stresses associated with them.

Mental side effects: Other

The proven cognitive side effects of ECT are temporary, but it is possible that ECT causes some persistent loss of memory dating from before the onset of depression. Recent study shows that, at two months after ECT, memory related to personal concerns (i.e., "autobiographical") is not lost, but there is a small and nonsignificant trend ($p = 0.07$) for decreased memory of nonpersonal events (Lisanby et al., 2000). Because the comparison group comprised normal persons rather than psychiatrically ill patients, even this trend is questionable. The amnestic effect is suspected more for bitemporal ECT than for other placements, and particularly with high-stimulus dosage, long ECT courses, and comorbid cerebrovascular disease or early dementia.

However, antipsychotic drugs can cause loss of personal memory (Harrison and Therrien, 2007). The hypofrontal effects of antipsychotics noted earlier can contribute to this loss, particularly through somnolence (and consequent impaired concentration) and abulia. Anticholinergic antipsychotics should have still greater amnestic effects; going beyond this expectation, initial data suggest that anticholinergic drugs induce and accelerate dementia (Tsao et al., 2008). This side effect of anticholinergic drugs is analogous to cholinesterase inhibitors slowing and perhaps postponing the development of dementia, just in the opposite direction.

At ordinary doses all clinically effective antipsychotics (whether new or old) cause profound disregard of previously learned warning signals, for as long as they are continued. Perceptions of overeating, weight gain, disordered grooming, uncleanliness, and health alerts on cigarette packs are examples of warning signals. Disregard of warning signals is a blunt and massive impairment of human cognition. In technical terms, antipsychotics selectively disrupt conditioned avoidance (Samaha et al., 2008). Disruption of conditioned avoidance occurs along with the other temporary cognitive side effects of ECT, but there is no evidence of persistence after convalescence from ECT.

Medical adverse effects

Among the most well-known adverse neurological effects of antipsychotics are tardive movement disorders such as dyskinesia and dystonia. These are observable as involuntary movements. Dyskinetic movements include chewing, lip clenching or smacking, tongue protruding, and writhing of the arms or trunk. Grimacing, pelvic thrusting, and neck rotating and hyperextending can also occur. These involuntary movements resemble rude gestures and are markedly stigmatizing. Higher doses and longer exposure to antipsychotic drugs increases the likelihood that these involuntary movements will continue permanently, even if the drug is stopped. These disorders are common, afflicting about one third of patients after five years and nearly 60% after 15 years (Glazer et al., 1993). Tardive dyskinesia is yet more common in elderly patients, with 43% incidence after just six months of low-dose perphenazine (average 10 mg/d) for psychotic depression in patients with an average age of 72 years (Meyers et al., 2001). Another group reported a 7% yearly rate of tardive dyskinesia onset in elderly depressed patients taking antipsychotics (Yassa et al., 1992). In incidence, tardive psychosis and other tardive phenomena should parallel tardive dyskinesia. ECT is not known to cause movement disorders.

Each of the classic cardiac risk factors is caused or exacerbated by antipsychotic drugs. These same factors also pose risks for stroke and Alzheimer's disease. In a prospective study, within three months of starting a second generation antipsychotic drug, 4.4% of patients developed new-onset diabetes (van Winkel et al., 2008). Particularly potent in this regard were olanzapine, clozapine, and quetiapine. Olanzapine and clozapine also increased triglyceride levels and suppressed "good lipid" high-density lipoprotein (HDL) cholesterol (Birkenaes et al., 2008).

New-onset hypertension developed within five years in 27% of patients on clozapine, 9% of those on other second generation antipsychotics, and 4% of those on first generation neuroleptics (Henderson et al., 2004). Olanzapine increased body weight by more than 7% in 30% of patients within 18 months or less (Lieberman et al., 2005); quetiapine, risperidone, and perphenazine did likewise in about 15% of patients. ECT does not affect cardiac risk factors.

Adverse medical conditions caused by antipsychotic drugs include weight gain, which in turn increases risks of diabetes, hypertension, atherosclerotic coronary vascular disease, myocardial infarction, stroke, and further weight gain. The lethal risks of antipsychotic drugs are illustrated by the 50% higher death rate within 12 weeks of beginning antipsychotic drugs (3.5%) in comparison with placebo (2.3%). These results came from a randomized study of more than 5,000 elderly patients with dementia (Schneider et al., 2005). This study involved patients taking only the second generation antipsychotic drugs olanzapine, risperidone, ziprasidone, aripiprazole, quetiapine, and clozapine. The death rate was not influenced by variations in drug, severity of illness, or type of dementia. The excess occurrence of stroke led to a mandatory "black box warning" in the FDA-approved prescribing information about these drugs, analogous to the health warning printed on cigarette packs. Until proven otherwise, this excess death rate should be expected in all elderly patients, not just those diagnosed with dementia.

Aspiration pneumonia was increased in ambulatory elderly patients with dementia who had received antipsychotic drugs (Wada et al., 2001). Logically, the combination of antipsychotic drugs and ECT should also have some risk for this. Propofol anesthesia brings a small risk of aspiration pneumonia, but other ECT anesthetics do not. Otherwise, aspiration pneumonia is not a palpable risk from ECT, even for morbidly obese patients (Kadar et al., 2002).

In addition to having higher risks for tardive dyskinesia, stroke, and pneumonia, elderly patients are particularly sensitive to neuroleptic malignant syndrome (NMS). I observed fatal NMS in two 89-year-old men after they received a total of 6 to 14 mg of haloperidol over one to two weeks, so this is surely not rare. ECT does not cause NMS and might mitigate it.

Patients who take even low doses of antipsychotic drugs (e.g., 100 mg/d chlorpromazine equivalent) experience 2.4 times the normal rate of sudden cardiac death, on average. This risk ratio increases to 3.5 in patients with severe cardiac disease (Ray et al., 2001). The overall risk of death associated with the ECT procedure approximates that from anesthesia alone (about 1:20,000) and is less than the lifetime death risk from taking baths at home.

Antipsychotic drugs are carcinogenic in laboratory animals at doses comparable to clinical prescriptions; clozapine is the lone exception (Swartz, 2004a). Several studies have examined this issue in humans and found confirmatory evidence (e.g., Yamazawa et al., 2003); there are no data or reasons to argue against these results. This carcinogenic effect has been attributed to increased serum prolactin levels, but also occurs with second generation antipsychotic drugs that do not increase prolactin. The selective serotonin reuptake inhibitor (SSRI) paroxetine likewise increases serum prolactin and has been implicated in breast cancer in men (Wallace et al., 2001) as well as women (Cotterchio et al., 2000). ECT has no carcinogenic aspects.

Antipsychotic drugs inhibit libido and sexual function. The vast majority of men who receive antipsychotic drugs report sexual dysfunction (Plevin et al., 2007), which presumably results from both behavioral effects (e.g., somnolence, abulia) and chemical actions. Dopamine plays a central role in libido, and the dopamine antagonism of antipsychotic drugs should directly diminish it. Anticholinergic effects inhibit sexual arousal and cause erectile dysfunction, and many antipsychotic drugs are anticholinergic. Sympatholytic and serotonergic effects decrease, delay, or prevent orgasm, and most antipsychotic drugs show these effects. Severely (but not moderately) elevated blood prolactin levels are associated with loss of libido (Corona et al., 2007); most antipsychotics persistently and severely increase blood prolactin levels. ECT does not have these chemical or hormonal actions and does not appear to cause somnolence or abulia that persists past the ECT procedure itself.

The sedation, abulia, and akinesia induced by antipsychotic drugs diminish physical activity. With time this decreases muscle strength and endurance, which decreases physical activity further. Decreases in physical activity tend to promote blood clots in leg veins and thereby pulmonary emboli. Together with diminished initiative and weakened willpower, hypoactivity can promote exacerbations of pulmonary infections and development of pneumonia. After pneumonia starts, sedation, abulia, akinesia, and muscle rigidity tend to decrease ventilatory effort and so exacerbate the illness. They also inhibit the patient from requesting help.

Patient tolerance and compliance

The recent high-profile Clinical Antipsychotic Trials of Intervention Effectiveness (CATIE) multisite study of the outcome of antipsychotic drugs in managing schizophrenia provides insight that probably applies as well to any psychiatric condition in which these drugs are used (Lieberman et al., 2005; Stroup et al., 2006). This study found that the antipsychotic drugs perphenazine, quetiapine, ziprasidone, olanzapine, and risperidone relieve only a small fraction of patients' symptoms, although more than placebo. About two thirds of patients discontinued medication, from either nonresponse or dissatisfaction. The mean time to drug discontinuation averaged about six months with the first drug trial and four months with the second. We know that antipsychotic drug effect is sufficient to allow most patients with acute psychosis to be discharged from the acute hospital and most patients with chronic psychosis to live outside institutions. Still, we should avoid mistaking these benefits from antipsychotic drugs for remission or good health. These patients remain markedly impaired and dissatisfied with their condition. Their usual noncompliance with medication leads to relapse in troublesome circumstances and emergent hospital readmission. Even most patients who comply experience relapse.

Encouraging patient compliance and tolerance of ECT is a clinical art that falls well within psychiatric practice. That is, it involves faith, trust, and suggestion, along with technical knowledge and skill. The vast majority of patients complete the intended course of ECT. There is a basic difference in noncompliance between ECT and outpatient medication. With ECT noncompliance is obvious, but with outpatient medication it is commonly unrecognized and can be mistaken for resistance to medication and lead to poor outcome.

There is a false lore that relapse is more common after ECT than with medications. However, about one third of ECT patients relapse within a year, the same rate of relapse as after response to antidepressant medication in depression or antipsychotic medication in psychosis.

Therapeutic benefits

The goal of ECT is prompt, true remission, which is the standard for comparing ECT with antipsychotics. True remission is full restoration of the patient's persona, abilities, and performance at pre-illness levels. It differs from the remission criteria used in research studies looking for large effects, typically taken as 60% reduction in depression rating with a final score in normal range such as an HRSD score less than 8 or 10. For patients who were high functioning premorbidly, there is a basic difference between a large decrease in severity and a return to pre-illness performance and persona. The latter means no thought disorder or other observable psychopathology, no lingering impairment (whether from treatment or remaining illness), and no personality changes such as childlike behavior. A large decrease in severity does not specifically correspond to any of these aspects of full remission.

Studies of depression treatment judge remission according to decreases in severity. However, severity ratings are coarse, far more so than details of personality or psychological performance in complex situations. So are changes in depression rating scores (e.g., HRSD, MADRS, Clinical Global Impressions). They are not complete enough to serve the best interests of patients who were high functioning. Studies of treating depression in hospitalized patients are primarily concerned about the suitability of patients for discharge from supervised care in the hospital.

This is a worthy and practical goal but is no substitute for bona fide restoration of persona and performance. Studies of patients with schizophrenia show that antipsychotics improve their psychological performance; these results do not apply to premorbidly high-functioning patients with acute or episodic conditions such as mood disorders, brief psychosis, or schizophreniform disorder.

Surely, with sufficiently large dosing, antipsychotic drugs acutely diminish the severity of depressive, manic, psychotic, and anxious symptoms. These are the drugs psychiatrists depend on to defervesce activated behavior, including agitation and active suicidality. We are not concerned with the closely supervised use of antipsychotic drugs for a month or less, to acutely suppress such symptoms, because it has no persisting effects. The focus is on persistent use in high doses.

Overall, studies suggest that the preponderance of improvement in psychotic depression with the tricyclic–antipsychotic combination derives from the tricyclic unless massive doses of antipsychotic drug are administered. Summarization of 17 studies found that 82% of patients with psychotic depression responded to ECT versus 77% to an antipsychotic–tricyclic combination and 51% to antipsychotics alone (Spiker et al., 1985). In one trial of perphenazine alone at 64 mg/d ($=$ 800 mg/d chlorpromazine) for five weeks in psychotic depression, the response rate was 19% for perphenazine alone but 78% for perphenazine combined with amitriptyline (Spiker et al., 1985).

By interfering with elimination of tricyclic antidepressants from the body (through the cytochrome P450 metabolic pathways), perphenazine boosts tricyclic levels. Moreover, tricyclics do likewise to perphenazine. Accordingly, combination medication clinical trials need an additional step of controlling blood drug levels. In a study with controlled nortriptyline blood levels in patients older than 50 years, response rates after four weeks were 47% both for nortriptyline alone and with an average of 19 mg/d perphenazine (Mulsant et al., 2001). In other words, these large but lower perphenazine doses were equivalent to placebo. Similarly, decreasing high doses of antipsychotic drugs in patients who responded to a tricyclic–antipsychotic combination leads to rapid relapse (Perry et al., 1982).

During six weeks of treatment, depression severity (Bech-Rafaelsen Melancholia Scale score) decreased by 70% with amitriptyline 180 mg/d plus haloperidol averaging 9 mg/d. This decrease was significantly greater than the 50% decrease with risperidone averaging 7 mg/d. Response occurred in 38/51 (75%) of the former and 24/47 (51%) of the latter. These patients had a variety of conditions that included both psychotic and depressive symptoms (Müller-Siecheneder et al., 1998).Amitriptyline apparently contributed substantially to the clinical responses, but the antipsychotic drug doses were high in both groups.

Although such studies indicate that persistent high doses of antipsychotics are needed to substantially mitigate resistant mood disorders and acute psychoses, psychiatrists at a prominent academic medical center prescribed such high doses to only 6% of patients with psychotic depression (Andreescu et al., 2007). More impressive is that a survey from the same medical center 10 years prior reported the same results (Mulsant et al., 1997). This finding implies that faculty psychiatrists are reluctant to prescribe the high antipsychotic doses that they know are required to decrease severity.

There is no reason to expect that SSRI–antipsychotic combinations are any better than tricyclic–antipsychotic combinations. Because tricyclics are more appropriate to melancholia and psychotic depression than SSRIs are, combining an antipsychotic with an SSRI should be less effective than with a tricyclic. Of two separately conducted double-blind clinical trials in psychotic depression, one found no differences among placebo, olanzapine, and olanzapine–fluoxetine combination. The other found greater improvement with the combination than with the placebo; improvement with olanzapine alone was in-between (Rothschild et al., 2004). However, fluoxetine impedes olanzapine elimination and increases its blood levels (Nelson and Swartz, 2000); this factor was not controlled for and can explain the results. Moreover, improvement on the combination was only twice that of placebo. Placebo response in psychotic depression points away from melancholia and toward dissociative phenomena associated with an anxiety disorder, described as "pseudopsychosis" or false psychotic depression (Swartz and Shorter, 2007a). Overall, the results of these two clinical trials do not indicate reliable efficacy for using olanzapine or its combination with fluoxetine for psychotic depression. The drug advocacy in that article should be considered in view of co-authorship by several employees of the drug manufacturer. ECT efficacy in the most common types of psychotic depression is 83% to 95% (Swartz and Shorter, 2007b).

Several studies have purported to treat "treatment-resistant depression" with an SSRI–antipsychotic combination. There is a basic omission in this diagnostic-like classification – it is not a diagnosis. It does not have characteristic signs or symptoms. Does the particular patient have an endogenous type (e.g., melancholic, catatonic, psychotic) or atypical type depression? Even the DSM stipulates that the atypical and melancholic types are mutually exclusive, that is, fundamentally different. Treatment-resistant depression can be melancholia irrelevantly treated with an SSRI. It can be atypical depression, whether accompanied by prominent somatic tension anxiety (Swartz, 2004c) that does not respond to SSRIs or misfitted with a tricyclic or bupropion. It can be major depression with catatonic features that rarely responds to any medication. Even ECT would not do well against atypical depression (see Chapter 22). Without additional information we cannot interpret the results from studies of depression characterized without more detail about psychopathology than "treatment-resistant." Even bipolar I depression has this same problem, because many patients with bona fide melancholic episodes eventually develop an anxiety disorder (or atypical depression) when not in an an episode of mania or melancholia.

The rebuttal to this logic is that these patients have unsubtyped major depression, just as in most studies of antidepressant treatment, so the studies are as valid as are studies of depression not known to be resistant. In other words, their results are just as valid or invalid. They seem as valid as putting a malfunctioning pen into a pencil sharpener. What you get might dribble ink but it is not a reasonable approach.

Typical results state remission rates of 27% for olanzapine–fluoxetine combination, 17% for fluoxetine, and 15% for olanzapine over eight weeks, without compensation for the fluoxetine-induced olanzapine level boost (Thase et al., 2007). No placebo was given, but we know that fluoxetine by itself approximates placebo, so these results show low efficacy. A comparison among these three treatments for bipolar I and II depressions found no differences among them over eight weeks (Amsterdam and Shults, 2005). A drug company–run comparison in bipolar I depression claimed remission in 25% with placebo, 33% with olanzapine, and 49% with an olanzapine–fluoxetine combination, again without correcting for higher olanzapine levels in the lattermost group (Tohen et al., 2003). The high placebo response indicates that the patients studied were not candidates for ECT, and it also indicates low drug efficacy.

ECT versus benzodiazepines in catatonia

It is reassuring that catatonia can be relieved by an intramuscular or oral dose of lorazepam (Hatta et al., 2007; Rosebush et al., 1990) or a related medication (e.g., clonazepam, diazepam, zolpidem, amobarbital). The lorazepam response gives the physician a feeling of empowerment over the troublesome condition of catatonia. Sometimes this response is sudden, dramatic, and wide ranging. The catatonia can seemingly melt into mundane normality. The patient expresses a return to consciousness, surprise at where he is, and gratitude to the hero psychiatrist for his wonderful rescue. The patient's family feels relieved by this improvement and asserts that the patient is completely back to his or her normal self, so that there is absolutely no need for any ECT. They imagine that any medication that is powerful enough to bring such a rapid and vast improvement must bring a satisfactory outcome by itself. They too praise the psychiatrist for this miraculous cure. What is the psychiatrists' published response to receiving such acclaim? Do they longitudinally examine the clinical outcome of giving lorazepam? Do they compare lorazepam with something else? Or do they prefer to accept the praise, discharge the patient, and assume the patient lives happily henceforth? Most publication authors are medical school psychiatrists, and after they discharge the patient other physicians likely provide follow-up.

Indeed, aside from a couple of individual cases there has been no longitudinal study of lorazepam or any related drug in mitigating catatonia. There is no evidence that any of these drugs provide a stable remission. My experience is that, after a few weeks, lorazepam loses efficacy and catatonia starts returning, major depression becomes prominent, or psychosis appears. I have seen just one stable remission of episodic catatonia on lorazepam. Peculiarly, this patient showed apparently normal function with merely 0.25-mg lorazepam. With dosage greater than 1 mg/d he was noticeably obtunded. He remained well on 0.25 mg twice daily for the several months I could follow up.

Examined in more detail, even the acute effect of benzodiazepines can be disappointing. In one study of 41 patients, 21 showed no change, 19 showed disappearance of some but not all catatonic signs, and only 1 showed complete suppression of catatonia (Hatta et al., 2007).

Patients who take a benzodiazepine such as lorazepam usually experience several adverse effects. These include impairments in concentration, psychomotor performance (including driving), learning ability, and memory, and a disinhibiting change of personality (Buffett-Jerrott and Stewart, 2002; Hindmarch et al., 1993; O'Hanlon et al., 1982). These problems persist for as long as the benzodiazepine is taken. However, persistent cognitive impairments have been seen even six months after stopping benzodiazepines (Barker et al., 2004). Older patients experience cognitive function decline from benzodiazepines more commonly and severely, and to the extent of dementia (Paterniti et al., 2002). Although these same problems can occur with ECT, they fade within one to five weeks of the last ECT session. This distinction is obviously important to quality of life.

Until proven otherwise, the lorazepam response in catatonia is analogous to the Tensilon® (edrophonium) test for myasthenia gravis. The effects are useful as a diagnostic aid or temporary aid to patient management, but not as treatment. Lorazepam can help the patient participate in informed consent for ECT and cooperate with treatment for medical conditions (such as infections) and with ECT procedures.

In contrast, ECT reliably relieves catatonia (see Chapter 7). The remission is generally stable when ECT is followed by prophylaxis with an antimelancholic medication such as lithium, a tricyclic antidepressant, or bupropion (Swartz et al., 2001). In comparison, prophylaxis with an SSRI after ECT does not produce a good outcome.

Physician behavior

Why might physician preference go to antipsychotic drugs instead of ECT in treating first-episode psychosis or psychotic depression? There may be a clue within several publications focusing on psychotic depression. These publications did not express doubt about ECT efficacy; they expressed personal opinions. "ECT does not provide . . . for the large numbers of patients who prefer pharmacologic treatment" and "patients don't like ECT." Another author group dramatically exclaimed "[by] its very nature, the induction of an epileptic seizure can seem barbaric, and overtones of social control remain . . . its use is complicated by the . . . need to starve the patient." One psychiatrist one-sidedly asserted, "the availability, cost, stigma, and side effects associated with ECT have limited its use as a first-line treatment." However, these statements do not apply to the patients of psychiatrists who are proficient in ECT practice.

Doctors experienced with ECT generally appreciate that it is incomparably more cruel to allow patients to remain ill and impaired than to regain health and pre-illness persona with ECT or a specific treatment medication such as lithium, nortriptyline, or bupropion, despite any side effects of treatment. There is no barbarism, social control, or starvation in modern ECT. In comparison, antipsychotic drugs can easily be used for social control in people who are not psychotic. Indeed, their expanding indications for nonpsychotic conditions and predominant off-label use suggest social control. We all know psychiatrists who press antipsychotic drugs for virtually any behavioral deviance; I have seen several self-styled "medical police." ECT cannot work in this way. Of course, aspects of barbarism and starvation occur in surgery, behavior therapy, and weight loss treatment, but these are only incidental when these treatments are used with appropriate selectivity. The allegations noted against ECT can be interpreted as a defense against the question of what ethical reasons a psychiatrist could have in advocating antipsychotic drugs over ECT when ECT might well work and can be provided. Several reasons are possible, such as inability to comply with prophylactic treatment after the ECT course, but I doubt these apply in most circumstances.

Throughout this essay, and my professional career, the forces of habit and others' expectations have enforced my consistent use of the misnomer "antipsychotic" on this class of drugs. Just as the primary use of these drugs is not antipsychotic, neither is their primary action. Surely, mentioning "antipsychotic" to patients who are not psychotic and their families causes confusion, if not some loss of credibility. Rather, these drugs are primarily "thought simplifiers," a characterization that I have previously advocated (Swartz, 2003a, 2003b). Removing objects from a messy child's room incidentally lessens disorganization; these drugs operate likewise. A very empty room is an uninteresting place to dwell, and it can be a prison. The intent of thought simplification by giving medications differs fundamentally from the personal independence we aim to achieve with ECT.

I fervently wish that pills were available to make surgery unnecessary, but no pill can mend a hernia, remove a ruptured spleen, or excise a brain tumor. Surely I wish that medications or transcranial magnetic stimulation worked as safely, reliably, and well as ECT, but they do not. Pretending they do is harmful to patients. As turnabout is fair play, in an earlier medical era, Hemingway artfully blamed ECT for interfering with his writing: "it was a brilliant cure but we lost the patient." Hemingway had not tasted antipsychotics. If he had, he surely would have said nothing.

References

Amsterdam, J. D. and Shults, J. 2005. Comparison of fluoxetine, olanzapine, and combined fluoxetine plus olanzapine initial therapy of bipolar type I and type II major depression – lack of manic induction. J Affect Disord 87: 121–30.

Andreescu, C., Mulsant, B. H., Peasley-Miklus, C., et al. 2007. STOP-PD Study Group. Persisting low use of antipsychotics in the treatment of major depressive disorder with psychotic features. J Clin Psychiatry 68: 194–200.

Avery, D. and Winokur, G. 1976. Mortality in depressed patients treated with electroconvulsive therapy and antidepressants. Arch Gen Psychiatry 33: 1029–37.

Barker, M. J., Greenwood, K. M., Jackson, M., et al. 2004. Persistence of cognitive effects after withdrawal from long-term benzodiazepine use: A meta-analysis. Arch Clin Neuropsychol 19: 437–54.

Bassett, S. S. 2005. Cognitive impairment in Parkinson's disease. Prim Psychiatry 12: 50–5.

Bigelow, H. J. 1850. Dr. Harlow's case of recovery from the passage of an iron bar through the head. Am J Med Sci 20: 13–22.

Birkenaes, A. B., Birkeland, K. I., Engh, J. A., et al. 2008. Dyslipidemia independent of body mass in antipsychotic-treated patients under real-life conditions. J Clin Psychopharmacol 28: 132–7.

Birkenaes, A. B., Opjordsmoen, S., Brunborg, C., et al. 2007. The level of cardiovascular risk factors in bipolar disorder equals that of schizophrenia: A comparative study. J Clin Psychiatry 68: 917–23.

Buffett-Jerrott, S. E. and Stewart, S. H. 2002. Cognitive and sedative effects of benzodiazepine use. Curr Pharm Des 8: 45–58.

Capasso, R. M., Lineberry, T. W., Bostwick, J. M., et al. 2008. Mortality in schizophrenia and schizoaffective disorder: An Olmsted County, Minnesota cohort: 1950–2005. Schizophr Res 98(1–3): 287–94.

Carpenter, W. T. Jr. and Buchanan, R. W. 1994. Schizophrenia. N Engl J Med 330: 681–90.

Chouinard, G., Annable, L., and Ross-Chouinard, A. 1986. Supersensitivity psychosis and tardive dyskinesia: A survey in schizophrenic outpatients. Psychopharmacol Bull 22: 891–6.

Cohen, R. M., Nordahl, T. E., Semple, W. E., et al. 1997. The brain metabolic patterns of clozapine- and fluphenazine-treated patients with schizophrenia during a continuous performance task. Arch Gen Psychiatry 54: 481–6.

Cohen, R. M., Semple, W. E., Gross, M., et al. 1989. Evidence for common alterations in cerebral glucose metabolism in major affective disorders and schizophrenia. Neuropsychopharmacology 2: 241–54.

Corona, G., Mannucci, E., Fisher, A. D., et al. 2007. Effect of hyperprolactinemia in male patients consulting for sexual dysfunction. J Sex Med 4: 1485–93.

Cotterchio, M., Kreiger, N., Darlington, G., and Steingart, A. 2000. Antidepressant medication use and breast cancer. Am J Epidemiol 151: 951–7.

Crebbin, K., Mitford, E., Paxton, R., and Turkington, D. 2008. First-episode psychosis: An epidemiological survey comparing psychotic depression with schizophrenia. J Affect Disord 105: 117–24.

Downs, J. M., Akiskal, H. G., and Rosenthal, T. L. 1993. Neuroleptic-induced pseudoschizoaffective disorder [Abstract 146]. Proceedings of the American Psychiatric Association Annual Meeting, p. 153 (full program on audiotape).

Fors, B. M., Isacson, D., Bingefors, K., and Widerlöv, B. 2007. Mortality among persons with schizophrenia in Sweden: An epidemiological study. Nord J Psychiatry 61: 252–9.

Glazer, W. M., Morgenstern, H., and Doucette, J. T. 1993. Predicting the long-term risk of tardive dyskinesia in outpatients maintained on neuroleptic medications. J Clin Psychiatry 54: 133–9.

Gunne, L. M. and Andren, P. E. 1993. An animal model for coexisting tardive dyskinesia and tardive parkinsonism: A glutamate hypothesis for tardive dyskinesia. Clin Neuropharmacol 16: 90–5.

Harrison, B. E. and Therrien, B. 2007. Effect of antipsychotic medication use on memory in patients with Alzheimer's disease: Assessing the potential risk for accelerated recent autobiographical memory loss. J Gerontol Nurs 33: 11–20.

Hatta, K., Miyakawa, K., Ota, T., et al. 2007. Maximal response to electroconvulsive therapy for the treatment of catatonic symptoms. J ECT 23: 233–5.

Henderson, D. C., Daley T. B., Kunkel, L., et al. 2004. Clozapine and hypertension: A chart review of 82 patients. J Clin Psychiatry 65: 686–9.

Hindmarch, I., Sherwood, N., and Kerr, J. S. 1993. Amnestic effects of triazolam and other hypnotics. Prog Neuropsychopharmacol Biol Psychiatry 17: 407–13.

Joseph, K. S., Blais, L., Ernst, P., and Suissa, S. 1996. Increased morbidity and mortality related to asthma among asthmatic patients who use major tranquillisers. BMJ 312(7023): 79–82.

Kadar, A. G., Ing, C. H., White, P. F., et al. 2002. Anesthesia for electroconvulsive therapy in obese patients. Anesth Analg 94: 360–1.

Laursen, T. M., Munk-Olsen, T., Nordentoft, M., and Mortensen, P. B. 2007. Increased mortality among patients admitted with major psychiatric disorders: A register-based study comparing mortality in unipolar depressive disorder, bipolar affective disorder, schizoaffective disorder, and schizophrenia. J Clin Psychiatry 68: 899–907.

Lieberman, J. A., Stroup, T. S., McEvoy, J. P., et al. 2005. Effectiveness of antipsychotic drugs in patients with chronic schizophrenia. N Engl J Med 353(12): 1209–23.

Lisanby, S. H., Maddox, J. H., Prudic, J., et al. 2000. The effects of electroconvulsive therapy on memory of autobiographical and public events. Arch Gen Psychiatry 57: 581–90.

Lu, M. L., Pan, J. J., Teng, H. W., et al. 2002. Metoclopramide-induced supersensitivity psychosis. Ann Pharmacother 36: 1387–90.

Meyers, B. S., Klimstra, S. A., Gabriele, M., et al. 2001. Continuation treatment of delusional depression in older adults. Am J Geriatr Psychiatry 9: 415–22.

Miller, B. J., Paschall, C. B. 3rd, and Svendsen, D. P. 2006. Mortality and medical comorbidity among patients with serious mental illness. Psychiatr Serv 57: 1482–7.

Miller, R. and Chouinard, G. 1993. Loss of striatal cholinergic neurons as a basis for tardive and L-dopa-induced dyskinesias, neuroleptic-induced supersensitivity psychosis and refractory schizophrenia. Biol Psychiatry 34: 713–38.

Müller-Siecheneder, F., Müller, M. J., Hillert, A., et al. 1998. Risperidone versus haloperidol and amitriptyline in the treatment of patients with a combined psychotic and depressive syndrome. J Clin Psychopharmacol 18: 111–20.

Mulsant, B. H., Haskett, R. F., Prudic, J., et al. 1997. Low use of neuroleptic drugs in the treatment of psychotic major depression. Am J Psychiatry 154: 559–61.

Mulsant, B. H., Sweet, R. A., Rosen, J., et al. 2001. A double-blind randomized comparison of nortriptyline plus perphenazine versus nortriptyline plus placebo in the treatment of psychotic depression in late life. J Clin Psychiatry 62: 597–604.

Munk-Olsen, T., Laursen, T. M., Videbech, P., et al. 2007. All-cause mortality among recipients of electroconvulsive therapy: Register-based cohort study. Br J Psychiatry 190: 435–9.

Nelson, L. A. and Swartz, C. M. 2000. Melancholic symptoms from concurrent olanzapine and fluoxetine. Ann Clin Psychiatry 12: 167–70.

O'Hanlon, J. F., Blaauw, G. J., and Riemersma, J. B. J. 1982. Diazepam impairs lateral position control in highway driving. Science 217: 79–81.

Paterniti, S., Dufouil, C., and Alperovitch, A. 2002. Long-term benzodiazepine use and cognitive decline in the elderly: The Epidemiology of Vascular Aging Study. J Clin Psychopharmacol 22: 285–93.

Perry, P. J., Morgan, D. E., Smith, R. E., and Tsuang, M. T. 1982. Treatment of unipolar depression accompanied by delusions. ECT versus tricyclic antidepressant – antipsychotic combinations. J Affect Disord 4: 195–200.

Philibert, R. A., Richards, L., Lynch, C. F., and Winokur, G. 1995. Effect of ECT on mortality and clinical outcome in geriatric unipolar depression. J Clin Psychiatry 56: 390–4.

Plevin, D., Galletly, C., and Roughan, P. 2007. Sexual dysfunction in men treated with depot antipsychotic drugs: A pilot study. Sex Health 4: 269–71.

Potkin, S. G., Buchsbaum, M. S., Jin, Y., et al. 1994. Clozapine effects on glucose metabolic rate in striatum and frontal cortex. J Clin Psychiatry 55 Suppl B: 63–6.

Ray, W. A., Meredith, S., Thapa, P. B., et al. 2001. Antipsychotics and the risk of sudden cardiac death. Arch Gen Psychiatry 58: 1161–7.

Roemer, R. A., Dubin, W. R., Jaffe, R., et al. 1990. An efficacy study of single- versus double-seizure induction with ECT in major depression. J Clin Psychiatry 51: 473–8.

Rosebush, P. I., Hildebrand, A. M., Furlong, B. G., and Mazurek, M. F. 1990. Catatonic syndrome in a general psychiatric inpatient population: Frequency, clinical presentation, and response to lorazepam. J Clin Psychiatry 51: 357–62.

Rothschild, A. J., Williamson, D. J., Tohen, M. F., et al. 2004. A double-blind, randomized study of olanzapine and olanzapine/fluoxetine combination for major depression with psychotic features. J Clin Psychopharmacol 24: 365–73.

Saha, S., Chant, D., and McGrath, J. 2007. A systematic review of mortality in schizophrenia: Is the differential mortality gap worsening over time? Arch Gen Psychiatry 64: 1123–31.

Said, Q., Gutterman, E. M., Kim, M. S., et al. 2008. Somnolence effects of antipsychotic medications and the risk of unintentional injury. Pharmacoepidemiol Drug Saf 17: 354–64.

Samaha A. N., Reckless G. E., Seeman P., et al., 2008. Less is more: Antipsychotic drug effects are greater with transient rather than continuous delivery. Biol Psychiatry 64: 145–52.

Schneider, L. S., Dagerman, K. S., and Insel, P. 2005. Risk of death with atypical antipsychotic drug treatment for dementia. JAMA 294: 1934–43.

Spiker, D. G., Weiss, J. C., Dealy, R. S., et al. 1985. The pharmacological treatment of delusional depression. Am J Psychiatry 142: 430–6.

Stroup, T. S, Lieberman, J. A., McEvoy, J. P., et al. 2006. Effectiveness of olanzapine, risperidone and ziprasidone in patients with chronic schizophrenia following discontinuation of a previous atypical antipsychotic. Am J Psychiatry 163: 611–22.

Stueber, D. and Swartz, C. M. 2006. Carvedilol suppresses intractable hiccups. J Am Board Fam Med 19: 418–21.

Swartz, C. M. 1995. Tardive psychopathology. Neuropsychobiology 32: 115–19.

Swartz, C. M. 2001. Olanzapine-lithium encephalopathy. Psychosomatics 42: 370.

Swartz, C. M. 2002. Olanzapine-induced depression. J Pharm Technol 18: 321–3.

Swartz, C. M. 2003a, January 20. Antipsychotics as thought simplifiers. Psychiatric Times 1: 12–14.

Swartz, C. M. 2003b, February 20. Simplicity as a complication: Antipsychotics. Psychiatric Times 2: 44–6.

Swartz, C. M. 2004a, September 21. Iatrogenic cancer. Psychiatric Times 10: 21–4.

Swartz, C. M. 2004b, October 21. Antipsychotic psychosis. Psychiatric Times 11: 17–20.

Swartz, C. M. 2004c, April 21. Less anxiety but more violence? Psychiatric Times 4: 49–52.

Swartz, C. M., Morrow, V., Surles, L., and James, J. F. 2001. Long-term outcome after ECT for catatonic depression. J ECT 17: 180–3.

Swartz, C. M. and Shorter, E. 2007a. Psychotic depression. New York: Oxford University Press, Chapter 3, pp. 59–127.

Swartz, C. M. and Shorter, E. 2007b. Psychotic depression. New York: Oxford University Press, Chapter 7, pp. 192–234.

Thase, M. E., Corya, S. A., Osuntokun, O., et al. 2007. A randomized, double-blind comparison of olanzapine/fluoxetine combination, olanzapine, and fluoxetine in treatment-resistant major depressive disorder. J Clin Psychiatry 68: 224–36.

Tohen, M., Vieta, E., Calabrese, J., et al. 2003. Efficacy of olanzapine and olanzapine-fluoxetine combination in the treatment of bipolar I depression. Arch Gen Psychiatry 60: 1079–88.

Tsao, J., Shah, R., Leurgans, S., et al. 2008. Impaired cognition in normal individuals using medications with anticholinergic activity occurs following several years [Abstract S51.001]. Academy of Neurology, 60th Annual Meeting, April 17.

van Winkel, R., De Hert, M., Wampers, M., et al. 2008. Major changes in glucose metabolism, including new-onset diabetes, within 3 months after initiation of or switch to atypical antipsychotic medication in patients with schizophrenia and schizoaffective disorder. J Clin Psychiatry 69: 472–9.

Vythilingam, M., Chen, J., Bremner, J. D., et al. 2003. Psychotic depression and mortality. Am J Psychiatry 160: 574–6.

Wada, H., Nakajoh, K., Satoh-Nakagawa, T., et al. 2001. Risk factors of aspiration pneumonia in Alzheimer's disease patients. Gerontology 47: 271–6.

Wallace, W. A., Balsitis, M., and Harrison, B. J. 2001. Male breast neoplasia in association with selective serotonin re-uptake inhibitor therapy: A report of three cases. Eur J Surg Oncol 27: 429–31.

Weinberger, D. R., Bigelow, L. B., Klein, S. T., and Wyatt, R. J. 1981. Drug withdrawal in chronic schizophrenic patients: In search of neuroleptic-induced supersensitivity psychosis. J Clin Psychopharmacol 1: 120–3.

Whitty, P., Clark, M., McTigue, O., et al. 2005. Diagnostic stability four years after a first episode of psychosis. Psychiatr Serv 56: 1084–8.

Yamazawa, K., Matsui, H., Seki, K., and Sekiya, S. 2003. A case-control study of endometrial cancer after antipsychotics exposure in premenopausal women. Oncology 64: 116–23.

Yassa, R., Nastase, C., Dupont, D., and Thibeau, M. 1992. Tardive dyskinesia in elderly psychiatric patients: A 5-year study. Am J Psychiatry 149: 1206–11.

24

Informed consent

Peter B. Rosenquist

> Dear sir, to my endeavours give consent;
> Of heaven, not me, make an experiment.
> I am not an impostor that proclaim
> Myself against the level of mine aim;
> But know I think and think I know most sure
> My art is not past power nor you past cure.
> —William Shakespeare

In Shakespeare's comedy *All's Well That Ends Well*, Helena, the orphan daughter of a physician, heals the king of France and thereby earns her betrothal to Bertram. That she begs the king's consent before rendering treatment is evidence that even at the turn of the 17th century the royal treatment for patients embodied not only beneficence and nonmaleficence but also patient autonomy and the prior authorization of treatment. In a modern society in which so many live like royalty, the legal standard of informed consent applies to all, regardless of birthright or education.

The outcome of electroconvulsive therapy (ECT) includes all that does and does *not* end well – including treatment failure, early relapse, and the possibility of significant adverse effects. Our duty as physicians has evolved into an artful balancing act. Because patients have a right to effective treatment, the ECT physician must be appropriately persuasive. Because patients have the right to refuse treatment, the doctor must provide an honest and reasonably full disclosure and avoid coercion. Because illness and medications may affect understanding, the standard of care requires an assessment of capacity of each patient to consent for treatment. There is an ample (perhaps ponderous) literature articulating what is meant by "informed consent" and related concepts, divided among perspectives of law, medical ethics, and clinical care. There is a growing body of research addressing implications for consenters who are mentally ill. ECT practice includes a consistent methodology that conforms to the modern standard of informed consent.

Informed consent: Definitions and historical development

The defining ethical issue in the development of the legal doctrine of informed consent is the need to reconcile the competing values of autonomy and health (Appelbaum et al., 1987). The roots of autonomy are deeply embedded in Western civilization and manifest in the common law protections against assault, battery, and homicide and tort law protections against invasion of privacy. However, society has a competing interest in protecting the health of individuals and the public. The doctrine of *Parens Patriae* (father of his country) empowers the government as the guardian of persons unable to protect themselves legally. Therefore, we have compulsory quarantine and vaccination to prevent communicable diseases and involuntary commitment and treatment of persons adjudicated mentally ill and dangerous.

The earliest precedent for the individual's right to refuse treatment involves simple consent, satisfied by a single question: Does the patient agree to be treated? A "yes" satisfies simple consent, and a "no" means the physician may not treat. Today two more complex questions are required: "Did the physician provide the patient with adequate information?" and "Based on this information, did the patient give consent?"

A landmark ECT-related case in 1960 involving a plaintiff who received insulin coma therapy and ECT for the treatment of schizophrenia and fractured several vertebrae illustrates this additional duty. Although consent had been obtained, the court ruled that the physician was negligent for not fulfilling the affirmative duty to disclose risks of the treatment (*Mitchell v. Robinson*, 1960). A similar case involving burns secondary to radiation therapy decided that same year defined the need to disclose not only risk information, but also the nature of the illness, the nature of the proposed treatment, the probability of success, and possible alternative treatments (*Natanson v. Kline*, 1960). These five elements of disclosure should be familiar to anyone who has undergone or performed a procedure in the past 50 years. The quality and scope of the information needed for each of these elements has become far more comprehensive during this period.

Legal application of the doctrine of informed consent

Malpractice cases involving informed consent arise with an injurious outcome that does not result from negligence, whereas the patient alleges never being informed of the possibility of such harm. First it must be proven that the bad outcome was foreseeable but not communicated to the patient in advance. Second, it must be shown that, had the patient known of the particular negative outcome not disclosed, the patient would not have chosen that treatment or procedure and therefore would have avoided the injury.

In addition to challenging the evidence provided by the plaintiff, these circumstances may be reasonable exceptions to fully informed consent:

1. The injury is so exceedingly rare as to be unforeseeable.
2. Full informed consent was not possible because of time constraints and emergent circumstances.
3. The patient expressly deferred rights to the information and signed a waiver.
4. The physician invoked "therapeutic privilege" with the professional judgment that the patient would be harmed by the disclosure itself.

These situations are rare in ECT practice, although emergency need can occur (e.g., neuroleptic malignant syndrome, lethal catatonia). When patients are re-consented for maintenance ECT, they sign a new consent form and may decline in-depth repetition of all the informed consent information. However, the patient may not sufficiently remember the earlier discussion. By addressing at least briefly each element of informed consent and monitoring understanding with each re-consent, the duty is met and no exception is taken. Therapeutic privilege should not be invoked lightly. One cannot avoid specific topics because the patient may not receive this information favorably (Council on Ethical and Judicial Affairs, 1997).

The State of California Welfare and Institutions Code specifies that a patient contemplating ECT must undergo an informed consent review with a board-certified or eligible psychiatrist and sign a state-approved consent form. The California Superior Court ruled in 2005 that an ECT physician and psychiatric hospital were negligent in using an out-of-date consent form, as it did not warn of possible permanent memory loss. However, this negligence was determined to not be a factor in causing harm to memory or damages, as no out-of-pocket costs were incurred (*Atze Akkerman and Elizabeth Akkerman v. Joseph Johnson, Santa Barbara Cottage Hospital et al.*, 2005). A subsequent class action suit against ECT device manufacturer Mecta Corporation was also unsuccessful (*Atze Akkerman v. Mecta Corporation, Inc.*, 2007).

Practical strategies and methods to achieve informed consent

Informed consent is often raised during pre-ECT consultation (Klapheke, 1997), because all the elements of this consultation bear on it (McCall and Dickerson, 2001):

1. Confirmation of the psychiatric diagnosis;
2. Assessment of the severity of the psychiatric illness;

3. Documentation of the adequacy of previous treatment;
4. Assessment of the urgency of symptom relief;
5. Estimation of the likelihood of a good response to ECT versus alternative approaches;
6. Appraisal of the medical risk of ECT;
7. Examination of the patient's capacity to provide informed consent;
8. Recommendations regarding the need for additional tests or medical consultation prior to ECT; and
9. An overall recommendation for or against ECT.

Of patients enthusiastically recommended for ECT in a pre-ECT consultation, 92% received it, versus 52% of patients without enthusiastic recommendation and 7% for whom ECT was discouraged (McCall and Dickerson, 2001). Frequently, informed consent involves more than one meeting with the patient, and a variety of people can be involved. Informed consent decisions can be influenced by the referring physician, family members, nursing staff, and even other patients, and the consultant needs to consider how they have affected deliberations by asking, "What have you been told or what have you learned about ECT?" and "Is there anyone whom you plan to talk to before you make a decision?"

In one study, 69% of patients admitted to not reading the consent form before signing (Lavelle-Jones et al., 1993). Still, the formal consent form itself (typically abbreviated to a single page for inclusion in the medical record) is often accompanied by a separate detailed handout for the patient to keep. The Institute of Medicine has reported that consent documents frequently demand better reading skills than the majority of Americans have (Institute of Medicine Committee on Health Literacy, 2004). This finding implies that readability of these documents should be ensured by committee and that patients should have time to read the forms they sign.

Treatment may not proceed in the absence of a document signed by a patient deemed fully competent (or legally responsible proxy), the consenting physician, and usually a witness. Most written consent documents have the principal points grouped and summarized, but these should be seen as only the highlights simplified for the patient. Legally, the patient's signature ratifies the process and authorizes treatment. Some critics of the ECT informed consent process have suggested that the consent discussion be recorded so that each patient can be assured of the process even if memory of the proceedings is compromised (Donahue, 2000).

Discussion of the consent process

The informed consent process includes five basic elements (American Psychiatric Association [APA] Task Force on ECT, 1990) (See Figure 24.1). First, the patient

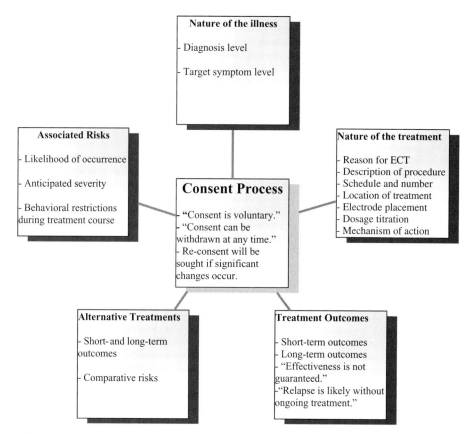

Figure 24.1 Informed consent criteria.

needs to understand the process of consent itself – that it is voluntary and can be withdrawn at any time. When compared with other procedures, ECT is less common by virtue of the consent being obtained for a course of treatment, which may include a number of individual treatments spread over several weeks or even months in the case of continuation or maintenance therapy. The consent is for a specified number of treatments, which should be included on the consent document. Sometimes the estimate of the number required will be more accurate because of prior experience with this patient. Lacking this, the clinician may estimate the median (typically, six treatments) or discuss how the number of treatments is determined, along with the usual range, agree with the patient on an initial number, and mention additional consent if more treatments are needed.

An offer should be extended to answer questions at any time, with names of individuals who can be contacted with such questions. Re-consent is advised any time that medical circumstances under which consent was given change substantially (e.g., an arrhythmia or some other health problem develops, whether ECT related or not).

When the process of information disclosure is shared with hospital staff or the patient views an instructional video (e.g., Dartmouth Hitchcock Medical Center Department of Psychiatry, 2001; Fink, 1986), the physician remains responsible for managing the quality of disclosure. This applies as well to any printed materials (Moll, 1986; Wohrm, 1994). Even with staff assistants and educational aid materials, an in-person meeting between patient and physician is needed to complete the informed consent process.

The patient should be made aware of the additional informed consent document and process with the anesthesiologist. The ECT physician should offer to field questions about ECT anesthesia and assist with definitive answers from the anesthesia team as needed.

Discussion of the nature of the illness

Rapport is facilitated when treatment goals are stated concretely, especially for patients with limited insight. The discussion can include ways the patient can regain independence, such as managing his own finances, making his own decisions, and leaving the hospital. The argument can be made that partial insight is evidence of incapacity. However, the patient may have an appreciation of the need for treatment without necessarily accepting the nomenclature. Swartz and Shorter (2007) offer a method for approaching ECT patients that builds insight on how the patient is perceived by others and the patient's personal concern for privacy:

"It starts with 'other people easily see that you are ill. You look ill, as if you have the flu.' Then you describe to the patient the signs of illness that other people see, such as: 'you look severely exhausted and worn out, you hardly move, you hardly speak, your voice sounds weak, your face looks stiff and wooden like a mask, you are drawn in to yourself and don't notice other people or try to help them.' Then continue, 'when other people see your movements and hear your speech they see that you are ill. They know your private business. There is a treatment that usually brings people back to looking normal and healthy, so that your health can be your private business again. This treatment is modern ECT.'"

Discussion of the reason for ECT and comparison with other treatment alternatives

The recommendation for ECT is made in the context of a discussion of all available treatment choices. For many hospitalized patients, ECT is an appropriate first-line treatment, but many prospective ECT patients will have already failed multiple medication trials. Therefore, the path of still another round of pharmacotherapy prior to ECT as per some algorithms might be chosen primarily by patients who wish to exhaust every conceivable alternative (Trivedi and Kleiber, 2001). Because

ECT is more effective for some conditions than for others, it is essential to clarify the diagnosis and the probable outcome to keep expectations realistic. Patients less likely to feel satisfied with the outcome (e.g., those with comorbid personality disorder) have the opportunity to choose with the understanding that ECT may not work as they hope. One colleague tells such patients, "I can't strongly recommend ECT, but there is a 50:50 chance that you will experience some temporary improvement." This is an acknowledgment of uncertainty about diagnosis and outcome. Many patients will respond to a noncommittal recommendation by requesting a stronger endorsement than warranted. Similarly, they may fixate on another treatment that is still less likely to be helpful.

Discussion of the nature of ECT treatment

Patients will frequently ask, "How does ECT work?" They may be asking about the procedural and technical aspects of treatment, but more likely this is a question about both the mechanism and stature of ECT. The short reply, "We don't know exactly how ECT works," does not really answer the question. Depending on the level of understanding, it may be appropriate to offer additional statements that convey the legitimacy of the treatment in relation to what is known about the state of illness (Wahlund and von Rosen, 2003). Andrade and Thyagarajan (2007) suggested using "politically correct" terminology to describe ECT, even going so far as to suggest an alternative name ("electrostimulatory therapy") that might be more easily accepted. They suggested this brief description:

"During electrostimulatory therapy, a . . . current is passed through the brain. The charge delivered is . . . commonly only about one tenth to one fifth of a coulomb. This current stimulates nerve cells across a wide range of brain territories and causes them to repeatedly signal in a synchronized fashion for about 1/2 to 1 minute. The stimulated nerve cells release chemicals which, in turn, elicit other changes in brain functioning. Antidepressant and other benefits are believed to result from some of these effects. The delivered current also stimulates the brain cells which control movement, resulting in brief contractions of the muscles of the body. As the muscular contractions are unnecessary for the therapeutic action of ECT, a muscle relaxant is administered before ECT. The entire treatment is conducted under brief general anesthesia so that there is no awareness of discomfort during the procedure. The procedure is painless."

This statement expects a lot. Few patients understand electricity, and "coulomb" is obscure. Patients sometimes ask "how many volts" are delivered, although they do not know what voltage is. A scientific term can be used if the doctor makes its meaning understood, by referring to what the patient does know. For example, regarding the electrical stimulus:

"The current that comes out of the wall socket is on continuously. In comparison, the electricity at ECT is given in brief pulses that each last about half of one-thousandth of a second. Then the current is off for about 20 times as long. Then another brief pulse is given, and so on. The current is off about 95% of the time. It is on for a total of about one-fifth of a second."

Discussion should also include where the procedure will be done, the time of day, how the stimulus dosage will be determined, the type of electrode placement, and the rationale for the recommended procedures. The discussion can be facilitated by having the patient view an instructional video (e.g., Fink, 1986; Dartmouth Hitchcock Medical Center Department of Psychiatry, 2001).

Discussion of risk

Understanding risk involves a basic comprehension of probability and uncertainty. Both frequency and severity of adverse outcomes must be described, along with their nature as temporary or permanent. Some patients do not understand percentages or fractions. Relative risk descriptions such as "likely," "common," "rare," and "extremely rare" should be used. *"About 1 in 10 people who get ECT experience a temporary state of confusion immediately following the treatment. This may last for several hours. For a few people this confusion may last longer."* The doctor can describe risk in his own experience (Tversky and Kahneman, 1974). *"I have not had a patient complain to me about (X side effect) in the 10 years I have been performing ECT, but there have been several cases described in the medical literature. It is possible, but I think this would be very unlikely."*

The patient should understand what will be done to minimize or mitigate risk but that these efforts are not guaranteed: *"We use muscle relaxant routinely to keep patients from feeling soreness after the treatment, but some still need medication for pain relief."* Risk mitigation is particularly important when the patient has a preexisting related condition, as with cardiovascular disease: *"You have high blood pressure, and ECT treatment may raise the pressure, so we recommend you take your blood pressure medication with a sip of water in the morning before you come for ECT. The anesthesiologist will also be monitoring your blood pressure and will use medications during the treatment, if needed."*

It is appropriate to admit uncertainty about adverse effects. For example, *"We don't know why some patients have more memory difficulty than others, and there have been a few individuals who complain that they have a permanent loss of memory for important events in their lives before ECT. However, psychiatric illness itself and many medications can lead to memory problems."*

Even clinically accurate terms can convey unintended meanings. Humans are taught to fear electricity, and even a static shock can provoke fear. It is natural for lack of knowledge to breed fear. Patients sometimes ask graphically, *"Doesn't ECT fry your brain?"* Questioning the patient about fears can identify misconceptions, and these can be directly refuted or clarified: *"Where did you learn this? To fry something you need heat, and ECT electricity does not put heat into the brain. Now there is a small chance of a burn on the skin if we don't clean it properly at the treatment. Our ECT instrument tests the connections to prevent skin burn."*

Opponents of ECT allege that practitioners of ECT ignore or suppress evidence of "brain damage"(Reisner, 2003). Citing Devanand et al. (1994), the APA Task Force report (2001) recommended that brain damage should not be stated as a potential risk, as neuropathological changes have not been found after ECT. Labeling the memory effects of ECT as "damage" is not appropriate and does not help patients understand the legitimate risks. Analogously, patients undergoing mitral valve repair are told specifically what can happen (e.g., stroke, infection, irregular rhythm), rather than nonspecific "heart damage." This is the standard of practice and it applies to ECT.

Obstacles to informed consent with a competent patient

Patients' recall of the elements of informed consent is faulty even when the information is straightforward and reinforced with visual aids (Hekkenberg et al., 1997; Mark and Spiro, 1990; Priluck et al., 1979). Poor recall is associated with advancing age, low IQ, depressed mood, and belief in having little control over personal health (Lavelle-Jones et al., 1993).

Preconceived notions about ECT are common. The process of informed consent routinely assumes that the patient has misconceptions and sets out to address them systematically, so the patient's mind will be open. Research into attitudes toward ECT has concerned both individuals naïve to treatment and patients who have completed ECT. Common preconceptions include that ECT is used to punish patients, is painful, and causes severe memory loss and brain damage (Dowman et al., 2005; Kerr et al., 1982). These impressions can be changed by education, including brochures and video programs (Andrews and Hasking, 2004; Battersby et al., 1993), and anxiety can be allayed by discussion with the physician (Kerr et al., 1982).

Patients who respond to ECT generally have a lasting favorable attitude toward it (Rosenquist et al., 2006; Sienaert et al., 2005). However, according to some consumer surveys (the "gray literature") and nonrandom internet "testimonies," half of ECT patients feel they were given insufficient information, and a third believed that they were coerced into ECT, although they had explicitly given written consent (Rose et al., 2003). Patient dissatisfaction about care received is certainly not new or confined to ECT; dissatisfaction occurs in about half of inpatients (Byrne et al., 1988). Patient dissatisfaction is part of many psychiatric disorders and is very common, so routine fulfillment of the tenets of informed consent is a cornerstone of ECT practice.

Competency

"It takes two to speak the truth – one to speak and another to hear."
—Henry David Thoreau, *A Week on the Concord and Merrimack Rivers*

"Capacity" and "competency" are bound to the consent process because mere disclosure, however well presented, can result in valid consent only if the patient is able to understand and decide. In the past mental illness was thought to invalidate consent. In the 19th century, patients were signed into the hospital by family and then received treatment as deemed appropriate by the medical staff (Appelbaum and Grisso, 1995). This approach changed with informed consent law and as courts began in the 1970s to require hearings for individualized determination of decision-making capacity. Determination of capacity is made first by a physician's assessment. It may be taken further to proceedings in which a judge determines competency. Without capacity or competency, both consent and refusal are disallowed, and a proxy must be identified to decide on the patient's behalf.

Usually a physician determines incapacity and seeks substituted decision making, sometimes assisted by a second medical opinion. There are no universally accepted criteria to determine capacity for consent, but four contributing abilities are frequently cited from case law (Appelbaum, 2007):

1. Understanding: The ability to comprehend relevant information;
2. Appreciation: The ability to apply information to one's own situation;
3. Reasoning: The ability to reflect on treatment options and consequences;
4. Communication of a choice: The ability to express one's decision.

Because the assessment by a physician can be questioned (Marson et al., 1997), standardized assessment tools to determine capacity to consent may be attractive. Sturman (2005) recently reviewed 10 such tools (one self-report and nine semistructured interviews). They were generally reliable, but varied in scope (measuring between one and all four of the competency criteria) and time for completion (10 to 20 minutes) (Sturman, 2005). The McArthur Competence Assessment Tool for Treatment (MacCAT-T) is a well-studied assessment tool with four subscales: understanding (scored 0 to 6), reasoning (0 to 8), appreciation (0 to 4), and expression of choice (0 to 2) (Grisso and Appelbaum, 1998).

Any diagnosis or condition affecting cognition may lead to impairments in capacity, for example, learning disability, stroke, dementia, and psychiatric disorders (Sturman, 2005). Lack of insight (about illness and need for treatment) was the strongest predictor of impaired capacity for psychiatric patients (Cairns et al., 2005). Across subscales, impairment varies widely. For the criterion of understanding, patients with dementia showed the most impairment (64.5%) followed by the schizophrenia (27.9%) and depression (17.1%) groups. For the reasoning component, the dementia and schizophrenia groups showed similar impairment (51.6% and 46.5%, respectively), whereas only 8.6% of patients with depression showed impairment. Impairment on the appreciation of disorder criterion occurred in no patients with depression, 22.6% of patients with dementia, and 16.3% of patients with schizophrenia. Only one depressed individual and three with schizophrenia failed to appreciate possible treatment benefits, compared with 32.3% of patients with dementia (Vollman et al., 2003).

There are a few reports about capacity for ECT consent. McCall and Dickerson (2001) reported that overall 13% of patients seen at first consultation needed further clarification about capacity to consent (specifically, 7% with unipolar depression, 13% with bipolar depression, and 13% with psychotic depression). Of depressed inpatients, most were competent, although repeated education and disclosure were sometimes needed (Roth et al., 1982). A group of 40 severely depressed individuals achieved high scores on the MacCAT-T, indicating adequate capacity to decide about ECT. Psychosis significantly decreased appreciation and reasoning subscores, and patients over 65 years old scored lower on understanding (Lapid et al., 2004a, 2004b). Overall, these reports indicate that most ECT patients are able to provide valid consent, but some have impaired capacity.

A semistructured approach is time consuming and can be disliked by highly educated patients, but can be useful in cases or groups of suspected incapacity. A typical first step is screening for dementia, psychosis, brain injury, or learning disability. Screening is followed by disclosure of ECT information and then by verification of understanding, appreciation, reasoning, and capacity for decision making. Appelbaum (2007) offered a questionnaire to assess competence with the expectation that "Any physician who is aware of the relevant criteria should be able to assess a patient's competence" (see Table 24.1). The National Quality Forum (2003) manual, "*Safe Practices for Better Healthcare*," recommends that clinicians "ask each patient or legal surrogate to teach back in his or her own words key information about the proposed treatments or procedures for which he or she is being asked to provide informed consent." Martin and Glancy (2007) described a questionnaire specific to ECT consent competency with 15 questions to measure patient understanding, appreciation, reasoning, and ability to make a choice.

The incapacitated ECT patient

In each case, the source of incapacity should be sought and attempts made to improve the patient's ability to consent. The medical evaluation is the same as for delirium, for example, dehydration, hypoxia, infection, sedating medications,

Table 24.1 Legally relevant criteria for decision-making capacity and approaches to assessment of the patient

Criterion	Patient's task	Physician's assessment approach	Questions for clinical assessment	Comments
Communicate a choice	Clearly indicate preferred treatment option	Ask patient to indicate a treatment choice	Have you decided whether to follow your doctor's (or my) recommendation for treatment? Can you tell me what that decision is? (If no decision) What is making it hard for you to decide?	Frequent reversals of choice because of psychiatric or neurologic conditions may indicate lack of capacity
Understand the relevant information	Grasp the fundamental meaning of information communicated by physician	Encourage patient to paraphrase disclosed information regarding medical condition and treatment	Please tell me in your own words what your doctor (or I) told you about: The problem with your health now The recommended treatment The possible benefits and risks (or discomforts) of the treatment Any alternative treatments and their risks and benefits The risks and benefits of no treatment	Information to be understood includes nature of patient's condition, nature and purpose of proposed treatment, possible benefits and risks of that treatment, and alternative approaches (including no treatment) and their benefits and risks

(continued)

Table 24.1 (*cont.*)

Criterion	Patient's task	Physician's assessment approach	Questions for clinical assessment	Comments
Appreciate the situation and its consequences	Acknowledge medical condition and likely consequences of treatment options	Ask patient to describe views of medical condition, proposed treatment, and likely outcomes	What do you believe is wrong with your health now? Do you believe that you need some kind of treatment? What is treatment likely to do for you? What makes you believe it will have that effect? What do you believe will happen if you are not treated? Why do you think your doctor has (or I have) recommended this treatment?	Courts have recognized that patients who do not acknowledge their illnesses (often referred to as "lack of insight") cannot make valid decisions about treatment Delusions or pathologic levels of distortion or denial are the most common causes of impairment
Reason about treatment options	Engage in a rational process of manipulating the relevant information	Ask patient to compare treatment options and consequences and to offer reasons for selection of option	How did you decide to accept or reject the recommended treatment? What makes (chosen option) better than (alternative option)?	This criterion focuses on the process by which a decision is reached, not the outcome of the patient's choice, because patients have the right to make "unreasonable" choices

Reprinted by permission: Appelbaum, 2007.

and medication withdrawal. Perhaps having someone else give the information can solve the problem, and family members can assist. For psychotic or catatonic patients, temporary medication (e.g., lorazepam) might allow the patient be able to understand and discuss treatment and consider informed consent. If a medication can temporarily substitute for ECT, it might be tried until the patient can consent. If these maneuvers are unsuccessful or if there is an emergency for ECT, consent by proxy should be sought without delay.

Court-ordered treatment and advance directives

There are several possibilities for patients who lack consent capacity. A difficult route is legal determination of incompetence and appointment of emergency guardianship. The guardian may be a family member or a guardian *ad litem* may be appointed. At the hearing, the judge will hear testimony from the treatment team and perhaps other witnesses. The patient has the right to oppose in person and to have representation. It may take one to three weeks to receive approval for court-ordered treatment. Proceeding through the courts can cause medically intolerable delay of treatment (Ottosson and Fink, 2004). The appointed guardian has the authority to consent for the patient. The process of disclosure is repeated, including examination of the guardian for capacity to consent.

This series of steps involving a guardian is skipped to the last step if the patient had authorized a health care power of attorney (POA). The clinician authorized to make the determination of incapacity may be specified in the advanced directive documents, but otherwise the attending physician makes the determination. The authorized POA is obliged to decide as the patient would if capable, and not according to the POA's own preferences. If the patient had demonstrated recent unrelenting informed refusal of ECT, so must the POA. Without clear guidance from history, the POA should consider consent according to the well-being of the patient.

Psychiatric advance directives (PADs) may include not just designation of a POA but provisions for "advance instructions" for common situations, such as preferences for or avoidances of specific medications, treatments, doctors, and hospitals. A survey of advance instructions from 106 patients in a mental health center reported that 72% declined ECT, 16% would consent, and 12% gave no instructions (Srebnik and Kim, 2006). The problem here is that there was no attempt to properly inform these patients about ECT, so there was no credible informed decision. Advance instructions may be helpful for patients who previously received ECT and wish to receive it again should they become incapacitated in an episode of psychiatric illness. To date, PADs have been completed by fewer than 5% of psychiatric patients (Swanson et al., 2006).

Summary

For patients the process of informed consent is a right. For physicians it is a duty and privilege. ECT practitioners are called on to demonstrate expertise in many aspects of the informed consent process, from skill in judging capacity for consent, to knowledge about the ECT procedure and ability to communicate clearly with candor and sensitivity.

References

American Psychiatric Association Committee on Electroconvulsive Therapy. 2001. The practice of electroconvulsive therapy: Recommendations for treatment, training and privileging. (A task force report of the American Psychiatric Association). Washington, DC: American Psychiatric Press.

American Psychiatric Association Task Force on ECT. 1990. The practice of ECT: Recommendations for treatment, training and privileging. Washington, DC: American Psychiatric Press.

Andrade, C. and Thyagarajan, S. 2007. The influence of name on the acceptability of ECT: The importance of political correctness. J ECT 23: 75–7.

Andrews, M. and Hasking, P. 2004. Effect of two educational interventions on knowledge and attitudes towards electroconvulsive therapy. J ECT 20: 230–6.

Appelbaum, P. S. 2007. Clinical practice. Assessment of patients' competence to consent to treatment. N Engl J Med 357: 1834–40.

Appelbaum, P. S. and Grisso, T. 1995. The MacArthur Treatment Competence Study. I. Law Hum Behav 19: 105–26.

Appelbaum, P. S., Lidz, C. W., and Meisel, A. 1987. Informed consent. New York: Oxford University Press.

Atze Akkerman and Elizabeth Akkerman v. Joseph Johnson, Santa Barbara Cottage Hospital et al. 2005. In 1069713 Superior Court of the State of California for the County of Santa Barbara.

Atze Akkerman v. Mecta Corporation, Inc. 2007. In 2d Civil No. B192109 Court of Appeal of the State of California Second Appellate District.

Battersby, M., Ben-Tovim, D. and Eden, J. 1993. Electroconvulsive therapy: A study of attitudes and attitude change after seeing an educational video. Aust N Z J Psychiatry 27: 613–19.

Byrne, D. J., Napier, A., and Cuschieri, A. 1988. How informed is signed consent? Br Med J (Clin Res Ed) 296: 839–40.

Cairns, R., Maddock, C., Buchanan, A., et al. 2005. Prevalence and predictors of mental incapacity in psychiatric in-patients. Br J Psychiatry 187: 379–85.

Council on Ethical and Judicial Affairs, 1997. Code of Medical Ethics. Chicago, IL.

Dartmouth Hitchcock Medical Center Department of Psychiatry. 2001. Electroconvulsive therapy. Hanover, NH.

Devanand, D.P., Dwork A.J., Hutchinson, E.R., et al. 1994. Does ECT alter brain structure? Am J Psychiatry 152: 1403.

Donahue, A. B. 2000. Electroconvulsive therapy and memory loss: A personal journey. J ECT 16: 133–43.

Dowman, J., Patel, A., and Rajput, K. 2005. Electroconvulsive therapy: Attitudes and misconceptions. J ECT 21: 84–7.

Fink, M. 1986. Informed ECT for patients and families (with Dr. Max Fink). Lake Bluff, IL: Somatics, LLC.

Grisso, T. and Appelbaum, P. S. 1998. The McArthur Competence Assessment Tool for Treatment (MacCAT-T). Sarasota, FL: Professional Resource Press.

Hekkenberg, R. J., Irish, J. C., Rotstein, L. E., et al. 1997. Informed consent in head and neck surgery: How much do patients actually remember? J Otolaryngol 26: 155–9.

Institute of Medicine Committee on Health Literacy. 2004. Health literacy: A prescription to end confusion. Washington, DC: National Academies Press.

Kerr, R. A., McGrath, J. J., O'Kearney, R. T., et al. 1982. ECT: misconceptions and attitudes. Aust N Z J Psychiatry 16: 43–9.

Klapheke, M. M. 1997. Electroconvulsive therapy consultation: An update. Convuls Ther 13: 227–41.

Lapid, M. I., Rummans, T. A., Pankratz, V. S., et al. 2004a. Decisional capacity of depressed elderly to consent to electroconvulsive therapy. J Geriatr Psychiatry Neurol 17: 42–6.

Lapid, M. I., Rummans, T. A., Poole, K. L., et al. 2004b. Decisional capacity of severely depressed patients requiring electroconvulsive therapy. J ECT 19: 67–72.

Lavelle-Jones, C., Byrne, D. J., Rice, P., and Cuschieri, A. 1993. Factors affecting quality of informed consent. BMJ 306: 885–90.

Mark, J. S. and Spiro, H. 1990. Informed consent for colonoscopy. A prospective study. Arch Intern Med 150: 777–80.

Marson, D. C., McInturrff, B., Hawkins, L., et al. 1997. Consistency of physician judgments of capacity to consent in mild Alzheimer's disease. J Am Geriatr Soc 45: 453–7.

Martin, B. A. and Glancy, G. D, 2007. Consent to electroconvulsive therapy: Investigation of the validity of a competency questionnaire. Convuls Ther 10: 279–86.

McCall, W. V. and Dickerson, L. A. 2001. The outcome of 369 ECT consultations. J ECT 17: 50–2.

Mitchell v. Robinson 1960. 334 S.W. 2d 11 Mo.

Moll, J. M. 1986. Doctor-patient communication in rheumatology: Studies of visual and verbal perception using educational booklets and other graphic material. Ann Rheum Dis 45: 198–209.

Natanson v. Kline 1960. 350 P. 2d 1093 Kan.

National Quality Forum. 2003. Safe practices for better health care: A consensus report. Washington, DC: National Quality Forum.

Ottosson, J. O. and Fink, M. 2004. Ethics in electroconvulsive therapy. New York: Brunner-Routledge.

Priluck, I. A., Robertson, D. M., and Buettner, H. 1979. What patients recall of the preoperative discussion after retinal detachment surgery. Am J Ophthalmol 87: 620–3.

Reisner, A. D. 2003. The electroconvulsive therapy controversy: Evidence and ethics. Neuropsychol Rev 13: 199–219.

Rose, D., Wykes, T., Leese, M., et al. 2003. Patients' perspectives on electroconvulsive therapy: Systematic review. Br Med J 326: 1–5.

Rosenquist, P. B., Dunn, A., Rapp, S., et al. 2006. What predicts patients' expressed likelihood of choosing electroconvulsive therapy as a future treatment option? J ECT 22: 33–7.

Roth, L. H., Lidz, C. W., Meisel, A., et al., 1982. Competency to decide about treatment or research. Int J Law Psychiatry 5: 29–50.

Sienaert, P., DeBecker, T., Vansteelandt, K., et al. 2005. Patient satisfaction after electroconvulsive therapy. J ECT 21: 227–31.

Srebnik, D. S. and Kim, S. Y. 2006. Competency for creation, use, and revocation of psychiatric advance directives. J Am Acad Psychiatry Law 34: 501–10.

Sturman, E. D. 2005. The capacity to consent to treatment and research: A review of standardized assessment tools. Clin Psychol Rev 25: 954–74.

Swanson, J. W., Swartz, M. S., Elbogen, E. B., et al. 2006. Facilitated psychiatric advance directives: A randomized trial of an intervention to foster advance treatment planning among persons with severe mental illness. Am J Psychiatry 163: 1943–51.

Swartz, C. M. and Shorter, E. 2007. Psychotic depression. New York: Cambridge University Press.

Trivedi, M. H. and Kleiber, B. A. 2001. Algorithm for the treatment of chronic depression. J Clin Psychiatry 62, Suppl 6: 22–9.

Tversky, A. and Kahneman, D. 1974. Judgement under uncertainty: Heuristics and biases. Science 185: 1124–31.

Vollman, J., Bauer, A., Danker-Hopfe, H., et al. 2003. Competence of mentally ill patients: A comparative empirical study. Psychol Med 33: 1471.

Wahlund, B. and von Rosen, D. 2003. ECT of major depressed patients in relation to biological and clinical variables: A brief overview. Neuropsychopharmacology 28, Suppl 1: S21–S26.

Wohrm, A. 1994. Educational illustrations as an aid in patient-doctor communication, exemplified by patients with dyspepsia. Scand J Prim Health Care 12: 84–7.

25

Electroconvulsive therapy in the medically ill

Keith G. Rasmussen and Paul S. Mueller

Introduction

This chapter focuses on prevention of electroconvulsive therapy (ECT-) related morbidity and mortality. There are three general steps in the management of medically ill patients receiving ECT. The first is careful pretreatment assessment and stabilization of medical problems. In addition to the obligatory medical history and physical examination, laboratory studies, electrocardiogram, chest x-ray, echocardiogram, and exercise stress test should be selectively considered. ECT may need to be delayed until decompensated medical concerns (e.g., angina pectoris, severe hypertension, asthma, poorly controlled diabetes mellitus) are stabilized. The ECT clinician should have access to specialist consultants, such as from internal medicine or cardiology, to advise on the pre-ECT evaluation.

The second step is planned management of medical concerns during ECT sessions. In addition to customary ECT anesthesia (see Chapter 26), additional medications, such as anticholinergics, beta blockers, or antiarrhythmics, can be selected for individual patient needs.

The third step is regularly repeated reevaluation during the ECT course to check for emerging medical complications. For example, a patient with congestive heart failure (CHF) may be stable enough to commence ECT but then decompensate after several treatments, so that further treatment must be postponed. Regular reevaluation can be made routine on the mornings of ECT.

Ordinarily, recommendations for evaluation and management of medically ill patients are based on systematic clinical trials. However, studies specific to ECT patients are lacking. Individual and series case reports are too numerous to compile here. Rather, we draw on selected literature together with extensive clinical experience in evaluating and treating medically complicated ECT patients. Our focus is ECT, and we do not review the management of complications that can emerge, such as myocardial ischemia. Those topics are in standard medical textbooks.

Cardiovascular disorders

There is increased stress on the heart during ECT treatments. There is a sharp increase in heart rate (see Chapter 30) and blood pressure during ECT seizure that normally returns to baseline within a few minutes postictally (Rasmussen et al., 1999). A variety of brief electrocardiogram (ECG) changes can occur during and shortly after the seizure, including P-R interval, QTc interval, and ST-T wave changes as well as premature atrial contractions, premature ventricular contractions (PVCs), paroxysmal supraventricular tachyarrhythmias, and short, non-hemodynamically significant runs of ventricular tachycardia (Rasmussen et al., 2004). Most of these rhythm disturbances are benign and require no treatment. Serious dysrhythmias or hemodynamic compromise necessitates immediate treatment. Finally, there are numerous reports in which transthoracic echocardiographic assessment was performed during or after ECT. Left ventricular systolic dysfunction (globally or regionally) can occur, is typically transient, and resolves spontaneously without adverse consequences (Rasmussen et al., 2004). ECT can pose some risk for patients with cardiac conditions such as coronary artery disease (CAD), dysrhythmias, or CHF. Although this risk has not been systematically and prospectively studied, practitioners should be conservative with the prospective ECT patient who has cardiac illness. An applicable practical reference is the 2007 American College of Cardiology/American Heart Association (ACC/AHA) *Guidelines on Perioperative Cardiovascular Evaluation and Care for Noncardiac Surgery* (ACC/AHA, 2007). The first step for such patients is to determine if the need for ECT is emergent, for example, catatonia, stupor, functional delirium, or mania. The second step is to determine if the patient has an active cardiac condition such as new, unstable, or severe angina pectoris; recent myocardial infarction (MI); decompensated CHF; significant dysrhythmia; severe aortic stenosis; or symptomatic mitral stenosis. Generally, medical stabilization should be accomplished before ECT. If the patient does not have an active cardiac condition, the third step is to determine the cardiac risk of the procedure. If it is low (e.g., less than 1%), ECT can be administered without further evaluation; indeed, no fatalities occurred in one large series of ECT patients (Nuttall et al., 2004). Cases in which the patient- or ECT-related cardiac risks are unclear should be referred to either an internal medicine or cardiology specialist. We now consider specific cardiac conditions.

CHF

Patients with CHF should be carefully assessed and monitored before and during ECT. As CHF patients are particularly sensitive to the sympathetic nervous system stimulation that routinely occurs during ECT, there may be an aggravation of compromised left ventricular function. The medical history should focus on symptoms of CHF such as dyspnea at rest or with minimal exertion and new or marked orthopnea. Physical examination may reveal pulmonary rales, jugular venous distention, an S3 gallop, peripheral edema, or other findings. The evaluation should also include sodium, potassium, creatinine, complete blood count, ECG, and a chest x-ray. Although assessing resting left ventricular function with echocardiography has not been a consistent predictor of periprocedure ischemic events (ACC/AHA, 2007), it can be helpful in the medical management (e.g., selection of medications) of patients with CHF. Patients with a history of CHF should undergo echocardiography if the study has not been done within two years of the planned ECT sessions or if symptoms and signs of CHF are new or have worsened.

Patients with decompensated CHF should not undergo ECT as they are at high risk for complications from the procedure and the anesthesia. Instead, the cardiac status of these patients should be optimized (e.g., diuresis, initiation of CHF-specific medications) before ECT treatment. Patients with stable or compensated CHF are much less likely to experience complications related to ECT and anesthesia, and with proper monitoring and management, they typically tolerate the procedures.

Cardiac medications should be administered in the morning before the treatment with a small amount of water. Sufficient time for absorption of the medication should be allowed. Recent practice guidelines caution against administration of diuretic agents in the morning of ECT to avoid bladder rupture or incontinence during the seizure (American Psychiatric Association Committee on ECT, 2001, p. 82). However, we recommend administering diuretics to patients to avoid pulmonary congestion and decompensation. Patients can be instructed to void their bladder just before treatment.

During the ECT session clinicians should pay particular attention to rhythm disturbances and be aware that they may be more difficult to treat in the CHF patient. Clinicians should also monitor for acute left or right ventricular failure, which can occur during ECT treatments. Such complications should be rapidly treated.

Anticholinergic agents such as glycopyrrolate or atropine help reduce bradyarrhythmias during ECT but also may increase myocardial workload. On balance, current practice is to at least start with a low dose and withhold it during future treatments if the patient experiences urinary hesitancy.

The use of β-adrenergic receptor antagonists, such as esmolol or labetalol, may help prevent sympathetic stimulation-induced hypertension and left ventricular decompensation as well as dysrhythmias. Such agents should be used with caution, however, because they can have deleterious effects on ventricular pump function.

The importance of intertreatment assessment in patients with CHF is demonstrated by the reported patient of Goldberg and Badger (1993), who died of congestive decompensation that began several days after the last ECT treatment.

Daily rounds should include assessment of breathing and physical examination for the signs of CHF. If any new significant findings occur, additional ECT treatments should be delayed until stabilization.

CAD/Post-MI

Cardiology consultation should probably be conducted before undertaking ECT in the patient with a history of CAD or MI. Such issues as risk assessment, advisability of pre-ECT cardiac testing, and adjustment of cardiac medications can be addressed by a cardiologist.

Cardiac medications should be administered in the morning before the treatment with a small amount of water. Sufficient time for medication absorption should be allowed. Risk-reduction strategies exist for the ECT patient with CAD, but none have been proven to reduce serious complications. For example, it is uncertain whether pretreatment with β-adrenergic receptor antagonists reduces morbidity associated with ECT. Pretreatment with antihypertensive agents reduces peak heart rate and blood pressure during seizures. Whether this reduction translates into protection against cardiac complications is unknown. Zvara et al. (1997) and Castelli et al. (1995), for example, found no evidence that use of β-adrenergic receptor antagonists at the time of treatment reduced evidence of myocardial ischemia despite robust reductions in peak heart rate and blood pressure with these agents. An echocardiogram study found that the use of esmolol did not appear to impact changes associated with ECT treatment (O'Connor et al., 1996). Nevertheless, it seems reasonable to use β-adrenergic receptor antagonists in selected cases during ECT depending on the patient's hemodynamic status, carefully weighing the risks and potential benefits of such treatment. In our practice, we prefer to use labetalol, a combined α-β blocker, which seems to have a more robust effect on increases in blood pressure than does esmolol.

According to the ACC/AHA guidelines (2007), recent MI (within one month) is an "active cardiac condition" of high risk. Before undergoing ECT, such patients should be evaluated by a cardiologist. Some patients being considered for ECT have undergone balloon angioplasty and stent placement for CAD. Coupled with medications, these intracoronary artery procedures maximize myocardial perfusion and therefore reduce risk of cardiac events. To prevent coronary thrombosis, especially stent thrombosis, it is crucial to continue antiplatelet agents in these patients during ECT sessions.

Dysrhythmias

The most common cardiac dysrhythmia in ECT patients is atrial fibrillation (AF). There are numerous case reports and small series of patients with AF receiving

ECT without complications as well as patients who develop AF or convert from AF to sinus rhythm during ECT (reviewed in detail in Rasmussen et al., 2004). For the patient who is known to have AF before undergoing ECT, evaluation should include assessment by an internal medicine specialist. Questions to be answered include whether to alter the patient's current regimen and whether to convert the patient to sinus rhythm just for ECT. The latter may not be helpful as the patient may return to AF during the ECT sessions. In the patient without contraindication, anticoagulation should be maintained. First, for the patient who is not on chronic anticoagulation, consideration should be given to short-term anticoagulation (e.g., with heparin) during the ECT course. Second, consideration should be given to performing a transesophageal echocardiogram to check if an atrial clot is present. Third, the patient's heart rate should remain well controlled. Fourth, one must take into account any associated cardiovascular comorbidities, such as CAD, CHF, or valvular disease. Fifth, consideration should probably be given to premedication with a β-adrenergic receptor antagonist before inducing the seizure to lessen sympathetic stimulation. ECG rhythm should be inspected prior to each treatment. Finally, the patient without a history of AF who develops this rhythm during ECT obviously should undergo a thorough cardiac evaluation before ECT is resumed.

Dysrhythmias other than AF are occasionally encountered in ECT practice. For example, baseline PVCs are quite common and usually benign, requiring no further evaluation unless there is some other indicator of cardiac dysfunction.

Pacemakers/Implantable cardioverter defibrillators

There are numerous case reports and case series of patients with pacemakers or implantable cardioverter defibrillators (ICDs) who have undergone safe ECT (Dolenc et al., 2004). With modern pacemakers and ICDs, there is no risk of electrical damage to the device during ECT, assuming proper grounding of the patient (Dolenc et al., 2004).

In our practice, pacemaker patients undergo device interrogation prior to the ECT course. Beyond that, no particular precautions are needed with modern pacemakers (e.g., we do not use a magnet to deactivate, or "turn off," the device). However, ICDs should be deactivated prior to each ECT treatment, and the ICD should be deactivated only after the patient is connected to ECG monitoring, which should be continued at least until the ICD is reactivated.

Vascular disease

It seems prudent to image known aneurysms before ECT, to consult the appropriate specialist for expert assessment of degree of risk during treatments, and to suggest risk-reduction strategies. Use of β-adrenergic receptor blockade is recommended for such patients during ECT treatments.

In patients with hypertension, it is not necessary to achieve perfect blood pressure control before ECT. High blood pressure can be managed rapidly and effectively during the treatments with the availability of short-acting antihypertensive agents. Also, it is reassuring that blood pressure does not increase during a course of ECT beyond the postictal recovery period (Albin et al., 2007).

Valvular disease

Presence of an implanted valve is not in itself a high risk for ECT. Such patients should be appropriately anticoagulated before ECT commences (assuming they already are anticoagulated). A patient with aortic stenosis should have an echocardiogram performed if one has not been obtained recently. Aortic stenosis can present with a sudden severe drop in cardiac output in the face of increased myocardial oxygen demand, as can occur at ECT. Preferably, if a patient needs an aortic valve replacement, this would be done before ECT. However, because of the severity of psychiatric status, this may not be feasible. A recent series attested to safe use of ECT in 10 patients with severe aortic stenosis (Mueller et al., 2007). The major management strategy is to monitor for and avoid hypotension and myocardial ischemia, if possible. Hypotension should be managed with phenylephrine (or similar agents) and intravenous fluids.

Anticoagulation

AF, deep venous thrombosis, and mechanical cardiac valve replacement are common circumstances encountered in ECT that need anticoagulation. Appropriate blood monitoring of anticoagulation indices, such as international normalized ratio (INR) or partial thromboplastin time (PTT), should be done before and periodically during courses of ECT. Maintaining therapeutic warfarin anticoagulation during courses of ECT appears to be safe (Mehta et al., 2004). We do not withhold anticoagulants during ECT, nor do we "bridge" patients on warfarin to heparin. Notably, if a patient has a deep venous thrombosis of the leg, that leg should not be cuffed during ECT.

Neurological disorders

In contrast to cardiac conditions, there is very little the ECT practitioner can do to assess neurologic risk status through imaging studies, nor are there specific neuroprotective strategies to use. However, there are pertinent clinical considerations for patients with certain neurological disorders who are undergoing ECT.

Dementia

Numerous case series indicate that ECT can be efficacious for depression or mania in patients with dementia (reviewed in Rasmussen et al., 2004). The question is whether ECT causes undue acute or long-term cognitive effects in such patients. To address this question scientifically, one would need a population of diagnostically well-characterized patients with dementia (e.g., elucidation of dementia subtype such as Alzheimer, Lewy body, vascular) with a psychopathological syndrome responsive to ECT (e.g., depression or mania) who are randomly assigned to receive ECT or some other treatment with blind assessments of both psychopathologic and cognitive outcomes, both acutely and over several months of follow-up. No such trial has been done, nor is it likely to be. In approaching the patient with dementia who is a candidate for ECT, there are a few technical considerations. First, elderly patients with depression often have cognitive impairment that is difficult to characterize as related solely to depression or part of a separate dementing syndrome. If severely depressed, such patients may need to be treated with ECT if their depression is highly medication refractory. Prudence probably dictates considering an electrode placement other than bitemporal to start with to try to minimize cognitive side effects (see Chapter 27). Additionally, use of twice rather than thrice weekly treatment frequency may be considered for the same reason.

As part of the pre-ECT workup, if the patient's dementia syndrome etiology is well characterized, there is no need to perform neurodiagnostic testing specifically in preparation for ECT. If, however, there is still diagnostic uncertainty about the dementia etiology, further workup may be appropriate.

Patients with dementia are often treated with cholinesterase inhibitors, which theoretically might prolong the action of succinylcholine. Rasmussen et al. (2003) have reported safe use of ECT in patients taking donepezil. A prudent recommendation would be discontinuing such medication when no clear benefit is obtained but otherwise continuing it, keeping in mind possible prolonged succinylcholine action.

Movement disorders

The most common movement disorder in ECT patients is Parkinson's disease (PD). There is a scarce case report literature on other rare movement disorders (reviewed in Rasmussen et al., 2004). Case reports, case series, and even one sham-controlled trial point to an anti-parkinsonian effect of ECT in some patients (reviewed in

Rasmussen et al., 2004). Common side effects of ECT in PD patients include delirium and treatment-emergent dyskinesia, which probably indicate a dopaminergic effect (Douyon et al., 1989). This can be reduced by cautious lowering of dopamine agonist dosage (e.g., l-DOPA), under guidance by a neurologist. The duration of ECT-related anti-parkinsonian effects has been variable in long-term follow-up studies. There are several case reports of PD patients given maintenance ECT to extend the initial motor improvement with index courses of treatment. Maintenance ECT seemed to prevent relapses. The frequency of such treatments was quite variable, depending on the period of improvement each patient sustained. Cognitive impairment was noticeable in some cases. We recommend twice weekly treatment and the use of electrode placements that may cause less cognitive impairment (see Chapter 27).

ECT can be lifesaving for patients with neuroleptic malignant syndrome or other forms of malignant catatonia caused by medical problems or occurring as part of the natural history of a psychiatric disorders (American Psychiatric Association Committee on ECT, 2001). A question occurs whether succinylcholine is safe in such patients, given the clinical similarity between malignant catatonia and malignant hyperthermia. Theoretically, the latter represents dysfunction at the neuromuscular junction and the former involves centrally mediated phenomena, so there should be no overlap. Some anesthesiologists, however, still prefer to use a nondepolarizing paralytic agent in such patients.

Cerebrovascular disease

In assessing the safety of ECT in a patient with poststroke status, one would consider time since stroke, the size of the stroke, and whether the stoke was a bleed or thromboembolic. Preferably, one would like to avoid ECT in poststroke patients. Although no scientifically driven data exist regarding a safe poststroke interval before commencing ECT if needed, prudence dictates waiting at least several weeks, or longer if the stroke was hemorrhagic. Consultation with the patient's attending neurologist in the poststroke time period would be essential to gauge vascular stability.

If ECT is used, risk-reduction strategies may involve use of antihypertensives at the time of treatment (although carefully avoiding hypotension, which might compromise cerebral circulation) and monitoring the appropriate coagulation indicator (e.g., INR, PTT) in patients who are anticoagulated. Intracerebral aneurysms probably represent high-risk situations for ECT. If they are known to be present, ECT should be undertaken only after other treatment measures have failed. Additionally, aggressive measures to prevent blood pressure spikes during the ECT seizures should be used.

Epilepsy

Pre-ECT neuroimaging in the patient with epilepsy is not necessary unless there is some other aspect of the patient's neurologic status that would indicate such (e.g., a new focal neurologic finding on examination). Lunde et al. (2006) recently reported a large series of patients with epilepsy who were undergoing ECT and found that most patients could be treated effectively without changes in anticonvulsant medication regimens. Occasionally, however, a patient with epilepsy will not seize during ECT, so then the question becomes whether the anticonvulsant medication regimen can be altered safely. One should undertake this in consultation with a neurologist. Lowering of anticonvulsant medication dosing may allow ECT seizures to be achieved but at the cost of increased risk of intertreatment spontaneous seizures.

Intracranial space-occupying lesions

The risks of ECT in patients with intracranial space-occupying lesions are probably small in the absence of focal neurologic signs, brain edema, mass effect, or papilledema. In a patient with a known intracranial mass, neurologic or neurosurgical consultation pre-ECT is suggested to assess the status of the mass, to consider whether a surgical procedure is indicated for the mass before ECT, and to suggest risk-reduction strategies that may be used during ECT. The latter might include use of corticosteroids, diuretics, or antihypertensive medications. Traditionally, a space-occupying brain lesion associated with increased intracranial pressure has been said to be an absolute contraindication to ECT, but a reasonable risk–benefit analysis may well indicate using ECT if the patient would otherwise die from severe psychopathology that is not responding to psychotropic medication. Moreover, medication may be able to lower intracranial pressure before ECT.

Pregnancy

In the first trimester of pregnancy, risk of fetal malformations is foremost on the minds of medical caregivers. In the case of ECT at this stage of gestation, the electrically induced seizure itself probably is harmless to the tiny fetus. The risks of anesthetic medications, which are probably small, must be compared with those of psychotropic medication. During the later stages of pregnancy, concerns about premature labor and placental abruption become more prominent. Noninvasive fetal monitoring should be undertaken, and ECT should be conducted in a facility having ready availability of specialist obstetric services should complications occur. As a matter of routine, any pregnant woman about to undergo ECT should have obstetric consultation beforehand.

Diabetes mellitus

Patients with diabetes should have blood glucose levels checked before each treatment. Patients with type 2 diabetes should not have orally administered antidiabetic medications or insulin administered until after ECT treatments but should be treated as early in the morning as feasible. Patients with type 1 diabetes, who by definition are insulin dependent and whose blood sugar tends to show large fluctuations, should either have insulin withheld but be given ECT in the morning promptly on awakening, then given insulin and breakfast, or should be given half their morning insulin before the treatment and the other half afterward along with breakfast. In either case, blood sugar needs to be closely monitored before and after the ECT treatment in patients with type 1 diabetes.

Miscellaneous conditions

Chronic obstructive pulmonary disease and asthma are common, and patients who are using inhalers should use them in the morning shortly before ECT treatment. Theophylline, rarely used for pulmonary disorders anymore, has been associated with a risk of prolonged seizures and status epilepticus at ECT. If a prospective ECT patient is being treated with theophylline, it should be discontinued if possible; if not possible, serial blood levels (i.e., before each treatment) should be obtained to consider postponing ECT if the theophylline level is unnecessarily high.

The patient who has sustained severe burns needs special attention to fluid and electrolyte balance before commencing ECT. Additionally, use of succinylcholine may be particularly dangerous, so a nondepolarizing paralytic agent may be considered (see Chapter 26). Similarly, spinal cord injuries predispose to extreme hyperkalemia with succinylcholine, and a nondepolarizing neuromuscular blocking agent should be used. Patients with severe osteoporosis should be carefully evaluated for relatively complete muscular paralysis so as to avoid bone fracture. Patients' mouths should be examined prior to ECT, and loose teeth removed prior to treatment. Patients with chronic headaches probably will have post-ECT headaches. We usually pretreat these patients with intravenous ketorolac. The morbidly obese patient may need special attention to airway management and may even need to be intubated during ECT treatments to prevent reflux. Benzodiazepine-dependent patients are commonly encountered in ECT practice. The desire to avoid anticonvulsant effects of these medications must be balanced against the need to not worsen the patient's psychiatric status by a too-abrupt withdrawal. Adequate ECT responses can usually be achieved even when patients are still receiving benzodiazepines during ECT.

References

Albin, S. M., Stevens, S. R., and Rasmussen, K. G. 2007. Blood pressure before and after ECT in hypertensive and non-hypertensive patients. J ECT 23(1): 9–10.

American College of Cardiology/American Heart Association (ACC/AHA). 2007. ACC/AHA 2007 guidelines on perioperative cardiovascular evaluation and care for noncardiac surgery. J Am Coll Cardiol 50(17): 1707–32.

American Psychiatric Association Committee on ECT. 2001. Electroconvulsive therapy: Recommendations for treatment, training, and privileging, 2nd edn. Washington, DC: American Psychiatric Press.

Castelli, I., Steiner, L. A., Kaufman, M. A., et al. 1995. Comparative effects of esmolol and labetalol to attenuate hyperdynamic states after electroconvulsive therapy. Anesth Analg 80(3): 557–61.

Dolenc, T. J., Barnes, R. D., Hayes, D. L., et al. 2004. Electroconvulsive therapy in patients with pacemakers and ICD's. PACE 27(9): 1257–63.

Douyon, R., Serby, M., Klutchko, B., et al. 1989. ECT and Parkinson's disease revisited: A "naturalistic" study. Am J Psychiatry 146: 1451–5.

Goldberg, R. K. and Badger, J. M. 1993. Major depressive disorder in patients with the implantable cardioverter defibrillator: Two cases treated with ECT. Psychosomatics 34(3): 273–7.

Lunde, M. E., Lee, E. K., and Rasmussen, K. G. 2006. Electroconvulsive therapy in patients with epilepsy. Epilepsy Behav 9(2): 355–9.

Mehta, V., Mueller, P. S., Gonzalez-Arriaza, H. L., et al. 2004. Safety of electroconvulsive therapy in patients receiving long-term warfarin therapy. Mayo Clin Proc 79(11): 1396–401.

Mueller, P. S., Barnes, R. D., Nishimura, R., et al. 2007. ECT in patients with aortic stenosis. Mayo Clin Proc 82(11): 1360–3.

Nuttall, G. A., Bowersox, M. R., Douglass, S. B., et al. 2004. Morbidity and mortality in the use of electroconvulsive therapy. J ECT 20(4): 237–41.

O'Connor, C. J., Rothenberg, D. M., Soble, J. S., et al. 1996. The effect of esmolol pretreatment on the incidence of regional wall motion abnormalities during electroconvulsive therapy. Anesth Analg 82(1): 143–7.

Rasmussen, K. G., Jarvis, M. R., Zorumski, C. F., et al. 1999. Low-dose atropine in electroconvulsive therapy. J ECT 15(3): 213–21.

Rasmussen, K. G., Russell, J. C., Kung, S., et al. 2003. ECT in major depression with probable Lewy Body dementia. J ECT 19(2): 103–9.

Rasmussen, K. G., Rummans, T. A., Tsang, T. S. M., and Barnes, R. D. 2004. ECT in the medically ill. In The American Psychiatric Publishing textbook of psychosomatic medicine (ed. Levenson, J.). Washington, DC: American Psychiatric Publishing, pp. 957–77.

Zvara, D. A., Brooker, R. F., McCall, W. V., et al. 1997. The effect of esmolol on ST-segment depression and arrhythmias after electroconvulsive therapy. Convuls Ther 13(3): 165–74.

26

Anesthesia for electroconvulsive therapy

Charles H. Kellner, Dongchen Li, and Limore Maron

Anesthesia for electroconvulsive therapy

Rationale for anesthesia in electroconvulsive therapy

Anesthesia has been a standard part of electroconvulsive therapy (ECT) for five decades because it ensures patient safety and comfort. ECT anesthesia is distinctive because it must not impede seizure induction. There may be no other procedure in which anesthetic technique is so intimately related to therapeutic outcome.

For many years after its invention in 1938, ECT was administered without anesthesia or muscle relaxants. In many countries around the world, it still is (Chapters 16 and 17; Andrade, 2003). In the United States and other Western countries, ECT unmodified by anesthesia is considered primitive and inappropriate. The World Psychiatric Association is considering issuing a policy statement denouncing unmodified ECT. Why is general anesthesia given at ECT? Although the answer may sound ridiculously obvious, it may not be. Years ago, the assertion was made that the electrical stimulus itself so quickly rendered the patient unconscious, sedation or anesthesia was unnecessary. It was asserted that the seizure ensured complete amnesia for the procedure. Only if muscle relaxants were given would sedation be necessary to prevent a terrifying awareness of being paralyzed and unable to breathe while fully conscious. Although some older practitioners may still believe this, it is certainly not in keeping with modern practice or earlier patient accounts of anticipatory fear of the procedure. Thus, the reasons to give general anesthesia with ECT are (a) to ensure patient comfort and prevent fear, and (b) to allow the use of systemic muscle relaxants to decrease motor activity and facilitate ventilation before and during seizure.

Several comprehensive review articles on the topic of anesthesia for ECT have appeared in recent years. The reader is recommended to consult them (Ding and White, 2002; Folk et al., 2000; Wagner et al., 2005).

History

ECT was invented before modern anesthesia techniques were introduced, so it was inevitable that ECT began in "unmodified" form. Despite being relatively safe, because of the fairly primitive way in which it was initially delivered, ECT frightened many patients. Bone fracture and muscle soreness were not rare. The introduction of muscle relaxant drugs and barbiturate anesthesia markedly changed ECT and the experience of patients undergoing it.

Starting in the late 1930s with the discovery of curare and the synthesis of d-tubocurare by the drug manufacturer Squibb, the technique of ECT began to change (Shorter and Healy, 2007). The American psychiatrist A. E. Bennett is credited with the early use of curare in ECT patients in California. Although the incidence of bone fractures decreased, the use of curare was somewhat dangerous and cumbersome. In 1951, succinylcholine was introduced, and in 1952 it was patented by an Austrian company (Shorter and Healy, 2007). A Swedish psychiatrist, G. Holmberg, and his anesthesia colleague, Stephan Thesleff, pioneered the modern use of succinylcholine with barbiturate anesthesia in Sweden in 1951. They published an article in the May 1952 issue of the *American Journal of Psychiatry* describing their technique (Holmberg and Thesleff, 1952). Thus, the three major elements of modern ECT anesthesia – barbiturate induction, muscle relaxation, and oxygenation – were developed by the early 1950s.

What has occurred in ECT anesthesia since then have largely been minor modifications of the original techniques. Of course, it took some time for the modern techniques to be adopted widely, and unfortunately many practitioners continued to perform unmodified ECT for many years. The dramatic change from a "brutal" appearance to a modern, comfortable, minor surgical procedure with little to see is chronicled in the autobiographical novel *The Bell Jar* by Sylvia Plath (1971). Early in the book she describes receiving ECT without anesthesia as follows:

"Doctor Gordon was fitting two metal plates on either side of my head. He buckled them into place with a strap that dented my forehead, and gave me a wire to bite.

I shut my eyes. There was a brief silence, like an indrawn breath. Then something bent down and took hold of me and shook me like the end of the world. Whee-ee-ee-ee-ee, it shrilled, through an air crackling with blue light, and with each flash a great jolt drubbed me till I thought my bones would break and the sap fly out of me like a split plant. I wondered what terrible thing it was that I had done."

Later in the book, her psychiatrist tells her how she hopes she will experience ECT with modern anesthetic technique: "*I told Doctor Nolan about the machine, and the blue flashes, and the jolting and the noise. While I was telling her she went very still. "That was a mistake," she said then. "It's not supposed to be like that. I stared at her. "If it's done properly," Doctor Nolan said, "it's like going to sleep*" (Plath, 1971).

The anesthesia issues described here are in the service of making ECT safer, more effective, and more comfortable for the patient. Because anesthetic technique has a profound influence on the clinical outcome, anesthesia methods are an integral and essential part of ECT itself.

Anticholinergics

Anticholinergic premedication is common in ECT. The main reason an anticholinergic is given is to prevent vagally mediated bradyarrhythmias (Perrin, 1961). Another reason is to reduce airway secretions (Kramer, 1993). Whereas some practitioners routinely administer an anticholinergic, others consider it optional. Certain clinical circumstances argue in favor of the use of an anticholinergic. These include a preexisting cardiac conduction problem, use of β-adrenergic antagonists (Wagner et al., 2005) and seizure threshold titration determination (Kellner et al., 1997). The latter situation increases the risk of bradycardia because a subconvulsive electrical stimulus results in unopposed vagal outflow because there is no subsequent sympathetic activity from a seizure (Kramer, 1993).

Two anticholinergic agents, glycopyrrolate and atropine, are commonly used prior to ECT. They can be given subcutaneously, intramuscularly, or intravenously (IV) (Kramer, 1993; Kramer et al., 1986; Mayur et al., 1998). IV administration is usually favored; the two other routes are rarely used. When given IV, the agent should be administered two to three minutes prior to anesthesia induction. Given in this fashion, it will have the desired vagolytic effect but not the antisialagogue effect (Kramer et al., 1992). This route of administration provides greater patient comfort because the IV catheter is already in place. With intramuscular injection, the anticholinergic should be given at least 30 minutes prior to the procedure. This has the advantage of allowing time for the antisialagogue effect, but the disadvantages of an additional injection for the patient and an interval of uncomfortable dry mouth and possible palpitations or anxiety (Kramer et al., 1992).

Glycopyrrolate does not cross the blood–brain barrier (Proakis and Harris, 1978) and is believed to lack central nervous system activity. Logically then it should not contribute to cognitive impairment, but limited comparative studies have failed to show a cognitive advantage over atropine (Kelway et al., 1986). Glycopyrrolate causes mild tachycardia and can reduce oral and airway secretions if administered well prior to the procedure. It is considered a weaker vagolytic than atropine. The typical dose range in ECT is 0.2 to 0.4 mg IV. Onset of IV action occurs in less than one minute, and peak effect is reached in approximately five minutes. Overall duration of action is two to three hours for vagolysis and seven hours for antisialagogue properties (Folk et al., 2000). A recent study demonstrating that vagally mediated bradycardia during ECT is associated with a reduction in cerebral perfusion by as much as 50% also showed that glycopyrrolate can attenuate these hemodynamic effects (Rasmussen, 2007). The clinical significance of this finding is unclear.

Atropine is the alternative choice for anticholinergic premedication in ECT. In contrast to glycopyrrolate, atropine crosses the blood–brain barrier so theoretically could contribute to cognitive adverse effects and sedation (Kramer et al., 1992). As noted earlier in this chapter, atropine is a more potent vagolytic agent. The dose range for atropine is 0.4 to 0.8 mg IV (American Psychiatric Association [APA], 2001).

Because of the potential for adverse effects, many practitioners consider the use of an anticholinergic optional, unless one of the previously mentioned special circumstances is present. Potential adverse effects of premedication with an anticholinergic may be exacerbation of preexisting tachycardia, with resultant increase in cardiac workload and oxygen demand of the heart (Kramer, 1993). Other possible adverse effects include constipation and urinary retention. Because of these effects, it is advisable for someone from the ECT team to be in contact with the patient later in the day after the first treatment to make sure that he or she has been able to void without difficulty.

Induction agents

The choice of induction agent for ECT requires consideration of the anesthetic properties of the agent as well as its effect on seizure induction. To date, no perfect agent has been developed; all represent a compromise in some characteristic (see Table 26.1). Among the barbiturates, methohexital has been the agent of choice, and among more recently developed agents, propofol, despite its anticonvulsant properties (Folk et al., 2000).

The ideal anesthetic agent for ECT has rapid onset, short duration, and little effect on seizure threshold or even some seizure-enhancing effect. It would be inexpensive, readily available, painless on injection, and have a favorable cardiac side effect profile. In this section, we review the most commonly used anesthetic agents for ECT and compare their characteristics.

Since the late 1950s, general anesthesia has been used for ECT. Barbiturates were the first class of hypnotic used to induce anesthesia for ECT. The most commonly used barbiturates today are thiopental, methohexital, and thiamylal. They all are short acting. All barbiturates increase seizure threshold and decrease seizure duration, but methohexital appears to have the least impact on these factors (Fredman et al., 1994). Thus, methohexital remains the most widely used general anesthetic for ECT and is considered the "gold standard" to compare with other agents. The recommended dose is 0.75 to 1.0 mg/kg. Onset of action is a few seconds, and duration is two to eight minutes (APA, 2001). One report has suggested that dividing the dose of methohexital can minimize its anticonvulsant effect, leading to

Table 26.1 Comparison of intravenous anesthesia induction agents

Agents	Typical ECT dose (mg/kg)	Relative anticonvulsant effects	Remarks
Methohexital	0.75–1.0	1	Standard for ECT; rapid recovery; pain on injection
Thiopental	2.0–5.0	2	Cardiovascular depression
Propofol	1.0–2.0	3	Pain on injection; may shorten seizures or increase seizure threshold
Etomidate	0.2–0.3	0	Myoclonus; adrenal suppression; relative cardiovascular stability, pain on injection
Ketamine	0.5–2.0	−1	Proconvulsant; less respiratory depression; sympathetic activation; hallucinations
Alfentanil	0.010–0.015	1	Increased duration of apnea; reduced hypertension and tachycardia; reduced hypnotic dose
Remifentanil	0.001–0.008	−1	Proconvulsant; reduced hypnotic dose; attenuated hemodynamic response

Note: ECT, electroconvulsive therapy.

improved outcomes in ECT. This method has not been widely accepted (Gurmarnik et al., 1996). Methohexital causes pain on IV injection and is contraindicated in patients with any porphyria (Ding and White, 2002). Other reported side effects include hypotension, shivering, hiccoughing, and soft tissue necrosis at the injection site (Chanpattana, 2001).

Thiopental has greater anticonvulsant effect than does methohexital. Even though a previous study showed that the frequency of sinus bradycardia and premature ventricular contractions was increased with thiopental compared with methohexital (Mokriski et al., 1992), a newly published report found that thiopental, propofol, and etomidate were associated with similar cardiovascular effects (Rosa, 2007).

Compared with propofol, middle cerebral artery flow velocities immediately after ECT were significantly higher with thiopental in one study (Saito et al., 2000). Again, the clinical significance of this finding is unclear. As a very tightly controlled substance, thiopental requires more paperwork than do other anesthetics.

Thiopental and methohexital must be dissolved in 0.9% normal saline or sterile water to prepare 2.5% thiopental and 1.0% methohexital solutions. If barbiturates are added to Ringer's lactate, precipitation will occur and may occlude an IV catheter. Thiopental (2.5%) does not cause pain on injection, and irritation of the vein is rare. Methohexital (1%) frequently causes discomfort when injected into a small vein (Chiu and White, 2001).

Propofol is a rapid-onset, short-acting IV induction agent. Because of its antiemetic effect, patients may have less postoperative nausea and vomiting than they would with other IV anesthetics. Patients given propofol for ECT have more stable heart rates and blood pressures afterward than when they are given thiopental or methohexital (Chiu and White, 2001; Fredman et al., 1994; Geretsegger et al., 1998). Propofol has a greater anticonvulsant effect than other hypnotics have, increasing seizure threshold and decreasing seizure duration. Nevertheless, the use of propofol (at 0.75 mg/kg) was associated with seizure duration that was comparable with one with a standard induction dose of methohexital (Avramov et al., 1995). Propofol's anticonvulsant effect is dose dependent. ECT seizure duration after larger dosages of propofol (1.0 to 1.5 mg/kg) was significantly shorter than after methohexital, etomidate, or thiopental (Avramov et al., 1995; Saito et al., 2000). However, studies show that even the largest doses of propofol (1.5 mg/kg) result in clinically acceptable seizure activity (Fredman et al., 1994; Geretsegger et al., 1998). Because it can significantly shorten the duration of seizure activity, its effect on the antidepressant action of ECT has been questioned and investigated. In two studies, the long-term efficacy of ECT was similar between propofol and methohexital, although shorter seizure duration was seen with propofol induction (Malsch et al., 1994; Mitchell, 1991). Therefore, propofol is recommended only in patients requiring attenuated hemodynamic responses during treatment, those who have had pronged seizures, and those who are prone to postictal nausea and vomiting (Bailine et al., 2003). Recent preliminary evidence suggests that propofol may be associated with diminished cognitive effects of ECT, but this association requires further study (Geretsegger et al., 2007).

Etomidate is used in doses of 0.15 to 0.3 mg/kg (APA, 2001). It produces a rapid onset of anesthesia. Involuntary myoclonic movements are common during induction. This myoclonic activity is caused by subcortical disinhibition, and is not related to cortical seizure activity (Chiu and White, 2001). When compared with methohexital, thiopental, and propofol, anesthetic induction with etomidate is generally associated with longer seizure duration. Etomidate should be considered when previous ECT sessions have yielded short seizures. As a result of the benign cardiovascular profile of etomidate and its ability to enhance seizure activity, it can be used to induce anesthesia in medically ill patients. Recovery after etomidate can be delayed because of post-ECT confusion and an increased incidence of nausea compared with methohexital and propofol (Avramov et al., 1995).

Ketamine is a unique anesthetic with sedative and analgesic properties; it is associated with less respiratory depression than are other agents (Rasmussen et al.,

1996). Compared with methohexital, ketamine has slower onset, delayed recovery, and increased incidence of nausea, ataxia, hypersalivation, and hallucinations during recovery (McInnes and James, 1972). Because of its direct stimulation of the sympathetic nervous system, ketamine increases heart rate and blood pressure (Chiu and White, 2001). A recent study showed that seizure duration was increased with ketamine doses ranging from 0.7 to 2.8 mg/kg, when compared with methohexital. Ketamine enhances ictal electroencephalographic evidence of seizure intensity (Krystal et al., 2003). It has also been postulated to have antidepressant effects during ECT (Ostroff et al., 2005). It is used in patients with high seizure thresholds who may be refractory to seizure induction despite maximal device settings. Typical IV doses are 0.5 to 2 mg/kg (Chanpattana, 2001).

Recently, ultrashort-acting narcotics, such as alfentanil and remifentanil, have been used alone or combined with propofol, methohexital, or etomidate to induce anesthesia for ECT. In general, using an adjunctive narcotic reduces hypnotic dose, increases seizure duration, and attenuates acute hemodynamic responses to ECT (Recart et al., 2003). Adjunctive narcotic use does not increase recovery time or incidence of side effects (van den Broek, 2004). One study showed that etomidate–alfentanil induction prolonged apnea and that alfentanil itself had no proconvulsant effect (Sullivan et al., 2004). Remifentanil (4 to 8 μg/kg) has also been used as the sole agent to induce anesthesia in patients who had become completely or relatively refractory to seizure elicitation despite maximal settings on the ECT device with methohexital anesthesia (Toprak et al., 2005). Typical doses are 10 μg/kg for alfentanil and 1 μg/kg for remifentanil, when combined with reduced doses of the hypnotics.

Inhalational anesthesia with sevoflurane is reportedly a reasonable alternative in ECT (Rasmussen et al., 2006a). Using 6% to 8% sevoflurane, seizure duration and patient tolerance were acceptable and similar to those with thiopental (Ding and White, 2002). Although this volatile anesthetic can be used to produce an adequate anesthetic state for ECT, it is more time consuming and possesses no obvious advantage when compared with the commonly used IV anesthetics. An exception may be for women requiring ECT in the late stages of pregnancy, when sevoflurane may reduce post-ECT uterine contractions (Hodgson et al., 2004). Sevoflurane anesthesia may be helpful for patients with severe needle phobia or for those in whom the placement of an IV catheter while awake is very difficult (Rasmussen et al., 2005).

Muscle relaxants

Muscle relaxants have been a feature of ECT since the 1950s. The muscle relaxant aims to modify or "soften" the motor manifestations of the induced seizure, to prevent musculoskeletal injury. There is variability among practitioners as to the degree of paralysis desired, with some preferring nearly complete absence of muscle movement and others merely the elimination of major axial skeletal movement. The "cuff method," invented by Max Hamilton, MD, of Great Britain (Shorter and Healy, 2007) has become standard in ECT. It involves the exclusion of the muscle relaxant from the right foot by means of a blood pressure cuff inflated to above systolic pressure. The purpose of the method is to visually ensure that a generalized motor seizure has been induced. In this section, we discuss the characteristics of succinylcholine and alternate muscle relaxant agents.

Succinylcholine, the only depolarizing muscle relaxant available today, has been the most commonly used muscle relaxant in ECT for decades (Swartz, 1993). Its popularity is due to its rapid onset (30 to 60 seconds) and short action (usually less than 10 minutes), which matches the duration of IV anesthesia for ECT. The typical dose range used in clinical practice is 0.5 to 1.0 mg/kg, but the dose is adjusted individually. Higher doses may be needed in patients at risk for fractures during the seizure, such as those with osteoporosis, preexisting fracture, severe degenerative joint disease, herniated disk (Folk et al., 2000), or Harrington rod implant (Bhat et al., 2007). In patients with a history of post-ECT agitation (presumably associated with elevated plasma lactate), increasing the dose of succinylcholine may reduce the likelihood of this emergence agitation (Auriacombe et al., 2000; Swartz, 1990).

There is a long list of side effects related to succinylcholine. Because of its chemical structure's similarity to that of acetylcholine, succinylcholine has parasympathetic activity. It may produce sinus bradycardia and even asystole after a second dose. When injected rapidly, succinylcholine causes fasciculations; this is a benign phenomenon. Serum potassium increases by 0.5 to 1.0 mEq/L after injection, and patients with certain coexisting diseases or conditions may develop severe hyperkalemia (Folk et al., 2000). These include renal failure, major denervation injuries, spinal cord transection, stroke, crush injuries, extensive burns, prolonged immobility, and catatonia (Folk et al., 2000; Hudcova and Schumann, 2006). Patients who receive succinylcholine may report posttreatment myalgias. For patients distressed by myalgias, pretreatment with a small dose of curare (a so-called "defasciculating" dose) several minutes before the procedure can be considered. Succinylcholine increases intraocular, intragastric, and intracranial pressures and elevates the tone of the masseter muscles. Succinylcholine can trigger malignant hyperthermia, presenting with sudden tachycardia, acute metabolic or respiratory acidosis, hypercarbia, and hyperthermia. Patients with a family history of malignant hyperthermia, Duchenne's or other muscular dystrophies, King-Denborough syndrome, or Central Core Disease should not receive succinylcholine. Although the clinical presentation of neuroleptic malignant syndrome is similar to that of malignant hyperthermia, the etiology is completely different, and succinylcholine has been used safely for patients with neuroleptic malignant syndrome who are undergoing ECT (Trollor and Sachdev, 1999).

Succinylcholine is metabolized by pseudocholinesterase (plasma cholinesterase, butyrylcholinesterase). Patients with genetic defects of the enzyme (those with atypical pseudocholinesterase) have longer neuromuscular blockade and apnea with succinylcholine (Williams, 2007). One in 50 patients (heterozygous for the gene) will have a prolonged block of 20 to 30 minutes, and 1 in 3,000 patients (homozygous for the gene) may have four to eight hours of block, as the atypical enzyme has little or no affinity for succinylcholine. The laboratory test to detect atypical pseudocholinesterase is the dibucaine number. Dibucaine is an amide local anesthetic that, when added to a patient's blood sample, will inhibit normal plasma cholinesterase by 80%. Patients who are heterozygous have a dibucaine number between 40% and 70%. Those who are homozygous have a dibucaine number less than 30% (Williams, 2007). Routine screening of pseudocholinesterase level is not recommended because of false positives.

Short- or moderate-acting nondepolarizing muscle relaxants – such as rapacuronium (Kadar et al., 2001), mivacurium (Burnstein and Denny, 1993; Gitlin et al., 1993; Janis et al., 1995), rocuronium (Williams, 2007), atracurium (Dwersteg and Avery, 1987; Hickey et al., 1987; Lui et al., 1993), and vecuronium (Herriot et al., 1996; Sakamoto et al., 1999; Vallance and McConachie, 1993) – have been used as alternatives for those patients who have contraindications to the use of succinylcholine. Rapacuronium has rapid onset and short action comparable to succinylcholine, but was found to increase risk of bronchospasm, and was withdrawn from clinical use in U.S. hospitals.

Mivacurium is the only short-acting drug more than rarely given as an alternative to succinylcholine during ECT. Compared with succinylcholine, mivacurium has a slower onset (2.5 to 3.0 minutes) and a longer duration (15 to 20 minutes). Patient recovery time is longer, but shorter than with atracurium or vecuronium (Swartz, 1993). The common dose for ECT is 0.15 to 0.2 mg/kg. As with succinylcholine, mivacurium is metabolized by pseudocholinesterase. To avoid prolonged paralysis, patients with this enzyme deficiency should not receive mivacurium. Mivacurium triggers histamine release and causes tachycardia and hypotension. Slow injection over one minute may minimize these side effects. If reversal of neuromuscular blockade is necessary after ECT, edrophonium is a better choice than neostigmine, as the latter inhibits the activity of pseudocholinesterase. Recently, some hospitals have stopped carrying mivacurium on formulary because of little usage in operating rooms.

Atracurium is an intermediate-duration muscle relaxant, with a typical dose range of 0.3 to 0.5 mg/kg, an onset of action in 2.5 to 3.0 minutes, and a duration of 30 minutes. Patients who received atracurium at 0.5 mg/kg IV have had more complete muscle block and longer recovery time than have those who received it at 0.3 mg/kg (Lui et al., 1993). Atracurium has been used for ECT in patients with atypical pseudocholinesterase who need to avoid succinylcholine and mivacurium. Atracurium causes dose-dependent histamine release, and should not be given to patients with asthma. It is largely metabolized by the Hofmann reaction, which is nonenzymatic degradation that is independent of renal and liver function. Thus, patients with renal or liver failure may receive atracurium. Atracurium has been largely replaced by one of its two stereoisomer components, cisatracurium. Cisatracurium is four times more potent than atracurium, does not increase plasma histamine levels, and lacks cardiovascular side effects at high dose (Sparr et al., 2001). Because of its long onset (3.0 minutes) and intermediate duration (40 minutes), cisatracurium has very limited usage in ECT.

Rocuronium is a rapid-onset and intermediate-duration nondepolarizing muscle relaxant. When given at high dose (0.9 to 1.2 mg/kg), onset time approaches that of succinylcholine, but it has a longer duration of action. Low doses (0.4 mg/kg) may allow reversal as soon as 25 minutes. In one report, a 90-kg patient with prolonged paralysis after ECT was found to be homozygous for atypical pseudocholinesterase (dibucaine number 19.2%). This patient received 30 mg of rocuronium at subsequent ECT treatments without side effects (Williams, 2007). This drug should be seriously considered as a newer alternative to succinylcholine, mivacurium, and atracurium. Vecuronium has a profile similar to that of rocuronium, but has slower onset (two to three minutes). There is no clear indication for, or advantage to, its use in ECT.

When patients receive a muscle relaxant, they should be monitored with a peripheral nerve stimulator to evaluate neuromuscular function. Common locations for its placement are the wrist (to observe adductor pollicis response) and the facial, posterior tibial, peroneal, or lateral popliteal nerves. The "train of four" – four electric stimuli at a frequency of 2 Hz, repeated every 10 seconds – is probably the most useful pattern of stimulation for monitoring. When the patient is completely paralyzed by the muscle relaxant, the "train of four" should give no response. Muscle response fades during partial paralysis with a nondepolarizing muscle relaxant. It is helpful to assess recovery from blockade by observation of the strength of twitches. The "train of four" is also used to indicate reversal time. The reversal drug should be given only after at least one twitch returns on the "train of four" stimulation. The most common reversal drug for nondepolarizing blockade is neostigmine at 0.05 mg/kg. Salivation, bradycardia, and bronchoconstriction (mediated by muscarinic receptors) are minimized by giving glycopyrrolate 0.01 mg/kg at the same time (Campagna, 2006).

Airway management

Airway management is necessary in ECT anesthesia. It involves not only the maintenance of a patent airway and adequate oxygenation, but may contribute to seizure quality and sometimes to complications. For the vast majority of patients, tracheal intubation is not necessary for ECT. Ventilation is carried out by the bag-valve face mask. Intubation may be needed in patients with high risk of pulmonary aspiration, such as those with full stomachs, morbid obesity, late pregnancy, and those who present difficulties with mask ventilation. One study showed that, in 50 obese patients under anesthesia for a total 660 ECT treatments (including 97 consecutive procedures in nine morbidly obese patients), there were no cases of aspiration as assessed clinically with patients managed using a face mask (Kadar et al., 2002).

Recently, successful use of the laryngeal mask airway (LMA) has been reported in patients with face mask difficulty. These include patients with obesity, mandibular protrusion, or dental abnormalities (Nishihara et al., 2003), and one with a 20- to 22-week pregnancy with a known difficult airway (Brown et al., 2003). Patients ventilated with facial masks had lower $PaCO_2$ and longer seizure duration than did those ventilated with LMAs (Nishihara et al., 2003). Because the LMA does not occlude the trachea as does a cuffed endotracheal tube, it does not afford the same degree of aspiration protection.

Before anesthesia, the patient's airway should be carefully evaluated and fasting status reconfirmed. Close attention should be paid to dental abnormalities, particularly loose teeth that may become dislodged during ECT. Dental consultation may be needed before ECT. Poor dentition can require special precautions (e.g., a custom bite block) or postponement of ECT.

Typically, an anesthesia machine is not required for ECT anesthesia, but equipment and devices for airway management must be immediately available. These include suction, oxygen supply, bag-valve face mask, oral and nasal airways, LMA, endotracheal tubes, and laryngoscope. Monitoring electrocardiogram, blood pressure, and pulse oximetry is now standard (Ding and White, 2002; Folk et al., 2000).

Optimally, patients should be asked to take deep breaths of 100% oxygen for several minutes before the start of the procedure. Then general anesthesia is induced, and when the patient becomes unconscious ventilation with the face mask is started and confirmed by visualizing chest movements. After the patient is paralyzed with the muscle relaxant and does not respond to "the train of four" stimulation, the bite block should be inserted by the ECT nurse or the anesthetist. The bite block is inserted into the patient's mouth prior to the delivery of the electrical stimulus to protect the tongue, teeth, and other oral structures. It is important to use bite blocks specifically designed for ECT to ensure proper protection; they are made of hard rubber or dense foam. The oxygen mask is removed, and the ECT nurse or anesthetist inserts the bite block. Proper technique involves pushing the tongue inferiorly and posteriorly into the throat behind the teeth. The bite block should then be held against the upper teeth and the lower teeth and jaw held up firmly to the bottom surface of the bite block. The patient's lips should be pulled over the bite block and the chin pushed upward with firm pressure during the stimulus. The bite block can be removed immediately after the delivery of the stimulus or left in place with the mask repositioned over it.

Studies on animals and humans have demonstrated that hypocapnia and hyperventilation increase seizure duration (Bergsholm et al., 1984; Chater and Simpson, 1988; Crawford et al., 1987). To increase seizure duration and perhaps improve the efficacy of ECT, hyperventilation is preferred both before and during the seizure. After the seizure, controlled ventilation with the face mask should be continued until spontaneous respiration resumes. Secretions in the upper airway should be suctioned as needed. When awake, alert, and showing both stable vital signs and satisfactory oxygen saturation, the patient can be moved to the recovery room.

Concomitant medications

ECT practitioners explicitly determine which medications the patient will continue taking during the course of ECT and which will be discontinued. This determination is part of the initial ECT consultation. At that time a plan should be written describing how to taper or discontinue selected medications, and the patient should be given instructions about how to take medications that are to be continued. It is beyond the purview of this chapter to consider all medications, but several specific types are reviewed.

Any medication with anticonvulsant effects has the potential to interfere with the efficacy of ECT. Benzodiazepines and the anticonvulsant mood stabilizers should be tapered and discontinued if at all possible. One important exception is when the patient is taking medication to treat epilepsy. For most patients who are taking valproic acid, carbamazepine, or other commonly prescribed antiepileptic medications for mood-stabilizing effects, these medications can be tapered and discontinued over one to four days prior to the first ECT treatment. Although there is no evidence that rapid withdrawal of these agents leads to rebound seizures in patients without epilepsy, it is always prudent to taper rather than abruptly discontinue them, whenever time permits. With benzodiazepines, the dose should be lowered to the minimal acceptable for control of anxiety. If the patient is taking a long-acting benzodiazepine such as clonazepam, many practitioners advocate switching to a shorter-acting preparation such as lorazepam several days before ECT. This practice will theoretically allow for lower serum levels of benzodiazepine at the time of ECT. Generally, long-standing benzodiazepines require a 10-day taper to discontinue.

There is a substantial literature about continuing lithium with ECT. This was recently well reviewed by Dolenc and Rasmussen (2005). Although many practitioners are leery of using this combination, the accumulated evidence suggests that, for most patients, it is quite safe. The concern is that, at therapeutic or high serum levels of lithium, patients may be at risk for both prolonged seizures and increased incidence of delirium. This concern has led to the generally recommended practice of ensuring that lithium levels are low at the time of ECT. This can be accomplished by having the patient discontinue lithium at least 24, and preferably 48, hours before each treatment. To completely avoid risk, some practitioners discontinue lithium throughout the acute course of ECT; however, abrupt lithium discontinuation has its own risks. With maintenance ECT, a patient may be requested to omit one or several doses of lithium prior to each ECT.

Patients taking l-dopa for Parkinson's disease may be at increased risk for developing delirium with ECT (Rasmussen and Abrams, 1991). Therefore, many practitioners routinely decrease or discontinue l-dopa during the course of ECT. As patients with severe Parkinson's disease must continue to take some l-dopa, a general rule of thumb is to try to decrease the dose by 50% during the course of ECT. This decrease may be adjusted up or down, to manage parkinsonian motor symptoms while monitoring for cognitive effects from ECT.

Patients with diabetes require special attention during ECT. Part of the pre-ECT planning should be deciding on a strategy of glucose control during the acute course of ECT. Patients with mild diabetes may require no special intervention other than taking their standard oral agents after the ECT procedure. Patients with more severe or brittle diabetes may require more specialized intervention. For example, patients on insulin may require split doses of insulin before and after the procedure (Rasmussen et al., 2006b). It may be advisable to request an endocrinology consultation prior to ECT in such patients, to design an appropriately individualized treatment plan. Pretreatment and posttreatment blood glucose monitoring may also be recommended.

Theophylline is relatively contraindicated in patients starting ECT because of a risk for prolonged seizures. Patients with chronic obstructive pulmonary disease or asthma who are taking theophylline should be reassessed for the need to continue it. If it is deemed necessary for them to continue, it should be maintained at the lowest therapeutic level possible (Fink and Sackeim, 1998).

Issues related to the collaboration between anesthesiology and psychiatry

The relationship between specialists in anesthesia and psychiatry is vital in the delivery of proper ECT care. Ideally, practitioners should know each other well, and have strong respect for the expertise and skill of the other. The roles of each member of the ECT team should be clearly defined, yet there should be enough flexibility so that there is optimal cooperation between team members at all times. In general, procedures go most smoothly when it is clear that one person is in charge of the team. In ECT, this should be the ECT psychiatrist. Communication between team members is crucial for optimal patient care. The treating psychiatrist should review with the anesthesia provider the plan for each patient's care in advance. This review should include specification of the induction agent and reexamination of the previously used doses of anticholinergic, induction agent, and muscle relaxant, if this information is available. The patient's medical history should be reviewed. Any special needs or requests of the patient should be considered. The team member responsible for placing the bite block should be determined in advance. Our preference is for the ECT nurse to assume this responsibility. Decisions about when to intervene to treat hypertension or tachycardia should be made collaboratively between the ECT psychiatrist and the anesthesia provider. Although many hospitals require that an anesthesiologist be present, nurse anesthetists are often the front-line providers of anesthesia care in ECT. We believe that what matters most is the quality and experience of the individual, not his or her degree. When a trainee is present in an academic or teaching hospital setting, it is imperative that the attending physicians be responsible for full supervision of the trainee's activities. As the team leader, the ECT psychiatrist should make it clear that a trainee may perform only what it is known that the trainee is fully competent to do, and under attentive and direct supervision. As always, the privilege of leading the team carries with it the responsibility for the clinical outcome.

In addition to helping patients, one of the most gratifying things about ECT practice is the development of close working relationships with respected anesthesia colleagues. It is truly a heartening experience to see them learn about psychiatric illness, as we learn modern anesthesia concepts from them.

As noted earlier, the ECT suite is a fertile training ground. Psychiatric residents, anesthesia residents, nurse anesthetist students, other nursing students, medical students, psychology interns, and various other health professionals may all rotate through the ECT suite in an academic center. It is up to the health care team to ensure that the atmosphere in the ECT suite is respectful of our patients and provides an environment in which junior colleagues can learn about ECT and its impact on psychiatric illness.

References

American Psychiatric Association. The practice of ECT: Recommendations for treatment, training, and privileging, 2nd edn. Washington, DC: American Psychiatric Press, 2001.
Andrade, C. 2003. Unmodified ECT: Ethical issues. Issues Med Ethics 11(1): 9–10.

Auriacombe, M., Reneric, J. P., Usandizaga, D., et al. 2000. Post-ECT agitation and plasma lactate concentrations. J ECT 16(3): 263–7.

Avramov, M. N., Husain M. M., and White, P. F. 1995. The comparative effects of methohexital, propofol, and etomidate for electroconvulsive therapy. Anesth Analg 81(3): 596–602.

Bailine, S. H., Petrides, G., Doft, M., and Lui, G. 2003. Indications for the use of propofol in electroconvulsive therapy. J ECT 19(3): 129–32.

Bergsholm, P., Gran, L., and Bleie, H. 1984. Seizure duration in unilateral electroconvulsive therapy. The effect of hypocapnia induced by hyperventilation and the effect of ventilation with oxygen. Acta Psychiatr Scand 69(2): 121–8.

Bhat, T., Pande, N., Shah, N., and Andrade C. 2007. Safety of repeated courses of electroconvulsive therapy in a patient with Harrington rods. J ECT 23(2): 106–8.

Brown, N. I., Mack, P. F., Mitera, D. M., and Dhar, P. 2003. Use of the ProSeal laryngeal mask airway in a pregnant patient with a difficult airway during electroconvulsive therapy. Br J Anaesth 91(5): 752–4.

Burnstein, R. M. and Denny, N. 1993. Mivacurium in electroconvulsive therapy. Anaesthesia 48(12): 1116.

Campagna J. A. 2006. Development of the neuromuscular junction. Int Anesthiol Clin 44(2): 1–20.

Chanpattana, W. 2001. Anesthesia for ECT. German Journal of Psychiatry 4: 33–9.

Chater, S. N. and Simpson, K. H. 1988. Effect of passive hyperventilation on seizure duration in patients undergoing electroconvulsive therapy. Br J Anaesth 60(1): 70–3.

Chiu, J. W. and White, P. F. 2001. Non opiod intravenous anesthesia. In Clinical anesthesia, 4th edn. (eds. Barash, P. G., Cullen, B. F., and Stoelting, R. K.).

Crawford, C. D., Butler, P., and Froese, A. 1987. Arterial PaO$_2$ and PaCO$_2$ influence seizure duration in dogs receiving electroconvulsive therapy. Can J Anaesth 34(5): 437–41.

Ding, Z. and White, P. F. 2002. Anesthesia for electroconvulsive therapy. Anesth Analg 94(5): 1351–64.

Dolenc, T. J. and Rasmussen, K. G. 2005. The safety of electroconvulsive therapy and lithium in combination: A case series and review of the literature. J ECT 21(3): 165–70.

Dwersteg, J. F. and Avery, D. H. 1987. Atracurium as a muscle relaxant for electroconvulsive therapy in a burned patient. Convuls Ther 3(1): 49–53.

Fink, M. and Sackeim, H. A. 1998. Theophylline and ECT. J ECT 14(4): 286–90.

Folk, J. W., Kellner, C. H., Beale, M. D., et al. 2000. Anesthesia for electroconvulsive therapy: A review. J ECT 16(2): 157–70.

Fredman B., d'Etienne, J., Smith, I., et al. 1994. Anesthesia for electroconvulsive therapy: Effects of propofol and methohexital on seizure activity and recovery. Anesth Analg 79: 75–9.

Geretsegger, C., Nickel, M., Judendorfer, B., et al. 2007. Propofol and methohexital as anesthetic agents for electroconvulsive therapy: A randomized double-blind comparison of electroconvulsive therapy seizure quality, therapeutic efficacy, and cognitive performance. J ECT 23(4): 239–43.

Geretsegger, C., Rochowanski, E., Kartnig, C., and Unterrainer, A. F. 1998. Propofol and methohexital as anesthetic agents for electroconvulsive therapy (ECT): A comparison of seizure-quality measures and vital signs. J ECT 14(1): 28–35.

Gitlin, M. C., Jahr, J. S., Margolis, M. A., and McCain, J. 1993. Is mivacurium chloride effective in electroconvulsive therapy? A report of four cases, including a patient with myasthenia gravis. Anesth Analg 77(2): 392–4.

Gurmarnik, S., Young, R., and Alesker, E. 1996. Divided doses of methohexitone improves ECT outcome. Can J Anaesth 43(5 Pt 1): 535.

Herriot, P. M., Cowain, T., and McLeod, D. 1996. Use of vecuronium to prevent suxamethonium-induced myalgia after ECT. Br J Psychiatry 168(5): 653–4.

Hickey, D. R., O'Connor, J. P., and Donati, F. 1987. Comparison of atracurium and succinyl-choline for electroconvulsive therapy in a patient with atypical plasma cholinesterase. Can J Anaesth 34(3 Pt 1): 280–3.

Hodgson, R. E., Dawson, P., Hold, A. R., et al. 2004. Anaesthesia for electroconvulsive therapy: A comparison of sevoflurane with propofol. Anaesth Intensive Care 32(2): 241–5.

Holmberg, G., and Thesleff, S. 1952. Succinyl-choline-iodide as a muscular relaxant in elec-troshock therapy. Am J Psychiatry 108(11): 842–6.

Hudcova, J. and Schumann, R. 2006. Electroconvulsive therapy complicated by life-threatening hyperkalemia in a catatonic patient. Gen Hosp Psychiatry 28(5): 440–2.

Janis, K., Hess, J., Fabian, J. A., and Gillis, M. 1995. Substitution of mivacurium for succinylcholine for ECT in elderly patients. Can J Anaesth 42(7): 612–13.

Kadar, A. G., Ing, C. H., White, P. F., et al. 2002. Anesthesia for electroconvulsive therapy in obese patients. Anesth Analg 94(2): 360–1.

Kadar, A. G., Kramer, B. A., Barth, M. C., and White, P. F. 2001. Rapacuronium: An alternative to succinylcholine for electroconvulsive therapy. Anesth Analg 92(5): 1171–2.

Kellner, C. H., Pritchett, J. T., Beale, M. D., and Coffey, E. C. 1997. Handbook of ECT, 1st edn. Washington, DC: Amercan Psychiatric Press, Inc.

Kelway, B., Simpson, K. H., Smith, R. J., and Halsall, P. J. 1986. Effects of atropine and glycopy-rrolate on cognitive function following anaesthesia and electroconvulsive therapy (ECT). Int Clin Psychopharmacol 1(4): 296–302.

Kramer, B. A. 1993. Anticholinergics and ECT. Convuls Ther 9(4): 293–300.

Kramer, B. A., Afrasiabi, A., and Pollock, V. E. 1992. Intravenous versus intramuscular atropine in ECT. Am J Psychiatry 149(9): 1258–60.

Kramer, B. A., Allen, R. E., and Friedman, B. 1986. Atropine and glycopyrrolate as ECT preanes-thesia. J Clin Psychiatry 47(4): 199–200.

Krystal, A. D., Weiner, R. D., Dean, M. D., et al. 2003. Comparison of seizure duration, ictal EEG, and cognitive effects of ketamine and methohexital anesthesia with ECT. J Neuropsychiatry Clin Neurosci 15(1): 27–34.

Lui, P. W., Ma, J. Y., and Chan, K. K. 1993. Modification of tonic clonic convulsions by atracurium in multiple-monitored electroconvulsive therapy. J Clin Anesth 5(1): 16–21.

Malsch, E., Gratz, I., Mani, S., et al. 1994. Efficacy of electroconvulsive therapy after propofol and methohexital anesthesia. Convuls Ther 10(3): 212–19.

Mayur, P. M., Shree, R. S., Gangadhar, B. N., et al. 1998. Atropine premedication and the cardiovascular response to electroconvulsive therapy. Br J Anaesth 81(3): 466–7.

McInnes, E. J. and James, N. M. 1972. A comparison of ketamine and methohexital anesthesia with ECT. Med J Aust 1(20): 1031–2.

Mitchell, P. 1991. Propofol as an anaesthetic agent for electroconvulsive therapy (ECT): Effect on outcome length of course. Aust N Z J Psychiatry 25(2): 255–61.

Mokriski, B. K., Nagle, S. E., Papuchis, G. C., et al. 1992. Electroconvulsive therapy-induced cardiac arrhythmias during anesthesia with methohexital, thiamylal, or thiopental sodium. J Clin Anesth 4(3): 208–12.

Nishihara, F., Ohkawa, M., Hiraoka, H., et al. 2003. Benefits of the laryngeal mask for airway management during electroconvulsive therapy. J ECT 19(4): 211–16.

Ostroff, R., Gonzales, M., and Sanacora, G. 2005. Antidepressant effect of ketamine during ECT. Am J Psychiatry 162(7): 1385–6.

Perrin, G. 1961. Cardiovascular aspects of electroconvulsive therapy (ECT). Acta Psychiatr Scand 36(7): 43.

Plath, S. 1971. The bell jar. New York: Bantam Windstone Books, pp. 117–18, 155.

Proakis, A. G. and Harris, G. B. 1978. Comparative penetration of glycopyrrolate and atropine across the blood–brain and placental barriers in anesthetized dogs. Anesthesiology 48(5): 339–44.

Rasmussen, K. and Abrams, R. 1991. Treatment of Parkinson's disease with electroconvulsive therapy. Psychiatr Clin North Am 14(4): 925–33.

Rasmussen, K. G., Jarvis, M. R., and Zorumski, C. F. 1996. Ketamine anesthesia in electroconvulsive therapy. Convuls Ther 12(4): 217–23.

Rasmussen, K. G., Laurila, D. R., Brady, B. M., et al. 2006a. Seizure length with sevoflurane and thiopental for induction of general anesthesia in electroconvulsive therapy: A randomized double-blind trial. J ECT 22(4): 240–2.

Rasmussen, K. G., Ryan, D. A., and Mueller, P. S. 2006b. Blood glucose before and after ECT treatments in type 2 diabetic patients. J ECT 22(2): 124–6.

Rasmussen, K. G., Spackman, T. N., and Hooten, W. M. 2005. The clinical utility of inhalational anesthesia with sevoflurane in electroconvulsive therapy. J ECT 21(4): 239–42.

Rasmussen, P. 2007. Glycopyrrolate prevents extreme bradycardia and cerebral deoxygenation during electroconvulsive therapy. J ECT 23(3): 147–52.

Recart, A., Rawal, S., White, P. F., et al. 2003. The effect of remifentanil on seizure duration and acute hemodynamic responses to electroconvulsive therapy. Anesth Analg 96(4): 1047–50.

Rosa, M. A. 2007. Cardiovascular effects of anesthesia in ECT: A randomized, double blind comparison of ethomidate, propofol, and thiopenthal. J ECT 23(1): 6–8.

Saito, S., Kadoi, Y., Nara, T., et al. 2000. The comparative effects of propofol versus thiopental on middle cerebral artery blood flow velocity during electroconvulsive therapy. Anesth Analg 91(6): 1531–6.

Sakamoto, A., Hoshino, T., Suzuki, H., et al. 1999. Repeated propofol anesthesia for a patient with a history of neuroleptic malignant syndrome. J Nippon Med Sch 66(4): 262–5.

Shorter, E. and Healey, D. 2007. Shock therapy: A history of electroconvulsive treatment in mental illness. New Brunswick, NJ: Rutgers University Press.

Sparr, H. J., Beaufort, T. M., and Fuchs-Buder, T. 2001. Newer neuromuscular blocking agents: How do they compare with established agents? Drugs 61(7): 919–42.

Sullivan, P. M., Sinz, E. H., Gunel, E., and Kofke, W. A. 2004. A retrospective comparison of remifentanil versus methohexital for anesthesia in electroconvulsive therapy. J ECT 20(4): 219–24.

Swartz, C. M. 1990. Electroconvulsive therapy emergence agitation and succinylcholine dose. J Nerv Ment Dis 178(7): 455–7.

Swartz, C. M. 1993. Anesthesia for ECT. Convuls Ther 9(4): 301–16.

Toprak, H. I., Gedik, E., Begec, Z., et al. 2005. Sevoflurane as an alternative anaesthetic for electroconvulsive therapy. J ECT 21(2): 108–10.

Trollor, J. N. and Sachdev, P. S. 1999. Electroconvulsive treatment of neuroleptic malignant syndrome: A review and report of cases. Aust N Z J Psychiatry 33(5): 650–9.

Vallance, H. and McConachie, I. 1993. Neuroleptic malignant syndrome and ECT. Br J Hosp Med 49(1): 50.

van den Broek, W. W. 2004. Double blind placebo controlled study of effects of etomidate-alfentanil anesthesia in electroconvulsive therapy. J ECT 20(2): 107–11.

Wagner, K. J., Mollenberg, O., Rentrop, M., et al. 2005. Guide to anaesthetic selection for electroconvulsive therapy. CNS Drugs 19(9): 745–58.

Williams, J. 2007. Pseudocholinesterase deficency and electroconvulsive therapy. J ECT 23(3): 198–200.

27

Stimulus electrode placement

Conrad M. Swartz

Introduction

The effectiveness and cognitive side effects of electroconvulsive therapy (ECT) depend somewhat on the location of the electrical stimulus on the head. This location must correspond to the path of the electrical stimulus through the brain. The therapeutic benefits presumably reflect the generalization of the induced seizure through the brain and its intensity, that is, the quality of the seizure. Several chapters in this volume elucidate seizure quality, including those on electroencephalogram (EEG, Chapter 29) and heart rate (Chapter 30). ECT cognitive and behavioral side effects (Chapter 31) probably correspond to temporary interference with brain function. Functional brain structures in the path of the electrical stimulus should be exposed to the most intense seizure activity. Interruption of the particular duties of these structures should correspond to the side effects specific to each type of electrode placement.

Accordingly, an electrode placed over one anterior temporal lobe should disrupt memory. Analogous to the Klüver-Bucy syndrome (Lilly et al., 1983), electrodes placed symmetrically over both hemispheres (as with bitemporal ECT) should produce greater disruption than asymmetrical stimulation. Several other functional brain regions are relevant to electrode placement. The left dorsolateral prefrontal cortex assembles environmental information into sets of short-term memory for problem solving and orientation. The parietal lobe participates in spatial processing. The orbitofrontal cortex, above the eye on the forehead, identifies and manages the complexity of social interactions. Although disruptions of these regions are temporary, some seem more problematic and less desirable than others. Moreover, insofar as aesthetics and semantics are important considerations, so are the side effects of electrode placements.

The four figures show the elements of the four modern electrode placements. Figure 27.1 shows the right-sided electrode for traditional bitemporal and LART (left anterior right temporal) placements. For bitemporal ECT, the left-sided electrode is located symmetrically. For LART ECT, the left-sided electrode is on the

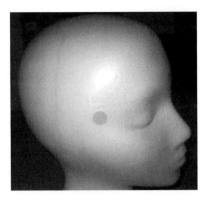

Figure 27.1 Right-sided electrode for bitemporal and left anterior right temporal (LART) placements.

forehead above the left eye, as in Figure 27.2. For right unilateral (temporal vertex) placement, both electrodes are shown in Figure 27.3; the lower electrode is in the same location as in Figure 27.1. Figure 27.4 shows the right-sided electrode for bifrontal placement; the left-sided electrode is located symmetrically.

With one electrode over each hemisphere, bitemporal, LART, and bifrontal placements are bilateral. Differences in outcome among these placements documented by controlled studies vary from minor to nonexistent. Even some of these few differences can be attributed to differing stimulus doses. The absence of proof of differing outcomes does not prove that there are no differences. This situation is analogous to that of antidepressant medications, in which large clinical trials usually identify little or no difference in benefits or side effects. Yet variations in antidepressant effects have long been clinically appreciated and seem important

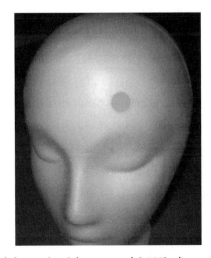

Figure 27.2 Left-sided electrode for left anterior right temporal (LART) placement.

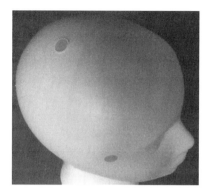

Figure 27.3 Right unilateral electrode placement.

in everyday practice. Just as expertise in medicating depression is based on direct clinical experience with a wide variety of methods and their effects, so is ECT proficiency.

Traditional discussion of electrode placement focuses on differences between bitemporal and right unilateral placements. Instead, we begin by asking why the same electrode placement should be used for every ECT session that a responding patient receives. The side effects of any particular electrode placement are primarily associated with the specific location of the electrodes, and these side effects accumulate along the course of treatment. It stands to reason that side effect aggregation should be diminished by decreasing the repetition of any particular placement. Why not rotate among the four modern electrode placements until the ECT course is concluded?

Perhaps the reason that rotation has not been done is because electrode placement is largely chosen by tradition and habit (Prudic et al., 2004), the cornerstones

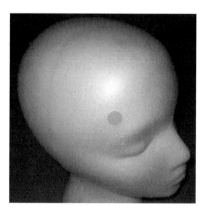

Figure 27.4 Right-sided electrode for bifrontal placement. The other electrode is placed symmetrically.

of medical practice. Changing electrode placement in reaction to nonresponse or side effects is a different issue, analogous to switching antidepressant medications. The only known report of planned electrode rotation along the course of ECT is in the Russian literature, by V. A. Rozhnov of the former USSR (Rozhnov, 1951). Rozhnov rotated among 12 different symmetrical bilateral placements, never repeating a placement for a patient. He reported benefit by the clinical impression that, of 11 patients, 4 remitted, 1 responded, 2 improved somewhat, and 4 were unchanged. Regarding side effects, he reported that no patient experienced harm; although vague, this sounds good for a course of 12 bilateral sine wave ECT treatments.

So, the starting point for electrode placement is that the best is yet to come. Our present practices are rooted in tradition and habit, rather than experience and evidence. The state of evidence does not compel any particular ECT method for electrode placement or for the stimulus-dosing plan that goes with it. Rather, its inconclusiveness suggests that practitioners accumulate experience with a variety of methods.

Just as no one antidepressant medication is best for all patients, no single ECT method suits every circumstance. The emergency of lethal catatonia generally calls for the most effective method, and potential side effects become unimportant. Conversely, an elderly patient with mild depression who has risky behavior and several medical problems is a candidate for an ECT method with diminished side effects, even if it has moderately less efficacy. The clinical balance is matching the individual patient to an electrode placement.

Studies comparing electrode placements incidentally bear on the basic issue of showing that ECT is more effective than sham treatment or doing nothing. Insofar as a study shows one ECT method to be more effective than another for patients who were randomized to the ECT treatment method they received, it shows that ECT is more effective than placebo because the lesser method is no less effective than sham treatment. Of course, insofar as the lesser method is superior to placebo, the comparison understates ECT efficacy.

Differences between tricyclic antidepressants such as desipramine and doxepin are primarily understood from clinical experience and pharmacological concepts because clinical trial comparisons have generally identified no differences. Similarly, therapeutic differences among selective serotonin-reuptake inhibitors (SSRIs) such as escitalopram and fluvoxamine have not been found. More impressive is that differences in clinical application and efficacy between tricyclics and SSRIs are usually not detected in clinical trials. Only a few focused studies have identified clinically important differences (e.g., Robinson et al., 2000; Roose et al., 1994).

Similarly, only minor variations in efficacy among the four placements have been reported. In many instances in which larger differences were reported, the placement with lower efficacy (or fewer side effects) was generally applied at lower stimulus dose. Again, there are a few exceptions.

Efficacy

We will consider electrode placement outcomes in view of these reasonable expectations for good efficacy: (a) median course of ECT no more than eight sessions, (b) remission in 80% of patients, and (c) low relapse, for example, less than 20% at one-month post-ECT. Studies should disqualify patients with comorbid conditions that increase depression ratings such as anxiety disorders, alcoholism, substance abuse, and substantial medical illness. Relapse occurring more than one month after ECT is probably related to insufficient prophylaxis rather than ECT method weakness.

Low efficacy can result from electrical stimulus underdosing. Any electrode placement can be underdosed. Low efficacy attributable to underdosing is identifiable for bitemporal (Christensen and Hedemand, 1983; Robin and de Tissera, 1982), unilateral (Letemendia et al., 1993; Sackeim et al., 1993), and bifrontal electrode placements (Heikman et al., 2002). Of course, underdosing a placement does not properly test it and can lead to no clinical implications about it. Occasional or mild underdosing will increase the number of ECT sessions needed. Marked underdosing decreases the remission rate and increases the relapse rate. Still, it is easier to underdose unilateral ECT than bilateral ECT because seizure can be induced by a lower dose; in other words, unilateral ECT has lower seizure threshold.

A problem analogous to underdosage is nonpenetrance of the stimulus, caused by inadequate pulse width. Nonpenetrance can occur with ultrabrief stimuli and any placement. It is explained in Chapter 1.

From the opposite perspective, higher stimulus dosage increases cognitive side effects for every electrode placement (UK ECT Review Group, 2003). Overdosing can decrease or erase cognitive advantages associated with any placement. Physiologically, an unnecessarily high stimulus dose increases the size of the brain region that the stimulus directly affects. It defocuses and diffuses the stimulus. The stimulus gradually loses its identity and specific characteristics as the dose increases. Differences among geometrically close electrode placements should vanish at moderate overdosage, such as among the three bilateral placements (bitemporal, LART, and bifrontal). At high overdosage, wide spread of the stimulus through the brain makes all electrode placements equivalent and indistinguishable in effects.

Cognitive issues

We will also consider electrode placement outcomes in view of reported observations. ECT cognitive side effects are temporary, and there is no persistent effect on the ability to learn. So, its cognitive side effects are a relatively small matter. After a course of ECT, a desirable and reasonable average Mini Mental State Examination (MMSE) score is at least 27, of course for patients who have no underlying cognitive impairment. These patients should also be able to manage their own personal care without supervision.

Cognitive side effects from ECT can be separated into three different types: gradual cumulative disorientation, acute-onset delirium, and retrograde memory loss. Cognitive dysfunction from ECT does not correspond to adverse neuronal effects. Rather, neurochemical and anatomical evidence shows that neuronal injury does not occur from ECT (Coffey et al., 1991; Zachrisson et al., 2000). Although adverse cognitive effects are often milder than pre-ECT cognitive impairment by the illness under treatment, they can require specific attention. Marked cognitive dysfunction does not have a desirable appearance, and patients with any cognitive dysfunction remaining from ECT or illness can exhibit impaired judgment. These are the reasons that every ECT patient does not receive bitemporal electrode placement and that alternatives are considered. Still, electrode placement and stimulus dosing are not the only alterable aspects of ECT method that influence cognitive side effects. Others include the frequency of ECT sessions, stimulus efficiency (mostly stimulus pulse width, see Chapter 1), and probably the anesthetic used and concurrent medications (e.g., intravenous caffeine).

Gradual cumulative disorientation is the ordinary form of ECT cognitive side effects. When it occurs, it is usually first noticeable after three or four ECT treatments and accumulates with additional ECT sessions. It is reflected by the decrease of MMSE scores along the course of treatment (Calev et al., 1991; Folstein et al., 1975). It varies among patients in both severity and duration, from negligible to substantial, and lasts up to a month. The largest and longest disorientations tend to occur in elderly patients and in patients with bitemporal electrode placement. Nevertheless, I have seen octogenarians receive full courses of ECT without any cognitive side effects and state surprise that I would ask. Despite their temporary nature, ECT cognitive side effects can delay the return of some patients home and necessitate nursing support for personal care. In some patients, they can obscure the observation of a bona fide therapeutic response that has occurred.

Acute-onset delirium from ECT is seen as sudden onset of marked confusion after a particular treatment. It can occur either after the first ECT or not until after several. Although temporary and unusual, acute-onset delirium is usually severe and requires staff supervision. This delirium can be mistaken for catatonia (Swartz, 2002a), but ECT mitigates (not causes) catatonia. When acute delirium occurs after ECT, nonconvulsive status epilepticus should be considered and a standard neurological EEG checked. Although it is uncommon, its severity is a reason to routinely monitor the EEG during ECT for signs that the seizure has terminated.

Presumably, some concurrent neurological illnesses (e.g., cerebrovascular disease, Lewy body dementia) pose risks for acute-onset delirium, which is not known to depend on electrode placement.

For some patients, cognitive side effects occur regardless of ECT method. In one report of elderly patients with depression, 5/34 (15%) receiving unilateral brief-pulse ECT but only 1/29 (3%) receiving bitemporal brief-pulse ECT experienced severe disorientation (Coffey et al., 1988). There is no rationale for greater disorientation from unilateral ECT, so severe disorientation should have occurred in these particular patients with any placement. The high 10% overall incidence of severe disorientation suggests that it tends to occur primarily in elderly patients. That it was severe and common with unilateral ECT suggests that these patients experienced acute-onset delirium rather than gradual cumulative disorientation, but sufficient details were not provided.

Permanent memory loss dating from before the onset of depression specifically caused by ECT is controversial. A demonstration of permanent memory loss from ECT would have to clearly separate it from cognitive dysfunction resulting from medications, psychiatric illness, comorbid medical illness, comorbid anxiety disorder, and subjective dissatisfaction from suffering with psychiatric illness and other life events. For example, cognitive dysfunction can persist for well beyond six months after discontinuing benzodiazepines (Barker et al., 2005), and anticholinergic drugs may cause permanent cognitive dysfunction (Tsao et al., 2008). As of two months post-ECT personal memory is not lost, but there is a nonsignificant trend ($p = .07$) for lost memory about nonpersonal events (Lisanby et al., 2000). Personal memory loss has been claimed to occur more frequently with bitemporal than with unilateral placement. Of course, bitemporal ECT is preferentially used in more severe and resistant forms of illness, which can themselves generate greater impairment of memory. Of course, a temporary disruption of learning and memory can produce a persisting gap in memories, and this occurs with ECT. It also occurs from psychiatric illness itself, anesthesia, heavy drinking, or the use of antipsychotic drugs (Harrison and Therrien, 2007), anticholinergic medications, or benzodiazepines. Referring to this temporary effect as permanent seems an exaggeration. Still, it seems reasonable to suppose that high-stimulus doses and long ECT courses can produce some persisting retrograde memory loss, especially in patients who experience acute-onset delirium, and perhaps more with bitemporal ECT.

Neurobiology

Please see Chapter 1 for background. The brain regions of highest current density with the electrical stimulus (i.e., the current path) should experience the most intense seizure activity, and so the strongest and longest interference with normal brain function. This current path depends on several aspects of geometry and anatomy: separation distance between electrodes, depth difference between electrodes, and electrode proximity to skull foramina and sutures, in addition to the particular sites and the stimulus dose.

A basic electrical consideration is that wider separation distance spreads the current over a larger volume, diluting it. Electrode separation by an additional 25% approximately doubles the volume. Larger depth distance between electrodes does the same thing. Moving two electrodes apart in the same plane spreads the current over two dimensions, but moving them apart depthwise spreads it over three dimensions, increasing the volume far more. To induce a seizure, this stimulus dilution over brain volume needs to be compensated for by increasing the stimulus dose, either the charge or the current. At the same time, raising the stimulus dose defocuses and spreads it over a larger volume. With electrodes that are spaced more widely or have larger depth distances, the brain volume in which the seizure begins (i.e., the volume of seizure foci) will be larger. This is probably why bilateral ECT placements have much higher seizure threshold than right unilateral placements, and also why they are more generalized through the brain (Swartz and Larson, 1986).

Electrical resistance through skull sutures and foramina is of course much lower than through unperforated skull bone. The skull sutures and foramina are essentially electrical short-circuits through the skull. If an electrode is placed on top of a suture, current density should be much higher in brain regions near the inside of the suture. Proximity to foramina and skull sutures focuses the stimulus into these regions and is also equivalent to a higher stimulus dose, both of which should cause more intense seizure and interruption of function within these brain regions. The proximity to skull sutures varies widely among electrode placements and is discussed later in this chapter. Placing stimulus electrodes near a surgical skull defect (e.g., a conductive metal plate or hole in the skull) requires unusual precautions and generally should be avoided when possible. Of course a hole in the skull is usually filled with extracellular fluid that conducts electricity well.

Both hemispheres contribute to many basic functions, including speech, memory, and cognition, although in somewhat different manners (Bragina and Dobrokhotova, 1981; Luria and Simernitskaya, 1975). Each side can compensate for a deficit in the other, so that bilateral deficits can cause far greater impairment of performance than a deficit on one side alone (Lilly et al., 1983). This greater toxicity of bilateral deficits suggests that asymmetry of an electrode placement should be associated with milder cognitive side effects.

The electrode placements are described one at a time. Bilateral and unilateral electrode placements have separate stimulus-dosing strategies. The three bilateral placements should have similar dosage. For background and principles of stimulus dosing and its effects, please see Chapters 1, 28, 30, and 31.

Bitemporal ECT

Bitemporal placement, also called bifrontotemporal, is the traditional bilateral placement. Some clinicians who use it exclusively say they turn to ECT because of reliable high efficacy. They aim to avoid any decrease in efficacy and consider bitemporal side effects to be tolerable. However, other clinicians use bitemporal placement solely for unusually severe cases and patients who do not respond to other electrode placements.

Bitemporal placement consists of one electrode on the flat of each temple, placed symmetrically. Of the four electrode placements, it has the largest depth distance and it geometrically includes the largest volume of brain between the two electrodes. Two skull sutures criss-cross the bitemporal site, shaping an "X" in the skull bone under it. This suggests focused stimulus penetration into the brain areas directly underneath the temple, the dorsolateral prefrontal cortex, and the anterior temporal lobe. Brain imaging study results are consistent with this expectation (Chapter 5). Each characteristic noted in this paragraph probably contributes to the mildly higher levels of seizure generalization (Swartz and Larson, 1986), efficacy, and cognitive side effects associated with bitemporal placement.

One of the best reported clinical outcomes for bitemporal ECT used a mean initial dose of 170 mC at 800 mA in patients with depression who were, on average, 55 years old. The initial dose was 1.5 times the seizure threshold, and equivalent to about 120 mC at 900 mA, which conforms to the method of half-age dosing (Petrides and Fink, 1996). Remission occurred in 95% of patients, average course length was six treatments, and average posttreatment MMSE score was 26/30. According to the results, about 1/6 of patients would score 20 or less on the MMSE (Bailine et al., 2000). This clinical outcome is desirable.

A clearly less desirable outcome was seen in patients with depression who received a much higher stimulus dose and a longer ECT course. These patients had a strong sense of chronicity, with illness onset about 15 years prior and current episode almost a year in duration. This long-standing pattern of illness suggests high levels of comorbid anxiety disorders. At an average dose of 260 mC at 800 mA in patients with an average age of 56 years (2.5 times seizure threshold, and equal to about 186 mC at 900 mA, which is dosing at 2/3 of age), response occurred in 65% with an average course length of 8.3 treatments (Sackeim et al., 2000). This result of "response" was not as good as remission and included patients who remained moderately ill, with a Hamilton Rating Scale for Depression score up to 16 points. The average decrease in MMSE score as a percentage of maximum possible score was 15.4%, corresponding to 4.6 points on a 30-point test. This indicates that half the patients scored fewer than 24 points, which is in the impaired range. The MMSE standard deviation implies that about one sixth of patients scored below 18 points. These high levels of side effects presumably reflect the high stimulus dose, higher than routinely desirable for bitemporal ECT. This report did not state that anxiety disorders were examined or accounted for, and neither did a similar earlier report (Sackeim et al., 1993). Accordingly, the investigators did not show that their post-ECT results were free from large effects by comorbid anxiety disorders. For more discussion about anxiety disorders and ECT, please see Chapter 22.

Overall, bitemporal placement is the reference for maximal ECT efficacy, but also for maximal side effects. It is the clear choice when efficacy is urgent and when avoiding side effects of the extent described above is not nearly as important as prompt efficacy. Dosing is more straightforward than for unilateral ECT, just as it is with other bilateral placements.

Right unilateral ECT

Several forms of right unilateral ECT have been in clinical use. The modern form, described by d'Elia (1980), has wider spacing between the electrodes than the previous Lancaster method had. In the d'Elia placement, one electrode is on the flat of the right temple, as with bitemporal placement. The other is just to the right of the vertex, which is the highest point on the skull.

A common variation relocates this upper electrode backward, midway between the vertex and the occiput, over the parietal lobe. The location of this variation is just to the right of the point where male pattern baldness begins. This point is diagonally across the skull from the chin. This location is notable because during the stimulus the jaw is normally held closed at the chin. With one hand on the chin and the other on the unilateral electrode handle it is natural to press the electrode down diagonally across from the chin. This pressure stabilizes the electrode location, the jaw closure, and the position of the patient's head. Probably most unilateral ECT in the United States is given with this variation rather than the actual d'Elia placement. With its spacing wider than that of the d'Elia placement, it should be at least as effective.

The rationale for placing both electrodes over the right hemisphere is that the left hemisphere is dominant in speaking and problem solving for the vast majority of patients whether right-handed or left-handed. The left hemisphere is dominant in 95% of right-handers and in 80% of left-handers. There is no practical way to identify the few right-brain–dominant patients, even for those who are left-handed. Giving ECT over the right hemisphere when it is dominant is not dangerous, because it still does not stimulate the right hemisphere as much as bitemporal ECT does.

Among the four electrode placements, unilateral ECT has the smallest depth distance and geometrical brain volume between its two electrodes. The minimum charge needed to induce a seizure with unilateral placement is about half that needed for bilateral placement (Sackeim et al., 1993), which suggests that the brain volume of seizure foci generated by a unilateral ECT stimulus is half that from a bilateral ECT stimulus. The temporal electrode is over a confluence of skull sutures, just as with bitemporal ECT. The edge of the upper electrode is on top of the sagittal skull suture, both for d'Elia unilateral and the common variation. Unilateral ECT is asymmetrical, of course.

The reason for the existence of unilateral ECT is to aim to decrease side effects to milder than those of bitemporal ECT. Indeed, the consensus has long been that bitemporal placement provokes stronger cognitive side effects and unilateral placement is less effective, with fewer remissions and more relapses (Sackeim et al., 1993, 2000; UK ECT Review Group, 2003). The contrast in side effects between bitemporal and unilateral ECT was much larger and thereby more important when 50- to 60-Hz sine wave stimuli and other inefficient waveforms were commonly used. The cognitive side effects of both placements are much lower with more efficient waveforms such as brief-pulse stimuli (see Chapter 1).

The differences between bitemporal and right unilateral ECT depend sensitively on the stimulus dose used with unilateral ECT. These differences are greatest with minimal unilateral doses and are negligible at high doses. At low stimulus dose (e.g., 85 mC average), therapeutic response to unilateral ECT is quite low, for example, 17% versus 65% for bitemporal ECT (Sackeim et al., 1993). Likewise, the lowest level of cognitive side effects for unilateral ECT appears at this low dosage (Sackeim et al., 2000). In the middle dose range (e.g., 130 to 175 mC average), the response rate to unilateral ECT increases to 30% to 45% (Sackeim et al., 1993, 2000). Both therapeutic and side effect differences between unilateral and bitemporal ECT fade at high unilateral doses (e.g., about 375 mC), with remission rates of 65% to 80% (Abrams et al., 1991; McCall et al., 2000, 2002).

Those statistics are for groups of patients. Best clinical practice is not to use one uniform dose for all patients; it is to match the dose to the patient. To illustrate, there is no dispute that low-dose right unilateral ECT has mild side effects. With remission rate one third that of bitemporal ECT (Sackeim et al., 1993), it brings remission in one third of patients who could respond to ECT. How do we identify these patients who respond to low dose? To medium dose? To nothing less than high dose? Not knowing how to set the dose for right unilateral ECT individually for patients is a problem that has not yet been solved.

Specifically, in the "seizure threshold multiple" method of dosing unilateral ECT, the multiple is associated with group response rates, not the need of the individual patient. Giving every patient high-dose unilateral placement (e.g., 5 to 6 times threshold) is analogous to giving everyone the same extra-large-size clothing to wear; everyone will fit in but smaller people will experience unnecessary difficulties. It is analogous to giving every patient with chronic schizophrenia 16 mg/d risperidone and no less because it has a higher response rate than any lower dose. Good practice is identifying which patients should respond well to a treatment with milder side effects than those that appear with high-dose right unilateral or bitemporal ECT. How can we identify the multiple to use with an individual patient? As yet no method is established. The "Benchmark Method" for adjusting stimulus dose along the course of ECT was used only in bilateral placement (Swartz, 2002b) and not tested for unilateral ECT.

The overall view of right unilateral ECT is less clear than for other placements. The essence of any electrode placement occurs at low dosage; at higher dosages, the stimulus path broadens. At low dosage, right unilateral ECT has weak effects, with long courses needed and low remission rate but negligible side effects. For reliable efficacy, clinicians must use a high stimulus dose, but then unilateral differs little from bitemporal ECT in efficacy or side effects. The advantages of unilateral ECT should largely be in middle-sized doses but there still is no clear method to match the dose to the individual patient. This uncertainty decreases the desirability of unilateral placement. Unilateral placement at less than high dosage is a first consideration for patients who previously responded well and enduringly to it and for those who experienced marked disorientation with other placements and have no special urgency for response. For most patients, dosing is less straightforward for unilateral ECT than for the three bilateral placements.

LART ECT

With LART placement, the left electrode is moved forward to be on the forehead (superior to the left eye), about 5 cm anterior on the skin to the location for bitemporal ECT. Just as the eye faces forward, so does this electrode. The right electrode is over the right temple, at the same site for bitemporal and right unilateral ECT.

LART was constructed as a modification of bitemporal ECT, with the expectation that moving the left electrode forward would decrease side effects but not diminish efficacy (Swartz, 1994). The first names used for it (bilateral frontal-frontotemporal and asymmetric bilateral) were not specific, so were changed. The discrepancy in naming is that for electrode placement "frontal" is not fully anterior, but the LART left electrode faces entirely forward. Its anterior location clearly separates it from the left temporal lobe and dorsolateral prefrontal cortex. It is over the orbitofrontal cortex.

Thanks to the experience and teaching of Alexander Nelson, LART is used in about 10% of ECT treatments in Russia; some hospitals there use LART in 80% of

ECT treatments (Nelson, 2005). LART has been consistently used at a variety of hospitals in the United States. At East Carolina University (Pitt County Memorial Hospital), consistent use of LART resulted from the clinical appearance of my LART ECT patients and the favorable impressions they made on the staff and private practice psychiatrists. My preference of LART is for all patients except emergencies such as lethal catatonia.

The depth distance and distance between electrodes of LART placement are intermediate between bitemporal and unilateral ECT, and about the same as for bifrontal placement. The geometric volume of brain between the two electrodes is about the same as in bifrontal placement and about 3/4 that in bitemporal ECT. Because seizure thresholds of bifrontal and bitemporal ECT are equal (Bailine et al., 2000), they and LART should have similar seizure thresholds and actual brain volumes of seizure foci. The left electrode of LART is not above any suture or foramen, so there should be no high concentration of current anywhere in the left hemisphere. LART is plainly asymmetric.

The initial study of LART was an open trial of 10 women. All patients achieved remission; 90% continued in remission on 6 to 10 weeks of follow-up. At the end of the ECT course, their MMSE scores averaged 28.4, markedly higher than the pretreatment average of 11. The median course length was seven ECT treatments (Swartz, 1994). The pre-ECT average of MMSE scores was low because the patients were severely ill with mania or psychotic depression. The good results for patients with mania suggest robust efficacy for this placement. In a double-blinded pilot study of eight subjects, LART tended to produce greater efficacy and lower cognitive side effects than did bitemporal ECT in both right- and left-hemisphere functions (Swartz and Evans, 1996). In an open trial of LART of 24 depressed patients, 88% achieved remission and 100% showed response (Swartz, 2000); the median course length was six ECT treatments. The stimulus dose was 2.5 mC per year of age at the beginning of the course at 900 mA (i.e., half-age dosing method) and it gradually increased to about 5 mC per year (i.e., full age) by the sixth ECT. The Benchmark Method describes how to adjust the stimulus dose of LART along the entire course of ECT without need to identify seizure threshold (Swartz, 2002b); it should apply in the same way to other bilateral placements.

Overall, LART placement seems to have fewer side effects than bitemporal placement with similar efficacy, when used at similar doses. Dosing is more straightforward for LART and the other bilateral placements than for unilateral ECT.

Bifrontal ECT

Despite its name, bifrontal electrodes do not face forward. The name corresponds to the location over the frontal cortex. In particular, both electrodes are over the dorsolateral prefrontal cortex, just anterior to the temporal lobe. Each electrode is located 2.5 cm forward of the site used for bitemporal ECT, one over each hemisphere. Because the typical diameter or length of an ECT electrode is 5 cm, each bifrontal electrode site overlaps halfway with the bitemporal electrode site. In other words, if both bifrontal and bitemporal electrodes were applied, one would cover half the other. Here is another way of describing the location: Many people have a bony ridge at the lateral edge of the forehead, where the forehead joins the temple. This bony ridge bisects (runs across the center of) the electrode. Anatomically, the bifrontal site is the least flat (most convex) of the electrode sites mentioned here.

Bifrontal placement was introduced by James Inglis and initially tested by his colleagues at Queens University in Ontario (Lawson et al., 1990; Letemendia et al., 1993). Its use is probably increasing, as clinicians become aware of alternatives to bitemporal and unilateral placements.

The bifrontal placement electrode depth distance and distance between electrodes are intermediate between bitemporal and unilateral ECT and about the same as for LART placement. The geometric brain volume between the two electrodes is about 3/4 that of bitemporal ECT and about the same as with LART. The seizure threshold with bifrontal ECT is the same as for bitemporal (Bailine et al., 2000), so the bifrontal brain volume of seizure foci apparently equals that for bitemporal ECT. Half of each bifrontal electrode is on top of two skull sutures; this is half the exposure to sutures of bitemporal electrodes. The bifrontal placement is inherently symmetrical.

Perhaps the best reported outcome for bifrontal ECT was remission in 95% of patients with depression, with a mean course length of six treatments and a post-ECT MMSE average score of 28/30. These outcomes were observed in patients with an average age of 55 years and with an average initial stimulus of 170 mC at 800 mA (1.5 times seizure threshold, equivalent to 120 mC at 900 mA, and consistent with half-age dosing). The mean and standard deviations imply that an MMSE score less than 20 should be rare with bifrontal ECT (Bailine et al., 2000). This is plainly a desirable clinical outcome. The Bailine report stated that elderly patients showed lower MMSE scores. This raises the possibility that the cognitive advantage of bifrontal over bitemporal ECT applies primarily to elderly patients, who are the same patients who receive the highest stimulus doses, because the dose needed increases with age.

Other studies reported lower efficacy or greater cognitive side effects with bifrontal placement. A study using the same stimulus dose reported only 12 of 46 (26%) patients responding to bifrontal ECT (with a 50% decrease in depression rating). The average MMSE score remained 26/30. Right unilateral ECT had the same outcome (Eschweiler et al., 2007). Another study reported an average post-ECT MMSE score of 24.1 and a standard deviation of 4.5; this implies that 1/6 of patients had an MMSE score less than 20. Results for bitemporal and right unilateral ECT were close to this, and all three produced similar post-ECT depression ratings. Unfortunately, the seizure thresholds and stimulus doses in this study were not properly reported (Ranjkesh et al., 2005).

In a small comparison of seven patients receiving bifrontal ECT at an average dose of 120 mC at 900 mA (equivalent to 170 mA at 800 mA), an average of 12 ECT sessions was needed, 3 of 7 patients responded, and the post-ECT MMSE average score was 26 (Heikman et al., 2002). This is an undesirably large number of ECT sessions. In comparison, patients receiving high-dose unilateral ECT (252 mC at 900 mA, equivalent to 85% of age) needed an average of 7 ECT sessions, 7/8 patients responded, and the post-ECT MMSE average score was 25.

The first comparisons among bifrontal, bitemporal, and unilateral placements used low stimulus doses, averaging 148 mC for bitemporal, 164 mC for bifrontal, and 107 mC for unilateral ECT, all at 800 mA (Lawson et al., 1990; Letemendia et al., 1993). The dosage was reflected in the outcomes, especially the underdosing of unilateral ECT. The course lengths for bifrontal, bitemporal, and unilateral ECT averaged 10.3, 11.5, and 15.7 sessions, respectively. These are unusually long courses for bitemporal and unilateral ECT, apparently because of underdosage. This underdosage prevents the study results from applying to clinical circumstances of proper (higher) dosing. The result that some depression scores were marginally lower with bifrontal than bitemporal ECT is attributable to the higher stimulus dose used with bifrontal placement. The low effectiveness of unilateral ECT reported in these studies is similarly explained by marked underdosage. Regarding side effects, only post-ECT verbal memory scores were better with bifrontal than with bitemporal ECT. However, there was no pre-ECT baseline measurement, and the difference between bifrontal and bitemporal ECT persisted for three months. This is far longer than an electrode placement effect should persist. Logically it is reasonable to take the three-month score as the baseline. Doing this leaves no side effect advantage of bifrontal ECT over bitemporal.

Overall, bifrontal placement usually tends to have moderately lower side effects than bitemporal placement with similar efficacy, when used at similar doses. As with other bilateral placements, dosing is more straightforward than for unilateral ECT.

In conclusion, for electrode placement just as with medications, selection and dosage are matters for individual consideration with each patient. Experience with each placement should help the clinician in making these decisions.

References

Abrams, R., Swartz, C. M., Vedak, C. 1991. Antidepressant effects of high-dose right unilateral ECT. Arch Gen Psychiatry 48: 746–8.

Bailine, S. H., Rifkin, A., Kayne, E., et al. 2000. Comparison of bifrontal and bitemporal ECT for major depression. Am J Psychiatry 157: 121–3.

Barker, M. J., Greenwood, K. M., Jackson, M., Crowe, S. F. 2005. An evaluation of persisting cognitive effects after withdrawal from long-term benzodiazepine use. J Int Neuropsychol Soc 11: 281–9.

Bragina, N. N. and Dobrokhotova, T. A. 1981. Human functional asymmetries. Moscow: Meditsina (Russian).

Calev, A., Cohen, R., Tubi, N., et al. 1991. Disorientation and bilateral moderately suprathreshold titrated ECT. Convuls Ther 7: 99–110.

Christensen, P. and Hedemand, E. 1983. EEG and EMG monitored electroconvulsive therapy. Psychopharmacol Bull 19: 20–2.

Coffey, C. E., Figiel, G. S., Djang, W. T., et al. 1988. Leukoencephalopathy in elderly depressed patients referred for ECT. Biol Psychiatry 24: 143–61.

Coffey, C. E., Weiner, R. D., Djang, W. T., et al. 1991. Brain anatomic effects of electroconvulsive therapy. A prospective magnetic resonance imaging study. Arch Gen Psychiatry 48: 1013–21.

d'Elia, G. 1980. Unilateral electroconvulsive therapy. Acta Psychiatr Scand Suppl 215: 1–98.

Eschweiler, G. W., Vonthein, R., Bode, R., et al. 2007. Clinical efficacy and cognitive side effects of bifrontal versus right unilateral electroconvulsive therapy (ECT): A short-term randomised controlled trial in pharmaco-resistant major depression. J Affect Disord 101: 149–57.

Folstein, M. R., Folstein, S. E., and McHugh, P. R. 1975. "Mini-Mental State": A practical method of grading the cognitive state of patients for the clinician. J Psychiatr Res 12: 189–98.

Harrison, B. E. and Therrien, B. 2007. Effect of antipsychotic medication use on memory in patients with Alzheimer's disease: Assessing the potential risk for accelerated recent autobiographical memory loss. J Gerontol Nurs 33: 11–20.

Heikman, P., Kalska, H., Katila, H., et al. 2002. Right unilateral and bifrontal electroconvulsive therapy in the treatment of depression: a preliminary study. J ECT 18: 26–30.

Lawson, J. S., Inglis, J., Delva, N. J., et al. 1990. Electrode placement in ECT: Cognitive effects. Psychol Med 20: 335–44.

Letemendia, F. J., Delva, N. J., Rodenburg, M., et al. 1993. Therapeutic advantage of bifrontal electrode placement in ECT. Psychol Med 23: 349–60.

Lilly, R., Cummings, J. L., Benson, F., and Frankel, M. 1983. The human Klüver-Bucy Syndrome. Neurology 33: 1141–5.

Lisanby, S. H., Maddox, J. H., Prudic, J., et al. 2000. The effects of electroconvulsive therapy on memory of autobiographical and public events. Arch Gen Psychiatry 57: 581–90.

Luria, A. R. and Simernitskaya, E. G. 1975. Interhemispheral relations and functions of the right hemisphere. Report I. About functional interaction of brain hemispheres in organization of verbal-mnesic functions [in Russian]. Fiziol Cheloveka 1: 411–16.

McCall, V. W., Dunn, A., Rosenquist, P. B., and Hughes, D. 2002. Markedly suprathreshold right unilateral ECT versus minimally suprathreshold bilateral ECT: Antidepressant and memory effects. J ECT 18: 126–9.

McCall, W. V., Reboussin, D. M., Weiner, R. D., and Sackeim, H. A. 2000. Titrated moderately suprathreshold vs fixed high-dose right unilateral electroconvulsive therapy. Arch Gen Psychiatry 57: 438–44.

Nelson, A. I. 2005. A national survey of electroconvulsive therapy use in the Russian Federation. J ECT 21: 151–7.

Petrides, G. and Fink, M. 1996. The "half-age" stimulation strategy for ECT dosing. Convuls Ther 12: 138–46.

Prudic, J., Olfson, M., Marcus, S. C., et al. 2004. Effectiveness of electroconvulsive therapy in community settings. Biol Psychiatry 55: 301–12.

Ranjkesh, F., Barekatain, M., and Akuchakian, S. 2005. Bifrontal versus right unilateral and bitemporal electroconvulsive therapy in major depressive disorder. J ECT 21: 207–10.

Robin, A. and de Tissera, S. 1982. A double-blind controlled comparison of the therapeutic effects of low and high energy electroconvulsive therapies. Br J Psychiatry 141: 357–66.

Robinson, R. G., Schultz, S. K., Castillo, C., et al. 2000. Nortriptyline versus fluoxetine in the treatment of depression and in short-term recovery after stroke: A placebo-controlled, double-blind study. Am J Psychiatry 157: 351–9.

Roose, S. P., Glassman, A. H., Attia, E., and Woodring, S. 1994. Comparative efficacy of selective serotonin reuptake inhibitors and tricyclics in the treatment of melancholia. Am J Psychiatry 151: 1735–9.

Rozhnov, V. A. 1951. Electroconvulsive therapy with the changing electrode position [in Russian]. Kirghiz State Medical Institute Proceedings, Frunze, VII, pp. 365–71.

Sackeim, H. A., Prudic, J., Devanand, D. P., et al. 1993. Effects of stimulus intensity and electrode placement on the efficacy and cognitive effects of electroconvulsive therapy. N Engl J Med 328: 839–46.

Sackeim, H. A., Prudic, J., Devanand, D. P., et al. 2000. A prospective, randomized, double-blind comparison of bilateral and right unilateral electroconvulsive therapy at different stimulus intensities. Arch Gen Psychiatry 57: 425–34.

Swartz, C. M. 1994. Asymmetric bilateral right frontotemporal left frontal stimulus electrode placement. Neuropsychobiology 29: 174–8.

Swartz, C. M. 2000. Physiological response to ECT stimulus dose. Psychiatr Res 97: 229–35.

Swartz, C. M. 2002a. Delirium or catatonic disorder due to general medical condition. J ECT 18: 167–8.

Swartz, C. M. 2002b. ECT dosing by the Benchmark method. German J Psychiatry 5: 1–4. Available at http://www.gjpsy.uni-goettingen.de.

Swartz, C. M. and Evans, C. M. 1996. Beyond bitemporal and right unilateral electrode placements. Psychiatr Ann 26: 705–8.

Swartz, C. M. and Larson, G. 1986. Generalization of the effects of unilateral and bilateral ECT. Am J Psychiatry 143: 1040–1.

Tsao, J., Shah, R., Leurgans, S., et al. 2008. Impaired cognition in normal individuals using medications with anticholinergic activity occurs following several years [Abstract S51.001]. Academy of Neurology, 60th Annual Meeting, April 17.

UK ECT Review Group. 2003. Efficacy and safety of electroconvulsive therapy in depressive disorders: A systematic review and meta-analysis. Lancet 361(9360): 799–808.

Zachrisson, O. C., Balldin, J., Ekman, R., et al. 2000. No evident neuronal damage after electroconvulsive therapy. Psychiatry Res 96: 157–65.

28

Stimulus dosing

W. Vaughn McCall

Introduction

Decision making regarding the choice of stimulus dose for a session of electroconvulsive therapy (ECT) has become increasingly complicated, making it difficult to make specific recommendations in selecting a stimulus dose. Variability in ECT provider awareness of new data, and differences between early adopters and late adopters of new information, will add to the already great variability in the practice of ECT, at least in the short term (Prudic et al., 2004). Still, some general recommendations can be made, and these are presented at the end of this chapter. Unless stated otherwise, all comments in this chapter pertain to the acute treatment of depressive disorders.

Questions about the proper management of the electrical stimulus have been central to the science and practice of ECT since the inception of the treatment. Problems in stimulus dosing include (a) whether the stimulus should be subconvulsive or convulsive; (b) defining the optimal stimulus waveform; (c) if a convulsive stimulus is desired, to what degree should the stimulus intensity be in excess of the convulsive threshold; and (d) which physiological parameters, if any, provide useful feedback to continuously refine stimulus dosing throughout the ECT course.

Units of measure in defining the stimulus dose

Two equations describe most of what an ECT practitioner needs to know about the magnitude of the stimulus: $V = IR$ and $Q = IT$. $V = IR$, also known as Ohm's law, states that electromotive force (V) is equal to current (I) multiplied by the impedance (R) to current flow. The unit of measure for V is volts, for I is amperes, and for R is ohms. In the case of ECT, the patient becomes part of a biological electrical circuit, and within this circuit the patient provides most of the impedance (R). Given that the patient's R cannot be controlled or even confidently predicted, R will vary continuously. If R is allowed to vary, then the equation $V = IR$ dictates

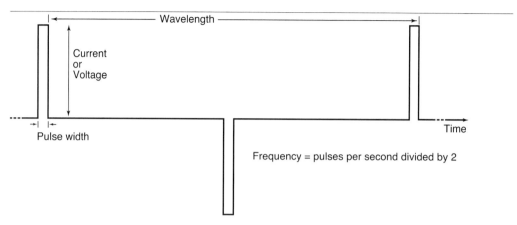

Figure 28.1 The components of the brief-pulse stimulus.

that *V* may be held constant while *I* varies inversely to *R*. Alternatively, *I* may be held constant while *V* varies proportionately to *R*. This implies that two basic types of ECT devices are possible: constant current and constant voltage. The constant-current machines are preferred and dominate American ECT devices, as constant-current machines are less likely to pose danger to the patient. Finally, although ECT stimulus-dosing parameters are sometimes reported in units of energy (i.e., joules), (a) energy is a function of impedance, and (b) impedance cannot be fixed in ECT; therefore, constant-current machines cannot deliver a fixed-energy stimulus. Instead, constant-current machines will deliver a stimulus of fixed electrical charge. The unit of measure for charge (*Q*) is coulombs, or more precisely (in the world of ECT), millicoulombs (mC).

When an ECT practitioner is setting the stimulus parameters on a constant-current device, he or she has only two considerations that influence the charge: (a) the magnitude of the current, and (b) the total duration of time that the current is flowing. Multiplied together, these two variables determine the total stimulus charge. For this reason, most ECT studies conducted within the past 20 years have reported the stimulus dose in millicoulombs.

The ECT practitioner has considerable latitude in controlling the pattern and timing of current flow. Modern ECT devices use brief-pulse waveforms, which break the stimulus up into small bits, spread out over time. Brief-pulse machines typically have a biphasic stimulus, meaning that the current alternates its direction of flow (see Figure 28.1). ECT providers then have the option of controlling the width of each pulse, the frequency of pulse pairs per second, and the duration of the entire stimulus train. It is important to emphasize that current is not actually flowing for the entire time that the ECT provider is pressing the stimulus button on the device and delivering the stimulus. The ECT practitioner's decisions regarding the magnitude of the stimulus current, and the magnitude and patterning of the timing of the stimulus delivery, will ultimately have an impact on the clinical outcome. For more information about the electrical stimulus and its dose, see Chapter 1.

Convulsive, subconvulsive, and sham stimulation

The development of modified ECT (including muscle relaxation and general anesthesia) raised questions as to whether the seizure was central to the antidepressant efficacy of ECT or whether anesthesia alone would be just as effective. The Northwick Park trial (Johnstone and Deakin, 1980) and the Leicestershire trial (Brandon et al., 1984) are examples of two "sham" ECT studies in which anesthesia alone was compared with real ECT. It was convincingly demonstrated that real ECT was more effective, especially for the most severe forms of depression (Brandon et al., 1984; Johnstone and Deakin, 1980; UK ECT Review Group, 2003). The effectiveness of ECT was clearly linked to the production of a seizure. Neither anesthesia alone without the electrical stimulus nor the use of subconvulsive stimuli appears to have real merit in the treatment of depression, at least in the context of ECT.

Stimulus waveform morphology

Given that a convulsive stimulus is necessary for the antidepressant effects of ECT, a nearly infinite number of variations were available for formulating the stimulus waveform. The earliest ECT devices delivered a sinusoidal stimulus, similar to what is delivered from a U.S. wall socket. Other waveforms available on early ECT devices included the "chopped" sine wave, the unidirectional-pulse square wave, and the alternating brief-pulse square wave. Sine wave stimulation has been discredited by a randomized study showing that sine wave ECT produced more memory side effects than brief-pulse ECT did, irrespective of the placement of the stimulating electrode (Weiner et al., 1986). This finding was recently replicated in an effectiveness study using a prospective cohort study, this time showing that, compared with brief-pulse stimulation, sine wave stimulation was associated with a slowing of reaction time that persisted for at least six months after ECT (Sackeim et al., 2007). "Standard" brief-pulse stimuli are defined by pulse duration of 0.5 to 2 ms, whereas ultrabrief-pulse stimuli are defined by pulse duration of less than 0.5 ms. In 1980, Weiner (1980) showed that standard brief-pulse stimuli could provoke a seizure with only one third of the energy required by sine wave stimuli. In the next 15 years, standard brief-pulse ECT devices replaced sine wave devices in the United States (Farah and McCall, 1993). New devices using ultrabrief stimuli may have the advantage of improving the efficiency of seizure induction. Abrams (2002) estimated that it takes only about 0.25 ms to initiate neuronal depolarization, and wider pulse widths are inefficient and waste electrical charge. The total energy output of these ultrabrief-pulse modalities is the same as the total energy output of the standard pulse widths; thus, as the stimulus pulse widths are shortened, the stimulus trains may be correspondingly lengthened. Ultrabrief-pulse widths may have an advantage because shorter pulse widths and longer pulse trains have been shown to elicit seizures with a smaller electrical charge and therefore may have fewer cognitive side effects (Sackeim et al., 2001). For a review of ultrabrief stimuli, see Chapter 1. Similarly, decreasing the frequency of pulses with a corresponding lengthening of the stimulus train will improve the efficiency of seizure induction (Kotresh et al., 2004).

Krystal et al. (2000a) reported that 5% of patients, especially older men, were nearly untreatable with standard American brief-pulse devices because the maximal output of the machine was not sufficient to induce an adequate seizure. The maximal charge of any device sold in the United States is 572 mC, whereas European devices can deliver twice as much.

Antidepressant efficacy and the magnitude of the stimulus dose

The consensus regarding the need for convulsive (as opposed to subconvulsive) stimuli and brief-pulse waveforms would seem to make stimulus dosing in ECT a straightforward process, leaving only the question, "By what degree should the stimulus exceed the convulsive threshold?" For years, ECT practitioners were satisfied that the answer to this question was found in the work of Ottosson (1962), who compared routine ECT with ECT modified by pretreatment intravenous lidocaine. He found that seizures induced by lidocaine-modified ECT were shorter than those induced by routine ECT, and an inverse relationship was found between seizure duration and antidepressant effect. From this work, it was widely accepted that stimulus doses producing seizures longer than 25 to 30 seconds had an antidepressant effect (American Psychiatric Association [APA] Task Force on Electroconvulsive Therapy, 1978). Still, there are multiple dosing strategies that will produce seizures of longer than 25 seconds. The various strategies can be grouped into three categories: (a) titrated dosing, (b) formula-based dosing, and (c) fixed dosing.

Titrated dosing

Sackeim et al. (1993) reported that, if the magnitude of the electrical stimulus was just barely greater than the convulsive threshold, then ECT was ineffective with right unilateral electrode placement, despite the production of electrographic seizures typically in excess of 25 seconds. In contrast, bilateral ECT was fully effective with stimuli minimally greater than or 2.5 times the seizure threshold, but excess memory side effects accrued at the higher stimulus dose.

In practice, measurements of the seizure threshold require a willingness to intentionally expose the patient to one or more subconvulsive stimuli in quick succession. The procedure of a stimulus-dose titration is carried out usually at the first treatment, as a reference for dosing at subsequent treatment sessions. The patient is first anesthetized and given muscle relaxation as at any other ECT session, perhaps with the exception of erring somewhat toward higher doses of both anesthetic and relaxant. The first stimulus delivered in a stimulus-dose titration sequence is chosen on the probable basis that is will be lower than the seizure threshold, and then a second stimulus is given at a higher dose. If the second stimulus also fails to induce a seizure, then a third or fourth stimulus could be given. How many stimuli can be given in a single session of general anesthesia depends on (a) how long the anesthetic and relaxant can be expected to last, and (b) how much time elapses between stimuli. As for the former, no more than two minutes (120 seconds) can reasonably expected from a single bolus of intravenous barbiturate anesthesia. As for the latter, a seizure that is induced very close to the seizure threshold may take 10 or more seconds to develop. Therefore, most research paradigms for stimulus-dose titration suggest a 20-second period of observation between successive stimuli to allow for sufficient time for barely suprathreshold seizures to develop. Given these considerations, there is sufficient time to deliver perhaps four stimuli in rapid succession, separated by 20 seconds each. The stimulus-dose titration is of course interrupted as soon as there is unequivocal evidence that a seizure has been produced. The peripheral motor convulsion is somewhat less equivocal than the electrographic seizure, so this writer sometimes uses the term "convulsive threshold" preferentially over "seizure threshold." Stimulus-dosing strategies during a stimulus-dose titration require that the practitioner know (a) the minimal dose to begin the titration sequence, and (b) what should be the incremental difference in stimulus-dose magnitude between "steps" in the dosing sequence. A truly informative stimulus-dosing sequence will produce a subconvulsive stimulus for the first stimulus given, and a guaranteed convulsion by a possible fourth and final stimulus, thus ensuring that the seizure threshold can be assumed to be higher than the first stimulus given and lower than the last. At best, this produces an estimate of the convulsive threshold. The convulsive threshold is dependent in part on the age and gender of the patient (higher for men, and higher for older persons), and dependent on electrode placement (higher for bilateral than for unilateral) (McCall et al., 1993b). A young woman receiving unilateral ECT might be recommended to receive 25 mC as her first stimulus dose in a stimulus-dose titration sequence, whereas an elderly man receiving bilateral ECT might receive a first stimulus of 100 mC. If the first stimulus is subconvulsive, then the next stimulus should be 50% to 100% greater than the first. These increments represent a compromise designed to preserve some rough

Table 28.1 Stimulus-dosing schedule for a device with a %Energy stimulus dial, using 50% to 100% increments between steps

Step	%Energy on the stimulus dial
1	5%
2	10%
3	15%
4	25%
5	40%
6	80%
7	100%

estimate of seizure threshold while ensuring that most (if not all) patients reach a convulsive dose by the fourth stimulus in the titration sequence.

The ECT practitioner should have a clear strategy in mind before beginning a titration sequence, as time passes much too quickly during a titration sequence to think it through "on the fly." There is no one best titration schedule, but various dosing schedules with which the writer has had some firsthand experience are presented in Tables 28.1 and 28.2.

The dose–response relationship of right unilateral ECT reflects the extent that the stimulus exceeds the convulsive threshold for a given patient and is not related to the absolute magnitude of the stimulus dose. The efficacy of right unilateral ECT follows a nearly linear relationship to the degree that the stimulus dose exceeds the seizure threshold, at least through 12 times the seizure threshold (McCall et al., 2000). This relationship is analogous to the pharmacological treatment of

Table 28.2 Stimulus-dosage schedule for a device with individual manipulation of stimulus parameters, using standard brief pulse with 50% increments

Step	Pulse width (ms)	Frequency (Hz)	Stimulus train duration (s)	Current (amp)	Charge (mC)
Step 1	1.0	40	0.5	0.8	32
Step 2	1.0	40	0.75	0.8	48
Step 3	1.0	40	1.25	0.8	80
Step 4	1.0	40	2.0	0.8	128
Step 5	1.0	60	2.0	0.8	192
Step 6	1.0	90	2.0	0.8	288
Step 7	1.4	90	2.0	0.8	403
Step 8	2.0	90	2.0	0.8	576

depression with tricyclic antidepressants in which serum blood levels are more important than the absolute oral dose in determining both efficacy and side effects. The newest reports consistently show that standard brief-pulse right unilateral ECT, at 5 to 12 times the seizure threshold, yields antidepressant results that are fully comparable to bilateral ECT (Haskett et al., 2007). The immediate post-ECT antidepressant remission rates are in the 70% to 80% range in the high-dose (more than five times the seizure threshold) treatment condition.

There have been fewer studies examining the speed of antidepressant response from ECT, but the available information suggests that higher doses produce quicker antidepressant results, at least for bilateral ECT (Sackeim et al., 1993). Indeed, speed of response may explain some of the overall differences in antidepressant efficacy previously observed for right unilateral versus bilateral placement. In a scenario that allows for an unlimited number of ECT sessions, it is possible that even low-dose right unilateral ECT would "catch up" and equal antidepressant response rates of bilateral ECT. Clinical urgency – coupled with the realities of modern, time-conscious managed care – does not allow for the luxury of a leisurely course of ECT; thus differences in speed of response accentuate the perceived final differences in antidepressant response rates. Higher stimulus dose may also speed the time to remission and reduce the number of treatments required when bilateral ECT is applied in the treatment of schizophrenia (Chanpattana et al., 2000a).

This discussion thus far has assumed that the stimulus dose is chosen early in treatment based on some strategy that considers the initial seizure threshold at the first treatment, whether it is directly measured or estimated through a proxy variable such as age. However, the reality is that seizure threshold is dynamic, and rises in some if not all patients during a course of ECT (Coffey et al., 1995). The field has not reached a consensus as to whether automatic small increments in stimulus dose (i.e., 25 mC) should be included at each treatment to offset an increasing threshold or whether to set the stimulus dose after the first or second treatment, and only increase it based on clinical circumstances of observations of ictal physiology (see the subsequent section on Adjusting the stimulus dose in response to dynamic physiology: "Benchmarking").

Formula-based dosing

A review of investigations of predictors of seizure threshold will show that age is the most consistent predictor. To this end, some authors state that titrating the stimulus dose is unnecessarily cumbersome, and that the correct stimulus dose can be estimated with an age-based mathematical formula (Petrides and Fink, 1996). Petrides and Fink noted that setting the ECT stimulus "%Energy" equal to half a patient's age produced a value similar to what would be found by stimulus-dose titration with bilateral ECT, and that 98% of patients have a seizure with the first stimulus under these conditions with bilateral ECT using a Thymatron device at 900 mA. Similarly, Gangadhar et al. (1998) found that the formula mC = age × 1.67 + 48.7 succeeded in eliciting a seizure with bilateral placement 80% of the time. In contrast, four sets of authors advocated stimulus-dose titration in right unilateral electrode placement after observing that age-based or half-age formulas either underdose (Colenda and McCall, 1995; Heikman et al., 1999; Tiller and Ingram, 2006) or overdose (Girish et al., 2000) patients with depression. Using a bilateral electrode placement, Chanpattana et al. (2000b) found that the half-age method led to missed seizures in 32% of patients with schizophrenia, but in a subsequent article comparing the efficiency of bilateral ECT seizure induction with the MECTA SR1 versus the Thymatron DGx device, they concluded that the half-age method was a "reasonable" dosing strategy for bilateral ECT using the Thymatron DGx for persons with acute psychotic illnesses, whereas no recommendation was made regarding dosing for the MECTA device (Chanpattana, 2001). Some of the differences observed between different dosing strategies are related to the choice of ECT device and the magnitude of current. For example, MECTA devices commonly deliver up to 800 mA whereas Thymatron devices deliver 900 mA; and the choice of stimulus parameters such as the magnitude of the current will influence ease of seizure induction, and hence the success of half-age versus age versus other formula-driven strategies. (See Chapter 1 for electrical current effect on stimulus dose.)

Although a substantial minority of ECT practitioners rely on formula-based dosing (Farah and McCall, 1993), there are no parallel-design efficacy comparisons of formula-based dosing versus titrated dosing, nor are there any parallel-design comparisons of efficacy of one formula versus another. In this respect, the science of formula-based dosing is underdeveloped.

Fixed dosing

The clinical trials of fixed-dosed right unilateral ECT have included comparison with titrated right unilateral ECT at low multiples of the seizure threshold, and generally show high efficacy for fixed dose (more than 80%), but with greater short-term cognitive side effects (McCall et al., 1995, 2000). Although fixed-dose ECT had its supporters (Abrams et al., 1991; Kellner, 2001), it presently is not under active study, as most clinicians (Farah and McCall, 1993) and most investigators make some attempt to individualize treatment, either through stimulus dose titration or formula.

Cognitive side effects and the stimulus dose

The anterograde and retrograde memory loss attributed to ECT has a temporal gradient, being more profound around the time of the treatments and extending back months before the treatment and several weeks after the ECT course (see Chapter 21; APA Committee on Electroconvulsive Therapy, 2001; Sackeim et al., 2007). The degree of amnesia incurred during a course of ECT is greater with bilateral ECT than with unilateral ECT and is increased with the number of treatments administered and the higher stimulus intensity (McCall et al., 2000; Sackeim et al., 2000, 2007). Although unilateral ECT is associated with fewer memory problems, the cognitive deficits show a dose relationship and increase as the stimulus dose is increased to 8 to 12 times the threshold (McCall et al., 2000). Research comparing bilateral and unilateral ECT has not addressed the question of whether right unilateral ECT given at a dose 10 to 12 times the seizure threshold would cause more cognitive side effects than would bilateral ECT that is minimally higher than or 1.5 times the seizure threshold.

Sine wave stimulus produces greater amnestic deficits than does a brief or ultra-brief stimulus pulse. In addition, Sackeim et al. (1993) reported that, within a specific waveform, the magnitude by which an electrical dose exceeds the seizure threshold (rather than the absolute electrical dose) is related to the severity of cognitive defects that develop during ECT. In a prospective, naturalistic, longitudinal study of cognitive outcomes in patients with depression treated with ECT at seven facilities in the New York City metropolitan area (Sackeim et al., 2007), sine wave stimulation resulted in pronounced slowing of reaction time, both immediately and six months following ECT. As expected, bilateral ECT resulted in larger and longer-lasting retrograde amnesia than did right unilateral ECT. They found that several clinical variables also were associated with post-ECT memory problems including older age, lower premorbid intellectual function, and female gender. The possibility of long-term (months) retrograde amnesia is a point of sharp debate within the field. The strongest evidence for long-term deficits comes from the Sackeim et al. (2007) article, but this study was limited by the use of nonrandomized design, the influence of concurrent medications during follow-up, the impact of the mental disorder itself on cognitive function, and the lack of a non-ECT comparison group. Long-term retrograde amnesia after ECT, should it be proven, might vary with ECT technique, including the choice of stimulus dose. Finally, any evidence of long-term cognitive side effects must be put in the context of the general improvement in quality of life that comes with treatment efficacy, as well as preservation of life through reduction in suicide risk (Kellner et al., 2005).

Generalizations regarding stimulus dosing for acute treatment of depression

These considerations lead to the following generalizations: (a) with standard brief-pulse stimulation delivered with right unilateral electrode placement, the stimulus should be substantially greater than the convulsive threshold to ensure the efficacy of ECT, and (b) with standard brief-pulse stimulation delivered with bilateral electrode placement, the stimulus should be only marginally greater than the convulsive threshold to avoid undue cognitive side effects.

So, in clinical practice, how is the practitioner to judge the convulsive threshold in a given patient? The convulsive threshold varies by a factor of at least 40-fold in large patient samples, thus making the mean threshold for a group of patients unhelpful for individual cases (Sackeim et al., 1991). It is clear that the convulsive threshold is related to age, sex, race, choice of stimulating electrode placement, and, perhaps, cranial dimensions (Chung, 2006; Colenda and McCall, 1996; McCall et al., 1993b; Sackeim et al., 1991). Still, these factors predict only a small amount of the variance in the convulsive threshold. Statistical models to predict the convulsive threshold, including age-based dosing approaches, fare poorly (Colenda and McCall, 1996; Tiller and Ingram, 2006). The field of ECT has been divided over whether estimates of the convulsive threshold are "good enough" for clinical practice (Kellner, 2001) versus whether it is necessary to empirically estimate the threshold at the first ECT session for each patient (Tiller and Ingram, 2006). The solution to this debate may depend on clinical circumstances; this is discussed later in this chapter in the form of clinical vignettes. In the meantime, approaches to selecting the stimulus dose over the course of ECT based on dynamic measurements made during an ECT session are presented (Tiller and Ingram, 2006).

Adjusting the stimulus dose in response to dynamic physiology: "Benchmarking"

Benchmarking has been described as a dynamic approach to stimulus dosing, and is conceptually different than titration, formula, or fixed dose. Benchmarking was described by Swartz (2002) as a technique of adjusting the stimulus dose to maintain physiologic markers of seizure intensity *for a given individual* within the bounds of what is observed during a vigorous ECT session. For example, if an ECT stimulus at the first session is delivered at a dose predicted to be much greater than an individual's seizure threshold, and indeed induces a vigorous seizure characterized by diffuse convulsive activity, high-amplitude electroencephalogram (EEG) discharge, significant acceleration of heart rate, and a sharp increase in blood pressure, then these observed correlates of "seizure intensity" can be used to document adequacy of treatment at subsequent sessions (see Chapter 30). The correlate's (i.e., increase in heart rate or EEG amplitude) failure to increase to the previously established level would signal a need to increase the stimulus intensity or otherwise change the treatment approach.

Benchmarking: Seizure morphology

The report of Sackeim et al. (1987) that threshold right unilateral ECT produced seizures of 25 seconds or longer without antidepressant efficacy cast into doubt the clinical wisdom that the stimulus dose was therapeutic if the electrographic seizure lasted 25 seconds. Investigators have sought to find a physiological marker of treatment adequacy to replace seizure duration. The most promising candidate is seizure morphology. Ottosson (1962) reported that lidocaine changed the shape of ECT seizures and affected duration, although the first finding is largely overlooked. Lidocaine-modified seizures, in addition to being less efficacious than standard ECT seizures, were characterized by loss of spike activity and poor postictal suppression.

This early finding is now extended by evidence that seizure morphology varies with ECT technique. That is, greater EEG seizure intensity corresponds to ECT techniques that progress from lower (right unilateral, low stimulus intensity) to higher (bilateral, high stimulus intensity) efficacy (Krystal et al., 1993). Electrode placement and stimulus intensity have independent and additive effects on seizure morphology. Seizures of greater intensity are characterized by higher peak ictal amplitudes, greater stereotypy (regularity) of the ictal discharge, greater symmetry and coherence between the left and right cerebral hemispheres, and more profound postictal suppression (see Figure 28.2). Preliminary evidence suggests that greater seizure intensity is predictive of greater likelihood of response or faster response (Krystal, 1998; McCall and Farah, 1995; Nobler et al., 1993).

The natural extension of this reasoning leads to the hope that seizure morphology could guide decisions about stimulus intensity as the course of ECT progresses. For example, if seizure intensity is poor in the middle of the treatment course, then treatment technique should be changed (by switching electrode placement or increasing the stimulus intensity) to optimize clinical outcome. Manufacturers of ECT devices now incorporate automated measures of seizure intensity onto the ECT chart recorder, and the accompanying owner's manual instructs the practitioner to increase the stimulus intensity if the seizure morphology appears to be degraded. Krystal et al. (2000b, 2000c) reported two theoretical experiments that conclude that use of a seizure morphology algorithm could predict which patients need a higher stimulus dose and which need a switch from right unilateral to bilateral placement to ensure antidepressant efficacy. Reliance on EEG seizure characteristics to make treatment decisions is complicated by the realization that (a) other factors, such as age, baseline convulsive threshold, and other intrinsic patient factors likely play an equal role in shaping the ictal EEG (McCall et al., 1996, 1998), and (b) dynamic changes in seizure duration and morphology during the course of ECT make it difficult to recommend a universal criterion value for ictal phenomena. For example, longer electrographic seizure durations coupled with greater EEG seizure regularity at either the second or fourth ECT session is predictive of better antidepressant outcome at the conclusion of a course of right unilateral ECT course, but the optimal values for seizure duration and seizure morphology change between the second and fourth sessions, as revealed in receiver operating curve analyses (Rosenquist et al., 2007).

Additionally, poor seizure morphology (e.g., in older patients with high thresholds) is little influenced by increasing the stimulus intensity above 2.5 times the seizure threshold (McCall et al., 1998). The importance of seizure morphology in predicting clinical outcome is far from being understood, and more work is needed to make it a practical tool for governing ECT technique. At the present time, the patient's clinical response should supersede EEG seizure characteristics in the choice of stimulus dose.

Benchmarking: Cardiovascular reactivity

Peak heart rate has been proposed by Swartz (2000) as an alternative physiological measure of treatment adequacy, with higher heart rate perhaps indicating better clinical outcomes. Swartz later stipulated that a peak heart rate of less than 140 bpm indicated either a suboptimal ECT session, intrinsic heart disease, or the effects of medications (Chapter 30). Saravanan and colleagues (2002) also observed that a greater degree of cardiac reactivity predicted earlier therapeutic response to ECT. Again, this approach has not been well examined by a wide audience of ECT investigators, and deserves more attention.

Augmentation strategies when the maximum stimulus dose is reached

ECT devices in the United States are limited to a maximum output of 100 Joules at 200 Ohms dynamic impedance. Also, it has been estimated that 5% of American ECT patients achieve seizures in fewer than 25 seconds despite maximum stimulus settings, and their clinical response is poorer (32% responder rate) than patients with seizures of longer than 25 seconds (66% responder rate) (Krystal et al., 2000a). In the absence of higher-output machines, a number of "augmentation" strategies have been suggested to counter short seizures at maximal stimulus settings.

- Reducing or eliminating anticonvulsant medications that are nonessential
- Switching the anesthetic from methohexital (a barbiturate) to ketamine (Krystal et al., 2003)
- Switching the anesthetic from thiopental (a barbiturate) to etomidate (Khalid et al., 2006)
- Switching the anesthetic from methohexital to remifentanil (Sullivan and Sinz, 2004)

- Vigorous assisted hyperventilation before stimulus delivery, to reduce pCO_2 (Bergsholm et al., 1984; Swartz, 1996)
- Intravenous caffeine two minutes before stimulus delivery (McCall et al., 1993a)
- Sleep depriving the patient the night before ECT (Gilabert et al., 2004)

Integrating the science of stimulus dosing with the choice of electrode placement

The most accurate means of measuring the convulsive threshold for a given patient is empirical observation – giving intentionally subconvulsive stimuli at the first treatment and then, in the same session, administering successively larger stimuli until a seizure is produced. Some ECT researchers have argued against titration of unilateral ECT and instead have encouraged practitioners to use fixed, high-dose unilateral ECT (Abrams, 2002) or fixed, moderate-dose bilateral ECT (Kellner, 2001). In fact, a survey of ECT practitioners in 1993 showed that only a minority perform titration of the stimulus dose (Farah and McCall, 1993). The reasons for this are unclear, but possible explanations include concerns that (a) the subconvulsive stimulation inherent in stimulus titration might be medically dangerous, (b) subconvulsive stimulation might add to memory side effects, or (c) producing a barely suprathreshold seizure with right unilateral placement is an ineffective treatment, thus "wasting" the first treatment.

It is true that subconvulsive stimulation transiently slows the heart rate (McCall et al., 1994), and if subconvulsive stimulation is given in the presence of β-blockers and no anticholinergic drug, there is a risk of asystole (McCall, 1996). Fortunately, atropine or glycopyrrolate pretreatment eliminates this risk. The possibility of excess acute cognitive side effects with subconvulsive stimuli has been examined and discounted (Prudic et al., 1994). The possibility of a sluggish antidepressant response when a titrated, "moderately" suprathreshold approach is combined with right unilateral placement, however, is a concern. Krystal et al. (1996) have countered this argument by noting that the first ECT session is different from all subsequent sessions in that the EEG seizure manifestations are more "intense," thus compensating for the relatively lower final stimulus that would result at the first treatment versus subsequent sessions.

Recommendations for stimulus dosing have been made with the following two caveats: (a) Recommendations can be made only in regard to major depression, as it is unknown whether dosing strategies for other diagnoses should be the same as those for depression, and (b) dosing recommendations can be made only in the context of the chosen electrode placement and the patient's clinical condition.

Those patients with the most serious complications of major depression (i.e., active suicidal behavior in the hospital, catatonia, or food refusal) merit an approach most likely to yield quick antidepressant results. In such circumstances, bilateral ECT with a relatively high, fixed dose (e.g., 50% of maximal output) could be justified; stimulus dose titration would not be required because concern about cognitive side effects becomes a purely secondary issue, based on the severity of the patient's clinical status. However, whether fixed, high-dose right unilateral ECT could provide an equally fast and effective response needs to be examined.

In contrast, a depressed patient for whom medication has failed but whose case is otherwise not urgent may be an appropriate candidate for right unilateral ECT at 5 to 6 times the seizure threshold, especially if cognitive side effects are a concern or the patient is being treated in an outpatient setting. The patient can start with right unilateral ECT and after five or six treatments change to bilateral ECT if he or she has not had an adequate response. Other special situations favoring titrated right unilateral ECT include depressed patients with comorbid dementia and other neurological conditions such as Parkinson's disease. The treatment of these patients should aim to minimize even transient memory side effects and may include starting at a conservative unilateral dose (i.e., 3.5 times the seizure threshold) and increasing the dose as tolerated. Other dosing strategies, such as titrated bilateral or high, fixed-dose right unilateral ECT, occupy the strategic middle ground between titrated right unilateral and fixed-dose bilateral ECT for patients whose condition is of intermediate acuity.

Stimulus dosing in continuation/maintenance ECT in major depression

The electrode placement and dose parameters used in the index course are usually maintained during continuation ECT (see Chapter 34). However, there is no science to support the practice of leaving the stimulus dose the same from acute to continuation treatment, and there are at least some theoretical reasons to change the magnitude of the stimulus dose after the patient is well into continuation therapy. Seizure threshold will increase during acute treatment (Coffey et al., 1995; Krystal et al., 1998), and the threshold might be expected to regress to the pre-ECT baseline as treatments are spaced out during continuation ECT. Indeed the seizure threshold was shown to decrease significantly when the treatments were separated by 60 days or more (Wild et al., 2004). These findings could produce contradictory positions regarding the stimulus dose during continuation therapy. On the one hand, a seizure threshold that is regressing back to baseline might imply that the stimulus dose could also be decreased to maintain a relative constant relationship between seizure threshold and stimulus dose. On the other hand, the ample opportunity for cognitive recovery between widely spaced continuation treatments, and the concern of waning ECT effects between widely spaced treatments, might argue for taking a more aggressive stance during continuation ECT than that which was

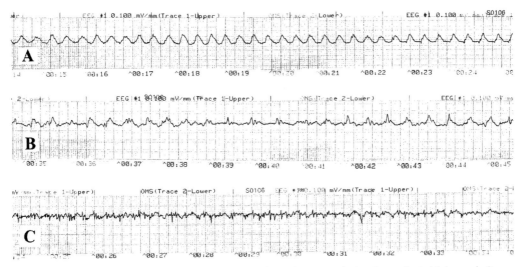

Figure 28.2 Examples of single channel, electrographic seizure regularity; Example A: high regularity, Example B: moderate regularity, Example C: low regularity.

used during acute treatment, including the possibility of a higher stimulus dose. This area is completely unstudied.

Examples of stimulus dosing with case vignettes

Case 1

A 30-year-old man with hypertalkativeness, hyperactivity, religiosity, and a history of bipolar disorder is admitted to a psychiatry unit. He receives antipsychotics, and within 48 hours he becomes inactive and rigid, with unresponsiveness, fluctuant blood pressure and pulse, and low-grade temperature. A diagnosis of catatonia/neuroleptic malignant syndrome is made. Concerns regarding risk for complications such as deep vein thrombosis lead the treatment team to quickly move to bilateral ECT, as the need for ensured efficacy and rapid response are paramount over concerns for cognitive side effects. The stimulus dose is titrated with bilateral electrode placement at treatment one, using a brief-pulse device with a %Energy dosing dial. Knowing that both male gender and bilateral placement are associated with higher seizure thresholds, the treating physicians elect to begin the stimulus titration sequence at step 2 (Table 28.1). The patient fails to have a convulsion at step 2, but has a robust seizure at step 3. All subsequent treatment session are given with bilateral placement at step 4, about 50% greater than the estimated seizure threshold. The EEG seizures at sessions 2 and beyond are exemplified by high ictal regularity (Figure 28.2) and abrupt, complete postictal suppression

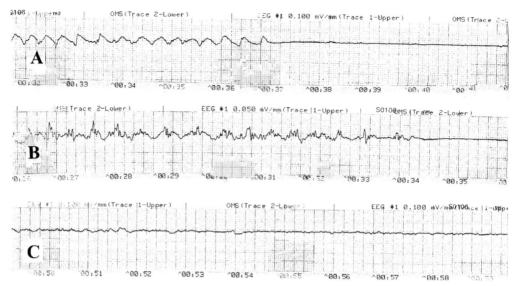

Figure 28.3 Examples of single channel, electrographic postictal suppression; Example A: abrupt, complete suppression; Example B: gradual, but complete suppression; Example C: poor (incomplete) suppression.

(Figure 28.3). The physician does not increment the stimulus dose beyond step 4, the patient makes excellent progress with six treatments, and the treatment course is concluded.

Case 2

A 40-year-old woman attorney has a serious depression that leaves her joyless, insomniac, and unresponsive to conventional medication therapy or psychotherapy. She would like to elect ECT, but asks that an approach be undertaken that will minimize cognitive side effects as she hopes to rapidly return to her practice. The treatment team decides to use right unilateral electrode placement at a moderate dose (4 times seizure threshold) as a good compromise between efficacy and side effects. Knowing that both female gender and right unilateral electrode placement are associated with low seizure thresholds, the treating physician decides to initiate the stimulus dose titration sequence at step 1 at the first treatment (Table 28.2). The patient does not have a seizure at steps 1 or 2, but has a robust seizure at step 3. The physician delivers her second and third treatment at step 5, approximately 2.5 times her right unilateral seizure threshold. Ictal EEG regularity is of a moderate level, and postictal suppression is poor at the third session. The patient shows no improvement after three sessions. The decision is made to advance the stimulus to step 6 at the fourth session, given the accumulated observation of poor clinical progress, lack of side effects, and poor physiologic response in the ictal EEG. The patient begins to improve after the fifth session.

Case 3

An 80-year-old man with treatment-resistant depression, weight loss, food refusal, and suicidality begins a course of bilateral ECT at 80% of maximum device output under methohexital anesthesia. The stimulus dose of 80% was picked to correspond to age-based dosing and to follow an aggressive treatment approach commensurate with the acuity of his illness. A 20-seconds EEG seizure at the first session leads to an increase in the stimulus dose to 100% at the second session, producing a 15-seconds EEG seizure with no motor manifestations. At this point the treatment team decides to eliminate all oral benzodiazepines, vigorously hyperventilate after induction of anesthesia, and switch from methohexital to ketamine; this decision produces a greater than 30-seconds EEG seizure at the third and all subsequent sessions. Intravenous caffeine was contemplated but did not become necessary, and the patient enjoys a full antidepressant response after eight sessions.

Conclusion

These three vignettes help to illustrate that decision making regarding the stimulus dose in ECT is a product of both science and clinical observation. The science serves as a starting point for approaching the patient's treatment plan, but the plan is tempered by common sense and clinical experience. The vignettes are fictional and serve as a guide to principles, and should not be construed as actual guidelines to patient care. Continued refinement of physics of stimulus delivery and new data from clinical trials are expected to lead to revisions of these principles.

Acknowledgment

Some portions of this chapter are reproduced (with permission) from McDonald, W. M., Thompson, T. R., McCall, W. V., and Zorumski, C. F. 2004. Electroconvulsive therapy. In *Textbook of Psychopharmacology* (eds. Schatzberg, A. F., and Nemeroff, C. B.). Washington, DC: American Psychiatric Publishing. pp. 685–714.

Editor's note

The mentioned 40-fold variation in seizure threshold becomes only fivefold if the pulse width is maintained at 1 ms (Petrides and Fink, 1996). This is because using a low efficiency wide pulse width when high stimulus doses are needed elevates seizure threshold. There is also about fivefold variation in age among ECT patients. This chapter should be considered together with Chapters 1, 27, and 31. –CMS

References

Abrams, R. 2002. Stimulus titration and ECT dosing. J ECT 18: 3–9.

Abrams, R., Swartz, C. M., and Vedak, C. 1991. Antidepressant effects of high-dose right unilateral electroconvulsive therapy. Arch Gen Psychiatry 48: 746–8.

American Psychiatric Association (APA) Committee on Electroconvulsive Therapy. 2001. The practice of electroconvulsive therapy: Recommendations for treatment, training and privileging, 2nd edn. Washington, DC: APA.

American Psychiatric Association (APA) Task Force on Electroconvulsive Therapy. 1978. Electroconvulsive therapy. Washington, DC: APA.

Bergsholm, P., Gran, L., and Bleie, H. 1984. Seizure duration in unilateral electroconvulsive therapy. The effect of hypocapnia induced by hyperventilation and the effect of ventilation with oxygen. Acta Psychiatr Scand 69: 121–8.

Brandon, S., Cowley, P., McDonald, C., et al. 1984. Electroconvulsive therapy: Results in depressive illness from the Leicestershire trial. Br Med J (Clin Res Ed) 288(6410): 22–5.

Chanpattana, W. 2001. Seizure threshold in electroconvulsive therapy: Effect of instrument titration schedule. German J Psychiatry 4: 51–6.

Chanpattana, W., Chakrabhand, M. L., and Buppanharun, W. 2000a. Effects of stimulus intensity in the efficacy of bilateral ECT in schizophrenia: A preliminary study. Biol Psychiatry 48: 222–8.

Chanpattana, W., Chakrabhand, S., Techakasem, P., et al. 2000b. Seizure threshold in ECT: Dose titration vs. age and half age methods. J Med Assoc Thai 3: 278–83.

Chung, K. 2006. Determinants of seizure threshold of electroconvulsive therapy in Chinese. J ECT 22: 100–2.

Coffey, C. E., Lucke, J., Weiner, R. D., et al. 1995. Seizure threshold in electroconvulsive therapy (ECT) II. The anticonvulsant effect of ECT. Biol Psychiatry 37: 777–88.

Colenda, C. C. and McCall, W. V. 1996. A statistical model predicting the seizure threshold for right unilateral ECT in 106 patients. Convuls Ther 12: 3–12.

Farah, A. and McCall, W. 1993. Electroconvulsive therapy stimulus dosing: A survey of contemporary practices. Convuls Ther 9: 90–4.

Gangadhar, B. N., Girish, K., Janakiramaiah, N., et al. 1998. Formula method for stimulus setting in bilateral electroconvulsive therapy: Relevance of age. J ECT 14: 259–65.

Gilabert, E., Rojo, E., and Vallejo, J. 2004. Augmentation of electroconvulsive therapy seizures with sleep deprivation. J ECT 20: 242–7.

Girish, K., Mayur, P., Saravanan, E., et al. 2000. Seizure threshold estimation by formula method: A prospective study in unilateral ECT. J ECT 16: 258–62.

Haskett, R. F., Rosenquist, P. B., McCall, W. V., et al. 2007. The role of antidepressant medications during ECT: New findings from OPT-ECT. J ECT 23: 56.

Heikman, P., Tuunainen, A., and Kuoppasalmi, K. 1999. Value of the initial stimulus dose in right unilateral and bifrontal electroconvulsive therapy. Psychol Med 29: 1417–23.

Johnstone, E. C. and Deakin, J. F. 1980. The Northwick Park electroconvulsive therapy trial. Lancet 2: 1317–20.

Kellner, C. H. 2001. Towards the modal ECT treatment. J ECT 17: 1–2.

Kellner, C. H., Fink, M., Knapp, R., et al. 2005. Relief of expressed suicidal intent by ECT: A consortium for research in ECT study. Am J Psychiatry 162: 977–82.

Khalid, N., Atkins, M., and Kirov, G. 2006. The effects of etomidate on seizure duration and electrical stimulus dose in seizure-resistant patients during electroconvulsive therapy. J ECT 22: 184–8.

Kotresh, S., Girish, K., Janakiramaiah, N., et al. 2004. Effect of ECT stimulus parameters on seizure physiology and outcome. J ECT 20: 10–2.

Krystal, A., Weiner, R., Dean, M., et al. 2003. Comparison of seizure duration, ictal EEG, and cognitive effects of ketamine and methohexital anesthesia with ECT. J Neuropsychiatry Clin Neurosci 15: 27–34.

Krystal, A. D. 1998. The clinical utility of ictal EEG seizure adequacy models. Psychiatr Ann 28: 30–5.

Krystal, A. D., Coffey, C. E., Weiner, R. D., et al. 1998. Changes in seizure threshold over the course of electroconvulsive therapy affect therapeutic response and are detected by ictal EEG ratings. J Neuropsychiatry Clin Neurosci 10: 178–86.

Krystal, A. D., Dean, M. D., Weiner, R. D., et al. 2000a. ECT stimulus intensity: Are present ECT devices too limited? Am J Psychiatry 157: 963–7.

Krystal, A. D., Holsinger, T., Weiner, R., et al. 2000b. Prediction of the utility of a switch from unilateral to bilateral ECT in the elderly using treatment 2 ictal EEG indices. J ECT 16: 327–37.

Krystal, A. D., Weiner, R., Coffey, C., et al. 1996. Effect of ECT treatment number on the ictal EEG. Psychiatry Res 62: 179–89.

Krystal, A. D., Weiner, R., Lindahl, V. H., et al. 2000c. The development and retrospective testing of an electroencephalographic seizure quality-based stimulus dosing paradigm with ECT. J ECT 16: 338–49.

Krystal, A. D., Weiner, R. D., McCall, W. V., et al. 1993. The effects of ECT stimulus dose and electrode placement on the ictal electroencephalogram: An intraindividual crossover study. Biol Psychiatry 34: 759–67.

McCall, W., Reid, S., Rosenquist, P., et al. 1993a. A reappraisal of the role of caffeine in ECT. Am J Psychiatry 150: 1543–5.

McCall, W. V. 1996. Asystole in electroconvulsive therapy: Report of four cases. J Clin Psychiatry 57: 199–203.

McCall, W. V., Farah, A., Reboussin, D., et al. 1995. Comparison of the efficacy of titrated, moderate-dose and fixed, high-dose right unilateral ECT in elderly patients. Am J Geriatr Psychiatry 3: 317–24.

McCall, W. V. and Farah, B. A. 1995. Greater ictal EEG regularity is associated with greater treatment efficiency. Convuls Ther 11: 69.

McCall, W. V., Reboussin, D. M., Weiner, R. D., et al. 2000. Titrated moderately suprathreshold vs fixed high-dose right unilateral electroconvulsive therapy: Acute antidepressant and cognitive effects. Arch Gen Psychiatry 57: 438–44.

McCall, W. V., Reid, S., and Ford, M. 1994. Electrocardiographic and cardiovascular effects of subconvulsive stimulation during titrated right unilateral ECT. Convuls Ther 10: 25–33.

McCall, W. V., Robinette, G. D., and Hardesty, D. 1996. Relationship of seizure morphology to the convulsive threshold. Convuls Ther 12: 147–51.

McCall, W. V., Shelp, F. E., Weiner, R. D., et al. 1993b. Convulsive threshold differences in right unilateral and bilateral ECT. Biol Psychiatry 34: 606–11.

McCall, W. V., Sparks, W., Jane, J., et al. 1998. Variation of ictal electroencephalographic regularity with low-, moderate-, and high-dose stimuli during right unilateral electroconvulsive therapy. Biol Psychiatry 43: 608–11.

Nobler, M. S., Sackeim, H. A., Solomou, M., et al. 1993. EEG manifestations during ECT: Effects of electrode placement and stimulus intensity. Biol Psychiatry 34: 321–30.

Ottosson, J. O. 1962. Seizure characteristics and therapeutic efficiency in electroconvulsive therapy: An analysis of the antidepressant efficiency of grand mal and lidocaine-modified seizures. J Nerv Ment Dis 135: 239–51.

Petrides, G. and Fink, M. 1996. The "half age" simulation strategy for ECT dosing. Convuls Ther 12: 138–46.

Prudic, J., Olfson, M., Marcus, S., et al. 2004. Effectiveness of electroconvulsive therapy in community settings. Biol Psychiatry 55: 301–12.

Prudic, J., Sackeim, H. A., Devanand, D. P., et al. 1994. Acute cognitive effects of subconvulsive electrical stimulation. Convuls Ther 10: 4–24.

Rosenquist, P. B., Kimball, J. N., and McCall, W. V. 2007. Prediction of antidepressant response in both 2.25 X threshold RUL and fixed high dose RUL ECT. J ECT 23: 55.

Sackeim, H., Prudic, J., Fuller, R., et al. 2007. The cognitive effects of electroconvulsive therapy in community settings. Neuropsychopharmacology 32: 244–54.

Sackeim, H. A., Decina, P., Kanzler, M., et al. 1987. Effects of electrode placement on the efficacy of titrated, low-dose ECT. Am J Psychiatry 144: 1449–55.

Sackeim, H. A., Devanand, D. P., and Prudic, J. 1991. Stimulus intensity, seizure threshold, and seizure duration: Impact on the efficacy and safety of electroconvulsive therapy. Psychiatr Clin North Am 14: 803–43.

Sackeim, H. A., Prudic, J., Devanand, D. P., et al. 1993. Effects of stimulus intensity and electrode placement on the efficacy and cognitive effects of electroconvulsive therapy. N Engl J Med 328: 839–46.

Sackeim, H. A., Prudic, J., Devanand, D. P., et al. 2000. A prospective, randomized, double-blind comparison of bilateral and right unilateral electroconvulsive therapy at different stimulus intensities. Arch Gen Psychiatry 57: 425–34.

Sackeim, H. A., Prudic, J., Nobler, M. S., et al. 2001. Ultra-brief pulse ECT and the affective and cognitive consequences of ECT [abstract]. J ECT 17(1): 77.

Saravanan, E., Gangadhar, B., Janakiramaiah, N., et al. 2002. Does higher cardiovascular response to ECT predict early antidepressant effect? J Affect Disord 69: 101–8.

Sullivan, P. and Sinz, E. 2004. The use of remifentanil anesthesia for electroconvulsive therapy in patients with high seizure thresholds. J ECT 20: 278.

Swartz, C. M. 1996. Obstruction of ECT seizure by submaximal hyperventilation: A case report. Ann Clin Psychiatry 8: 31–4.

Swartz, C. M. 2000. Physiological response to ECT stimulus dose. Psychiatry Res 97: 229–35.

Swartz, C. M. 2002. ECT dosing by the benchmark method. German J Psychiatry 5: 1–14.

Tiller, J. W. and Ingram, N. 2006. Seizure threshold determination for electroconvulsive therapy: Stimulus dose titration versus age-based estimations. Aust N Z J Psychiatry 40: 188–92.

UK ECT Review Group. 2003. Efficacy and safety of electroconvulsive therapy in depressive disorders: A systematic review and meta-analysis. Lancet 361: 799–808.

Weiner, R. 1980. ECT and seizure threshold: Effects of stimulus wave form and electrode placement. Biol Psychiatry 15: 225–41.

Weiner, R. D., Rogers, H. J., Davidson, J. R., et al. 1986. Effects of stimulus parameters on cognitive side effects. Ann NY Acad Sci 462: 315–25.

Wild, B., Eschweiler, G., and Bartels, M. 2004. Electroconvulsive therapy dosage in continuation/maintenance electroconvulsive therapy: When is a new threshold titration necessary? J ECT 20: 200–3.

29

Electroencephalogram monitoring and implications

Hideki Azuma

History of electroencephalogram monitoring

Pioneering studies on monitored electroconvulsive therapy (ECT) were performed in the mid-1960s (Blachly and Gowing, 1966), shortly followed by the introduction of an ECT device with built-in electroencephalogram (EEG) and electrocardiogram (ECG) monitoring (Blachly, 1976). In the 1990s and 2000s, the American Psychiatric Association (APA) Task Force on ECT recommended routine EEG monitoring for several reasons (APA, 2001). First, ictal motor responses may not always be detectable, and EEG monitoring may prevent unnecessary restimulation. Second, EEG seizures generally persist after termination of the motor convulsion. Third, prolonged seizure can be detected only by EEG monitoring. Finally, the ictal EEG may eventually help to judge therapeutic adequacy. The APA recommends the use of the cuff method along with EEG monitoring.

Recording electrode placement

Typically one or two EEG channels are monitored. Two types of recording electrode placements at ECT are commonly used: left hemispheric (for single-channel ictal EEG monitoring) or left and right hemispheric placement (for two-channel monitoring). Two-channel monitoring is preferable. In both cases, the reference electrodes for the prefrontal electrodes are positioned over the ipsilateral mastoid (Weiner et al., 1991). Prefrontal positioning can be accomplished with either a template incorporating the proportions of the patient's actual head measurements ("the 10–20 system" for clinical EEG) or the placement of the recording electrode one inch above the midpoint of the eyebrow (APA, 2001). Left prefrontal mastoid electrode placement is helpful for identifying interhemispheric spread of ictal discharge in right unilateral ECT. A disadvantage of prefrontal-mastoid electrode placement is artifactual electrical noise transmitted from the carotid artery. It can be

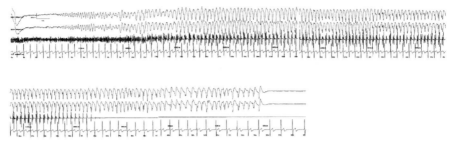

Figure 29.1   Time course of ictal electroencephalogram (EEG), two-channel EEG (left and right frontal-mastoid electrode placement), electromyogram (EMG), and electrocardiogram (ECG). EEG started just after the termination of the electrical stimuli, preictal fast rhythm intermingled with low-amplitude epileptic recruiting rhythm for about four seconds, and gradually 5- to 6-Hz middle- or high-amplitude theta wave emerged and changed from polyspike phase to slow-wave phase. Slow-wave burst and spike and slow-wave complex burst continued and gradually changed to slower frequency. Then ictal EEG stopped abruptly and showed postictal suppression.

minimized by concurrent ECG monitoring to avoid misinterpreting pulse artifacts as continued seizure activity (Weiner et al., 1991).

When using left and right prefrontal-mastoid electrode placement, the practitioner should consistently use channel 1 for left and channel 2 for right. Bilateral single-channel recordings made from two recording electrodes both in the prefrontal region have much lower amplitudes at low frequencies because what is displayed is the difference between left and right hemispheres. In the low-frequency range, the activity in both hemispheres is usually equal, so the difference is zero (Weiner et al., 1991). Inadequate recordings of seizures generally result from loose electrode attachment, defective lead wires, or unsuitable recording electrodes. In preparation the prefrontal and mastoid recording sites are rubbed with an alcohol swab and wiped dry (APA, 2001). After starting EEG monitoring it is helpful to check the quality of the EEG recording and consider adjusting the sensitivity. If the sensitivity is too low, the baseline EEG recording will be flat. Typically the baseline EEG activity should be clearly seen, and then ictal changes will be large enough to identify.

Time course of ictal EEG

The ECT grand mal seizure is illustrated in Figure 29.1. The EEG of the awake adult usually consists of low-amplitude alpha and beta activities mixed with movement and muscle activity artifacts. In anesthetized patients, baseline EEG usually consists of mixed fast and slow activities, the degrees of which depend on the depth of anesthesia. Typically, EEG recording is automatically started by the ECT device just after termination of the electrical stimulus.

Rarely the seizure is preceded by a brief period (1–3 s) of EEG flattening (desynchronization) or low-amplitude fast activity at about 20 Hz showing progressive synchronization. The seizure usually begins with a rhythm at about 10 Hz, with amplitude increasing rapidly over a few seconds. This rhythm is fundamental to tonic–clonic attacks, and is known as the epileptic recruiting rhythm (Gastaut and Broughton, 1972). The recruiting rhythm changes to polyspike activity (bursts of spike discharges) concurrent with the tonic and early clonic portions of the motor convulsion. This phase typically lasts 10 to 15 seconds but may be shorter or longer. The polyspikes become combined with an apparently separate rhythm of slow waves, which increases in amplitude and decreases in frequency. This separate rhythm corresponds to the intermediate oscillatory period, the appearance of which ends the tonic phase. In practice, polyspike activity may be impossible to distinguish from electromyogram activity, particularly when low doses of succinylcholine are given. The polyspike phase of the seizure is generally defined as the period from the offset of electrical stimulation to the point at which visually discernible slow activity fully replaces early chaotic polyspike activity (Nobler et al., 1993).

The EEG slow rhythm becomes increasingly intermingled with polyspikes, and when the slow activity reaches a frequency of about 4 Hz each slow wave interrupts the polyspike activity. This interruption gives rise to polyspike and wave complexes that decrease in frequency. Each burst of sharp waves (polyspikes) is associated with the massive bilateral myoclonus of grand mal seizure. Each slow wave is associated with a decrease or abolition of muscle tone, representing the recurrent flaccidity between myoclonic contractions. Each polyspike and wave complex lasts 0.3 to 1 seconds until the termination of myoclonus. Together, these are the characteristic phenomena of the clonic phase. The clonic phase consists of high-amplitude paroxysmal complexes of one or more spikes followed by a slow wave. These clonic EEG phenomena always occur during a clonic motor convulsion, although these classical characteristics are not always displayed. Typically, frequencies of 5 Hz or higher appear at the beginning of the clonic phase and decrease to 1 to 3 Hz during the latter portions of the convulsion. The slow-wave phase is defined as the period from the end of the polyspike phase until seizure termination.

The postictal phase begins immediately on seizure termination. After the final polyspike and slow-wave burst, the EEG becomes flat or isoelectric for several seconds. This is the phase of postictal cortical extinction. Increasing diffuse slow activity then begins, initially in the delta band. This EEG accelerates to include predominantly theta activity and then changes into alpha activity. The degree of postictal suppression varies considerably from patient to patient and is influenced by the ECT method, whether bilateral or unilateral stimulus placement, sine or pulse wave stimuli, and sometimes the stimulus dose. The end point is easily detected if postictal suppression emerges abruptly. When minimal suppression is present, the immediate postictal EEG is characterized by a mixture of low-amplitude fast and slow activities; such activities may obscure the seizure end point. One method to identify the seizure end is to pick the most likely point at which the immediate postictal baseline can be said to begin. This procedure is admittedly arbitrary and may require a more extended recording period to ensure that what appears to be the postictal baseline is actually so (rather than extended seizure).

Scalp distribution of ictal EEG

Using the 10–20 system for electrode placement for ictal EEG, ECT seizure begins with a low amplitude. Although EEG activity is present in all scalp areas, its amplitude varies considerably (Weiner et al., 1991). In monopolar montage, the amplitudes of the polyspike and slow-wave complexes appear to reach a maximum in the central regions. Amplitude asymmetry in the anterior areas can also be seen in right unilateral ECT, with substantially greater amplitude in the right frontal and anterior temporal regions than in the corresponding regions on the left.

Ictal EEG interpretation

Seizure duration

Generally, stimulus intensity is associated with seizure duration, but seizure duration is not sufficient evidence for the efficacy of ECT (Kales et al., 1997; Nobler et al., 1993; Sackeim et al., 1987, 1991). EEG recordings of shorter than 15 seconds imply an insufficient electrical stimulus and efficacy (APA, 2001). Adequate seizure duration is commonly considered to be 20 to 25 seconds. Seizures induced by a near-threshold unilateral stimulus produce low-amplitude EEG and are not followed by clear postictal suppression. Unilateral stimuli moderately higher than threshold produce shorter convulsions but higher-amplitude EEG and stronger postictal suppression. A similar pattern is sometimes but less frequently seen with bilateral ECT. Older age is also associated with shorter seizure duration.

Seizure expression

Manually rated seizure expression in clinical studies consists of polyspike phase, slow-wave phase, and postictal suppression (McCall et al., 1996b; Nobler et al., 1993; Weiner and Krystal, 1993). The evaluated parameters included the maximal amplitude (in millivolts [mV]) of the polyspike phase, the duration of the polyspike phase, the maximum amplitude (mV) of the slow-wave phase, the duration of the slow-wave phase, the regularity (global seizure strength), the stereotypy (global seizure patterning), and the postictal suppression (degree of postictal bioelectric suppression). The maximal amplitudes during the polyspike and slow-wave phases are defined as the largest peak-to-peak deflections in the relevant phase, and the mean maximal amplitude is determined for each patient. Seizures are rated as more stereotypic if a clear progression from low-amplitude chaotic polyspike activity to high-amplitude slow activity is seen, without the reappearance of chaotic polyspike activity or marked variability in the amplitude during the phases. Seizures are rated as having greater regularity if slow activity with a high amplitude predominates during the slow-wave phase. Postictal suppression is rated as follows: High scores indicate good seizure suppression (very flat), and low scores indicate ambiguous seizure suppression, in which the seizure end point is clear but the suppression is weak (far from flat). EEG power spectral analysis includes each EEG band, i.e., alpha, beta, theta, and delta, and coherence (Nobler et al., 2000; Perera et al., 2004).

Relationship to clinical changes, adverse effects, and depression

Seizure adequacy is the most important and interesting issue in interpreting ECT seizure monitoring. EEG signs of intense seizure and postictal suppression were associated with good clinical outcome in patients treated with high-dose right unilateral and bilateral ECT (Folkerts, 1996; Krystal et al., 1995; Luber et al., 2000; Nobler et al., 1993, 2000; Suppes et al., 1996). In general, unequivocal EEG evidence of seizure occurrence consists of clear or repetitive polyspikes and slow-wave discharges. When such seizure evidence is not seen, the patient might have received inadequate treatment. These seizure findings are associated with patient age, treatment course, initial seizure threshold, and drugs administered (Boylan et al., 2000; McCall et al., 1996a, 1996b; Sackeim et al., 1987). Studies have reported possible EEG signs of stronger seizure with increases in relative stimulus intensity (Krystal et al., 1996, 2000). Interictal EEG recordings suggest that prefrontal slow-wave activity is associated with greater efficacy in treating depression, although it did not distinguish between effective and ineffective treatments (see Figure 29.2) (Sackeim et al., 1996).

Although ECT can produce an anterograde amnesia that rapidly resolves and a limited retrograde amnesia that persists, ictal EEG is not correlated with cognitive changes after the final ECT of the course (Perera et al., 2004). Preliminary results suggest that ictal EEG changes might correlate with improvements in anterograde memory two weeks after the last bitemporal ECT (Azuma et al., 2007). Disorientation immediately following right unilateral ECT correlated with accentuated delta power in anterior frontal and temporal regions (Sackeim et al., 2000). Marked delta

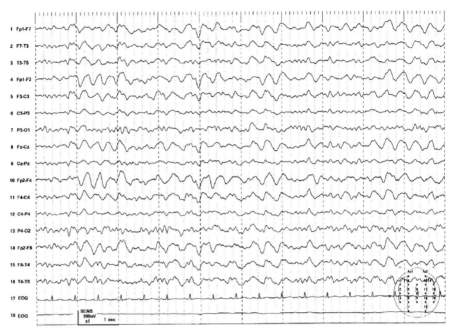

Figure 29.2   Interictal delta waves, nine days after 11 sessions of bilateral electroconvulsive therapy. Bipolar recording (the 10–20 system). Time constant, 0.3 second; sensitivity, 10 μV/mm. In the frontal area, 3- to 5-Hz high-amplitude slow waves were seen; in the occipital area, 9- to 10-Hz middle-amplitude alpha waves were seen.

and theta waves globally across the cortex correlated with global cognitive function represented by modified Mini-Mental State Examination scores. Retrograde amnesia, particularly for autobiographical memories, correlated with increased theta activity in the left frontotemporal region. Further studies of the effects of cognitive changes on depression rating after ECT are needed to more accurately rate the clinical outcome of ECT and the effects of treatment modifications on it.

Missed seizure

When there is no evidence of seizure occurrence after the electrical stimulus, the situation is identified as a missed seizure (APA, 2001). Missed seizures occur when the stimulus dose is not sufficient to reach the threshold, the electrode attachment is inadequate, ventilation is insufficient, the patient is dehydrated or has another acute medical problem, or the medications given have an anticonvulsant effect. These seizures can be remedied by restimulation at a higher electrical dose, reduction of medications with anticonvulsant effects, possibly using flumazenil in patients exposed to benzodiazepines (Bailine et al., 1994; Berigan et al., 1995; Doering and Ball, 1995; Krystal et al., 1998), more vigorous hyperventilation, or change of anesthetic, for example, to etomidate (Christensen et al., 1986; Saffer and Berk, 1998; Trzepacz et al., 1993) or ketamine (Rasmussen et al., 1996). Restimulation is generally administered after about 45 seconds, because a seizure can start with onset delayed up to 45 seconds (APA, 2001).

Abortive or brief seizure

Seizures sometimes stop abruptly. A duration of fewer than 15 seconds is generally identified as an abortive seizure and generally indicates an insufficient stimulus dose. This determination is not always easy to make because the presence of low-amplitude signals, artifacts, or atypical EEG responses may seriously confound the EEG display. If a patient requires restimulation, the addition of an additional dose of muscle relaxant or anesthetic agent should be considered, but a repeated dose of succinylcholine is associated with arrhythmias. With further treatment sessions, the seizure duration will likely shorten and the seizure threshold increase (Kales et al., 1997).

Prolonged seizure

Occasionally prolonged seizure occurs, which generally refers to an EEG seizure lasting for at least two minutes (Abrams, 1997; Royal College of Psychiatrists, 1995) or three minutes (APA, 2001). After treatment, nonconvulsive status epilepticus is rare but possible, so EEG monitoring is required to ensure that the signs of EEG seizure have stopped (Mayur et al., 1999; Parker et al., 2001; Scott and Riddle, 1989). When prolonged EEG (or motor) seizure occurs, an anesthetic with anti-convulsant effect (e.g., methohexital, propofol) or an intravenous benzodiazepine should be promptly administered to terminate the seizure. Because of exceptional anticonvulsant effects, propofol is particularly effective for status epilepticus. If the seizure still does not stop, the status epilepticus protocol should be followed (Lowenstein and Alldredge, 1998; Treiman et al., 1998).

References

Abrams, R. 1997. Electroconvulsive therapy, 3rd edn. New York: Oxford University Press.

American Psychiatric Association. 2001. Practice of electroconvulsive therapy: Recommendations of treatment, training, and privileging, 2nd edn. A task force report of the American Psychiatric Association. Washington, DC: American Psychiatric Association.

Azuma, H., Fujita, A., Otsuki, K., et al. 2007. Ictal electroencephalographic correlates of post-treatment neuropsychological changes in electroconvulsive therapy: A hypothesis-generation study. J ECT 23(3): 163–8.

Bailine, S. H., Safferman, A., Vital-Herne, J., et al. 1994. Flumazenil reversal of benzodiazepine-induced sedation for a patient with severe pre-ECT anxiety. Convuls Ther 10: 65–8.

Berigan, T. R., Harazin, J., and Williams, H. L. 2nd. 1995. Use of flumazenil in conjunction with electroconvulsive therapy. Am J Psychiatry 152: 957.

Blachly, P. 1976. New developments in electroconvulsive therapy. Dis Nerv Syst 37: 356–8.

Blachly, P. and Gowing, D. 1966. Multiple monitored electroconvulsive treatment. Compr Psychiatry 7: 100–9.

Boylan, L. S., Haskett, R. F., Mulsant, B. H., et al. 2000. Determinants of seizure threshold in ECT: Benzodiazepine use, anesthetic dosage, and other factors. J ECT 16(1): 3–18.

Christensen, P., Kragh-Sorensen, P., Sorensen, C., et al. 1986. EEG-monitored ECT: A comparison of seizure duration under anesthesia with etomidate and thiopentone. Convuls Ther 2: 145–50.

Doering, E. B. and Ball, W. A. 1995. Flumazenil before electroconvulsive therapy: Outstanding issues. Anesthesiology 83: 642–3.

Folkerts, H. 1996. The ictal electroencephalogram as a marker for the efficacy of electroconvulsive therapy. Eur Arch Psychiatry Clin Neurosci 246: 155–64.

Gastaut, H. and Broughton, R. 1972. Epileptic seizures. Springfield, IL: Thomas.

Kales, H., Raz, J., Tandon, R., et al. 1997. Relationship of seizure duration to antidepressant efficacy in electroconvulsive therapy. Psychol Med 27: 1373–80.

Krystal, A. D., Watts, B. V., Weiner, R. D., et al. 1998. The use of flumazenil in the anxious and benzodiazepine-dependent ECT patient. J ECT 14: 5–14.

Krystal, A. D., Weiner, R. D., and Coffey, C. E. 1995. The ictal EEG as a marker of adequate stimulus intensity with unilateral ECT. J Neuropsychiatry Clin Neurosci 7(3): 295–303.

Krystal, A. D., Weiner, R. D., Coffey, C. E., and McCall, W. V. 1996. Effect of ECT treatment number on the ictal EEG. Psychiatry Res 62(2): 179–89.

Krystal, A. D., Weiner, R. D., Lindahl, V., and Massie, R. 2000. The development and retrospective testing of an electroencephalographic seizure quality-based stimulus dosing paradigm with ECT. J ECT 16(4): 338–49.

Lowenstein, D. H. and Alldredge, B. K. 1998. Status epilepticus. N Engl J Med 338: 970–6.

Luber, B., Nobler, M. S., Moeller, J. R., et al. 2000. Quantitative EEG during seizures induced by electroconvulsive therapy: Relations to treatment modality and clinical features. II. Topographic analyses. J ECT 16(3): 229–43.

Mayur P. M., Gangadhar B. N., Janakiramaiah N., et al. 1999. Motor seizure monitoring during electroconvulsive therapy. Br J Psychiatry 174: 270–2.

McCall, W. V., Colenda, C. C., and Farah, B. A. 1996a. Ictal EEG regularity declines during a course of RUL ECT. Convuls Ther 12(4): 213–16.

McCall, W. V., Robinette, G. D., and Hardesty, D. 1996b. Relationship of seizure morphology to the convulsive threshold. Convuls Ther 12(3): 147–51.

Nobler, M. S., Luber, B., Moeller, J. R., et al. 2000. Quantitative EEG during seizures induced by electroconvulsive therapy: Relations to treatment modality and clinical features. I. Global analyses. J ECT 16(3): 211–28.

Nobler, M. S., Sackeim, H. A., Solomou, M., et al. 1993. EEG manifestations during ECT: Effects of electrode placement and stimulus intensity. Biol Psychiatry 34(5): 321–30.

Parker, V., Nobler, M. S., Pedley, T. A., et al. 2001. A unilateral, prolonged, nonconvulsive seizure in a patient treated with bilateral ECT. J ECT 17: 141–5.

Perera, T. D., Luber, B., Nobler, M. S., et al. 2004. Seizure expression during electroconvulsive therapy: Relationships with clinical outcome and cognitive side effects. Neuropsychopharmacology 29(4): 813–25.

Rasmussen, K. G., Jarvis, M. R., and Zorumski, C. F. 1996. Ketamine anesthesia in electroconvulsive therapy. Convuls Ther 12: 217–23.

Royal College of Psychiatrists. 1995. The ECT handbook: The second report of the Royal College of the Psychiatrists' special committee on ECT. London: Royal College of Psychiatrists.

Sackeim, H., Decina, P., Prohovnik, I., and Malitz, S. 1987. Seizure threshold in electroconvulsive therapy. Effects of sex, age, electrode placement, and number of treatments. Arch Gen Psychiatry 44(4): 355–60.

Sackeim, H. A., Devanand, D. P., Prudic, J., et al. 1991. Stimulus intensity, seizure threshold, and seizure duration: Impact on the efficacy and safety of electroconvulsive therapy. Psychiatr Clin North Am 14(4): 803–43.

Sackeim, H. A., Luber, B., Katzman, G. P., et al. 1996. The effects of electroconvulsive therapy on quantitative electroencephalograms. Relationship to clinical outcome. Arch Gen Psychiatry 53(9): 814–24.

Sackeim, H. A., Luber, B., Moeller, J. R., et al. 2000. Electrophysiological correlates of the adverse cognitive effects of electroconvulsive therapy. J ECT 16(2): 110–20.

Saffer, S. and Berk, M. 1998. Anesthetic induction for ECT with etomidate is associated with longer seizure duration than thiopentone. J ECT 14: 89–93.

Scott, A. I. and Riddle, W. 1989. Status epilepticus after electroconvulsive therapy. Br J Psychiatry 155: 119–21.

Suppes, T., Webb, A., Carmody, T., et al. 1996. Is postictal electrical silence a predictor of response to electroconvulsive therapy? J Affect Disord 41(1): 55–8.

Treiman, D. M., Meyers, P. D., Walton, N. Y., et al. 1998. A comparison of four treatments for generalized convulsive status epilepticus. Veterans Affairs Status Epilepticus Cooperative Study Group. N Engl J Med 339: 792–8.

Trzepacz, P. T., Weniger, F. C., and Greenhouse, J. 1993. Etomidate anesthesia increases seizure duration during ECT. A retrospective study. Gen Hosp Psychiatry 15: 115–20.

Weiner, R. D., Coffey, C. E., and Krystal, A. D. 1991. The monitoring and management of electrically induced seizures. Psychiatr Clin North Am 14: 845–69.

Weiner, R. D. and Krystal, A. D. 1993. EEG monitoring and management of electrically induced seizures. In The clinical science of ECT (ed. Coffey, C. E.). Washington DC: American Psychiatric Press, pp. 93–109.

30

Heart rate and electroconvulsive therapy

Conrad M. Swartz

Heart rate (HR) changes during the electroconvulsive therapy (ECT) seizure are clinically useful, not merely a peculiarity or side effect. They can provide information about ECT efficacy, adequacy of the electrical stimulus dose, need to increase stimulus dose, and cardiovascular condition. Just as these are basic concerns, so are HR changes.

HR reflecting seizure activity

A variety of large and small changes occur in HR during ECT. The largest is ECT-induced HR elevation. A study of the highest peak HR within ECT courses for 87 men and 90 women found that it clustered within the range of 140 to 180 bpm and did not decrease with age (Swartz and Shen, 2007). This was with ordinary methohexital-succinylcholine anesthesia and hyperventilation with oxygen; high-dose propofol (e.g., more than 1 mg/kg) or less active ventilation should produce lower HR values. The HR values of a few patients lay below this range and showed age-related decrease. ECT peak HR exceeded the maximum HR in the cardiac treadmill test for patients older than 60 years, and more so in older people. This is a profound increase in HR.

The higher peak HR during ECT than during treadmill exercise suggests that exercise HR is limited by metabolic demand and humoral factors, and not the heart itself. Reasoning in the opposite direction does not point to the heart limiting ECT-induced HR because, in young people, treadmill peak HR exceeds ECT peak HR; if the heart limited ECT HR it would similarly limit treadmill HR.

What, then, limits ECT HR? With cardiac, metabolic, and humoral factors excluded, peak HR should primarily reflect brain activity and function. This might seem surprising. Nevertheless, it is consistent with what has been, until now, by far the strongest reported relationship between a physiologic measurement and clinical factors. Specifically, peak HR closely and significantly reflected both stimulus dose and clinical efficacy, as described later in this chapter.

There is a neuroanatomic rationale for ECT clinical outcome to correspond more closely to peak HR than to electroencephalogram (EEG). ECT peak HR largely reflects seizure activity in the medulla, deep in the brainstem. In comparison, EEG directly reflects primarily the outer cortex and motor activity reflects the cortical motor strip. Accordingly, HR changes should more closely and specifically reflect seizure activity in the deep brainstem (diencephalon) than EEG or motor activity do. This is important because the therapeutic effect of ECT on melancholia, catatonia, and psychosis might well be primarily subcortical (i.e., the diencephalic site of ECT therapeutic effect).

This rationale rests on neurogenic drive of ECT HR acceleration. This has been established in several different ways. Histologically, studies of artificial neurovirus spread along neural pathways reveal that brainstem nuclei in and around the reticular activating system in the upper medulla and lower pons mediate sympathetic nervous system activation of HR elevation and adrenal catecholamine release (Jansen et al., 1995). These central nervous system (CNS) neurons contain a preponderance of epinephrine, about 10 times as much as serotonin. This preponderance indicates epinephrinergic neurotransmission. Another component in this mechanism is corticotropin-releasing hormone (CRH), which acts as both a hormone (on the pituitary) and a neurotransmitter. As a neurotransmitter, CRH in the CNS directly stimulates cardiac acceleration (Brown and Fisher, 1984).

Physiologically, after the ECT electrical stimulus the HR accelerates and peaks well before one period of circulation time. Indeed, the peak HR typically occurs 10 to 20 seconds after the stimulus (Swartz et al., 1994). Accordingly, the peak HR cannot result from humoral factors, such as epinephrine in the bloodstream, but reflects CNS activity. Neuroanatomically, the peak HR is maintained longer with right unilateral ECT than with left unilateral ECT in the same patients (Swartz et al., 1994). This right cerebral hemisphere superiority in increasing HR correlates with observations in laboratory animals that direct stimulation of sites in the right medulla typically provokes cardioacceleration, whereas the left medulla more often generates bradyarrhythmias.

Right-sided superiority is further supported by comparable HR elevation during the seizure for both right unilateral and bitemporal ECT. Shortly after the seizure, HR is higher with bitemporal ECT (Lane et al., 1989). This apparently corresponds to both greater right hemisphere stimulation and greater catecholamine release into the peripheral circulation with bitemporal ECT, as catecholamines persist for several minutes after the seizure. This hormone pattern correlates with other reports, of greater release of prolactin (Swartz and Abrams, 1984) and cortisol (Swartz, 1992) into the bloodstream with bitemporal than with unilateral ECT.

Not only are the brain sites controlling HR in close proximity to the putative brain site of ECT therapeutic action, but they are far from the stimulus electrodes.

This is so for all modern electrode placements (see Chapter 27), and it is important because measuring seizure activity near the stimulus electrodes does not reflect seizure activity that has spread far from it. Measuring seizure activity distant from the stimulus site (e.g., with peak HR) is more suited to identifying how well seizure activity spread through the brain.

EEG channels with one or both electrodes close to the stimulus electrodes primarily reflect seizure activity near the stimulus sites. Seizure that is intense near the stimulus electrodes but does not spread well through the brain will appear to be intense according to the usual methods of EEG recording at ECT. Usually, anterior-to-mastoid or bi-anterior EEG recording electrodes are used. Their use probably explains why EEG recordings (for such phenomena as postictal suppression) were not substantially different among moderate-dose unilateral, high-dose unilateral, and bitemporal ECTs (McCall et al., 1998; Nobler et al., 1993). It also explains why associations between EEG findings and ECT efficacy have been weak, even if there was some statistical significance. Of course, the EEG is complex and involves specific training and experience to interpret. In contrast, peak HR is simple to measure and interpret.

Peak HR and seizure quality

As with virtually all physiological measurements, HR varies markedly from one patient to the next. This applies to ECT peak HR as well as resting HR. Allowing interpersonal variations to influence the expression of ECT-induced HR elevation should obscure trends and results by increasing random variations (i.e., noise). Specifically, should baseline HR be subtracted from peak HR, or not? To answer this question, HR values were measured for all successful ECT treatments on 24 patients. Within patients, the baseline HR mean variation was 7.7 bpm; of course, baseline HR does not reflect ECT seizure. Within patients again, the ECT peak HR mean variation was 4.6 bpm, significantly lower than the baseline HR variation (Swartz, 1999). This means that subtracting baseline from peak HR increases random variations more than subtracting one peak HR from another peak HR. There was no correlation between peak and baseline HR values, verifying that baseline HR does not reflect seizure changes by anticipating them.

This led to the Benchmark Method of expressing peak HR (and in turn to the Benchmark Method of stimulus dose regulation; see next section). In this, peak HR is stated as comparative peak HR, which is how much peak HR differs from highest peak HR seen recently in that patient, in other words, peak HR submaximality. This can be compared between patients or between ECT treatments within a patient. Of course, baseline HR is still important because if it is near peak HR there is no clear seizure-induced HR elevation and no valid peak HR.

Peak HR submaximality was found to reflect both stimulus dose and clinical efficacy. Half-age and full-age stimulus doses were given to each of 24 patients. Peak HR was 12 bpm higher with the higher dose, averaging 156 bpm. The mean peak HR submaximality was 4.2 bpm at the higher dose and 16.4 bpm at the lower dose. Even when the three patients who showed only EEG seizure but no motor seizure at the lower dose were excluded, peak HR was 6 bpm higher (still significant). Patients whose average peak HR submaximality was smaller needed fewer ECT treatments for remission than did the other patients ($p = .00003$). Peak HR submaximality averaged 6.5 bpm for patients who did not need more than the minimum of six ECT treatments, but it averaged 18.1 bpm for those who did. This relationship is much more robust than relationships reported between EEG measurements and ECT response. In this study, the only EEG measure to show sensitivity to stimulus dose was recruitment phase duration, but the effect and its significance ($p = .04$) were much weaker (Swartz, 2000).

In comparing four different ECT stimuli of the same charge but different pulse widths (0.5 ms or 1 ms) and frequencies (30 Hz or 60 Hz), peak HR was higher with 0.5 ms than with 1 ms. Peak HR submaximality at 0.5-ms pulse width averaged 10.7 and 11.0 bpm at 30 Hz and 60 Hz, respectively. At 1-ms pulse width, it averaged 18.0 and 21.3 bpm at 30 Hz and 60 Hz, respectively. This finding shows that the peak HR is sensitive enough to reflect the efficiency of different pulse widths at the same stimulus dose. The ability of peak HR to reflect changes in pulse width implies that its sensitivity to the stimulus is greater than reflecting only changes in stimulus dose. Frequency did not significantly affect peak HR (Swartz and Manly, 2000).

Hyperventilation during ECT anesthesia produced higher HR than less avid ventilation did, averaging 131 bpm and 113 bpm, respectively (Bergsholm et al., 1993). This result is attributable to lower carbon dioxide levels and higher oxygen levels promoting more intense seizure activity (Swartz, 1996). The resulting greater seizure intensity then produces higher peak HR. The statistical significance for the difference between the two peak HR values ($p < .001$) is further testimony to the high sensitivity of seizure HR in reflecting seizure intensity, because HR was measured only once during seizure at a seemingly random time. The seizure HR average with hyperventilation was 131 bpm, well below the expected 140- to 180-bpm range for peak HR measured with hyperventilation (Swartz and Shen, 2007). Determination of actual peak HR should produce an even stronger result.

These studies indicate that peak HR submaximality is influenced by the electrical stimulus dose and the location and intensity of the resulting seizure. It can be modified by the patient's cardiovascular condition, the anesthetics used, and background medications. Conversely, peak HR can reflect on the quality of the ECT seizure, and then guide ECT stimulus dosing along the course of treatment. A peak HR of less than 140 bpm can reflect cardiovascular impairment or exposure to cardioactive medications, such as propofol anesthesia dosed higher than 1 mg/kg. Still, unlike seizure quality, these cardiac effects usually do not vary along the course of ECT.

Benchmark Method of stimulus dose regulation

Based on this sensitivity of peak HR to seizure quality, monitoring peak HR along the course of ECT can indicate when the electrical stimulus should be increased and when a decrease may be possible. To date, this is the only published measurement-based technique to regulate the stimulus dose along the course of ECT (Swartz, 2002). At the first ECT treatment, a stimulus dose expected to produce an intense seizure is administered. For most patients, this dose might be 5 mC/year of age for unilateral ECT or 3 mC/year for bilateral ECT at 900-mA current, or 7 mC/year of age for unilateral ECT or 4 mC/year for bilateral ECT at 800-mA current. (For discussion of how current affects stimulus dose, see Chapter 1). The peak HR for this intense seizure becomes the benchmark for treatment efficacy. The initial peak HR should usually be in the range of 140 to 190 bpm (Swartz and Shen, 2007). If it is and a bilateral placement is being used, consider decreasing the stimulus dose by 0.5 mC/year of age at the next session. If it is lower than 140 bpm and there is no pharmacological or cardiopathological reason for this, consider increasing the stimulus dose at the next ECT session to try to obtain a peak HR in the range of 140 to 180 bpm.

At each of the following ECT sessions, if the peak HR is within 6 bpm of the benchmark, consider the treatment efficacy maximal. If it is higher than the benchmark, it replaces the benchmark. If it is 6 to 12 bpm lower than the benchmark, consider a small dose increase, for example, by 25 mC. If it is 12 bpm or more less than the benchmark, consider a moderate dose increase, for example, by 75 mC. If there is no sign of seizure, increase the dose by 100 to 125 mC. The same concepts can be used with other physiological signs such as EEG measurements.

Tachycardia duration

The archetypal pattern for ECT HR begins with slowing during the stimulus, presumably a vagal effect. Starting 1 to 3 seconds after the stimulus ends, the HR then accelerates rapidly into the range of 140 to 180 bpm, remains near the peak for 10 to 20 seconds, then slowly falls until near the end of the seizure. The HR then decelerates and returns to pre-ECT baseline. Occasional exceptions include a peak HR of less than 140 bpm, a brief bradyarrhythmia at the end of the seizure, and persistent tachycardia after seizure termination. Peak HR during an individual seizure of less than 140 bpm suggests weakness and the need to increase stimulus dose. A maximum peak HR of less than 140 bpm with a high-stimulus dose and vigorous seizure suggests cardiac disease or medication effect.

Despite this common pattern, there are wide variations from one physically healthy person to another. Although the duration of asystole immediately after the electrical stimulus is usually one to three seconds, it can last up to seven seconds. The HR at the end of the seizure can decrease to less than the baseline HR, with asystole as long as five to nine seconds observed (Bhat et al., 2002). One patient received precordial impact after nine seconds and was given no further ECT.

On average, the ECT HR elevation lasts about as long as the EEG seizure, but some individual patients show marked differences between durations of EEG seizure and tachycardia (Larson et al., 1984). The duration of ECT-induced tachycardia was measured in 203 seizures of 28 patients. The end point of this tachycardia was taken as the point of greatest decrease in the HR. Using ECG calipers, this is the midpoint of the interval between the QRS complexes during which the greatest decline in HR occurred. In 90% of ECT sessions, this tachycardia end point was quickly determinable by visual inspection to within five seconds of the value obtained with calipers. Timed from the end of the electrical stimulus, the tachycardia duration correlated highly with cuffed arm convulsion duration ($r = .79$) and EEG seizure duration ($r = .75$). The tachycardia end point was less frequently indeterminate than the EEG seizure end point (Larson et al., 1984). Accordingly, the duration of ECT-induced HR elevation can be used as a measure of seizure duration.

Tachycardia duration provides a way to compare the quality of ECT treatment among different ECT techniques. Specifically, tachycardia duration correlates more closely with EEG total seizure duration, duration of EEG spike activity, and motor convulsion duration with bitemporal ECT than with right unilateral ECT. This higher correlation presumably corresponds to more extensive generalization of the seizure through the brain, and presumably greater efficacy. This correlation was one of the earliest measurements to suggest that seizure quality is greater with bitemporal ECT than with unilateral ECT. Specifically, the Pearson correlation coefficient (r) was 0.77, 0.80, and 0.78 between tachycardia duration and total EEG duration, EEG spike duration, and motor convulsion duration, respectively, with bitemporal ECT. However, the correlation coefficient was 0.37, 0.02, and 0.40, respectively, with unilateral ECT. These large differences have a significance of at least $p < .02$ (Swartz and Larson, 1986).

Similarly, tachycardia duration correlates more closely with EEG and motor seizure durations for the first of two bitemporal ECT treatments given under the same anesthesia than for the second treatment. This result suggests that seizure generalization (and presumably efficacy) decreases with additional ECT treatments given in the same ECT session (Larson and Swartz, 1986).

The HR usually decreases to a level at or somewhat greater than baseline after the seizure. A few patients, particularly elderly ones, show marked post-ECT tachycardia (or hypertension) that can need mitigation by medication. Because the half-life of epinephrine and norepinephrine in the bloodstream is in the range of one to two minutes (Anton et al., 1977), changes substantially faster than this are not following humoral factors. Accordingly, an abrupt decrease in HR at the end of the seizure indicates little effect from humoral factors on HR. In a prospective study, 19 of 24 patients showed consistently abrupt endings of the ECT HR elevation, and the other five patients showed consistently gradual endings. The patients with abrupt endings had lower baseline HR (mean 88 bpm) than did those with gradual endings (mean 118 bpm). There was an apparent demarcation between these groups at 100 bpm. A gradual ending of the ECT-induced tachycardia might be associated with higher levels of circulating catecholamines, and higher baseline HR might signal greater risk for persistent post-ECT tachycardia (Swartz and Manly, 1999).

Most studies that examined the HR during the ECT session did so with a device that automatically measures HR and blood pressure once per minute. The availability of this device apparently spawned several similar studies that reported HR only after the seizure. These studies did not find substantial patterns. For example, one reported that pre-ECT lidocaine did not affect the post-ECT HR, although it greatly shortened the ECT seizure in a dose-dependent manner (Fu et al., 1997). The authors hypothesized that post-ECT HR primarily reflects circulating catecholamines liberated during the seizure, but they did not measure catecholamines. They found no relationship between post-ECT HR and seizure duration within patients, but this has no implications for catecholamine levels.

Studies measuring peak HR as representing clinical efficacy should help to clarify several aspects of ECT clinical methods. These include individualizing the stimulus dose for right unilateral ECT for each patient (according to the Benchmark Method previously described), and identifying possible clinically effective pulse widths that are narrower than 0.5 milliseconds separately for unilateral and bilateral ECT.

References

Anton, A. H., Uy, D. S., and Redderson, C. L. 1977. Autonomic blockade and the cardiovascular and catecholamine response to electroshock. Anesth Analg 56: 46–54.

Bergsholm, P., Bleie, H., Gran, L., and d'Elia, G. 1993. Cardiovascular response and seizure duration as determined by electroencephalography during unilateral electroconvulsive therapy. Acta Psychiatr Scand 88: 25–8.

Bhat, S. K., Acosta, D., and Swartz, C. M. 2002. Postictal asystole during ECT. J ECT 18: 103–6.

Brown, M. R. and Fisher, L. A. 1984. CRF: Integration of the neuroendocrine and autonomic nervous system responses to stress. In Endocrinology (eds. Labrie, F. and Proulx, F.). New York: Excerpta Medica International Congress Series 655, pp. 597–600.

Fu, W., Stool, L. A., White, P. F., and Husain, M. M. 1997. Acute hemodynamic responses to electroconvulsive therapy are not related to the duration of seizure activity. J Clin Anesth 9: 653–7.

Jansen, A. S. P., Nguyen, X. V., Karpitskiy, V., et al. 1995. Central command neurons of the sympathetic nervous system: Basis of the fight-or-flight response. Science 270: 644–6.

Lane, R. D., Zeitlin, S. B., Abrams, R., and Swartz, C. M. 1989. Differential effects of right-unilateral and bilateral ECT on heart rate. Am J Psychiatry 146: 1041–3.

Larson, G., Swartz, C., and Abrams, R. 1984. Duration of ECT-induced tachycardia as a measure of seizure length. Am J Psychiatry 141: 1269–71.

Larson, G. and Swartz, C. M. 1986. Differences between first and second ECTs given in the same session. Convuls Ther 2: 191–6.

McCall, W. V., Sparks, W., Jane, J., et al. 1998. Variation of ictal electroencephalographic regularity with low-, moderate-, and high-dose stimuli during right unilateral electroconvulsive therapy. Biol Psychiatry 43: 608–11.

Nobler, M. S., Sackeim, H. A., Solomou, M., et al. 1993. EEG manifestations during ECT: Effects of electrode placement and stimulus intensity. Biol Psychiatry 34: 321–30.

Swartz, C. M. 1992. Electroconvulsive therapy-induced cortisol release after dexamethasone in depression. Neuropsychobiology 25: 130–3.

Swartz, C. M. 1996. Obstruction of ECT seizure by submaximal hyperventilation. Ann Clin Psychiatry 8: 31–4.

Swartz, C. M. 1999. Variations of peak and baseline heart rates. J ECT 15: 222–5.

Swartz, C. M. 2000. Physiological response to ECT stimulus dose. Psychiatry Res 97: 229–35.

Swartz, C. M. 2002. ECT dosing by the benchmark method. German J Psychiatry 5: 1–4. Available at: http://www.gjpsy.uni-goettingen.de.

Swartz, C. M. and Abrams, R. 1984. Prolactin levels after bilateral and unilateral ECT. Br J Psychiatry 144: 643–5.

Swartz, C. M., Abrams, R., Lane, R., et al. 1994. Heart rate differences between right and left unilateral ECT. J Neurol Neurosurg Psychiatry 57: 97–9.

Swartz, C. M. and Larson, G. 1986. Generalization of the effects of unilateral and bilateral ECT. Am J Psychiatry 143: 1040–1.

Swartz, C. M. and Manly, D. T. 1999. The endpoint of ECT-induced elevation in heart rate. J ECT 15: 125–8.

Swartz, C. M. and Manly, D. T. 2000. Efficiency of the stimulus characteristics of ECT. Am J Psychiatry 157: 1504–6.

Swartz, C. M. and Shen, W. W. 2007. ECT generalized seizure drives heart rate above treadmill stress test maximum. J ECT 23: 71–4.

31

Cognitive side effects and psychological testing

James Stuart Lawson

Introduction

Concerns about the cognitive side effects of electroconvulsive therapy (ECT), particularly with regard to memory, have been reported almost from the introduction of the treatment in the late 1930s (Levy et al., 1942). Access to information stored before ECT (retrograde amnesia) and registration and recall of information presented after (anterograde amnesia) have been of particular clinical concern. This chapter reviews the elements of the clinical and neuropsychological examination pertinent to the investigation of putative cognitive side effects in ECT-treated patients. We also consider the seeming paradox that patients with untreated major depression can present with cognitive deficits that respond to ECT as the depression improves (Calev et al., 1995). This apparent paradox can also occur with illnesses treatable by ECT such as bipolar disorder and schizophrenia.

Several clinical, treatment, and demographic factors can influence post-ECT cognitive deficits. These include psychiatric diagnosis, concurrent medical condition or medication, anesthesia for ECT, electrode placement, stimulus dosing, stimulus waveform, age, sex, premorbid intelligence, and socioeconomic status. The first six of these have chapters devoted to them in this book (Chapters 22, 25, 26, 27, 28, and 1, respectively). In this chapter we discuss these modulating factors and gauge the extent of their influences on cognitive side effects to help the clinician to make sound decisions about treatment details.

Clinical evaluation: Mini Mental State Examination

When the Mini Mental State Examination (MMSE) was introduced more than 30 years ago (Folstein et al., 1975), it proved a welcome initiative to standardize and make objective what had until then been a highly variable assessment. The results of applying cognitive assessment procedures were informally and subjectively interpreted without regard to basic standards of test validity or reliability. Validity refers to the test measuring what is intended, and reliability refers to the stability of test scores when no real change occurs in the object of measurement (Nunnally and Bernstein, 1994). In contrast, the MMSE is constructed on sound psychometric principles incorporating validity and reliability information as well as norms for various groups including healthy individuals (Butler et al., 1996; Chatfield et al., 2007; Crum et al., 1993; Dufouil et al., 2000; Huppert et al., 2005; Tombaugh and McIntyre, 1992).

The MMSE is sufficiently sensitive to identify the cognitive deficits associated with untreated major depression, with ECT, and with variations in the ECT procedure. Nevertheless, the MMSE shows a lack of sensitivity in identifying individuals who experience mild cognitive deficits from ECT that continue more than several hours after the ECT session (Sackeim et al., 2007). This lack of detection can be important in studies that aim to detect any mild deficits that remain at long-term follow-up. Whatever the sensitivity of a test, the absence of detection does not prove the absence of an effect. In reviewing the results of MMSE testing in ECT patients, it is important to note that this test was designed primarily to aid differential diagnosis between major depression and dementia, where cognitive deficits are more salient than after ECT. Whether cognitive abilities are completely recovered at some point after ECT is better addressed by means of a battery of neuropsychological tests than by the MMSE alone.

Neuropsychological examination of patients treated with ECT

Postictal disorientation and confusion

"Postictal disorientation and confusion" refers to the short-lived impairment of consciousness during the time period between complete unconsciousness and the return of full consciousness after each ECT. The phenomenon of postictal disorientation in ECT has been studied extensively since the 1940s. Daniel and Crovitz (1982, 1983a, 1983b) have provided comprehensive reviews of the earlier literature on this topic. The experimental procedure in these studies differed somewhat from one study to the other, as did the procedural details. Still, their results showed remarkable agreement on the general structure of the deficits despite variations in electrode placement, stimulus dose and waveform, use of oxygenation, and unstated other details. The experimental paradigms involved the determination of the time point after seizure when consciousness returned, followed by questions at discrete intervals or continuously presented testing orientation for person, place, and time. In general, the studies agreed that orientation for person recovered first, followed by orientation for place, and then orientation for time. This illustrates what is known as Ribot's Law, named for the 19th-century philosopher and early neuropsychologist, Theodule Ribot (1882): "The dissolution of memory is inversely related to the recency of the event." This feature of retrograde amnesia (inability to access information previously stored) is commonly observed in the aftermath of acute insult to the brain (e.g., motor vehicle accident). Specifically, long-consolidated information can be accessed earlier than more recently stored material. In a later study, Daniel et al. (1987) found that patients' responses when asked their age and the current year were at first displaced backward in years from the correct response. This displacement diminished as recovery continued, finally vanishing when recovery was complete.

Studying disorientation after moderately suprathreshold bitemporal ECT, Calev et al. (1991) incorporated a novel design. Four of eight assessments following "sham" ECT revealed that disorientation increased sharply after the first real ECT, improved after the second, and remained at that level through the fourth treatment. Sham ECT was followed by the most rapid recovery of orientation and did not vary with ECT number. Disorientation to person, place, and time followed Ribot's Law. To assess interictal disorientation, the investigators evaluated orientation at baseline before each real ECT was given. There was a cumulative effect as the baseline orientation score declined through the course of 11 ECT treatments. A correlational analysis showed a reliable and independent association between both length of seizure and electrical stimulus intensity on the one hand and degree of disorientation on the other. The effects of these electrical stimulus variables were independent of demographic variables. Overall, this result supported the hypothesis of a direct effect of the stimulus dose on orientation.

Valentine et al. (1968) note that bitemporal pulse stimulation produced more disorientation than did nondominant unilateral placement, and sine wave substantially more than pulse. There appears to be an interaction between placement and waveform in the more difficult time orientation questions. The combination of sine wave stimulus with bitemporal placement apparently produced a severity of disorientation greater than the sum of the independent effects of waveform and placement, although the authors did not specifically test this hypothesis.

General intelligence

To clarify the role of assessment of general intellectual functions in evaluating the cognitive effects of ECT (or any biological perturbation of the brain), it is useful to consider the concept of general intelligence. The modern model proposed by Spearman (1904) was founded on the expectation that abilities for distinct mental tasks show substantial correlations within groups of people. In other words, abilities required for one intellectual task contribute somewhat to the performance of another. The correlations were not all equal, but if the test could reasonably be regarded as intellectual, they were never zero. This finding led Spearman to conjecture that any intellectual tests shared some variance with all the others, but also incorporated some test-specific variance that reflected abilities specific to the task. The shared variance he named "g" for general intelligence. The specific variance he called "s" for specific ability. There were many "s" abilities, but there was only one "g." Although the tests Spearman investigated were superseded by the formal test batteries of modern intelligence testing, his concepts formed the basis of the intelligence quotient (IQ). IQ now represents the standardized, normalized unweighted sum of scores from a broad sample of intellectual tests.

Why should we be interested in evaluating general intellectual ability in ECT patients? The answer is that it should permit us to distinguish between a general depression of subtest scores and impairment of particular specific abilities. The latter suggests dysfunction of particular brain structures or functions. Of course a general decrease must be compared with premorbid levels and expectations associated with demographic profile. General intellectual evaluation is the typical first step in the neuropsychological evaluation of individual patients who were exposed to a physical stress on the brain and provides a basis for more specific understanding of any deficits. Analogously, it provides a starting point for evaluating the cognitive sequelae of ECT.

Malloy et al. (1982) studied 231 patents with a variety of diagnoses who received ECT with bitemporal, right unilateral, or left unilateral ECT. The placement was changed if the treatments appeared ineffective. The diagnoses included schizophrenia, affective disorder, and schizoaffective disorder. A cognitive battery included the Wechsler Adult Intelligence Scale (WAIS) two or three days before and two to three weeks after treatment. Patients showed reliable *improvements* in performance IQ in one of the six verbal subtests and in four of the five performance subtests. None of the three IQ measures or the 11 subtests showed a reliable decline. An important feature of this study is the large sample size, which virtually guarantees avoidance of a type II error wherein a true difference is not detected. We can conclude from these results that, far from causing decline of general intellectual function, ECT improves scores during the time period studied. This finding is a powerful reminder that we should never underestimate the capacity of major mental illness to cause cognitive deficits. These deficits from illness may remit as a result of effective treatment despite the supposed iatrogenic side effects of the treatment. In other words, pathogenic cognitive deficits, particularly from melancholic major depression, may dwarf any adverse effects of ECT. In a study of 38 depressed patients treated with unilateral ECT, McKenna and Pratt (1983) showed reliable *improvement* in the Digit Symbol subtest (a measure of information processing speed) of the WAIS (Wechsler, 1955).

Lawson et al. (1990) studied a total of 59 patients suffering from major depression treated with bitemporal, right unilateral, or a novel bifrontal placement proposed by Inglis (1969, 1970). The brief-pulse stimulus dose was barely suprathreshold. In a novel analysis, they regarded the study patients before treatment as unable to follow testing instructions properly; the mean Hamilton Rating Scale for Depression score was 30. Pretreatment scores were constructed for general intelligence (WAIS-R) on the basis of demographic characteristics, using known correlations. These were compared with the observed scores after six ECT treatments, at seven days and at three months after the ECT course. After ECT treatment 6, the average verbal IQ of the bitemporal patients was 10 points less than expectancy, but those of the right unilateral and bifrontal groups were not reliably depressed. In contrast, performance IQ was less than expectancy in all three placement groups: 15 points for bitemporal, 15 points for right unilateral, and 10 points for bifrontal. At seven days posttreatment, only the bitemporal group continued to have a significantly low verbal IQ. The deficits were nine, three, and three points for bitemporal, right unilateral, and bifrontal, respectively. The performance IQ at seven days post- ECT, however, remained significantly less than expectancy (17, 11, and 9 points, respectively). At three months posttreatment, only the bitemporal group remained deficient in verbal IQ (6, 1, and 1 points, respectively). At this point also, only the bitemporal group showed significant depression of performance IQ (10, 4, and 2, respectively).

Sackeim et al. (1992) reported a study of WAIS-R verbal and performance IQ in 100 patients suffering from major depressive disorder (MDD). Before treatment, the mean verbal IQ proved comparable with that of matched healthy controls, but the mean performance IQ was significantly lower than that of the controls. Similar results from a patient subsample given the WAIS-R with unlimited time conditions implied that this result was probably not attributable to mental and motor retardation, as occurs in MDD. Subgroups of the ECT-treated patients were retested on the WAIS-R one or two weeks after treatment. Scores were generally improved, but the verbal/performance discrepancy persisted. The authors concluded that selective depression of performance IQ is a feature of MDD regardless of its current severity and cannot be attributed to ECT. In contrast, a study of the cognitive effects of right unilateral ECT at 2.5 times threshold (Ng et al., 2000) showed no reliable change in two verbal and two performance subtests of the WAIS-R from baseline to after ECT treatment 6, the end point of treatment, and at one-month follow-up. A persistent verbal/performance discrepancy similar to that found in the Sackeim et al. (1992) study is apparent from inspection of the reported subtest mean scores. Comparing maintenance ECT with pharmacotherapy after a full course of ECT, Vothknecht et al. (2003) found no difference in general intelligence or the WAIS Digit Symbol subtest after six months of maintenance. Although the sample sizes were small, the numbers indicate a substantive disconfirmation of the hypothesis of difference between the two groups in general intelligence.

The consensus of these studies is that there is little evidence to support the view that ECT produces any lasting deficits in general intellectual functions, particularly if due allowance is made for the cognitive deficits associated with MDD in the absence of ECT. Only one study (Lawson et al., 1990) provided any evidence of persistent deficit in performance IQ at three months post-ECT. It was specific to bitemporal electrode placement, and did not occur with either right unilateral or bifrontal placement.

Memory and new learning

Subjective memory complaints

This refers to patient complaints, spontaneously expressed or solicited after ECT. It is important to bear in mind that this differs from – and shows little correlation with – objectively assessed memory impairment. Patients' complaints of difficulty with memory are a primary source of information about adverse effects of ECT. Early investigators were aware that subjective memory complaints might be influenced by the changed clinical state of the patient. For example, Cronholm and Ottosson (1963) evaluated 35 patients suffering from "endogenous" depression (probably MDD with melancholic features) treated with three or four brief-pulse treatments at either "liminal" (near-threshold) or "supraliminal" levels. All results were combined in the analysis. Before- and after-treatment subjective and objective measures of memory function were obtained. Multiple regression analysis showed that subjective complaints were influenced *independently* by the objective measures of dysmnesia (the greater the objective deficits, the greater the complaints) and by the response to treatment (the better the response, the fewer the complaints). This neatly illustrated the independent role of clinical state (incomplete remission) in prompting complaints about memory. However, Squire and Chace (1975) found no relationship between clinical response to treatment and subjective estimates of memory function. For the 38 patients receiving bitemporal, unilateral, or no ECT, the rates of subjective complaints of impairment were 63%, 30%, and 17%, respectively. These results were about what we would expect if the complaints were founded in fact and patient expectancies played no role.

The 70 years since the inception of ECT have seen major advances in the technique of ECT treatment aimed at minimizing cognitive side effects without compromising therapeutic efficacy. These advances include the introduction of non-dominant unilateral, bifrontal, and other more novel electrode placements (e.g., left anterior right temporal [LART], see Chapter 27), the development of brief pulse and more recently, ultrabrief-pulse stimulation, to replace sine wave ECT (see Chapter 1). These methods have undoubtedly mitigated the worst memory effects of the older treatment methods. Cholinesterase inhibitors, which are used to treat memory dysfunction in dementia, show promise as adjuvant treatment for ECT-induced dysmnesia (Prakash et al., 2006). These advances have diminished the degree of actual memory side effects and they have possibly moderated the patients' subjective perception of memory problems. Coleman et al. (1996) used the Squire Subjective Memory Questionnaire (SSMQ; Squire et al., 1979) in depressed patients treated with either bitemporal or right unilateral placement at either low (threshold) or high (2.5 times threshold) dose. They found high correlations between SSMQ scores and depression levels at baseline. That is, more severely depressed patients rated their memory worse than did more moderately depressed patients before ECT was started. Immediately following the course of ECT, patients' assessments of memory improved dramatically, more so in responders than in nonresponders. Patients' SSMQ scores continued to improve through two months of follow-up, finally approaching the scores of the healthy control group. There was no association between SSMQ scores and objective memory test scores in the immediate post-ECT period. Still, after two months, objective testing for retrograde memory concerning autobiographical information was associated with self-rated greater memory impairment. When clinical improvement was statistically controlled there was evidence that high stimulus dose and bitemporal placement resulted in less improvement in self-ratings. The authors interpret differences between the results of their study and those of earlier researchers as attributable to "fundamental changes in ECT practice" involving more efficient electrical waveforms and electrode placement.

In a review of subjective memory complaints in ECT, Prudic et al. (2000) reported that, with modern treatment parameters, subjective memory improves with ECT. They found no clear evidence of an association between subjective and objectively measured memory but substantial evidence of a negative association between subjective memory complaints and mood state. They do concede that there may be aspects of memory impairment not measured by standard psychometric instruments. They note a lack of information about the number and characteristics of the patients who complain of severe memory impairment after ECT.

Retrograde amnesia

Retrograde amnesia refers to an inability to access memories already stored before the course of ECT begins. It does not mean an impairment in the ability to learn. Its presence can be a source of distress in some patients. Typically the loss is not permanent, and the period of amnesia shrinks with earlier memories returning first and those stored immediately before ECT recovering last, if at all. The issue of retrograde amnesia has already been touched on under the section heading of postictal disorientation and confusion.

In a major study of the effects of ECT on retrograde amnesia, Lisanby et al. (2000) examined differences between personal and public information in relation to electrode placement (bitemporal or right unilateral) and stimulus dose (barely suprathreshold or 2.5 times threshold). A matched healthy control group followed a test protocol that mimicked that of the patients. The results showed that retrograde amnesia for both personal and public (impersonal) information occurred for patients in the week after ECT. Compared with that of controls, the amount of retrograde amnesia in patients was much more marked for public information. The different results between personal and impersonal information may have been caused by better consolidation of personal information – that is, more robust encoding of memories in the brain. At two months after ECT, patients' retrograde amnesia had diminished but the recall of impersonal events remained reliably poorer than that of the controls. The more recent the event, the more likely it would not be recalled, following the classic retrograde amnesic pattern. Bitemporal ECT produced more profound retrograde amnesia than did right unilateral ECT, but there was no effect of electrical dose.

In a systematic review of the effects of ECT on autobiographical memory, Fraser et al. (2008) aimed at addressing inconsistencies in the literature about the extent and persistence of effects. They concluded that there was indeed compelling evidence of retrograde amnesia for autobiographical information after ECT, but the objectively measurable loss was brief (less than six months). Subjective complaints tended to last more than six months. More recent events were the worst affected, as is usual with retrograde amnesia. Memory loss was less for brief-pulse stimulation than for sinusoidal waveform, for unilateral electrode placement than for bitemporal, and for careful titration of the dose in relation to each patient's seizure threshold.

Sackeim et al. (2008) reported on a comparison of depressed patients treated with either brief (1.5-ms pulse width) or ultrabrief (0.3 ms) pulse in right unilateral electrode placement at 6 times threshold or bitemporal placement at 2.5 times threshold. Patients treated with ultrabrief-pulse width showed markedly less anterograde amnesia in the acute term immediately after each ECT. There were, however, no reliable differences in retrograde memory between electrode placements in the acute phase. In the short term (at the end of treatment) there were both pulse width (ultrabrief superior) and electrode placement (right unilateral superior) main effects but no interaction of pulse width and electrode placement (i.e., the effects of each variable were the same for all levels of the other variables). At two and six months of follow-up, the results in the two ultrabrief groups were superior to those in the two brief-pulse groups. At six months posttreatment, only the two ultrabrief-pulse groups had reverted to pretreatment levels in terms of retrograde amnesia. However, the stimulus used with bitemporal placement was twice the customary and desirable clinical dose, so comparisons made to it may have no practical clinical implications.

Anterograde amnesia

Anterograde amnesia refers to difficulty in recalling information presented after a course of ECT either because it has not been stored, or access to the memory trace (the physical storage in the brain) is not available. Unlike retrograde amnesia, anterograde amnesia may constitute a failure to learn, associated with a lack of any physical memory (trace). As in retrograde amnesia, anterograde loss can cause distress in some patients. Calev et al. (1989) reported a study in which anterograde memory function was assessed with a battery of verbal and nonverbal tests before and after seven ECT treatments in 16 unmedicated patients, and in 10 patients before and after 21 days of imipramine at 200 mg per day. Both groups showed comparable deficits in a verbal paired associate test but no deficit in immediate memory (digit span). This study is of particular interest as it shows that memory deficit, at least in the anterograde zone, is no worse with ECT than with antidepressant pharmacotherapy.

Lawson et al. (1990) compared bitemporally, right unilaterally, and bifrontally treated patients after ECT treatment 6, at one week after ECT and at three months after ECT with the Wechsler Memory Scale-Revised Logical Memory (verbal) and Visual Memory (nonverbal) subtests. The results of patients treated right unilaterally and bifrontally were superior to those treated bitemporally after ECT treatment 6 and seven days after ECT, but there was no difference between the groups three months after ECT. Thus the differential effects of ECT electrode placement on anterograde memory had disappeared after three months. Vakil et al. (2000) tested a group of right unilateral ECT-treated depressed patients before treatment and after ECT treatments 1 and 8 with tests of explicit (visual paired associates) and implicit (learning a skill) tests. The patients showed a persistent deficit in the explicit paired associate task, as has been shown in many studies, but there was no deficit in the implicit task.

Sackeim et al. (2008) reported the effects of pulse width and electrode placement on anterograde memory. These results were similar to those for retrograde memory, a substantial beneficial effect of ultrabrief-pulse width and a less robust electrode placement effect.

Executive functions

Executive functions comprise a loosely defined group of abilities that are important for the planning and control of sequences of behaviors to ensure that complex goals are achieved. Executive functions are important in the strategic deployment of well-learned skills in a possibly novel context to achieve desired results (Shallice, 1990). Hebb and Penfield (1940) showed that skills in planning, monitoring behavior, and correcting course could be severely damaged whereas general intellectual functions are preserved. This means that general intelligence tests sometimes give normal results when executive functions are markedly impaired. These authors also considered the frontal lobes to play a vital part in the execution of such "command and control" functions.

Few studies have addressed specifically the issue of the effect of ECT on executive functions. Many studies using comprehensive neuropsychological test batteries have included tests of some aspects of executive function as part of a standard battery. For example Goldstein et al. (1977) included two tests of executive function from the Halstead-Reitan Neuropsychological Test Battery (Reitan and Wolfson, 1985) in a study of the cognitive effects of sinusoidal and brief-pulse ECT. The tests were the Categories Test and the Trail Making Test; these tests evaluate concept formation and visuomotor planning, respectively. No differences between the two methods of treatment on those aspects of executive function were found. Lawson et al. (1990) included the Trail Making Test, suspecting that the bifrontal placement might adversely affect executive function. In fact the bifrontal patients performed better on this test than the bitemporal and right unilateral patients. However, testing executive function demands a comprehensive battery of tests, and the Trail Making Test is not sufficient by itself to establish preservation of executive function. No comprehensive evaluation of executive function in bifrontal ECT has yet been done.

Rami-Gonzalez et al. (2003) describe a study of 11 depressed patients treated with maintenance ECT compared with matched patients on pharmacological treatment. The "frontal" tests comprised Trail Making, letter fluency, digit span, Coding, and the Tower of Hanoi. Although ECT patients generally performed more poorly than controls, there was no significant correlation between any of the cognitive measures, including the frontal lobe tests, and the total number of ECT treatments administered. Therefore, there was no clear effect by ECT itself. In a study of cortisol levels as a predictor of ECT-induced cognitive impairment, Neylan et al. (2001) tested 16 right unilateral ECT patients. The results showed that executive functions were adversely affected by ECT, but the effect sizes were comparable to those in other aspects of the neuropsychological picture.

Language function

Despite a comment by d'Elia (1972) that *left* unilateral electrode placement produced signs of aphasia in the immediate postictal period, there have been no subsequent studies of language function in ECT. Particularly, there is no study of challenge object naming, the classic test for nominal aphasia. This gap in the literature may testify to the immunity of this aspect of cognition to the effects of ECT given with conventional electrode placements. It is obvious that patients treated with ECT do not show evidence of aphasia, and the use of clinical data is the logical starting point for investigation of the side effects of any treatment.

Editor's note

For complementary yet somewhat different approaches to the cognitive side effects of ECT please see Chapters 1, 23, 25, 27, 28, and 34. Cognitive effects are the primary adverse effect and risk of ECT. Under the magnification of scrutiny, the nature, extent, and persistence of these effects must always be compared to those of the untreated illness, medications, the consequences of treatment delay, and concurrent medical conditions. It is also notable that generalized seizure has temporary cognitive effects, even when not induced electrically.

In monitoring cognitive function along a course of ECT for clinical purposes, patients should be allowed at least three hours to recover from the anesthesia before testing. If they received a sympatholytic or sedating drug, a longer recovery is desirable. Patients vary widely in how quickly cognitive effects fade after a course of ECT. Although many patients seem intact immediately after ECT, a few geriatric patients do not fully recover for 30 days.

Subjective memory complaints can represent symptoms of dissatisfaction from an undertreated anxiety or personality disorder. Dissatisfaction is a core symptom of anxiety, and patients commonly attribute it to circumstances in their lives rather than to an anxiety state. Anxiety disorders are commonly comorbid with mood disorders, especially with patients long ill. Undertreated anxiety symptoms can seem to decrease the effectiveness of ECT and increase its cognitive side effects. Studies of ECT-related side effects have generally not accounted for effects from anxiety or personality disorders.

It is reasonable to expect that advances in clinical ECT methods will further reduce cognitive effects while preserving efficacy. The present chapter identifies the range and types of cognitive effects to examine when testing new clinical methods. –CMS

References

Butler, S. M., Ashford, J. W., and Snowdon, D. A. 1996. Age, education and changes in the Mini-Mental State Exam scores of older women: Findings from the Nun Study. J Am Geriatr Soc 44: 675–81.

Calev, A., Ben-Tzvi, E., Schapira, B., et al. 1989. Distinct memory impairments following electroconvulsive therapy and imipramine. Psychol Med 19: 111–19.

Calev, A., Cohen, R., Tubi, N., et al. 1991. Disorientation and bilateral moderately suprathreshold titrated ECT. Convuls Ther 7: 99–110.

Calev, A., Gaudino, E. A., Aquires, N. K., et al. 1995. ECT and non-memory cognition: A review. Br J Clin Psychol 34: 505–15.

Chatfield, M., Matthews, F. E., and Brayne, C. 2007. Medical Research Council Cognitive Function and Ageing Study. J Am Geriatr Soc 55: 1066–71.

Coleman, E. A., Sackeim, H. A., Prudic, J., et al. 1996. Subjective memory complaints prior to and following electroconvulsive therapy. Biol Psychiatry 39: 346–56.

Cronholm, B. and Ottosson, J. 1963. The experience of memory function after electroconvulsive therapy. Br J Psychiatry 109: 251–8.

Crum, R. M., Anthony, J. C., Basssett, S. S., Folstein, M. F. 1993. Population-based norms for the Mini-Mental State Examination by age and education level. JAMA 269: 2386–91.

Daniel, W. F. and Crovitz, H. F. 1982. Recovery of orientation after electroconvulsive therapy. Acta Psychiatr Scand 66: 421–8.

Daniel, W. F. and Crovitz, H. F. 1983a. Acute memory impairment following electroconvulsive therapy: I. Effects of electrical stimulus, waveform and number of treatments. Acta Psychiatr Scand 67: 1–7.

Daniel, W. F. and Crovitz, H. F. 1983b. Acute memory impairment following electroconvulsive therapy: II. Effects of electrode placement. Acta Psychiatr Scand 67: 57–68.

Daniel, W. F., Crovitz, H. F., and Weiner, R. D. 1987. Neuropsychological aspects of disorientation. Cortex 23: 169–87.

d'Elia, G. 1972. Memory studies in electroconvulsive therapy with different electrode placements. Brain Res 37: 364.

Dufouil, C., Clayton, D., Brayne, C., et al. 2000. Population norms for the MMSE in the very old: Estimates based on longitudinal data. Neurology 55: 1609–13.

Folstein, M. F., Folstein, S. E., and McHugh, P. R. 1975. "Mini-Mental State": A practical method of grading the cognitive state of patients for the clinician. J Psychiatr Res 12: 189–98.

Fraser, L. M., O'Carroll, R. E., and Ebmeier, K. P. 2008. The effect of electroconvulsive therapy on autobiographical memory: A systematic review. J ECT. 24: 10–17.

Goldstein, S. G., Filskov, S. B., Weaver, L. A., and Ives, J. O. 1977. Neuropsychological effects of electroconvulsive therapy. J Clin Psychol 33: 798–806.

Hebb, D. O. and Penfield, W. 1940. Human behaviour after extensive removal from the frontal lobes. Arch Neurol Psychiatry 44: 421–38.

Huppert, F. A., Cabelli, S. T. and Matthews, F. E. 2005. MRC Cognitive Function and Ageing Study. BMC Geriatr 5: 7.

Inglis, J. 1969. Electrode placement and the effect of ECT on mood and memory in depression. Can Psychiatr Assoc J 14: 463–71.

Inglis, J. 1970. Shock, surgery and cerebral asymmetry. Br J Psychiatry 117: 143–8.

Lawson, J. S., Inglis, J., Delva, N. J., et al. 1990. Electrode placement in ECT: Cognitive effects. Psychol Med 20: 335–44.

Levy, N. A., Serota, H. M., and Grinker, R. R. 1942. Disturbances in brain function following convulsive shock therapy. Arch Neurol Psychiatry 47: 1009–29.

Lisanby, S. H., Maddox, J. H., Prudic, J., et al. 2000. The effects of electroconvulsive therapy on memory of autobiographical and public events. Arch Gen Psychiatry 57: 581–90.

Malloy, F. W., Small, I. F., Miller, M. J., et al. 1982. Changes in neuropsychological test performance after electroconvulsive therapy. Biol Psychiatry 17: 61–7.

McKenna, P. and Pratt, R. T. C. 1983. The effects of unilateral non-dominant ECT on memory and perceptual functions. Br J Psychiatry 142: 276–9.

Neylan, T. C., Canick, J. D., Hall, S. E., et al. 2001. Cortisol levels predict cognitive impairment induced by electroconvulsive therapy. Biol Psychiatry 50: 331–6.

Ng, C., Schweitzer, I., Alexopoulos, P., et al. 2000. Efficacy and cognitive effects of right unilateral electroconvulsive therapy. J ECT. 16: 370–9.

Nunnally, J. C. and Bernstein, I. H. 1994. Psychometric theory, 3rd edn. New York: McGraw-Hill.

Prakash, J., Kotwal, A., Prabhu, H. R. A. 2006. Therapeutic and prophylactic utility of the memory-enhancing drug donepezil hydrochloride on cognition of patients undergoing electroconvulsive therapy: A randomized controlled trial. J ECT 22(3): 163–8.

Prudic, J., Peyser, S., Sackeim, H. A. 2000. Subjective memory complaints: A review of patient self-assessment of memory after electroconvulsive therapy. J ECT 16: 121–32.

Rami-Gonzalez, L., Salamero, M., Boget, T., et al. 2003. Pattern of cognitive dysfunction in depressive patients during maintenance electroconvulsive therapy. Psychol Med 33: 345–50.

Reitan, R. M. and Wolfson, D. 1985. The Halstein-Reitan neuropsychological test battery: Theory and clinical interpretation. Tucson, AZ: Neuropsychology Press.

Ribot, T. 1882. Diseases of memory: An essay in positive psychology. New York: D. Appleton and Co.

Sackeim, H. A., Freeman, J., McElhiney, M., et al. 1992. Effects of major depression on intelligence. J Clin Exp Neuropsychol 14: 268–8.

Sackeim, H. A., Prudic, J., Fuller, R., et al. 2007. Neuropsychopharmacology 32: 244–54.

Sackeim, H. A., Prudic, J., Nobler, M. S., et al. 2008. Effects of pulse width and electrode placement on the efficacy and cognitive effects of electroconvulsive therapy. Brain Stimulation 1: 71–83.

Shallice, T. 1990. From neuropsychology to mental structure. New York: Cambridge University Press.

Spearman, C. 1904. "General intelligence" objectively determined and measured. Am J Psychol 15: 201–93.

Squire, L. R. and Chace, P. M. 1975. Memory functions six to nine months after electroconvulsive therapy. Arch Gen Psychiatry 32: 1557–64.

Squire, L. R., Wetzel, C. D., and Slater, P. C. 1979. Memory complaint after electroconvulsive therapy: Assessment with a new self-rating instrument. Biol Psychiatry 14: 791–801.

Tombaugh, T. N. and McIntyre, N. J. 1992. The Mini-Mental State Examination: A comprehensive review. J Am Geriatr Soc 40: 922–35.

Vakil, E., Grunhaus, L., Nagar, I., et al. 2000. The effect of electroconvulsive therapy (ECT) on implicit memory: Skill learning and perceptual priming in patients with major depression. Neuropsychologia 38: 1405–14.

Valentine, M., Keddie, K. M. G., and Dunne, D. 1968. A comparison of techniques in electroconvulsive therapy. Br J Psychiatry 114: 989–96.

Vothknecht, S., Kho, K. H., van Schaick, H. W., et al. 2003. Effects of maintenance electroconvulsive therapy on cognitive functions. J ECT 19: 151–7.

Wechsler, D. 1955. Wechsler Adult Intelligence Scale. New York: The Psychological Corporation.

32

Electroconvulsive therapy in children and adolescents

Garry Walter, Colleen Loo, and Joseph M. Rey

Rates of use

Electroconvulsive therapy (ECT) is an uncommon treatment in adolescents and is rarely used in children. For example, it was estimated that approximately 500 of 33,384 (1.5%) patients who received ECT in the United States in 1980 were in the 11- to 20-year age range (Thompson and Blaine, 1987). On average, eight patients younger than 18 years received ECT each year in California from 1977 through 1983, 0.3% of all persons treated with ECT during those seven years (Kramer, 1985). The rate decreased to four per year between 1984 and 1994. In the period 1990 through 1999 in the Australian state of New South Wales, 72 adolescents aged 14 to 18 years received 826 ECT treatments in 84 courses (Walter and Rey, 2003a). The mean number of courses per year was 8.9, equivalent to 1.53/100,000 adolescents being treated with ECT per year. Adolescents received 0.89% of all ECT treatments. Between 1982 and 1992, the ECT Clinic at Royal Edinburgh Hospital in Edinburgh, Scotland – the only facility in Edinburgh where young people can be treated with ECT – treated an average of one patient younger than 18 years every two years (Scott et al., 2005). Between 1993 and 1998, the annual rate of ECT use among young people in Edinburgh was calculated to be 0.5 young patients per 100,000 total population, or 2.5 patients per 100,000 young people. No patient younger than 18 years was treated at the clinic in the period 1999 through 2004.

These findings are consistent with the results of practice surveys (e.g., Walter and Rey, 2003b), in which psychiatrists report low rates of ECT use in young people. It is also worth noting that some hospitals and governments set lower age limits for ECT.

ECT is rarely used in prepubertal children, but case reports of ECT in this age group sporadically appear. For example, in recent years, Russell et al. (2002) described a nine-year-old girl who was successfully treated with ECT for severe depression and catatonic features, and Esmaili and Malek (2007) described a six-year-old girl with similar clinical features and outcome. Notwithstanding the isolated use of ECT in young children, the remainder of this chapter will focus on ECT in adolescents.

Assessing adolescent patients for ECT

A competent assessment of adolescents for ECT ought to address three areas: (a) the need for treatment with ECT, (b) the patient's fitness to undergo the treatment, and (c) baseline evaluations that will assist appraisal of response and potential side effects.

Need for treatment with ECT

It should be noted that in some countries and jurisdictions there are legal requirements that evaluation of adolescents for ECT be conducted not only by the treating physician but also by an independent child psychiatrist not involved in the patient's care and preferably experienced in the therapy. To ascertain if an adolescent may benefit from ECT, it is necessary to conduct a comprehensive psychiatric history and examination (including interviews with the family and other relevant informants), and make a diagnosis to establish that he or she suffers from a disorder that may benefit from ECT, that previous treatments have not been effective, and that symptoms are of sufficient severity. According to the American Academy of Child and Adolescent Psychiatry (2004), patients should meet three criteria to be eligible for treatment with ECT. First, they should have major depression, mania, schizoaffective disorder, catatonia, schizophrenia, or neuroleptic malignant syndrome (Rey and Walter, 1997). Second, symptoms ought to be serious and disabling enough to threaten the patient's life (e.g., refusal to eat or drink, high and unrelenting suicide risk) or to cause persistent and grave disability. Third, the illness should be resistant to treatment or patients must be unable to tolerate medication because of serious side effects. It is necessary to ascertain not only that symptoms have not responded, but also that earlier therapies have been adequately given (i.e., with a drug shown to be effective for treating the illness, at a suitable dose, and for a satisfactory duration) and that patients have complied with these treatments; nonadherence to pharmacotherapy leading to nonresponse is often a problem in adolescents. The United Kingdom's National Institute for Health and Clinical Excellence (NICE) (2005) has similar but slightly narrower recommendations (e.g., ECT should only be used in specialist settings and not in children younger than 11 years). Comorbidity with personality problems, other psychiatric conditions (e.g., mental retardation, personality disorder), or drug and alcohol problems ought to be examined but is no contraindication, although response to ECT in patients with comorbid illnesses might not be as consistent as in those without co-occurring conditions (Walter and

Rey, 2003a); the presence of comorbidity needs to be kept in mind when estimating prognosis.

Patient's fitness to undergo ECT

The main risks of ECT are those associated with general anesthesia. Thus, evaluation of patients' fitness for ECT would require an assessment of their physical health status and whether they would tolerate a very short anesthesia, which should be assessed by the anesthetist. It is of note that, at least in adults, there are no absolute contraindications for ECT, which has been administered safely to frail elderly patients with cardiovascular problems and patients with craniotomy or brain tumors. Data for adolescents are limited, but there will be few contraindications as well. For example, Ghaziuddin et al. (1999) described a successful outcome in an adolescent female who had a complicated neurological history. The patient had undergone craniotomy for a brainstem astrocytoma and suffered extensive postsurgical neurological deficits. Despite her complicated neurological presentation, she achieved remission with eight treatments. Yet, to be fully aware of all potential risks and take preventive measures if necessary, a complete medical history and physical examination are necessary. Further investigations, such as blood tests, electroencephalogram, and radiological investigations, will be dictated by the findings of the history and physical examination.

It is important to elicit information about all medications that patients are taking at the time – prescribed, over the counter, and herbal drugs – as well as substances of abuse. Psychoactive substances can influence the ECT-induced seizure (e.g., benzodiazepines), or interact with the action or metabolism of drugs used in anesthesia.

Further baseline evaluations

Assessment also aims to establish a baseline to help appraise the outcome of ECT and to detect treatment-emergent side effects. This assessment usually entails completing rating scales to quantify the relevant symptoms (e.g., depression rating scales) by the clinician, nursing or other mental health staff, patient, and family, as relevant.

A proactive approach to detecting side effects starts with a systematic assessment of symptoms at baseline. Otherwise, it is impossible to determine if the symptom described is new, substantially different, slightly different, or essentially the same as before ECT. Open-ended questions alone are unlikely to provide reliable information (Kutcher et al., 2009). One useful instrument is the Mental Health Therapeutic Outcomes Tool (Kutcher et al., 2009), which includes a treatment-emergent adverse events detection scale and has the added advantage of including treatment outcome items, thus measuring both therapeutic outcomes and adverse effects with a single instrument.

Unless the patient is too ill or disorganized, baseline neuropsychological assessment should be performed. The minimum standard recommended by the American Academy of Child and Adolescent Psychiatry (2004) is a memory assessment, but a more comprehensive battery may be undertaken (Walter et al., 1999).

ECT technique

There have been no randomized controlled trials testing the relative benefits of different approaches to ECT treatment (electrode placement, dose, frequency of treatments, etc.) in adolescents specifically. Thus the recommendations here are drawn from extrapolation of adult data, reports in the available literature, and impressions from clinical experience.

General approach

In the absence of evidence to the contrary, it is recommended that ECT follow the recommendations for treatment in adults (Abrams, 2002; American Psychiatric Association, 2001). Thus, treatment should commence with nondominant electrode placement, switching to bilateral treatment if response is poor, unless there are reasons to begin with bilateral ECT (e.g., patient is catatonic). Similarly, treatment should be given two to three times per week, the lesser frequency being desirable if significant cognitive side effects occur (Lerer et al., 1995; McAllister et al., 1987).

Special considerations

Seizure threshold

Although controlled comparisons with the adult age group are not available, there are reasons to believe that seizure thresholds may be lower in children and adolescents. Age has been found to be a predictor of seizure threshold in adults; in other words, threshold increases with increasing age (e.g., Colenda and McCall, 1996; Weiner, 1980), and this relationship was also found in a sample 13 to 65 years old (Gangadhar et al., 1998). Many reports of ECT in persons younger than 18 years failed to measure or report seizure thresholds. In 20 adolescents 14 to 19 years old in whom seizure threshold was empirically determined, mean thresholds (female, 104 mC; male, 139 mC) were reported to be lower than those typically found in adults in the same ECT service, in other words, when comparable anesthetic and ECT techniques were used (Cohen et al., 1997).

Stimulus dose

There is little room for variation in the initial stimulus dose with adolescents and children. The half-age stimulus dosing method would prescribe 25 mC at 900 mA for all patients through age 15. Dosing methods based on seizure threshold have not been tested in this age group, but seizure threshold measurement would also start with 25 mC at 900 mA. Accordingly, it is reasonable and maximally conservative to initiate treatment with 25 mC charge at 900 mA current or with 35 mC at 800 mA, for any electrode placement.

Adverse events

Overall, adverse events with ECT in young people appear similar in type and frequency to those described in adults, and are generally minor and transient. However, reports on ECT use in young persons have seldom scrutinized them systematically or have not commented about them at all (Rey and Walter, 1997). In a whole population study of ECT in young persons (Walter and Rey, 2003a), adverse events included headache (61% courses), confusion (20%), subjective memory problems (19%), nausea or vomiting (15%), muscle aches (11%), and manic switch (4%). Kutcher and Robertson (1995) reported side effects following 28% of ECTs in their sample: headache, 15%; confusion, 5%; agitation, 3%; hypomanic symptoms, 2%; subjective memory loss, 2%; and vomiting, 1%.

Two areas that have attracted particular interest in young people pertain to (a) seizures, and (b) the influence of ECT on cognitive functioning.

Prolonged (treatment) seizures and tardive (posttreatment) seizures are risks associated with ECT. There is debate about whether the rate of prolonged seizures in children and adolescents is greater than in adults. The lack of uniform definition of prolonged seizures has complicated this matter. In their group of 16 patients, Kutcher and Robertson (1995) did not observe any prolonged seizures (defined as longer than 180 seconds). In the series described by Walter and Rey (2003b), prolonged seizures (longer than 180 seconds) occurred in 3 (0.4%) of the 826 treatments. Ghaziuddin et al. (1996) noted prolonged seizures, which they defined as longer than 150 seconds, in 7 of their 11 patients (9.6% of a total of 135 treatments). Prolonged seizures are important to identify because of their association with greater postictal confusion and amnesia, and hypoxia-related risks (cerebral and cardiovascular complications) (American Academy of Child and Adolescent Psychiatry, 2004).

Tardive seizures are thankfully rare. Schneekloth et al. (1993) observed a tardive seizure in 1 of 20 young patients, and Ghaziuddin et al. (1996) noted a tardive seizure in 1 of their 11 patients.

Two studies have examined cognitive effects of ECT in adolescents. The first (Cohen et al., 2000) measured cognitive status among 10 adolescents, who had received the treatment for severe mood disorders, on average 3.5 years after completion of ECT, and 10 psychiatric controls who had never had ECT. There were no significant group differences on tests of short-term memory, attention, new learning, and objective memory scores. The second study (Ghaziuddin et al., 2001) examined cognitive status among 16 adolescents prior to their ECT treatment, and at 7.0 ± 10.3 days and 8.5 ± 4.9 months posttreatment. There was significant impairment of attention and concentration, verbal and visual delayed recall, and verbal fluency at the first posttreatment session compared with baseline, but by the second posttreatment assessment there was complete return to pre-ECT functioning.

It follows from the above discussion that it is important to accurately record seizure length with ECT, to monitor for side effects systematically, and to measure cognitive function. Psychometric assessment should be performed at baseline, as noted, and also repeated on completion of the ECT course, and three to six months later.

Editor's note

Because children and adolescents should generally have a particularly low threshold to seizure induction and exhibit long convulsions, propofol might be a desirable anesthetic agent for these patients, at least during the first three or four sessions. Conversely, propofol is at a disadvantage with elderly patients. –CMS

References

Abrams, R. 2002. Electroconvulsive therapy, 4th edn. Oxford, UK: Oxford University Press.

American Academy of Child and Adolescent Psychiatry. 2004. Practice parameter for use of electroconvulsive therapy with adolescents. J Am Acad Child Adolesc Psychiatry 43: 1521–39.

American Psychiatric Association (APA). 2001. The practice of electroconvulsive therapy: Recommendations for treatment, training and privileging: A task force report of the American Psychiatric Association, 2nd edn. Washington, DC: American Psychiatric Association.

Cohen, D., Paillere-Martinot M.-L., and Basquin, M. 1997. Use of electroconvulsive therapy in adolescents. Convuls Ther 13: 25–31.

Cohen, D., Taieb, O., Flament, M., et al. 2000. Absence of cognitive impairment at long term follow-up in adolescents treated with ECT for severe mood disorders. Am J Psychiatry 157: 460–2.

Colenda, C. C. and McCall, W. V. 1996. A statistical model predicting the seizure threshold for right unilateral ECT in 106 patients. Convuls Ther 12: 3–12.

Esmaili, T. and Malek, A. 2007. Electroconvulsive therapy in a six-year-old girl suffering from major depressive disorder with catatonic features. Eur J Psychiatry 16: 58–60.

Gangadhar, B. N., Girish, K., Janakiramiah, N., et al. 1998. Formula method for stimulus setting in bilateral electroconvulsive therapy: Relevance of age. J ECT 14: 259–65.

Ghaziuddin, N., DeQuardo, J. R., Ghaziuddin, M., et al. 1999. Electroconvulsive treatment in an adolescent treated with craniotomy. J Child Adolesc Psychopharmacol 9: 63–9.

Ghaziuddin, N., King, C. A., Naylor, M. W., et al. 1996. Electroconvulsive treatment in adolescents with pharmacotherapy refractory depression. J Child Adolesc Psychopharmacol 6: 259–71.

Ghaziuddin, N., Laughrin, D., and Giordani, B. 2001. Cognitive side effects of electroconvulsive therapy in adolescents. J Child Adolesc Psychopharmacol 10: 269–76.

Kramer, B. A. 1985. Use of ECT in California, 1977–1983. Am J Psychiatry 142: 1190–2.

Kutcher, S., McDougall, A., and Murphy, A. 2009. Preventing, detecting and managing side effects of medications. In Treating depression in children and adolescents (eds. Rey, J. M. and Birmaher, B.). Baltimore MD: Lippincott Williams & Wilkins, pp. 190–3.

Kutcher, S. and Robertson, H. A. 1995. Electroconvulsive therapy in treatment resistant bipolar youth. J Child Adolesc Psychopharmacol 5: 167–75.

Lerer, B., Shapira, B., Calev, A., et al. 1995. Antidepressant and cognitive effects of twice-versus three-times-weekly ECT. Am J Psychiatry 152: 564–70.

McAllister, D. A., Perri, M. G., Jordan R. C., et al. 1987. Effects of ECT given two vs. three times weekly. Psychiatry Res 21: 63–9.

National Institute for Health and Clinical Excellence (NICE). 2005. Depression in children and young people: Identification and management in primary, community and secondary care. National Clinical Practice Guideline Number 28. Leicester, UK: The British Psychological Society. 131.

Rey, J. M. and Walter, G. 1997. Half a century of ECT use in young people. Am J Psychiatry 154: 595–602.

Russell, P. S., Tharyan, P., Kumar, A., et al. 2002. Electroconvulsive therapy in a pre-pubertal child with severe depression. J Postgrad Med 48: 290–1.

Schneekloth, T. D., Rummans, T. A., and Logan, K. M. 1993. Electroconvulsive therapy in adolescents. Convuls Ther 9: 159–66.

Scott, A. I. F., Gardner, M., and Good, R. 2005. Fall in ECT use in young people in Edinburgh. J ECT 21: 50.

Thompson, J. W. and Blaine, J. D. 1987. Use of ECT in the United States in 1975 and 1980. Am J Psychiatry 144: 557–62.

Walter, G. and Rey, J. M. 2003a. Has the practice and outcome of ECT in young persons changed? Findings from a whole population study. J ECT 19: 84–7.

Walter, G. and Rey, J. M. 2003b. How fixed are child psychiatrists' views about ECT in the young? J ECT 19: 88–92.

Walter, G., Rey, J. M., and Mitchell, P. 1999. Practitioner review: ECT in adolescents. J Child Psychol Psychiatry 40: 325–34.

Weiner, R. D. 1980. ECT and seizure threshold: Effects of stimulus wave form and electrode placement. Biol Psychiatry 15: 225–41.

33

Postelectroconvulsive therapy evaluation and prophylaxis

T. K. Birkenhäger and Walter W. van den Broek

Introduction

Electroconvulsive therapy (ECT) is one of the few psychiatric treatments that are stopped, often abruptly, after sufficient improvement has been achieved. However, most psychiatric illnesses require continuation treatment after response for months or years. Most research on the topic of prophylaxis after ECT has been performed with depression. This chapter reviews the post-ECT prophylaxis predominantly following ECT for depression. For other disorders, data on prophylactic treatment are presented when available.

Another important topic with treatment termination after ECT is the reevaluation of patients. Depression or other psychiatric conditions for which ECT is indicated may mask underlying psychiatric disorders. Depression can obscure the presence of a personality disorder or axis 1 disorders such as anxiety disorders. Conversely, depression can give the impression that a personality disorder is distinctly present, yet sometimes after successful ECT treatment the inaccuracy of this initial impression becomes obvious. Post-ECT reevaluation is clinically important because proper treatment of underlying or comorbid illness is essential for good outcome.

Continuation treatment after successful ECT

Depression

Patients without medication failure: post-ECT antidepressant

When ECT leads to remission of depression, the ECT course is usually terminated abruptly. Based on studies from the 1960s (Imlah et al., 1965; Kay et al., 1970; Seager and Bird, 1962), patients with unipolar depression often receive continuation treatment with antidepressants. Seager and Bird (1962) carried out a randomized double-blind study in which 43 patients received 150 mg of imipramine or placebo; simultaneously, they were treated with ECT. After patients had responded to combination treatment, the ECT course was stopped and patients received continuation treatment with either imipramine or placebo for six months. The relapse rate was 17% for patients using imipramine versus 69% for patients on placebo (Seager and Bird, 1962). Imlah et al. (1965) performed a randomized double-blind study comparing ECT plus imipramine, ECT plus phenelzine, and ECT plus placebo in a sample of 150 patients. Again, after the ECT course was terminated, patients received continuation treatment for six months with the pharmacologic agent they had taken during the ECT course. The relapse rate was 15% for phenelzine, 20% for imipramine, and 51% for placebo. Kay et al. (1970) conducted a similar double-blind randomized (seven-center) study combining ECT with either amitriptyline at 50 to 150 mg or diazepam at 4 to 12 mg in a sample of 132 patients; 8 patients on amitriptyline versus 21 patients on diazepam relapsed.

Although in these studies relapse rates for patients on antidepressants were substantially lower than those for patients on placebo or diazepam, interpretation of these results is difficult. Not only was ECT the first antidepressant treatment these patients received, they actually received a combination of ECT together with medication. An undetermined proportion presumably responded to the antidepressant drug and may have been less likely to relapse during continuation treatment with the same drug. Hypothetically, some individual patients might respond to antidepressant medication but not to ECT.

Krog-Meyer et al. (1984) performed a double-blind study comparing the effect of 25- to 200-mg amitriptyline with that of placebo in 24 ECT responders. Antidepressant treatment prior to ECT is not mentioned. The relapse was significantly lower in the patients who took amitriptyline (2 of 11) than those who took placebo (9 of 13 patients). Lauritzen et al. (1996) compared the effect of paroxetine with that of imipramine and placebo after successful ECT. Antidepressants were started prior to ECT; patients were randomized to placebo versus paroxetine if there was a contraindication for imipramine. Patients knew the treatment they were assigned to (placebo vs. paroxetine or imipramine vs. paroxetine). At the end of the ECT course, both the Hamilton Rating Scale for Depression (HRSD) and the Melancholia Scale scores were lower in the ECT–imipramine sample. Responders to ECT ($n = 74$) were admitted to the continuation treatment. The relapse rate in the six-month continuation phase was high for placebo (65%) and lower for imipramine (30%), but lowest for paroxetine (10%). In the paroxetine versus imipramine group, more than 50% were treated with a tricyclic antidepressant (TCA) prior to receiving ECT; in the other group, this rate was 16% to 35%. The imipramine dose (mean, 138 mg) was suboptimal in this study, which could account for the difference in relapse rate between paroxetine and imipramine.

Patients without medication failure: post-ECT lithium

In a retrospective chart review of 54 patients, Perry and Tsuang (1979) studied the effect of lithium after ECT versus a TCA after ECT. There was no difference in relapse rates between the two groups: Four of 20 (20%) patients on lithium relapsed versus 7 of 34 (21%) patients on a TCA.

Coppen et al. (1981) reported a double-blind, randomized study comparing lithium with placebo after response to ECT. During the first 15 weeks, the relapse rate was similar for both samples: 5 of 20 (25%) for placebo versus 4 of 18 (22%) for lithium. Only after nine months of continuation treatment did an advantage in favor of lithium emerge: 50% relapse on placebo versus 22% on lithium. After reanalyzing their data, the authors concluded that lithium treatment after successful ECT should be continued for at least one year (Abou-Saleh and Coppen, 1988).

In an open uncontrolled study, Shapira et al. (1995) treated 28 ECT responders with lithium for six months with an average lithium level of 0.65 mmol/L. During the six-month period, 33% of the patients suffered a relapse.

Patients with medication failure: post-ECT antidepressant

Many patients treated with ECT have received prior unsuccessful treatment with antidepressants. Several recent studies examined post-ECT relapse in such patients. Uncontrolled observational studies from the United States found high post-ECT relapse rates. In a sample consisting of patients with psychotic depression exclusively, Spiker et al. (1985) observed a relapse rate of 50% over one year; continuation treatment was given without a protocol.

In a similar patient population, Aronson et al. (1987) reported a relapse rate of 80% during one-year continuation treatment with either a TCA or a monoamine oxidase inhibitor (MAOI). In another observational study, Sackeim et al. (1990) found a considerably higher relapse rate (64%) in medication-resistant patients than in patients who had not received adequate pharmacotherapy prior to ECT (32%). Again, continuation pharmacotherapy was not performed with a protocol.

Sackeim et al. (2001) performed a three-center, double-blind, randomized study comparing 24-week continuation treatment with placebo, nortriptyline, and a nortriptyline–lithium combination. Doses of nortriptyline and lithium were adjusted according to predetermined plasma levels: The adequate plasma level for nortriptyline was 75 to 125 ng/mL and for lithium 0.5 to 0.9 mmol/L. During a six-year period, 84 patients were enrolled in the study. The relapse rates amounted to 84% for placebo, 60% for nortriptyline, and 39% for the nortriptyline–lithium combination. The difference in relapse rate between combination treatment and placebo was statistically significant. The authors concluded that post-ECT relapse is high, that without continuation treatment almost all patients relapse, and that monotherapy with a TCA is not sufficient.

In a randomized, double-blind study conducted in two centers in The Nether-lands, continuation treatment for six months with imipramine was compared with placebo (van den Broek et al., 2006). Included in this study were 27 depressed inpatients with a high degree of medication resistance. Twenty-two of those patients had been treated with a TCA with adequate plasma levels for four weeks, whereas five had received high doses (225 to 300 mg) of fluvoxamine. Furthermore, 24 of the 27 patients had also been treated with lithium in addition to the antidepressant, and the same proportion of patients had received treatment with 60 to 100 mg of a MAOI (tranylcypromine or phenelzine) for five weeks. In the placebo group, 12 of 15 (80%) patients relapsed compared with 2 of 11 (18%) patients on imipramine. This difference in relapse is significant. Analysis of the results when omitting the five patients treated with fluvoxamine showed a similar efficacy of imipramine in preventing relapse.

It is not easy to explain the difference in results between the studies of Sackeim et al. (2001) and van den Broek et al. (2006). In the earlier study, the prophy-lactic efficacy of nortriptyline was disappointing (60% relapse), whereas in the latter study the efficacy of imipramine continuation treatment was very good (18% relapse). Imipramine is an inhibitor of the reuptake of both serotonin and nora-drenaline, whereas nortriptyline inhibits mainly noradrenalin reuptake, but there is no evidence of difference in antidepressant efficacy between these TCAs. The more stringent relapse criteria of Sackeim et al. may explain in part the high relapse rate in their study.

Differences in the administration of ECT may also account for differences in relapse. In the study of van den Broek et al. (2006), a higher proportion of patients was treated with bilateral ECT and none of the patients received benzodiazepines during the ECT course. Moreover, all patients in the Dutch study were ECT naïve, whereas about half of the patients in the Sackeim et al. study had received a prior ECT course. If there is a phenomenon like "ECT resistance," it could account for the higher relapse in the Sackeim et al. study. However, there is no evidence for the existence of ECT resistance; it merely is an unverified hypothesis (Iodice and McCall, 2003).

Conclusions and recommendations regarding continuation pharmacotherapy for depression

Patients who did not receive adequate pharmacotherapy prior to ECT (patients without medication resistance) appear to benefit considerably from continuation pharmacotherapy following a successful ECT course. In these patients, continu-ation treatment with a TCA, using therapeutic drug monitoring, is probably the appropriate choice.

Uncontrolled observational studies show a very high post-ECT relapse among patients with medication resistance in the United States, and a moderately high relapse rate in The Netherlands. These studies do not provide data comparing the specific prophylactic efficacy of TCAs and lithium, respectively. Interestingly, the post-ECT relapse rate appears to be lower among patients with psychotic depression than among those with nonpsychotic depression (Birkenhager et al., 2005).

The efficacy of continuation treatment with a TCA after successful ECT among patients with medication-resistant depression varies between studies. A fairly large, double-blind, randomized study from the United States shows that continuation treatment with a TCA results in limited efficacy, although it is superior to placebo (Sackeim et al., 2001). A relatively small double-blind, randomized study from The Netherlands shows a low relapse rate for patients on imipramine, as compared with those on placebo (van den Broek et al., 2006).

The study by Sackeim et al. (2001) also shows that continuation treatment with a nortriptyline-lithium combination results in a lower relapse rate, as compared with nortriptyline monotherapy. The choice between monotherapy with a TCA and a TCA–lithium combination depends on the weighing of the pros and cons of a smaller chance of relapse and potential serious side effects.

If a patient has achieved a partial response during previous antidepressant treatment, it seems sensible to choose that specific antidepressant for continuation treatment. Sackeim et al. proposed two interesting strategies that may reduce post-ECT relapse. One is tapering ECT over a few weeks instead of the standard abrupt discontinuation of an ECT course. The other is starting continuation treatment with a TCA during the final two weeks of an ECT course, with the aim of attaining a therapeutic plasma level at the end of the ECT course. However, neither strategy has yet been studied.

Continuation ECT for depression

For patients who experience a post-ECT relapse, despite an adequate antidepressant continuation treatment, continuation ECT (cECT) might be helpful.

Until 2006, no randomized controlled study of cECT efficacy had been published. Since the 1940s, many case reports about cECT have been published, concerning a variety of diagnoses. Wijkstra et al. (2000) performed a literature search, selecting studies that included at least five patients who responded to ECT for a mood disorder and then received cECT for at least four months with a dropout rate of 20% or lower. These selection criteria led to only one study (Clarke et al., 1989); it had a prospective naturalistic design, included 29 patients receiving cECT for six months, and reported a relapse rate of 29%.

Wijkstra et al. (2000) performed an open prospective study in which 14 patients were treated with cECT for six months; they observed a relapse rate of 50%. Gagné et al. (2000) conducted a retrospective case-control study; they compared 29 patients who were treated with both cECT and antidepressants with 29 patients receiving medication only. After two years, the relapse rate in the combination group was 7%, versus 48% in patients receiving monotherapy with medication.

Indications for cECT

Based on the available studies on continuation treatment after successful ECT, it is not easy to provide recommendations regarding the choice between continuation pharmacotherapy and cECT. When choosing between these forms of continuation treatment, several factors should be taken into account.

Continuation ECT is a more demanding procedure than continuation pharmacotherapy, as it requires anesthesia and hospital admission for several hours. Furthermore, ECT can be emotionally demanding for the proportion of patients who are frightened of anesthesia or electricity. After the depressive episode has remitted during the first ECT course, administering continuation pharmacotherapy with a TCA or a TCA–lithium combination is a desirable choice.

If a patient achieves remission on ECT and relapses despite receiving adequate pharmacotherapy, cECT after the second ECT course should be considered. The patient should be willing to receive cECT and provide informed consent.

Praxis of cECT

At the end of an ECT course, when the illness has remitted, and ECT is chosen for continuation treatment, the actual cECT starts. Continuation ECT is commonly administered to patients in remission. With intertreatment intervals of one week or longer, it is usually given on an outpatient basis.

There has been considerable discussion about the preferred schedule of cECT, but there are no data on the comparative efficacy of different schedules (Abrams, 2002; Committee on Electroconvulsive Therapy, 2001; Fink et al., 1996). Most often, treatments are started on a weekly basis, extending the intertreatment interval to two weeks after one month. Two months after cECT has started, the interval is prolonged to three weeks, and after another one to two months the ECT frequency is set at once a month, if the patient is still in remission. Whenever symptoms reappear, one should consider shortening the intertreatment interval.

Whether cECT should be combined with pharmacotherapy is another unresolved question. Many patients who are treated with cECT suffer from treatment-resistant depression. Combining ECT with pharmacotherapy might be desirable, especially with patients who experience a relapse during an intensive cECT schedule.

The patient must be adequately informed as to what time he or she is expected to arrive at the hospital. A relative should accompany the patient to and from the hospital, and the patient must not drive. The patient must have nothing by mouth for at least six hours prior to ECT, and this must be explicitly verified before each treatment. Just prior to ECT, the patient is questioned about possible depressive symptoms and somatic problems. If necessary, a basic physical examination is done.

The clinical status, including cognitive functions, current medications, and the presence/absence of depressive symptoms, should be evaluated on a regular basis, for example, monthly. During that visit the next treatment can be planned.

The treatment procedure of cECT does not differ from that in a regular ECT course (see Chapter 34). Most authors advise the use of the same ECT method used to achieve remission, particularly the same electrode placement. Some authors prefer bilateral ECT because of reliable efficacy (Kellner et al., 1991).

Schizophrenia

Continuation ECT for schizophrenia

Several open uncontrolled studies suggest efficacy for cECT in schizophrenia (Chanpattana, 1997, 1998, 2000b; Chanpattana et al., 1999; Chanpattana and Kramer, 2003) (see also Chapters 7 and 22). In these studies, ECT was combined with an antipsychotic drug, similar to the recommended acute ECT treatment for schizophrenia.

Rami et al. (2004) published a study of 10 patients diagnosed with schizophrenia who were treated with cECT. They were compared with a matched control group of 10 patients with schizophrenia who had never received ECT. All patients received treatment with a second generationl antipsychotic drug. No differences in cognitive functioning were found between the groups.

Bipolar Disorder

ECT is well established as an effective and safe treatment of acute episodes of depressed and manic phases (Small et al., 1991) of bipolar disorder and of mixed mania (Ciapparelli et al., 2001). ECT is usually discontinued after the acute illness has been treated. The need for continued pharmacotherapy after successful treatment of acute illness is necessary to prevent relapse and recurrence (see Chapter 6).

Continuation ECT is ongoing ECT treatment after treatment of the index episode to prevent relapses, and it continues for as long as six months. Maintenance ECT (mECT) has no fixed end point and is designed to prevent a new episode of the illness. Most research on cECT and mECT has been done in a mixed population of patients including those with bipolar or unipolar mood disorder.

Several case reports suggest efficacy of cECT and mECT in bipolar disorder (Barnes et al., 1997; Chanpattana, 2000a; Gupta et al., 1998; Sienaert and Peuskens, 2006).

A review and retrospective chart survey of 13 patients with bipolar disorder manic type or schizoaffective disorder suggests that cECT and mECT can be efficacious (Vaidya et al., 2003). In the circumstance of medication failures or multiple hospitalizations but a good previous response to a course of ECT, a patient with bipolar disorder manic type or schizoaffective disorder should be a candidate for cECT or mECT. Concurrent psychotropic use and intertreatment intervals not greater than one to three weeks is generally desirable during cECT or mECT with these patients. If relapse occurs, a short course of three to four sessions is usually enough to regain response during cECT or mECT. Bilateral electrode placement is mostly used in these cases.

Usually in bipolar disorder the ECT course is combined with one or more mood stabilizers or other psychotropics, or a mood stabilizer is started toward the end of an index series. The practice of combining ECT with mood stabilizers is based on practical considerations, not on evidence. Lithium, as the most effective and most often used mood stabilizer, is sometimes combined with ECT.

Early reports cautioned against combining ECT with lithium, citing risks of excessive cognitive disturbances, prolonged apnea, and spontaneous seizures. A review and case series of 12 patients concluded that this combination is not obviously unsafe (Dolenc and Rasmussen, 2005). If the chance of a toxic reaction is definite but rare, proof of its existence requires a large prospective randomized controlled trial. Such a study of the lithium and ECT combination will probably never be conducted. Generally the combination should be avoided, but there may be circumstances warranting it. One possible such circumstance is recurrence of lithium-responsive mania during mECT that has been clearly effective in preventing depressive relapse.

Editor's note

Comorbid anxiety disorder may have contributed to several study outcomes mentioned in this chapter, as it was not accounted for. The higher post-ECT relapse rate reported by Sackeim et al. (2001) than van den Broek et al. (2006) in patients who had failed medication before ECT may have resulted from exceptionally high incidence and severity of comorbid anxiety disorders. The Sackeim et al. patients were chronically ill and so probably had relatively severe anxiety comorbidity, which should predispose to worse outcome. Likewise, the Lauritzen et al. (1996) observation of better six-month outcome with paroxetine than imipramine may have resulted from comorbid anxiety disorder, as anxiety disorder is more responsive to paroxetine than imipramine. –CMS.

References

Abou-Saleh, M. T. and Coppen, A. J. 1988. Continuation therapy with antidepressants after electroconvulsive therapy. Convuls Ther 4: 263–8.

Abrams, R. 2002. Electroconvulsive therapy. Oxford: Oxford University Press.

Aronson, T. A., Shukla, S., and Hoff, A. 1987. Continuation therapy after ECT for delusional depression: A naturalistic study of prophylactic treatments and relapse. Convuls Ther 3: 251–9.

Barnes, R. C., Hussein, A., Anderson, D. N., and Powell, D. 1997. Maintenance electroconvulsive therapy and cognitive function. Br J Psychiatry 170: 285–7.

Birkenhager, T. K., van den Broek, W. W., Mulder, P. G., and De Lely, A. 2005. One-year outcome of psychotic depression after successful electroconvulsive therapy. J ECT 21: 221–6.

Chanpattana, W. 1997. Continuation electroconvulsive therapy in schizophrenia: A pilot study. J Med Assoc Thai 80: 311–18.

Chanpattana, W. 1998. Maintenance ECT in schizophrenia: A pilot study. J Med Assoc Thai 81: 17–24.

Chanpattana, W. 2000a. Combined ECT and clozapine in treatment-resistant mania. J ECT 16: 204–7.

Chanpattana, W. 2000b. Maintenance ECT in treatment-resistant schizophrenia. J Med Assoc Thai 83: 657–62.

Chanpattana, W., Chakrabhand, M. L., Sackeim, H. A., et al. 1999. Continuation ECT in treatment-resistant schizophrenia: A controlled study. J ECT 15: 178–92.

Chanpattana, W. and Kramer, B. A. 2003. Acute and maintenance ECT with flupenthixol in refractory schizophrenia: Sustained improvements in psychopathology, quality of life, and social outcomes. Schizophr Res 63: 189–93.

Ciapparelli, A., Dell'osso, L., Tundo, A., et al. 2001. Electroconvulsive therapy in medication-nonresponsive patients with mixed mania and bipolar depression. J Clin Psychiatry 62: 552–5.

Clarke, T. B., Coffey, C. E., Hoffman, G. W. Jr., and Weiner, R. D. 1989. Continuation therapy for depression using outpatient electroconvulsive therapy. Convuls Ther 5: 330–7.

Committee on Electroconvulsive Therapy. 2001. The practice of electroconvulsive therapy: Recommendations for treatment, training and privileging. Washington, DC: American Psychiatric Association Committee on Electroconvulsive Therapy.

Coppen, A., Abou-Saleh, M. T., Milln, P., et al. 1981. Lithium continuation therapy following electroconvulsive therapy. Br J Psychiatry 139: 284–7.

Dolenc, T. J. and Rasmussen, K. G. 2005. The safety of electroconvulsive therapy and lithium in combination: A case series and review of the literature. J ECT 21: 165–70.

Fink, M., Abrams, R., Bailine, S., and Jaffe, R. 1996. Ambulatory electroconvulsive therapy: Report of a task force of the association for convulsive therapy. Association for Convulsive Therapy. Convuls Ther 12: 42–55.

Gagné, G. J., Furman, M., Carpenter, L., and Price, L. 2000. Efficacy of continuation ECT and antidepressant drugs compared to long-term antidepressants alone in depressed patients. Am J Psychiatry 158: 1933–4.

Gupta, S., Austin, R., Devanand, D. P. 1998. Lithium and maintenance electroconvulsive therapy. J ECT 14: 241–4.

Imlah, N., Ryan, E., and Harrington, J. 1965. The influence of antidepressant drugs on the response to electroconvulsive therapy and on subsequent relapse rates. Neuropsychopharmacology 1: 38–442.

Iodice, A. J. and McCall, W. V. 2003. ECT resistance and early relapse: Two cases of subsequent response to venlafaxine. J ECT 19: 238–41.

Kay, D., Fahy, T., and Garside, R. 1970. A seven-month double-blind trial of amitriptyline and diazepam in ECT-treated depressed patients. Br J Psychiatry 117(541): 667–71.

Kellner, C. H., Burns, C. M., Bernstein, H. J., and Monroe, R. R. Jr. 1991. Electrode placement in maintenance electroconvulsive therapy. Convuls Ther 7: 61–2.

Krog-Meyer, I., Kirkegaard, C., Kijne, B., et al. 1984. Prediction of relapse with the TRH test and prophylactic amitriptyline in 39 patients with endogenous depression. Am J Psychiatry 141: 945–8.

Lauritzen, L., Odgaard, K., Clemmesen, L., et al. 1996. Relapse prevention by means of paroxetine in ECT-treated patients with major depression: A comparison with imipramine and placebo in medium-term continuation therapy. Acta Psychiatr Scand 94: 241–51.

Perry, P. and Tsuang, M. T. 1979. Treatment of unipolar depression following electroconvulsive therapy. Relapse rate comparisons between lithium and tricyclics therapies following ECT. J Affect Disord 1: 123–9.

Rami, L., Bernardo, M., Valdes, M., et al. 2004. Absence of additional cognitive impairment in schizophrenia patients during maintenance electroconvulsive therapy. Schizophr Bull 30: 185–9.

Sackeim, H. A., Haskett, R. F., Mulsant, B. H., et al. 2001. Continuation pharmacotherapy in the prevention of relapse following electroconvulsive therapy: A randomized controlled trial. JAMA 285: 1299–307.

Sackeim, H. A., Prudic, J., Devanand, D. P., et al. 1990. The impact of medication resistance and continuation pharmacotherapy on relapse following response to electroconvulsive therapy in major depression. J Clin Psychopharmacol 10: 96–104.

Seager, C. and Bird, R. 1962. Imipramine with electrical treatment in depression: A controlled trial. J Ment Sci 108: 704–7.

Shapira, B., Gorfine, M., and Lerer, B. 1995. A prospective study of lithium continuation therapy in depressed patients who have responded to electroconvulsive therapy. Convuls Ther 11: 80–5.

Sienaert, P. and Peuskens, J. 2006. Electroconvulsive therapy: An effective therapy of medication-resistant bipolar disorder. Bipolar Disord 8: 304–6.

Small, J. G., Milstein, V., and Small, I. F. 1991. Electroconvulsive therapy for mania. Psychiatr Clin North Am 14: 887–903.

Spiker, D. G., Stein, J., and Rich, C. L. 1985. Delusional depression and electroconvulsive therapy: One year later. Convuls Ther 1: 167–72.

Vaidya, N. A., Mahableshwarkar, A. R., and Shahid, R. 2003. Continuation and maintenance ECT in treatment-resistant bipolar disorder. J ECT 19: 10–16.

van den Broek, W. W., Birkenhager, T. K., Mulder, P. G., et al. 2006. Imipramine is effective in preventing relapse in electroconvulsive therapy-responsive depressed inpatients with prior pharmacotherapy treatment failure: A randomized, placebo-controlled trial. J Clin Psychiatry 67: 263–8.

Wijkstra, J., Nolen, W. A., Algra, A., et al. 2000. Relapse prevention in major depressive disorder after successful ECT: A literature review and a naturalistic case series. Acta Psychiatr Scand 102: 454–60.

34

Ambulatory and maintenance electroconvulsive therapy

Charles H. Kellner and Unnati D. Patel

Introduction

"Ambulatory electroconvulsive therapy (ECT)" refers to performing the treatment on an outpatient basis. This was common in the early days of ECT and has again become common. "Maintenance ECT" refers to administering treatment for preventing symptom recurrence in a remitted patient. They are presented together because both are usually provided on an outpatient basis.

Ambulatory ECT

The venue in which ECT is performed has been subject to change during the nearly seven decades since ECT was invented. The history of the oscillation between inpatient and outpatient venues is an interesting one that parallels how ECT was regarded. Invented in a hospital setting in 1938 in Rome, Italy, the treatment quickly spread across Europe and the world, and was soon being performed on both an inpatient and outpatient basis. In its original form, no anesthesia or oxygen was given, so it was a simple matter for the psychiatrist and an assistant to perform ECT. Hospital facilities were unnecessary, and the common practice evolved of performing ECT in an outpatient psychiatric office. This early era of ambulatory ECT is chronicled by Shorter and Healy (2007). Even when anesthesia and muscle relaxation became commonplace, ECT continued to be provided in both inpatient wards and outpatient office settings. Psychiatrists would give the medications themselves and ventilate the patient with oxygen using a face mask.

When the trends toward increased medical specialization and malpractice concern arrived in the 1970s, it became much more difficult for this relatively informal way of performing ECT to continue. Standards mandated that an anesthesiologist be present to administer the medications and control the patient's airway. Concerns about the ability to deal with possible medical emergencies, even though they rarely occurred, made practitioners more reluctant to give ECT in facilities without full capacity to deal with such emergencies. Thus, ECT moved from the private psychiatrist's office back into either the freestanding psychiatric hospital or the general medical hospital setting. This move took place during a time when the revolution that eventually transformed many medical or surgical procedures into outpatient procedures was not even imagined. It became the norm to associate the need for ECT with the necessity of being an inpatient in a psychiatric hospital. In other words, if a patient was sick enough to require ECT, that patient was sick enough to require inpatient psychiatric care.

By the early 1990s, pressures brought to bear by managed care companies were forcing changes in the way that medical care was delivered. Inpatient hospital stays are both expensive and restrictive for patients, so practice patterns began to include more and more reliance on ambulatory settings. For ECT, this meant a resurgence of outpatient care, not in private psychiatrists' offices, but either in the hospital itself or in a so-called "same day" surgical procedure suite. If the patient's psychiatric illness could be managed on an outpatient basis, he or she could get ECT, even complete acute courses of ECT, without needing to be kept in the hospital. Thus was born the modern era of ECT in the United States, in which much of the ECT (probably the majority, in fact, although good data are lacking) is done on outpatients, whenever possible.

Sensing the need to promote standards of care for ambulatory ECT, the Association for Convulsive Therapy (ACT) convened a task force in 1995 to consider the following questions (Shorter and Healy, 2007): (a) For which conditions is it acceptable or preferable for psychiatric patients to receive ECT in ambulatory care settings? (b) Does such treatment warrant special considerations? (c) In which circumstances is inpatient care indicated? The report was published in *Convulsive Therapy* (now the *Journal of ECT*) in 1996 (Fink et al., 1996). It provided guidelines about diagnostic indications, venue ("Hospital or Home"), ECT management, facilities and personnel, and fees. Here, we briefly summarize the contents of the guidelines.

The ACT Task Force report simply stated that indications for inpatient and ambulatory ECT are identical, also referring back to the American Psychiatric Association (APA) Task Force Report of 1990 (APA, 1990) and its definitions of "primary" (for urgent situations) and "secondary" (after medication failure) indications. In considering where the treatment is best performed, the ACT Task Force report listed four conditions that weighed *against* outpatient ECT: suicide risk, states of adverse behaviors (e.g., delirium, stupor, catatonia), systemic disease (e.g., dementia, inanition), and lack of a caretaker to bring the patient back and forth for the treatment. The authors noted that many depressed patients who initially require an inpatient setting will improve to the point that outpatient treatment is possible after only a few ECT treatments.

In the "ECT Management" section, consent issues were noted to be identical with those for acute inpatient ECT, with additional attention paid to the renewal of consent on a timely basis, depending on local policies and procedures. The importance of the pretreatment psychiatric assessment to establish the indications for treatment as well as documentation of the mental status examination findings were noted. Administration of the Mini Mental State Examination was suggested. The pretreatment physical examination and medical assessments were noted to be identical with those for inpatients. Likewise, treatment techniques were deemed identical, and the availability of different electrode placements and stimulus-dosing strategies individualized to patient need was recommended.

The role of the caretaker was stressed, and specific patient instructions were spelled out: nothing to eat or drink for eight hours before the procedure, specified medicines to be taken with one ounce or less of water on awakening, shampoo of the hair the night before or the morning of treatment, no smoking the morning of treatment, and the request to bring a change of clothing, in case of incontinence. The caretaker's responsibility to bring the patient to the treatment suite, wait as long as necessary, and supervise the patient during the convalescent period was duly noted. The issue of number and temporal spacing of ECT was addressed, with the guidance that typical continuation courses begin with weekly treatments, with gradual lengthening to monthly or even bimonthly intervals. "Breakthrough" symptoms were said to be indicators useful in tailoring the treatment schedule.

Standard guidance for the management of concurrent medications was given (e.g., withholding one or two doses of lithium, minimizing medications with anticonvulsant properties). Lines of authority between the treating and referring psychiatrist were outlined, and the ready availability of someone from the ECT team to answer questions for the caretaker, patient, or other members of the health care team was suggested. A minimum requirement of renewal of laboratory studies every six months in stable patients was noted, with more frequent repetition in patients with unstable or complex medical illnesses. Documentation standards were noted to be the same as for inpatient treatments, and the facility requirement for waiting and changing areas was specified. Appendices to the ACT report included the section on outpatient ECT from the 1990 APA Task Force Report and an information sheet for outpatients.

Almost all of the guidance provided in the ACT Task Force Report on Ambulatory ECT (Fink et al., 1996) remains relevant. Many facilities offer both acute and continuation/maintenance treatments on an ambulatory basis. This is a boon for patients, as it allows for much less disruption of their lives than would an inpatient hospital stay. It is of paramount importance for the success of outpatient ECT that the patients and caretakers fully understand the specific requirements for treatment days as well as the restrictions on nontreatment days. We recommend the frequent repetition of the admonition to refrain from driving during the entire acute course of ECT. We also let patients know that they will be prohibited from driving for a variable time period after the completion of the index course of ECT, depending on several variables, including how much memory impairment they sustain and how closely they can be monitored by family members when they first resume driving. For individual maintenance ECT treatments that are spaced apart by one week or longer, we generally prohibit driving for 24 hours after the treatment. Finally, because considerable time may have elapsed since the treating psychiatrist has last seen the patient, outpatient ECT schedules should provide adequate time on the morning of treatment for the treatment team to assess the patient, gather any necessary information, or perform any needed tests. If the treating psychiatrist is not comfortable that the indication for the treatment is clear or feels that there is a safety or consent issue that needs to be resolved, then the option to postpone or cancel the treatment should, of course, be considered.

As suggested above, ambulatory ECT represents a considerable cost savings compared with inpatient ECT. If patients either have their entire ECT course on an outpatient basis or transition to outpatient ECT after a small number of inpatient treatments, potential cost savings could be in the range of $1,000 per treatment. A small literature attests to the potential financial benefits of ambulatory and maintenance ECT, particularly when compared with long inpatient stays (Aziz et al., 2005; Fink and Bailine, 1998; Kramer, 1990a; Steffens et al., 1995).

Maintenance ECT

Maintenance ECT has become an increasingly important and integral part of contemporary ECT practice in the United States. Although many practitioners use the terms "continuation" and "maintenance" interchangeably, referring generically to any treatment after the acute course, the two words actually have specific and different meanings. Continuation treatment refers to treatment during the six-month period following remission from an index episode of psychiatric illness. Maintenance treatment, as defined by the APA in its Task Force Report on ECT, refers to "the prophylactic use of psychotropics or ECT longer than 6 months past the end of the index episode." The authors of the APA Task Force Report further state: "Conceptually, maintenance therapy aims to protect against recurrence, and thus is distinct from continuation therapy, which aims to prevent relapse" (APA Committee on Electroconvulsive Therapy, 2001). Referring to the increasingly common practice of tapering, rather than abruptly stopping, an acute course of ECT as "continuation ECT" is one particularly helpful use of the term. In this chapter, we use the term maintenance ECT unless the author(s) of a study to which we are referring used the term "continuation ECT."

The need for maintenance ECT arises from the high relapse rate after successful acute ECT without prophylaxis (Bourgon and Kellner, 2000). In one study (Sackeim et al., 2001), the post-ECT relapse rate for patients on placebo was 84%. The period of greatest risk is the first month after remission. The reasons for the high relapse rate are not fully understood, although it seems logical that recurrent illnesses recur, and that the abrupt withdrawal of the successful therapy would leave the patient vulnerable. That notwithstanding, very quick relapse may have something to do with the characteristics of the ECT itself or the changes that ECT produces in the brain. Unfortunately there are no biological markers to reliably determine when a sufficient number of ECT treatments has been delivered in an acute course. Practitioners must depend on clinical judgment to determine treatment endpoints. Current practice tends toward treating to full symptomatic remission, followed by the previously mentioned taper of the acute course into the continuation period. Continuation and maintenance pharmacotherapy after successful ECT, still the mainstay of postacute ECT treatment, are dealt with elsewhere.

Maintenance ECT has been a feature of clinical practice for many decades. A considerable literature over the last several decades suggests that it is effective against depressive relapse and that it is well tolerated. Most of this literature consists of retrospective case reports and case series, the overwhelming majority of which conclude that maintenance ECT reduces relapse rates (Bozkurt et al., 2007; Buhl et al., 2007; Clarke et al., 1989; Dubin et al., 1989, 1992; Fox, 2001; Grunhaus et al., 1990; Gupta et al., 1998; Jaffe et al., 1990; Kramer, 1990b, 1999a, 1999b; Loo et al., 1991; Petrides et al., 1994; Russell et al., 2003; Scott et al., 1991; Stewart, 2000; Stiebel, 1995; Thienhaus et al., 1990; Thornton et al., 1990; Vanelle et al., 1994; Wijkstra and Nolen, 2005). Although some of these reports used comparisons with patient groups not receiving ECT (Gagne et al., 2000; Schwarz et al., 1995), methodological weaknesses of the study designs did not allow for definitive conclusions about the effectiveness of maintenance ECT. Reviews by Andrade and Kurinji (2002) and Frederikse et al. (2006) are excellent summaries of the recent literature. The Andrade and Kurinji review (2002) is particularly helpful for its inclusion of reports on schizophrenia (very limited evidence, but good results) and Parkinson's disease (favorable results in a small subset of patients), as well as a section on cognitive function and maintenance ECT. The Frederikse review was a response to the National Institute for Clinical Excellence (NICE) Technology Appraisal, "Guidance on the Use of Electroconvulsive Therapy," a report from the British National Health Service that appeared in 2003. The NICE report was anything but, and took an extreme and negative view of maintenance ECT (see Chapter 14). It concluded that ECT is "*not recommended as a maintenance therapy in depressive illness*" largely because "*longer-term benefits and risks of ECT have not been clearly established.*" It also stated, "*there was no conclusive evidence to support the effectiveness of ECT beyond the short term or that it is more beneficial as a maintenance therapy in depressive illness than currently available pharmacological alternatives.*" The radical conclusions of the NICE report flew in the face of decades of clinical practice and the unpleasant reality that there are many patients with severe, recurrent mood disorders for whom "pharmacological alternatives" are not really viable alternatives, because they do not work.

The evidence base for the effectiveness of maintenance ECT in mood disorders continues to grow and improve. Swoboda et al. (2001) reported on a prospective controlled trial in which 42 patients with depression or schizoaffective disorder who had responded to an acute course of ECT were either treated with maintenance ECT plus pharmacotherapy ($n = 21$) or with pharmacotherapy alone ($n = 21$). At 12 months, the maintenance ECT group had a rehospitalization rate of 33%, compared with 67% for the other group, as well as significantly longer time to rehospitalization (mean, 9.14 months) than the other group (mean, 5.71 months). In the subset of patients with schizoaffective disorder, although a significant difference in survival time was found in favor of the maintenance ECT group, overall outcome was poorer compared to those patients with depression.

Recognizing the need for prospectively collected randomized trial data on maintenance ECT, the Consortium for Research in ECT (CORE) designed a study to compare continuation ECT with pharmacotherapy during a six-month period (Kellner et al., 2006). The study was designed to be comparable with a previous study (Sackeim et al., 2001), in which acute ECT responders were randomized to receive placebo, monotherapy with the tricyclic antidepressant nortriptyline, or combination pharmacotherapy with nortriptyline and lithium as continuation treatments. Results were relapse rates of 84%, 60%, and 39%, respectively. Missing from that study was the maintenance ECT arm, and the CORE study aimed to provide these data.

The CORE study was a multicenter, National Institute of Mental Health (NIMH)-funded, randomized, and controlled trial carried out between 1997 and 2005. Five hundred thirty-one patients with unipolar major depression were treated with three-times-per-week bitemporal ECT until they met remitter criteria (Hamilton Rating Scale for Depression score of less than or equal to 10 on two consecutive measures and reduction from baseline score by more than 60%). Remitters remained medication-free for one week, and were then randomized to either a fixed schedule of continuation ECT (C-ECT) (weekly for four weeks, biweekly for eight weeks, and monthly for two months, for a total of 10 treatments over five months, with no concurrent medications) or pharmacotherapy (C-Pharm) of combination nortriptyline and lithium. One hundred eighty-four patients were randomized, 89 to C-ECT and 95 to C-Pharm. Forty-six percent of both the C-ECT and C-Pharm groups remained relapse-free for the full six-month period. Thirty-seven percent of the C-ECT group relapsed, compared with 32% of the C-Pharm group (nonsignificant difference). Seventeen percent of the C-ECT group dropped out compared with 22% of the C-Pharm group (nonsignificant difference). Both groups tolerated the treatments well.

Conclusions from this study were that maintenance ECT is a viable relapse-prevention treatment option, comparable to that of the best-studied, aggressive pharmacotherapy regimen, but that better treatments are urgently needed. Limitations of the study include the fact that the maintenance ECT was fixed, not flexible, and that no concurrent medications were allowed for the ECT patients. The similar relapse rate in the combination pharmacotherapy arm to that of the same arm in the Sackeim et al. (2001) study is also noteworthy.

Further research on maintenance ECT is needed to optimize the way this type of ECT is performed. Data on treatment schedules, electrode placement, stimulus dosing strategies, and cognitive effects need to be collected. Very importantly, studies need to be conducted using combined modalities, that is, maintenance ECT in patients who are also taking concurrent pharmacotherapy regimens.

The current state of practice of maintenance ECT is well summarized in guidelines from both the APA (1990, 2001) and the Royal College of Psychiatrists (2005). Indications are listed by the APA as follows: "1) a history of illness that is responsive to ECT, 2) either a patient preference for continuation ECT or resistance or intolerance to pharmacotherapy alone, and 3) the ability and willingness of the patient (or surrogate consentor) to receive continuation ECT, provide informed consent, and comply with the overall treatment plan, including any necessary behavioral restrictions."

The specific schedule for continuation and maintenance ECT has been widely commented on in the literature, but there are few data to support any particular scheme. The guiding concept is to declare an end to the acute treatment course, and then begin spacing the treatments farther apart, which might mean decreasing initially from three to two treatments per week, but more commonly it means going directly to weekly treatment for a few weeks, followed by gradual increase in the intertreatment interval to one month or more (Abrams, 2002). "Pure" maintenance ECT involves treating patients who remain remitted, but in practice it is not uncommon to use early symptom reemergence to help decide on timing of the subsequent treatment.

Periodic reassessment of the need for ongoing maintenance ECT is important, and risk–benefit discussions should be held with the patient and family, as appropriate. Although caution must be exercised in stopping maintenance ECT for patients with histories of severe affective recurrences, and although no lifetime "maximum" number of treatments has been established, uncritically continuing maintenance ECT interminably is a potential abuse (Abrams, 2002; Fink et al., 1996).

Monitoring of cognitive function during maintenance ECT is important, as it is in acute ECT. Generally, it is believed that cognitive effects are less severe with maintenance ECT because of the greater intertreatment interval (Abraham et al., 2006; Barnes et al., 1997; Rami et al., 2004; Rami-Gonzalez et al., 2003; Vothknecht et al., 2003). Data from the CORE study (reported earlier) showed that cognitive effects from the previously completed index course of ECT were slightly greater in the C-ECT group than in the C-Pharm group at three months, but were not different at six months (personal communication, G. Smith, 2008).

Typically, the electrode placement and stimulus-dosing strategy that were effective in inducing initial remission are continued in the maintenance phase. An argument for using bilateral electrode placement preferentially in maintenance ECT has been offered, given the relative importance of ensuring efficacy and the lower risk of cognitive effects, but there are no data to support this suggestion (Kellner et al., 1991).

As the field continues to grapple with the large public health problem of relapse of depression, it is likely that maintenance ECT will continue to play an important, and perhaps increasing, role in treatment planning. Further research is needed to optimize treatment schedules and technical aspects of the administration of the treatment. Combining treatment modalities is likely to be helpful. As the evidence base for the efficacy and tolerability of maintenance ECT builds, it is our hope that published treatment algorithms will include this important strategic option.

References

Abraham, G., Milev, R., Delva, N., and Zaheer, J. 2006. Clinical outcome and memory function with maintenance electroconvulsive therapy: A retrospective study. J ECT 22(1): 43–5.

Abrams, R. 2002. Electroconvulsive therapy, 4th edn. New York: Oxford University Press.

American Psychiatric Association (APA). 1990. The practice of electroconvulsive therapy: Recommendations for treatment, training, and privileging. Washington, DC: APA Press.

American Psychiatric Association (APA) Committee on Electroconvulsive Therapy. 2001. The practice of electroconvulsive therapy: Recommendations for treatment, training, and privileging Washington, DC: APA.

Andrade, C. and Kurinji, S. 2002. Continuation and maintenance ECT: A review of recent research. J ECT 18(3): 149–58.

Aziz, M., Mehringer, A. M., Mozurkewich, E., and Razik, G. N. 2005. Cost-utility of 2 maintenance treatments for older adults with depression who responded to a course of electroconvulsive therapy: Results from a decision analytic model. Can J Psychiatry 50(7): 389–97.

Barnes, R. C., Hussein, A., Anderson, D. N., and Powell D. 1997. Maintenance electroconvulsive therapy and cognitive function. Br J Psychiatry 170: 285–7.

Bourgon, L. N. and Kellner, C. H. 2000. Relapse of depression after ECT: A review. J ECT 16(1): 19–31.

Bozkurt, A., Karlidere, T., Isintas, M., et al. 2007. Acute and maintenance electroconvulsive therapy for treatment of psychotic depression in a pregnant patient. J ECT 23(3): 185–7.

Buhl, C., Riaux, A., Andraud, F., et al. 2007. Nine-year prophylactic maintenance electroconvulsive therapy in an 89-year-old woman with recurrent psychotic major depressive disorder. Am J Geriatr Psychiatry 15(4): 357.

Clarke, T. B., Coffey, C. E., Hoffman, G. W. Jr., and Weiner, R. D. 1989. Continuation therapy for depression using outpatient electroconvulsive therapy. Convuls Ther 5(4): 330–7.

Dubin, W. R., Jaffe, R., Roemer, R., et al. 1992. The efficacy and safety of maintenance ECT in geriatric patients. J Am Geriatr Soc 40(7): 706–9.

Dubin, W. R., Jaffe, R. L., Roemer, R. A., et al. 1989. Maintenance ECT in coexisting affective and neurologic disorders. Convuls Ther 5(2): 162–7.

Fink, M., Abrams, R., Bailine, S., and Jaffe, R. 1996. Ambulatory electroconvulsive therapy: Report of a task force of the association for convulsive therapy. Association for Convulsive Therapy. Convuls Ther 12(1): 42–55.

Fink, M. and Bailine, S. 1998. Electroconvulsive therapy and managed care. Am J Manag Care 4(1): 107–12; quiz 13–14.

Fox, H. A. 2001. Extended continuation and maintenance ECT for long-lasting episodes of major depression. J ECT 17(1): 60–4.

Frederikse, M., Petrides, G., and Kellner, C. 2006. Continuation and maintenance electroconvulsive therapy for the treatment of depressive illness: A response to the National Institute for Clinical Excellence report. J ECT 22(1): 13–17.

Gagne, G. G. Jr., Furman, M. J., Carpenter, L. L., and Price, L. H. 2000. Efficacy of continuation ECT and antidepressant drugs compared to long-term antidepressants alone in depressed patients. Am J Psychiatry 157(12): 1960–5.

Grunhaus, L., Pande, A. C., and Haskett, R. F. 1990. Full and abbreviated courses of maintenance electroconvulsive therapy. Convuls Ther 6(2): 130–8.

Gupta, S., Austin, R., and Devanand, D. P. 1998. Lithium and maintenance electroconvulsive therapy. J ECT 14(4): 241–4.

Jaffe, R., Dubin, W., Shoyer, B., et al. 1990. Outpatient electroconvulsive therapy: Efficacy and safety. Convuls Ther 6(3): 231–8.

Kellner, C. H., Burns, C. M., Bernstein, H. J., and Monroe, R. R. Jr. 1991. Electrode placement in maintenance electroconvulsive therapy. Convuls Ther 7(1): 61–2.

Kellner, C. H., Knapp, R. G., Petrides, G., et al. 2006. Continuation electroconvulsive therapy vs pharmacotherapy for relapse prevention in major depression: A multisite study from the Consortium for Research in Electroconvulsive Therapy (CORE). Arch Gen Psychiatry 63(12): 1337–44.

Kramer, B. A. 1990a. Outpatient electroconvulsive therapy: A cost-saving alternative. Hosp Community Psychiatry 41(4): 361–3.

Kramer, B. A. 1990b. Maintenance electroconvulsive therapy in clinical practice. Convuls Ther 6(4): 279–86.

Kramer, B. A. 1999a. A naturalistic review of maintenance ECT at a university setting. J ECT 15(4): 262–9.

Kramer, B. A. 1999b. A seasonal schedule for maintenance ECT. J ECT 15(3): 226–31.

Loo, H., Galinowski, A., De Carvalho, W., et al. 1991. Use of maintenance ECT for elderly depressed patients. Am J Psychiatry 148(6): 810.

National Institute for Clinical Excellence (NICE). 2003. Guidance on the use of electroconvulsive therapy (Technology Appraisal 59). London: NICE.

Petrides, G., Dhossche, D., Fink, M., and Francis, A. 1994. Continuation ECT: Relapse prevention in affective disorders. Convuls Ther 10(3): 189–94.

Rami, L., Bernardo, M., Boget, T., et al. 2004. Cognitive status of psychiatric patients under maintenance electroconvulsive therapy: A one-year longitudinal study. J Neuropsychiatry Clin Neurosci 16(4): 465–71.

Rami-Gonzalez, L., Salamero, M., Boget, T., et al. 2003. Pattern of cognitive dysfunction in depressive patients during maintenance electroconvulsive therapy. Psychol Med 33(2): 345–50.

Royal College of Psychiatrists' Committee on ECT. 2005. The ECT handbook. London: The Royal College of Psychiatrists.

Russell, J. C., Rasmussen, K. G., O'Connor, M. K., et al. 2003. Long-term maintenance ECT: A retrospective review of efficacy and cognitive outcome. J ECT 19(1): 4–9.

Sackeim, H. A., Haskett, R. F., Mulsant, B. H., et al. 2001. Continuation pharmacotherapy in the prevention of relapse following electroconvulsive therapy: A randomized controlled trial. JAMA 285(10): 1299–307.

Schwarz, T., Loewenstein, J., and Isenberg, K. E. 1995. Maintenance ECT: Indications and outcome. Convuls Ther 11(1): 14–23.

Scott, A. I., Weeks, D. J., and McDonald, C. F. 1991. Continuation electroconvulsive therapy: Preliminary guidelines and an illustrative case report. Br J Psychiatry 159: 867–70.

Shorter, E. and Healy, D. 2007. Shock therapy: A history of electroconvulsive treatment in mental illness. New Brunswick, NJ: Rutgers University Press.

Steffens, D. C., Krystal, A. D., Sibert, T. E., et al. 1995. Cost effectiveness of maintenance ECT. Convuls Ther 11(4): 283–4.

Stewart, J. T. 2000. Lithium and maintenance ECT. J ECT 16(3): 300–1.

Stiebel, V. G. 1995. Maintenance electroconvulsive therapy for chronic mentally ill patients: A case series. Psychiatr Serv 46(3): 265–8.

Swoboda, E., Conca, A., Konig, P., et al. 2001. Maintenance electroconvulsive therapy in affective and schizoaffective disorder. Neuropsychobiology 43(1): 23–8.

Thienhaus, O. J., Margletta, S., and Bennett, J. A. 1990. A study of the clinical efficacy of maintenance ECT. J Clin Psychiatry 51(4): 141–4.

Thornton, J. E., Mulsant, B. H., Dealy, R., and Reynolds, C. F. 3rd. 1990. A retrospective study of maintenance electroconvulsive therapy in a university-based psychiatric practice. Convuls Ther 6(2): 121–9.

Vanelle, J. M., Loo, H., Galinowski, A., et al. 1994. Maintenance ECT in intractable manic-depressive disorders. Convuls Ther 10(3): 195–205.

Vothknecht, S., Kho, K. H., van Schaick, H. W., et al. 2003. Effects of maintenance electroconvulsive therapy on cognitive functions. J ECT 19(3): 151–7.

Wijkstra, J. and Nolen, W. A. 2005. Successful maintenance electroconvulsive therapy for more than seven years. J ECT 21(3): 171–3.

Part VI

Neuromodulation treatment

35

Transcranial magnetic stimulation

Oded Rosenberg and Pinhas N. Dannon

Introduction

Transcranial magnetic stimulation (TMS) is a relatively new treatment in psychiatry. In this chapter we present the updated studies of TMS in various psychiatric disorders and selected neurological disorders. We review safety and efficacy issues in TMS. Finally we discuss recent advances and future directions in TMS.

The public image of TMS is unknown, but it surely appears less threatening than other somatic treatments in psychiatry because it does not involve anesthesia, unconsciousness, or surgical implantation. Moreover, TMS can be administered in private doctors' offices or clinics, and exposure to hospitals and surgical environments can be avoided.

In TMS, a rapidly changing magnetic field is applied to the head and passes through the skull. It induces a weak electrical current in the superficial cortex of the brain that lasts as long as the series of current pulses in the coil (Barker, 2002). The induced electrical activity causes cortical neurons to discharge action potentials. This superficial field stimulates nervous tissue only within about two centimeters from the scalp (Lisanby et al., 2000). New experimental coils are claimed to stimulate deeper tissues (Levkovitz et al., 2007).

TMS guidelines for treating different psychopathologies are difficult to establish. Until now, TMS has been more of a research tool than a clinical treatment procedure like electroconvulsive therapy (ECT). TMS researchers around the world have used different treatment parameters with variations in anatomic locations, stimulation frequencies (1 to 20 Hz), pulse intensity, time period, and numbers of sessions in the treatment course (Gross et al., 2007; Post and Keck, 2001).

Neurobiological background

TMS can be used to generate either excitation or inhibition of the brain, depending on technique. These responses are related to the anatomic structure stimulated and the frequency of magnetic pulses. High-frequency ($\geq$3 Hz) TMS (referred to as rapid TMS [rTMS]) applied to the motor cortex generates motor-evoked potentials of progressively increasing amplitude (Pascual-Leone et al., 1994). Cortical excitability varies with rTMS frequency and intensity (Pascual-Leone et al., 1994) and correlates with increased regional cerebral blood flow (Speer et al., 2000). Conversely, low-frequency TMS ($\leq$3 Hz) decreases cortical excitability (Chen et al., 1997, Wassermann et al., 1996) and lowers regional blood flow (Chen et al., 1997, Speer et al., 2000; Wassermann et al., 1998).

Excitability apparently follows reduction of intracortical inhibition (gamma-aminobutyric acid [GABA] receptor based) or enhancement of intracortical excitation (glutamate receptor based) or both (Ragert et al., 2004). Several neurophysiological changes were demonstrated after TMS:

1. Increased firing rate of dopaminergic neurons in the ventral tegmental area and in the substantia nigra (Crawley and Corwin, 1994),
2. Elevated taurine, serine, and aspartate in the hypothalamic paraventricular nucleus (Keck et al., 2000),
3. Release of monoamines in the hippocampus (Holsboer, 2001),
4. Increased hippocampal serotonin and 5-hydroxyindoleacetic acid (Post and Keck, 2001),
5. Selectively increased 5-HT1A binding sites in frontal cortex, cingulate cortex, and anterior olfactory nucleus (Kole et al., 1999), and
6. Down-regulation of cortical β-adrenergic receptors (Fleischmann et al., 1996; Zyss et al., 1997).

TMS treatment

Major depression

The largest clinical literature about TMS is published about major depression. Several variations of TMS treatment have been used in treatment. The major key points of the different TMS procedures were:

1. Low-frequency (1- to 3-Hz) TMS versus high-frequency (3- to 20-Hz) rTMS,
2. Anatomical orientation of the coil: left prefrontal cortex (usually rTMS) versus right prefrontal cortex (usually low-frequency TMS),
3. Variable number of TMS pulses per session,
4. Magnetic intensity, expressed as percentage of motor threshold,
5. Duration of each session, and
6. Total number of sessions

Most studies demonstrated efficacy with (high-frequency) rTMS over the left prefrontal cortex in major depression (Berman et al., 2000; Eschweiler et al., 2000;

Figiel et al., 1998; George et al., 1995, 1997, 2000; Grunhaus et al., 2000, 2003; Janicak et al., 2002; Pascual-Leone et al., 1996; Pridmore et al., 2000; Triggs et al., 1999). In a review of 139 patients treated with rTMS at this anatomic location, 41% were full responders. Response corresponded to a 50% decrease in Hamilton Rating Scale for Depression (HRSD) score, and a full response corresponded to a final HRSD score of less than eight points (Gershon et al., 2003).

Low-frequency (1-Hz) TMS applied to the right prefrontal cortex has also shown encouraging results. Klein et al. (1999) reported that 17 of 35 patients (49%) treated with low-frequency TMS to the right prefrontal cortex experienced a greater than 50% decrease in depression rating score after 10 treatments. These results were significantly better than those from sham treatment, to which eight of 32 patients (25%) responded.

Studies comparing long courses of (high-frequency) rTMS to ECT show comparable effectiveness in certain patient populations, specifically nonpsychotic depression (George et al., 2000; Grunhaus et al., 2000, 2003). Grunhaus et al. reported two different studies on the effectiveness of rTMS in nonpsychotic patients with major depression. ECT and rTMS obtained similar rates of achieving ECT response, with 60% of patients responding to ECT and 64% to rTMS (George et al., 2000; Grunhaus et al., 2000).

Hausmann et al. (2004a) in a prospective, randomized, double-blind study of depressed patients showed no augmentative effects of TMS to antidepressants. Implications and drug usage in this study were not completely explained. The effectiveness of augmenting antidepressants with TMS remains unresolved.

Recently, a meta-analysis of 19 studies of a major depressive episode treated with rTMS concluded that rTMS was not more effective than sham TMS in treating major depression. The authors stated that the power of the studies to detect a difference between real and sham rTMS was generally low (Couturier, 2005).

These mixed results do not answer the question of whether TMS should be used as a treatment in major depression. To resolve this question, future studies need to focus on using verifiable, observable evidence in selecting patients for TMS study and evaluating the outcome. They also need to resolve questions about technique, including identifying the anatomic regions for magnetic stimulation that provide greatest clinical efficacy. Patients with global cerebral hypometabolism respond better to excitatory treatment, whereas cerebral hypermetabolism responds to inhibitory TMS (Kimbrell et al., 1999). Previous brain function studies demonstrated hypometabolism in the cerebellum, temporal lobes, and the occipital and anterior cingulate regions in depression. Accordingly, regions of hypometabolism might be treated with 20-Hz stimuli whereas regions of hypermetabolism are treated with 1-Hz stimuli.

Bipolar depression

There are few reports of bipolar depressive episode. In the only published pilot study, patients were randomly treated with daily left prefrontal rTMS (5 Hz, 110% motor threshold, 8 seconds on, 22 seconds off, over 20 minutes) or sham. TMS failed to demonstrate effectiveness (Nahas et al., 2003).

Dysthymic disorder

A few case reports with small samples reported effectiveness of rTMS in treating dysthymic disorder. The single study of dysthymia with Parkinson's disease showed effectiveness (Dragasevic et al., 2002). Future studies with larger samples could clarify this issue.

Schizophrenia

Auditory hallucinations

In a double-blind study of schizophrenia, patients with treatment-refractory auditory hallucinations were treated daily with TMS at 1 Hz for 20 minutes per day. TMS was performed for 10 treatment days over the left or right temporoparietal lobes. At the end of the session, patients achieved significant changes in the frequency of auditory hallucinations, in positive symptoms of Positive and Negative Syndrome Scale (PANSS), and in the Clinical Global Impression (CGI-I) rating (Lee et al., 2005).

Hoffman et al. (2003) applied TMS to the left temporoparietal cortex at 1 Hz for 9 days in 24 patients with schizophrenia or schizoaffective disorder with medication-resistant auditory hallucinations. Patients achieved substantial improvement in hallucination frequency and attentional salience. In 52% of the patients, improvement was maintained for another 15 weeks. Brunelin et al. (2006) had performed low-frequency (1-Hz) TMS to the left temporoparietal cortex over five consecutive working days. They achieved improvement in Auditory Hallucinations Rating Scale scores as well as in source monitoring.

A double-blind crossover study in patients with schizophrenia and resistant auditory hallucinations applied five days of low-frequency TMS (1 Hz) over the left temporoparietal cortex. Authors reported diminution of 56% in hallucinations, with reduction of all seven items of the Auditory Hallucinations Rating Scale and the Scale for Assessment of Positive Symptoms (SAPS) (Poulet et al., 2005).

Preliminary clinical experience with auditory hallucinations raises the possibility that transcranial magnetic stimulation will be a useful ancillary treatment in schizophrenia. Similarly, it might be useful in isolated auditory hallucinosis or hallucinosis secondary to a medical condition such as stroke.

Catatonia

Only a few case reports describe TMS treatment for catatonia. Grisaru et al. (1998a) reported a 24-year-old woman with a history of an acute psychotic episode; she was treated with 20-Hz rTMS over the right prefrontal cortex in a 10-day course. The intensity of the stimulus was 80% of patient motor threshold. Marked improvement was noticed in psychotic mutism, negativism, waxy flexibility, and rigidity. She started to show concern for personal hygiene, participate in ward activities, and cooperate with the staff and her family (Grisaru et al., 1998a).

In another case report, TMS to the left dorsolateral prefrontal cortex was administered over two weeks to an 18-year-old catatonic patient. This treatment produced marked improvement (Saba et al., 2002).

Negative symptoms of schizophrenia

According to the literature, TMS studies produced conflicting results in treating negative symptoms. Hajak et al. (2004) studied 20 patients with schizophrenia treated with high-frequency 10-Hz rTMS for 10 days. They observed a significant reduction of negative symptoms and a nonsignificant trend for improvement in depressive symptoms. These observations led them to conclude that high-frequency rTMS could have beneficial effects on negative and depressive symptoms.

In another study, 22 patients taking antipsychotic medication were randomized to two groups. Eleven were treated with effective TMS, and 11 with sham rTMS. Stimulation was applied to the left dorsolateral prefrontal cortex. This study reported a statistically significant decrease in negative symptoms (Prikryl et al., 2007).

However, Mogg et al. (2007) found no difference between sham and real rTMS in 17 patients with prominent negative symptoms. All were randomized to a 10-day course of real or sham rTMS applied to the left dorsolateral prefrontal cortex. Novák et al. (2006) treated 16 schizophrenia patients taking antipsychotic medication. TMS treatment was performed as 20-Hz rTMS (90% of motor threshold, 2,000 stimuli per session to left dorsolateral prefrontal cortex) with 10 sessions in two weeks. This treatment did not improve the negative symptoms of schizophrenia (Novák et al., 2006).

Bipolar mania

TMS was used to treat manic episodes (of bipolar disorder) in a few preliminary studies with small samples. Michael and Erfurth (2004) treated with right prefrontal rTMS in an open study of nine bipolar manic (type I) hospitalized patients. Eight of nine patients received TMS as add-on treatment to an insufficient or only partially effective drug. The pharmacological treatment regimen included mood stabilizers as well as antipsychotics. During the four weeks of TMS treatment, a sustained reduction of manic symptoms as measured by the Bech-Rafaelsen Mania Scale was observed. The investigators concluded that right prefrontal rTMS is safe and efficacious as an add-on treatment for bipolar mania (Michael and Erfurth, 2004).

Promising results were achieved in a study of 16 patients who completed a 14-day double-blind, controlled trial of right versus left prefrontal TMS at 20 Hz (two-second duration per train, 20 trains per day, for 10 treatment days). In this study, significantly more improvement was observed with patients given right rather than left prefrontal TMS (Grisaru et al., 1998b).

Post-traumatic stress disorder

Post-traumatic stress disorder (PTSD) treatment is less studied with TMS. In a double-blind, placebo-controlled study, 24 patients received 10 daily treatments of low-frequency (1-Hz) or high-frequency (10-Hz) rTMS at 80% motor threshold over the right dorsolateral prefrontal cortex. PTSD core symptoms (re-experiencing, avoidance) markedly improved with TMS. Moreover, high-frequency rTMS over the right dorsolateral prefrontal cortex alleviated anxiety symptoms (Cohen et al., 2004).

Obsessive-compulsive disorder

There are few published studies in the treatment of obsessive-compulsive disorder (OCD) with TMS. Greenberg et al. (1997) demonstrated in 12 patients with OCD the partial effectiveness of TMS treatment. TMS was given randomly as repetitive TMS (80% motor threshold, 20 Hz, two seconds per minute for 20 minutes) to the right lateral prefrontal, the left lateral prefrontal, and the midoccipital regions on separate days. Compulsive urges decreased significantly for eight hours after right lateral prefrontal repetitive TMS, but there were no changes in compulsive urges after rTMS of the midoccipital site. In contrast to stimulation of the right lateral prefrontal area, no significant reduction in compulsive urges occurred after stimulation of the left lateral prefrontal area. Mood improved during the session and at 30 minutes after right lateral prefrontal stimulation. These preliminary results suggest that right prefrontal rTMS might affect prefrontal mechanisms involved in OCD (Greenberg et al., 1997).

In another double-blind, sham-controlled study, 13 patients were randomly assigned to 13 sessions of 20 minutes. TMS frequency was 1 Hz, and the intensity was 110% of motor threshold. No significant changes in OCD were detected in either group, suggesting that low-frequency TMS of the right prefrontal cortex does not treat OCD (Alonso et al., 2001).

A study of 33 patients randomly assigned participants to 10 sessions of either active TMS or sham TMS. The active TMS was administered at 1 Hz and 110% of motor threshold over the left dorsolateral prefrontal cortex. Both groups improved during the study with no difference between the sham and active TMS group (Prasko et al., 2006).

Panic disorder

Several case reports described using TMS in treating panic disorder. A 52-year-old woman suffering from panic disorder with six panic attacks per week was treated for two weeks with slow TMS on the right dorsolateral prefrontal cortex. After two weeks, the patient reported a marked improvement in her anxiety. Her score on the Hamilton Anxiety Scale decreased from 27 to 6 (−78%), and her score on the Panic and Agoraphobia Scale decreased from 34 to 14 (−59%). Her maximum scores on the Acute Panic Inventory and the Panic Symptom Scale decreased from 34 to 20 (−41%) and from 38 to 26 (−32%), respectively. The patient did not require further pharmacotherapy (Zwanzger et al., 2002a).

Tinnitus

Tinnitus has long been an untreatable and sometimes disabling disorder. It can be accompanied by anxiety and unstable mood when it becomes a subchronic or chronic condition (Kleinjung et al., 2007; Rossi et al., 2007). The prevalence of tinnitus is 8.2% in persons older than 50 years. In elderly populations, it is frequently associated with deafness (Kleinjung et al., 2007).

TMS was used to treat tinnitus (Kleinjung et al., 2007). Tinnitus was shown to respond to modulations of cortical activity by high- and low-frequency repetitive TMS (Plewnia et al., 2007). Sixteen patients with chronic tinnitus underwent a randomized, double-blind, crossover, placebo-controlled trial of 1-Hz TMS (120% of motor threshold; 1,200 stimuli per day for five days) of the left temporoparietal region. Significant improvement was achieved in 8 of 14 participants, although tinnitus worsened in two patients (Rossi et al., 2007).

Another study treated 15 participants with sham or real TMS at an intensity of 100%. Participants received trains of 30 pulses at 10 Hz delivered every minute for five minutes. TMS caused partial suppression of tinnitus for six participants. The decrease ranged from 19% to 86% (average 50%). Tinnitus suppression persisted for between 20 minutes and four days (Folmer et al., 2006).

Six patients with chronic tinnitus were enrolled in a positron emission tomography–assisted rTMS, sham-controlled, and crossover study. In five of six patients, rTMS induced a greater reduction of rated tinnitus than did sham stimulation (Plewnia et al., 2007). In another study, 14 patients received neuronavigated low-frequency TMS (110% motor threshold, 1 Hz, 2,000 stimuli per day over five days) or sham TMS. Patients were followed up for six months. The five days of TMS demonstrated significant improvement of the tinnitus score whereas the sham treatment did not show any changes. The treatment outcome after six months still demonstrated significant reduction of tinnitus (Eichhammer et al., 2003). Similarly, two of three patients treated with 1-Hz TMS using positron emission tomography–guided neuronavigation achieved considerable improvement in tinnitus (Eichhammer et al., 2003).

Khedr et al. (2008) conducted the largest study of chronic tinnitus to date, involving 66 patients. The participants were randomized into four treatment groups. Each group received a different frequency of TMS (1 Hz, 10 Hz, 25 Hz, or sham). TMS and rTMS produced greater improvement than did sham. However, there was no significant difference in response rates at different TMS frequencies. Patients with tinnitus for the longest duration were the least likely to respond to treatment.

TMS comparison with ECT

Grunhaus et al. (2000, 2003) conducted two randomized studies in patients with medication-resistant nonpsychotic major depression. They received an average of 10 treatments with either unilateral ECT or rTMS, applied over the left dorsolateral prefrontal cortex with an intensity of 100%, a frequency of 10 Hz and 20 to 30 trains of two-second duration per treatment session. Patients were assessed for objective and subjective cognitive impairments before and a week after treatment. Treatment response was comparable: Forty-six percent of the ECT group and 44% of the rTMS group showed a reduction of 50% or more in HRSD scores. In patients treated with rTMS, cognitive performance remained constant or improved, and memory complaints decreased, whereas in the ECT group memory recall deficits emerged and memory complaints remained (Schulze-Rauschenbach et al., 2005).

Eranti et al. (2007) reported a study of 46 patients with major depression referred for ECT. Patients were randomly assigned to either a 15-day course of rTMS of the left dorsolateral prefrontal cortex or a standard course of ECT. Each session entailed 20 trains at 10 Hz for five seconds. A full course comprised 15 daily sessions with a total of 15,000 magnetic pulses. HRSD scores at the end of treatment were significantly lower for ECT, with 13 patients (59.1%) achieving remission in the ECT group and four (16.7%) in the rTMS group. However, at six months the HRSD scores did not differ between groups. Beck Depression Inventory, visual analogue mood scale, and Brief Psychiatric Rating Scale scores were lower for ECT at the end of treatment and remained lower after six months. Self-rated and observer-rated cognitive measures were similar in the two groups.

Some possibilities for treating with TMS are to administer it to patients who have not responded well to medications and to use it along with nonpharmacological therapies. Other TMS candidates are patients who fulfill criteria for ECT but are unwilling to receive ECT. Similarly, patients who are not physically stable enough for ECT or its general anesthesia (e.g., patients with severe heart failure, severe chronic obstructive pulmonary disease) might be able to tolerate TMS.

Likely responders to TMS treatment include patients with a shorter duration of depressive episode (Holtzheimer et al., 2004), with deeper sleep disturbances (Brakemeier et al., 2007), with response to left lateral visual field stimulation (Schiffer et al., 2002), relatively younger patients, and treatment-naive patients (Fregni et al., 2006).

Safety issues

Low-/high-frequency/repetitive TMS

Risk for seizures

TMS treatment is generally well tolerated and safe in humans (Wassermann et al., 1998). Low rates of headache and dizziness have been reported. No serious adverse effects are known. There is no evidence that rTMS causes brain injury or irreversible changes.

TMS can induce seizures, but the occurrence of seizure has been rare. Seizures are a risk only with high-frequency rTMS. However, high-frequency rTMS has rarely precipitated seizure, even in people with epilepsy. (Tassinari et al., 2003). TMS has caused seven known cases of seizure since 1996 (Wassermann, 1998). These seizures were usually brief and without persisting physical sequelae (Wassermann, 1998). Although the risk is low, prior history of one or more seizures is considered a relative contraindication for TMS administration (Hoffman et al., 2005). Combining data from 17 studies in which TMS was used for a variety of disorders found no evidence of seizure induction regardless of frequency. No seizures occurred in 58 patients treated with TMS at a frequency of 1 Hz (Hoffman et al., 2003; McIntosh et al., 2004; Poulet et al., 2005; Rosenberg et al., 2002; Saba et al., 2006), in 101 patients treated with TMS at a frequency of 10 Hz (Fitzgerald et al., 2006; Loo et al., 2008; Padberg et al., 2002; Saba et al., 2004; Wassermann, 1998), or in 48 patients treated with TMS at a frequency of 20 Hz (George et al., 1997; Greenberg et al., 1997; Grisaru et al., 1998b; Michael and Erfurth, 2004). The risk of seizures seems to be relatively small, but it still needs to be mentioned orally and in writing in obtaining informed consent to perform TMS.

Treatment-emergent mania/hypomania

TMS treatment of depression has a theoretical risk of treatment-emergent mania or hypomania (TEM). A review of literature published from 1966 through 2007 concluded that the rate of TEM was 0.84% for the TMS group and 0.73% for the sham group. The difference was not statistically significant. A total of 13 cases of

TEM associated with rTMS have been published. Because of these cases it appears that TEM is a slight possible risk of TMS (Dolberg et al., 2001; Hausmann et al., 2004b; Xia et al., 2007).

Occurrence of delusions

Zwanzger et al. (2002a) reported that a patient experienced a first onset of severe delusions after receiving 13 daily sessions of rTMS monotherapy for treating nonpsychotic major depression. These psychotic symptoms remitted quickly with antipsychotic medication. No other reports of induced delusions are known. Because TMS can increase excretion of dopamine metabolites and mitigate Parkinson's disease, it probably increases central nervous system dopamine levels and so might possibly although rarely provoke psychosis.

Contraindications to TMS treatment

An absolute contraindication for TMS is the presence of metal particles. Accordingly, history of metal in the head (outside the mouth), known history of any metallic particles in the eye, implanted neurostimulators or medical pumps, and known history of cochlear implants or iron-containing surgical clips are contraindications to TMS. Modern surgical clips are compatible with magnetic resonance imaging and so are not necessarily contraindicated. A thorough investigation of any specific clip is needed before administration of TMS. A cardiac pacemaker or intracardiac line might be a contraindication. Relative contraindications include history of epilepsy or seizure in first-degree relatives and history of head injury.

Precautions should be taken to avoid hearing damage caused by the magnetic stimulator. Patients generally wear noise protection earmuffs.

Future prospects

As a new treatment tool, TMS requires further investigations in various psychiatric conditions. Five major questions need to be clarified about TMS.

1. How should treatment parameters be established for most psychopathologies?
2. What is the possibility of maintenance treatment with TMS in various psychiatric conditions or post-ECT?
3. What are the connections between anatomical structure and TMS efficacy?
4. What are the connections between cerebral blood flow and the clinical utility of TMS?
5. What are the augmentative effects of TMS?

Deep TMS

Deep TMS has been studied in Israel with promising results in patients with major depression. A recent safety study found no major side effects (Levkovitz et al.,

2007). If it truly penetrates deeper into brain tissues, it might be more effective than standard rTMS. Deeper penetration should produce greater action on nerve fibers connecting the prefrontal cortex to the limbic system.

Editor's note

In clinical treatment studies, there is no replacement for using verifiable, observable evidence in selecting patients for study and in evaluating their response to treatment. Diagnosing major depression does not require observable evidence – even with Diagnostic and Statistical Manual of Mental Disorders *melancholic features. Neither does rating depression with the HRSD. Evaluating subjective major depression is usually equivalent to a patient satisfaction survey, and this is what depression evaluation in treatment studies are unless they provide additional details of psychopathology. Unfortunately, because details of verifiable observable features of depression were not included in studies of TMS, there is no reliable way to compare the studied patients with any other patients including those we see in our own clinics. Studies reporting similar outcomes for TMS and ECT have presented only subjective results. Patients with psychotic depression treated with TMS probably had observable psychopathology, but even these were not detailed.*

Logically, TMS and rTMS resemble subthreshold unilateral ECT. TMS and rTMS should be much less effective than regular ECT for those conditions we know to respond well to ECT. However, TMS might be most useful for a different group of conditions, for which ongoing long-term outpatient treatment is appropriate. These include anxiety disorders (PTSD, generalized anxiety disorder, OCD, social phobia), chronic atypical depression, seasonal affective disorder, tinnitus, borderline personality disorder, impulse control disorders, eating disorders, and perhaps chronic psychotic conditions such as delusional disorder. In October 2008, the U.S. Food and Drug Administration approved the commercial availability of rTMS. –CMS.

References

Alonso, P., Pujol, J., Cardoner, N., et al. 2001. Right prefrontal repetitive transcranial magnetic stimulation in obsessive-compulsive disorder: A double-blind, placebo-controlled study. Am J Psychiatry 158: 1143–5.

Barker, A. T. 2002. The history and basic principles of magnetic nerve stimulation. In Handbook of transcranial magnetic stimulation, 1st edn. (eds. Pascual-Leone, A., Davey, N., Rothwell, J., et al.). New York: Oxford University Press, pp. 3–17.

Berman, R. M., Narasimhan, M., Sanacora, G., et al. 2000. A randomized clinical trial of repetitive transcranial magnetic stimulation in the treatment of major depression. Biol Psychiatry 47: 332–7.

Brakemeier, E. L., Luborzewski, A., Danker-Hopfe, H., et al. 2007. Positive predictors for antide-pressive response to prefrontal repetitive transcranial magnetic stimulation (rTMS). J Psychiatr Res 41(5): 395–403.

Brunelin, J., Poulet, E., Bediou, B., et al. 2006. Low frequency repetitive transcranial magnetic stimulation improves source monitoring deficit in hallucinating patients with schizophrenia. Schizophr Res 81(1): 41–5. Epub 2005 November 28.

Chen, R., Classen, J., Gerloff, C., et al. 1997. Depression of motor cortex excitability by low frequency. Schizophr Res 81: 41–5.

Cohen, H., Kaplan, Z., Kotler, M., et al., 2004. Repetitive transcranial magnetic stimulation of the right dorsolateral prefrontal cortex in posttraumatic stress disorder: a double-blind, placebo-controlled study. Am J Psychiatry. 161: 515–24.

Couturier, J. L. 2005. Efficacy of rapid-rate repetitive transcranial magnetic stimulation in the treatment of depression: A systematic review and meta-analysis. J Psychiatry Neurosci 30(2): 83–90.

Crawley, J. N. and Corwin, R. L. 1994. Biological actions of cholecystokinin. Peptides 5: 731–55.

Dolberg, O. T., Schreiber, S., and Grunhaus, L. 2001. Transcranial magnetic stimulation-induced switch into mania: A report of two cases. Biol Psychiatry 49(5): 468–70.

Dragasevic, N., Potrebić, A., Damjanović, A., et al. 2002. Therapeutic efficacy of bilateral pre-frontal slow repetitive transcranial magnetic stimulation in depressed patients with Parkinson's disease: An open study. Mov Disord 17(3): 528–32.

Eichhammer, P., Langguth, B., Marienhagen, J., et al. 2003. Neuronavigated repetitive transcranial magnetic stimulation in patients with tinnitus: A short case series. Biol Psychiatry 54(8): 862–5.

Eranti, S., Mogg, A., Pluck, G., et al. 2007. A randomized, controlled trial with 6-month follow-up of repetitive transcranial magnetic stimulation and electroconvulsive therapy for severe depression. Am J Psychiatry 164: 1.

Eschweiler, G. W., Wegerer, C., Schlotter, W., et al. 2000. Left prefrontal activation predicts therapeutic effects of repetitive transcranial magnetic stimulation (rTMS) in major depression. Psychiatry Res 99: 161–72.

Figiel, G. S., Epstein, C., McDonald, W. M., et al. 1998. The use of rapid-rate transcranial magnetic stimulation (rTMS) in refractory depressed patients. J Neuropsychiatry Clin Neurosci 10: 20–5.

Fitzgerald, P. B., Benitez, J., de Castella, A., et al. 2006. A randomized, controlled trial of sequential bilateral repetitive transcranial magnetic stimulation for treatment-resistant depression. Am J Psychiatry 163: 88–94.

Fleischmann, A., Sternheim, A., Etgen, A. M., et al. 1996. Transcranial magnetic stimulation downregulates beta-adrenoreceptors in rat cortex. J Neural Transm 103: 1361–6.

Folmer, R. L., Carroll, J. R., Rahim, A., et al. 2006. Effects of repetitive transcranial magnetic stimulation (rTMS) on chronic tinnitus. Acta Otolaryngol Suppl (556): 96–101.

Fregni, F., Marcolin, M. A., Myczkowski, M., et al. 2006. Predictors of antidepressant response in clinical trials of transcranial magnetic stimulation. Int J Neuropsychopharmacol 9(6): 641–54.

George, M. S., Nahas, Z., Molloy, M., et al. 2000. A controlled trial of daily left prefrontal cortex TMS for treating depression. Biol Psychiatry 48: 962–70.

George, M. S., Wassermann, E. M., Kimbrell, T. A., et al. 1997. Mood improvement following daily left prefrontal repetitive transcranial magnetic stimulation in patients with depression: A placebo-controlled crossover trial. Am J Psychiatry 154: 1752–6.

George, M. S., Wassermann, E. M., Williams, W. A., et al. 1995. Daily repetitive transcranial magnetic stimulation (rTMS) improves mood in depression. Neuroreport 6: 1853–6.

Gershon, A. A., Dannon, P. N., and Grunhaus, L. 2003. Transcranial magnetic stimulation in the treatment of depression. Am J Psychiatry 160: 835–45.

Greenberg, B. D., George, M. S., Martin, J. D., et al. 1997. Effect of prefrontal repetitive transcranial magnetic stimulation in obsessive-compulsive disorder: A preliminary study. Am J Psychiatry 154: 867–9.

Grisaru, N., Chudakov, B., Yaroslavsky, Y., and Belmaker, R. H. 1998a. Catatonia treated with transcranial magnetic stimulation. Am J Psychiatry 155: 1626.

Grisaru, N., Chudakov, B., Yaroslavsky, Y., and Belmaker, R. H. 1998b. Transcranial magnetic stimulation in mania: A controlled study. Am J Psychiatry 155: 1608–10.

Gross, M., Nakamura, L., Pascual-Leone, A., and Fregni, F. 2007. Has repetitive transcranial magnetic stimulation (rTMS) treatment for depression improved? A systematic review and meta-analysis comparing the recent vs. the earlier rTMS studies. Acta Psychiatr Scand 116: 165–73.

Grunhaus, L., Dannon, P. N., Schreiber, S., et al. 2000. Repetitive transcranial magnetic stimulation is as effective as electroconvulsive therapy in the treatment of nondelusional major depressive disorder: An open study. Biol Psychiatry 47: 314–24.

Grunhaus, L., Schreiber, S., Dolberg, O. T., et al. 2003. A randomized controlled comparison of electroconvulsive therapy and repetitive transcranial magnetic stimulation in severe and resistant nonpsychotic major depression. Biol Psychiatry 53: 324–31.

Hajak, G., Marienhagen, J., Langguth, B., et al. 2004. High-frequency repetitive transcranial magnetic stimulation in schizophrenia: a combined treatment and neuroimaging study. Psychol Med. 34: 1157–63.

Hausmann, A., Kemmler, G., Walpoth, M., et al., 2004a. No benefit derived from repetitive transcranial magnetic stimulation in depression: a prospective, single centre, randomised, double blind, sham controlled "add on" trial. J Neurol Neurosurg Psychiatry 75: 320–2.

Hausmann, A., Kramer-Reinstadler, K., Lechner-Schoner, T., et al. 2004b. Can bilateral prefrontal repetitive transcranial magnetic stimulation (rTMS) induce mania? A case report. J Clin Psychiatry 65(11): 1575–6.

Hoffman, R. E., Gueorguieva, R., Hawkins, K. A., et al. 2005. Temporoparietal transcranial magnetic stimulation for auditory hallucinations: Safety, efficacy and moderators in a fifty patient sample. Biol Psychiatry 58: 97–104.

Hoffman, R. E., Hawkins, K. A., Gueorguieva, R., et al. 2003. Transcranial magnetic stimulation of left temporoparietal cortex and medication-resistant auditory hallucinations. Arch Gen Psychiatry 60: 49–56.

Holsboer, F. 2001. Neuroendocrinology of mood disorders. In Psychopharmacology: The fourth generation of progress (eds. Bloom, F. E. and Kupfer, D. J.). New York: Raven Press, pp. 957–68.

Holtzheimer, P. E. III, Russo, J., Claypoole, K. H., et al. 2004. Shorter duration of depressive episode may predict response to repetitive transcranial magnetic stimulation. Depress Anxiety 19(1): 24–30.

Janicak, P. G., Dowd, S. M., Martis, B., et al. 2002. Repetitive transcranial magnetic stimulation versus electroconvulsive therapy for major depression: Preliminary results of a randomized trial. Biol Psychiatry 51: 659–67.

Keck, M. E., Sillaber, I., Ebner, K., et al. 2000. Acute transcranial magnetic stimulation of frontal brain regions selectively modulates the release of vasopressin, biogenic amines and amino acids in the rat brain. Eur J Neurosci 12: 3713–20.

Khedr, E. M., Rothwell, J. C., Ahmed, M. A., and El-Atar, A. 2008. Effect of daily repetitive transcranial magnetic stimulation for treatment of tinnitus: Comparison of different stimulus frequencies. J Neurol Neurosurg Psychiatry 79(2): 212–15.

Kimbrell, T. A., Little, J. T., Dunn, R. T., et al. 1999. Frequency dependence of antidepressant response to left prefrontal repetitive transcranial magnetic stimulation (rTMS) as a function of baseline cerebral glucose metabolism. Biol Psychiatry 46: 1603–13.

Klein, E., Kreinin, I., Chistyakov, A., et al. 1999. Therapeutic efficacy of right prefrontal slow repetitive transcranial magnetic stimulation in major depression: A double-blind controlled study. Arch Gen Psychiatry 56: 315–20.

Kleinjung, T., Steffens, T., Londero, A., and Langguth, B. 2007. Transcranial magnetic stimulation (TMS) for treatment of chronic tinnitus: Clinical effects. Prog Brain Res 166: 359–67.

Kole, M. H. P., Fuchs, E., Ziemann, U., et al. 1999. Changes in 5-HT1A and NMDA binding sites by a single rapid transcranial magnetic stimulation procedure in rats. Brain Res 816: 309–12.

Lee, S. H., Kim, W., Chung, Y. C., et al. 2005. A double blind study showing that two weeks of daily repetitive TMS over the left or right temporoparietal cortex reduces symptoms in patients with schizophrenia who are having treatment-refractory auditory hallucinations. Neurosci Lett 376(3): 177–81.

Levkovitz, Y., Roth, Y., Harel, E. V., et al. 2007. A randomized controlled feasibility and safety study of deep transcranial magnetic stimulation. Clin Neurophysiol 118: 2730–44.

Lisanby, S. H., Luber, B., Perera, T., and Sackeim, H. A. 2000. Transcranial magnetic stimulation: Applications in basic neuroscience and neuropsychopharmacology. Int J Neuropsychopharmacol 3: 259–73.

Loo, C. K., McFarquhar, T. F., and Mitchell, P. B. 2008. A review of the safety of repetitive transcranial magnetic stimulation as a clinical treatment for depression. Int J Neuropsychopharmacol (1): 131–47.

McIntosh, A. M., Semple, D., Tasker, K., et al. 2004. Transcranial magnetic stimulation for auditory hallucinations in schizophrenia. Psychiatry Res 127: 9–17.

Michael, N. and Erfurth, A. 2004. Treatment of bipolar mania with right prefrontal rapid transcranial magnetic stimulation. J Affect Disord 78(3): 253–7.

Mogg, A., Purvis, R., Eranti, S., et al. 2007. Repetitive transcranial magnetic stimulation for negative symptoms of schizophrenia: A randomized controlled pilot study. Schizophr Res 93(1–3): 221–8. Epub May 2.

Nahas, Z., Kozel, F. A., Li, X., et al. 2003. Left prefrontal transcranial magnetic stimulation (TMS) treatment of depression in bipolar affective disorder: A pilot study of acute safety and efficacy. Bipolar Disord 5(1): 40–7.

Novák, T., Horácek, J., Mohr, P., et al. 2006. The double-blind sham-controlled study of high-frequency rTMS (20 Hz) for negative symptoms in schizophrenia: Negative results. Neuro Endocrinol Lett 27(1–2): 209–13.

Padberg, F., Zwanzger, P., Keck, M. E., et al. 2002. Repetitive transcranial magnetic stimulation (rTMS) in major depression: Relation between efficacy and stimulation intensity. Neuropsychopharmacology 27: 638–45.

Pascual-Leone, A., Half-Sole, J., Wassermann, E. M., and Hallett, M. 1994. Responses to rapid-rate transcranial magnetic stimulation of the human motor cortex. Brain 117: 847–58.

Pascual-Leone, A., Rubio, B., Pallardo, F., and Catala, M. D. 1996. Rapid-rate transcranial magnetic stimulation of left dorsolateral prefrontal cortex in drug-resistant depression. Lancet 348: 233–7.

Plewnia, C., Reimold, M., Najib, A., et al. 2007. Moderate therapeutic efficacy of positron emission tomography-navigated repetitive transcranial magnetic stimulation for chronic tinnitus: A randomised, controlled pilot study. J Neurol Neurosurg Psychiatry 78(2): 152–6.

Post, A. and Keck, M. E. 2001. Transcranial magnetic stimulation as a therapeutic tool in psychiatry: What do we know about the neurobiological mechanisms? J Psychiatr Res 35: 193–215.

Poulet, E., Brunelina, J., Bedioua, B., et al. 2005. Slow transcranial magnetic stimulation can rapidly reduce resistant auditory hallucinations in schizophrenia. Biol Psychiatry 57(2): 188–91.

Prasko, J., Pasková, B., Záleský, R., et al. 2006. The effect of repetitive transcranial magnetic stimulation (rTMS) on symptoms in obsessive compulsive disorder. A randomized, double blind, sham controlled study. Neuro Endocrinol Lett 27(3): 327–32.

Pridmore, S., Bruno, R., Turnier-Shea, Y., et al. 2000. Comparison of unlimited numbers of rapid transcranial magnetic stimulation (rTMS) and ECT treatment sessions in major depressive episode. Int J Neuropsychopharmacol 3: 129–34.

Prikryl, R., Kasparek, T., Skotakova, S., et al. 2007. Treatment of negative symptoms of schizophrenia using repetitive transcranial magnetic stimulation in a double-blind, randomized controlled study. Schizophr Res 95(1–3): 151–7.

Ragert, P., Becker, M., Tegenthoff, M., et al. 2004. Sustained increase of somatosensory cortex excitability by 5 Hz repetitive transcranial magnetic stimulation studied by paired median nerve stimulation in humans. Neurosci Lett 356: 91–4.

Rosenberg, P. B., Mehndiratta, R. B., Mehndiratta, Y. P., et al. 2002. Repetitive transcranial magnetic stimulation treatment of comorbid posttraumatic stress disorder and major depression. J Neuropsychiatry Clin Neurosci 14: 3.

Rossi, S., De Capua, A., Ulivelli, M., et al. 2007. Effects of repetitive transcranial magnetic stimulation on chronic tinnitus: A randomised, crossover, double blind, placebo controlled study. J Neurol Neurosurg Psychiatry 78(8): 857–63. Epub February 21.

Saba, G., Rocamora, J. F., Kalalou, K., et al. 2002. Catatonia and transcranial magnetic stimulation. Am J Psychiatry 159: 10–12.

Saba, G., Rocamora, J. F., Kalalou, K., et al. 2004. Repetitive transcranial magnetic stimulation as an add-on therapy in the treatment of mania: A case series of eight patients. Psychiatr Res 128: 199–202.

Saba, G., Verdon, C. M., Kalalou, K., et al. 2006. Transcranial magnetic stimulation in the treatment of schizophrenic symptoms: A double blind sham controlled study. J Psychiatr Res 40: 147–52.

Schiffer, F., Stinchfield, Z., and Pascual-Leone, A. 2002. Prediction of clinical response to transcranial magnetic stimulation for depression by baseline lateral visual-field stimulation. Neuropsychiatry Neuropsychol Behav Neurol 15(1): 18–27.

Schulze-Rauschenbach, S. C., Harms, U., Schlaepfer, T. E., et al. 2005. Distinctive neurocognitive effects of repetitive transcranial magnetic stimulation and electroconvulsive therapy in major depression. Br J Psychiatry 186: 410–16.

Speer, A. M., Kimbrell, T. A., Wassermann, E. M., et al. 2000. Opposite effects of high and low frequency rTMS on regional brain activity in depressed patients. Biol Psychiatry 48: 1133–41.

Tassinari, C. A., Cincotta, M., Zaccara, G., and Michelucci, R. 2003. Transcranial magnetic stimulation and epilepsy. Clin Neurophysiol 114: 777–98.

Triggs, W. J., McCoy, K. J., Greer, R., et al. 1999. Effects of left frontal transcranial magnetic stimulation on depressed mood, cognition, and corticomotor threshold. Biol Psychiatry 45: 1440–6.

Wassermann, E. M. 1998. Risk and safety of repetitive transcranial magnetic stimulation: Report and suggested guidelines from the International Workshop on the Safety of Repetitive Transcranial Magnetic Stimulation. Electroencephalogr Clin Neurophysiol 108: 1–16.

Wassermann, E. M., Grafman, J., Berry, C., et al. 1996. Use and safety of a new repetitive transcranial magnetic stimulator. Electroencephalogr Clin Neurophysiol 101: 412–17.

Wassermann, E. M., Wedegaertner, F. R., Ziemann, U., et al. 1998. Crossed reduction of human motor cortex excitability by 1-Hz transcranial magnetic stimulation. Neurosci Lett 250: 141–4.

Xia, G., Gajwani, P., Muzina, D. J., et al. 2008. Treatment-emergent mania in unipolar and bipolar depression: Focus on repetitive transcranial magnetic stimulation. Int J Neuropsychopharmacol 11(1): 119–30. Epub 2007, March 5.

Zwanzger, P. A., Minov, C., Ella, R., et al. 2002b. Transcranial magnetic stimulation for panic disorder. Am J Psychiatry 159: 2.

Zwanzger, P., Ella, R., Keck, M. E., et al. 2002a. Occurrence of delusions during repetitive transcranial magnetic stimulation (rTMS) in major depression. Biol Psychiatry 51(7): 602–3.

Zyss, T., Gorka, Z., Kowalska, M., and Vetulani, J. 1997. Preliminary comparison of behavioral and biochemical effects of chronic transcranial magnetic stimulation and electroconvulsive shock in the rat. Biol Psychiatry 42: 920–4.

36

Vagus nerve stimulation: Indications, efficacy, and methods

Shawn M. McClintock, Kenneth Trevino, and Mustafa M. Husain

Introduction and background

Vagus nerve stimulation (VNS) therapy is a relatively new form of neuromodulation. The U.S. Food and Drug Administration (FDA) has allowed the commercial availability of VNS devices for patients with treatment-resistant depression (TRD) or intractable epilepsy. The VNS system is an implantable device, similar to the size and shape of a cardiac pacemaker. It provides brief intermittent amounts of electrical stimulation to the left vagus nerve.

Neuroanatomy of the vagus nerve

The vagus nerve is the tenth and longest cranial nerve in the human body. In the neck it is located between the carotid arteries and the jugular vein. The vagus nerve is a mixed cranial nerve that consists of both efferent fibers sending impulses to extracranial areas, and afferent fibers bringing impulses to the brain. The majority (80%) are afferent fibers.

Mechanisms of action

Although the exact mechanisms by which VNS therapy works are currently unknown, the antidepressant and anticonvulsant effects of stimulating the vagus nerve may be related to its neuroanatomical pathways. The cell bodies of the afferent fibers that comprise the vagus nerve are located in the nodose ganglion. They project impulses to the nucleus tractus solitarius (NTS) (Sackeim, 2004). These incoming sensory impulses are then projected by the NTS through three main pathways that include (a) an autonomic feedback loop, (b) direct projections to the reticular formation in the medulla, and (c) ascending projections to the forebrain mainly through the parabrachial nucleus (PB) and the locus ceruleus (LC) (George et al., 2000). The PB and LC provide direct connections to multiple regions of the forebrain, including the hypothalamus and thalamic regions that modulate activity in the insula, orbitofrontal, and prefrontal cortices. The PB/LC ceruleus complex also has connections to the amygdala and the red nucleus of the stria ter-minalis. These regions have been implicated in mood regulation (Sackeim, 2004). Through this path, VNS may have antidepressant properties.

In addition to neurophysiological changes through VNS, changes in neurochem-ical activity that develop during stimulation of the vagus nerve may contribute to antidepressant effects. These include increases in γ-aminobutyric acid (GABA) and decreases in glutamate, both of which can produce anticonvulsant effects and perhaps mood stabilization (Walker et al., 1999). Stimulation of the vagus nerve may also enhance transmission of the neurotransmitters norepinephrine and sero-tonin, which have been associated with antidepressant treatments. Stimulation of the LC increases release of norepinephrine, possibly contributing to both the anticonvulsant and antidepressant effects of VNS (Krahl et al., 1998). Stimulation of the vagus nerve increases the major metabolite of serotonin in cerebrospinal fluid – 5-hydroxyindoleacetic acid – implying increased serotonergic activity (Ben-Menachem et al., 1995).

Positron emission tomography (PET) scans indicate that VNS increases regional cerebral blood flow (rCBF) in the rostral medulla, thalamus, hypothalamus, insula, and postcentral gyrus. Other PET studies show decreased blood flow in the hip-pocampus, amygdala, and cingulate gyrus (Henry et al., 1998). Single-photon emission computed tomography (SPECT) demonstrated similar patterns of rCBF changes in many of the same cortical areas (Zobel et al., 2005). Comparable changes in rCBF have been observed in depressed patients who benefited from treatment with selective serotonin reuptake inhibitors (SSRIs) (Kennedy et al., 2001; Mayberg et al., 2000). This similarity suggests that VNS therapy may have antidepressant properties.

VNS therapy system and surgical implant procedure

The VNS therapy system consists of an implantable VNS Therapy Pulse Generator (Cyberonics, Inc., Houston, TX), a lead, and a programming wand. The pulse generator is a multiprogrammable device hermetically sealed in a titanium case. The power supply is provided by a single battery with an estimated life span of three to eight years, but can vary depending on the stimulation delivered (Cyberonics, Inc., 2003).

The brief intermittent electrical pulses produced by the generator are sent directly into the vagus nerve through a lead that is attached by three helical contacts (cathode, anode, and anchor).

The VNS generator is implanted subcutaneously in the left chest wall (Fig-ure 36.1). A small incision in the neck allows for the wrapping of the three helical contacts around the left vagus nerve. The lead is then tunneled subcutaneously

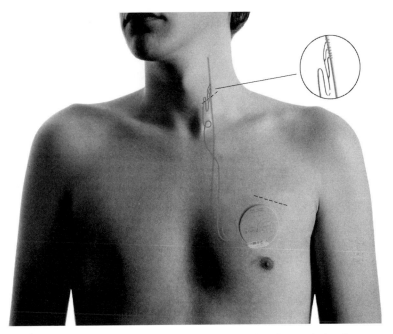

Figure 36.1   The Vagus Nerve Stimulation Therapy System. Reproduced with permission from
Cyberonics, Inc.

to the infraclavicular incision and connected to the generator. The VNS Therapy
System is briefly activated during the implant procedure to verify that the device is
functioning properly and that there is no impedance in the lead connection. The
implant procedure takes one to two hours to complete and is usually performed as
an outpatient procedure. The VNS device is not activated for at least 14 days after
implantation (Cyberonics, Inc., 2003).

Noninvasive programming of the pulse generator is accomplished with a programming wand that is connected to a handheld computer. To set the stimulation
parameters of the generator, the programming wand is first held evenly over the
VNS device and typically over the patient's clothes. The programming wand is used
to interrogate (i.e., communicate with) the device, which involves retrieving and
storing the current treatment parameters of the VNS pulse generator. Upon successful interrogation, the physician is able to activate and adjust different treatment
parameters. Output current, frequency, pulse width, and stimulation on and off
time are the most commonly adjusted parameters. The pulse generators (Models
102 and 102R) currently used for VNS therapy deliver an output current between
0.25 and 3.5 mA, with a signal frequency between 1 and 30 Hz, and a pulse width
from 130 to 1,000 ms. The range of stimulation-on time is from 7 to 60 seconds,

and from 0.2 to 180 minutes for the stimulation-off time. The computer-controlled programming wand can also perform diagnostic tests on the generator and the contact lead to verify proper functioning.

Although the interrogation and programming of the VNS Therapy System is typically performed in a medical setting with trained personnel, the patient can deactivate the device by placing a handheld magnet over it. The pulse generator deactivates automatically if placed under a constant magnetic field, and then resumes stimulation on removal of the magnet. The patient may choose to temporarily deactivate the device to avoid certain side effects (e.g., voice alteration, dyspnea) that can occur during stimulation and might be inconvenient at certain times (e.g., public speaking, exercising).

Indications for the use of VNS

VNS for the treatment of epilepsy

The therapeutic application of VNS was first used as a treatment for patients who were diagnosed with intractable seizures after demonstration that stimulation of the vagus nerve produced anticonvulsant effects (Zabara, 1985a, 1985b, 1992). In laboratory animal studies, direct stimulation was applied to the vagus nerve to assess effects on artificially induced seizures. Zabara's research indicated that stimulation of the vagus nerve was able to interrupt and even terminate seizure activity induced in canines.

The first clinical investigation of VNS for treating intractable partial seizures was conducted in 1988 (Penry and Dean, 1990). Based on the positive results, additional large-scale trials were conducted (Ben-Menachem et al., 1994; George et al., 1994; Ramsay et al., 1994). These additional trials examined the safety and efficacy of both acute and long-term VNS therapy in patients who experienced treatment-recalcitrant seizures. The results demonstrated that VNS therapy significantly reduced frequency and severity of seizures. Relatively mild and limited side effects support the safety of VNS therapy.

VNS therapy was approved in the European Union for the therapeutic application of intractable epilepsy in 1994. In July 1997, the FDA approved the commercial availability of VNS devices in adjunctive treatment to reduce seizures in adults and adolescents older than 12 years with medically refractory partial-onset seizures. A total of 32,065 VNS therapy devices were implanted for treating epilepsy between 1997 and 2004.

Rationale for VNS in depression

The application of VNS in treating depression is consistent with the use of anticonvulsant medications (e.g., carbamazepine, gabapentin, lamotrigine, and valproate) in treating severe mood disorders (George et al., 2003; Post et al., 1998). Additional evidence for using VNS in depression is related to the neuroanatomy of the vagus nerve, proposed mechanisms of action during stimulation of the vagus nerve, and various positive clinical reports from epileptic patients who received VNS therapy (Nemeroff et al., 2006).

Regarding neuroanatomy, there are many regions of the brain related to depression that have monosynaptic and polysynaptic connections with the NTS, to which the afferent fibers of the vagus nerve project (Drevets, 2000; George et al. 2000; Sackeim, 2004). PET imaging has demonstrated that stimulation of the vagus nerve influences the functioning of various structures within the brainstem and limbic system (Henry et al., 1998) in a manner similar to the effects of antidepressant medications (Mayberg et al., 1997; Schlaepfer and Kosel, 2005), as VNS alters the concentration of serotonin, norepinephrine, GABA, and glutamate (Ben-Menachem et al., 1995; Walker et al., 1999).

The most compelling evidence for VNS antidepressant effects comes from case reports of improved mood in patients who participated in VNS trials for the treatment of epilepsy. Interestingly, this mood effect was independent of changes in the frequency or intensity of the patients' seizure activity (Sackeim, 2004; Schlaepfer and Kosel, 2005). Based on these clinical observations, a small pilot study was conducted and the results suggested VNS had antidepressant properties (Harden et al., 2000). To confirm these findings, two trials were conducted over the course of nine years to investigate the therapeutic benefits of VNS therapy for patients with depression.

Pilot study of VNS in depression

The initial trial was an open-label pilot study of feasibility and safety of VNS in patients with major depressive disorder (MDD) or bipolar type I or II disorder (Rush et al., 2000). Required were a current major depressive episode (MDE) lasting for a minimum of two years or at least four lifetime MDEs, with failure to benefit from two or more antidepressant treatments. The pilot study was conducted at four university medical centers. Of the first 30 participants completing the acute phase, 40% to 50% showed a significant (at least 50%) decrease in depression severity, and 17% experienced remission (defined as a 28-item HRSD score of 10 or less) (Hamilton, 1960). Unfortunately, the second set of 30 patients showed less favorable results, with response and remission rates of 20.7% and 13.8%, respectively. Collectively, 37.3% showed improvement per the Clinical Global Impression scale (Guy, 1976), 57.7% showed no change, and the remainder showed worsening (Sackeim et al., 2001a).

The pilot trial showed both acute and long-term benefits (Marangell et al., 2002). After nine months of active stimulation, 46% and 29% of the initial 30 participants

Table 36.1 Vagus nerve stimulation parameters for the pilot and pivotal trials

	Pilot trial	Pivotal trial
Output current	0.25–3.0 mA	0.75–1.0 mA (range: 0.00–2.25 mA)
Signal frequency	20 or 30 Hz	20 Hz (range: 2–30 Hz)
Pulse width	250–500 ms	500 ms (range: 130–750 ms)
Signal-on time	30 s	30 s (range: 7–60 s)
Signal-off time	5 min	5 min (range: 0.20–180 min)

showed response and remission, respectively. Clinical benefit increased from the acute phase to the long-term phase, suggesting that VNS may be more effective in the long term (Husain et al., 2006). General quality of life was improved, and as patients developed tolerance to stimulation, adverse effects decreased.

Pivotal trial of VNS to treat depression

Next was a double-masked trial to determine the efficacy in treating depression at 21 sites across the United States. A total of 235 patients with MDD or bipolar type I or II disorder were randomized 1:1 to receive either sham or active VNS. After two weeks of surgical recovery, patients in the active group received stimulation for 10 weeks. At the end of the acute phase, the sham and active groups showed no significant difference in clinical outcome (Rush et al., 2005a).

The different outcomes between the pilot and pivotal trials may have been due to methodological differences, perhaps in stimulation parameters (see Table 36.1). The mean output current in the pivotal trial (0.67 mA) was lower than the mean output current in the pilot trial (0.96 mA). To address the clinical effects of VNS current output, a double-masked clinical investigation is currently studying three different settings: low dose (0.25 mA), moderate dose (0.5 to 1.0 mA), and high dose (1.25 to 1.5 mA).

As in the pilot trial, the pivotal trial showed additional clinical benefit following long-term VNS stimulation (Rush et al., 2005b). Decreases in depression severity scores were observed each month. After 12 months of active stimulation, the response and remission rates increased to 29.8% and 17.1%, respectively. A longitudinal observational investigation of patients enrolled in the pivotal trial who did not receive the VNS implant found that 12.5% responded to treatment as usual at the 12-month follow-up (George et al., 2005).

Treatment-Resistant Depression (TRD)

Currently VNS has the FDA indication of adjunctive long-term treatment of patients with recurrent or chronic major depressive disorders who have failed to respond to at least four separate antidepressant medication trials. Between 29% and 46% of depressed patients fail to fully respond to treatment with antidepressant medication at adequate dose and duration, and 19% to 34% show no response (Fava and Davidson, 1996).

Although TRD has been accepted as a type of depression, it is not codified in the *Diagnostic and Statistical Manual of Mental Disorders* (DSM-IV-TR) (American Psychiatric Association, 2000) and so remains incompletely defined. The number of treatment courses that a patient must fail for the patient's depression to qualify as TRD is not established. It has been proposed that at least two monotherapy trials of antidepressant medications from different pharmacological classes should be attempted (Trivedi, 2000). The medication should be administered at an adequate dose for a sufficient duration, typically at least six weeks (Fava and Davidson, 1996). After multiple failed antidepressant trials and a chronic and debilitating pattern of depression, VNS therapy may be considered as an adjunctive treatment.

Separate from depression severity, severity of treatment resistance is rated for VNS candidates. This rating follows the number of unsuccessful medication trials: mild after two or three, moderate after four or five, and severe after six or more.

Suggested guidelines for VNS applications

Patient selection

Highly selective clinical decision making is appropriate for VNS prescription. There is limited empirical research regarding selection of patients for this treatment. The depressive episode at entry into the pilot and pivotal trials was rated severe on both objective and subjective structured scales. Accordingly, VNS should be used as an adjunctive treatment in only patients with severe, chronic TRD.

Analyses of 59 patients in the pilot trial found that patients were more likely to improve with VNS if they had never received ECT, as were those whose treatment resistance was rated as moderate rather than severe (Sackeim et al., 2001a). VNS might initially be ineffective for patients with severe treatment resistance, but following long-term use may become effective. Indeed, at two-year follow-up in the pilot trial, Nahas et al. (2005) found no significant relationship between severity of treatment resistance and clinical outcome. Patients with low to moderate treatment resistance showed a trend for better response than did those with severe TRD, but differences between the groups did not reach statistical significance.

VNS may be a beneficial treatment alternative for patients who are intolerant to antidepressants or when antidepressants are contraindicated. Particularly, VNS

Table 36.2 Vagus nerve stimulation
device parameters

Output current	Signal-on time
Signal frequency	Signal-off time
Pulse width	Magnet current

can be used with patients who also receive ECT and those who are planning to become pregnant. In the pivotal trial, 14 patients received ECT along with VNS, and there were no complications (Burke and Husain, 2006). Just before ECT was administered, the VNS device was turned off. After ECT, the same stimulation settings were restarted. The VNS device was unaffected by ECT (Burke and Husain, 2006). This lack of effect by VNS exposure on ECT is notable, as several psychotropic drugs interfere with ECT.

For pregnant patients, VNS may provide an alternative to antidepressant medications, given their risks to the pregnancy (Chambers et al., 1996; Moses-Kolko et al., 2005). There is one case report that documents the use of VNS therapy in a pregnant woman (Husain et al., 2005). The woman had started VNS therapy three years prior to pregnancy. She received active VNS stimulation throughout her pregnancy, including labor and delivery, without complication to herself or her baby. However, more data in addition to the one case report are needed before an experienced-based recommendation can be made.

In general, there is limited research to guide clinical decision making in selecting VNS therapy for patients. From the data available, clinicians may prescribe the use of VNS therapy only for patients with severe major depressive disorders that are clearly chronic and moderately treatment resistant.

VNS stimulation parameter settings

The VNS device parameter settings (see Table 36.2) can be set and adjusted by a trained medical professional with the programming wand. Initially, when the device is first activated (typically two weeks postimplantation), the output current should be set at 0.25 mA to allow for the patient to acclimate to stimulation. Thereafter, parameter settings may be adjusted to maximize efficacy and tolerability. At the present time, there is limited information to guide clinical decision making about stimulation dosing at low, moderate, or high currents. Empirical investigations are in progress to resolve this issue and provide guidance for determining therapeutic treatment parameters.

To ensure that the VNS device is properly functioning, it should be interrogated at each patient assessment with the programming wand. This interrogation ensures appropriate parameter settings and assesses for device changes between visits.

Table 36.3 Vagus nerve stimulation (VNS) therapy-associated adverse effects

VNS device implantation related	VNS stimulation related
Incision pain	Most common: voice alteration, increased cough
Incision site reaction (i.e., itching)	Least common: Dyspnea, neck pain, dysphagia,
Voice alteration	laryngismus, paresthesia

Annual or biannual device diagnostic evaluations are also important to assure proper output, desirable lead impedance, and battery reserve. The diagnostic evaluation assesses device and lead integrity at amplitudes of 0.25 mA to 1.00 mA. For patients who are unable to tolerate moderate to high stimulation doses, the diagnostic test may produce mild pain sensations. These sensations usually terminate upon test completion in about 30 seconds.

Patient safety and adverse effects

Patients should be monitored regularly throughout the course of treatment with VNS for adverse effects (see Table 36.3). There are two categories of adverse effects associated with VNS therapy: surgical implantation effects and VNS stimulation effects. It is common for patients to experience tenderness or pain around the incision site, but these typically dissipate over time. To reduce aggravation of incision-related discomfort, stimulation should be postponed for at least two weeks, until it is clinically determined that the surgical side effects are no longer present.

The VNS stimulation may produce some mild discomfort (Rush et al., 2005a). The two most common are voice alteration and increased cough. Most stimulation-related adverse effects decrease over time, and most patients develop tolerance except to voice alteration. These effects are reversible. During active stimulation, the patient who has difficulty talking should find return of his or her normal voice when stimulation ceases. To aid tolerance development, the VNS output current may be reduced or other stimulation parameters may be modulated (Sackeim, 2004).

There have been few documented cases of serious adverse events in VNS therapy. In the pilot study, serious adverse events that could have been related to VNS therapy included implantation-related infection, leg pain, worsening of depression, and agitation/panic (Sackeim et al., 2001a). In the pivotal trial, serious adverse events reported over a 12-month period included development of mania in three patients, suicide attempt in seven patients, and worsening of depression in 30 patients (which required hospitalization) (Rush et al., 2005b). Because the patients in these two trials had longstanding severe depression, and some had prior hospitalizations and suicide attempts, these severe adverse events were relatively small, and many were probably not actually related to VNS therapy (Rush et al., 2005b; Sackeim et al., 2001a).

There has been little research on the neuropsychological effects of VNS. Within the initial cohort of patients enrolled in the pilot study, 27 provided information related to their cognitive functioning before and after VNS (Sackeim et al., 2001b). No cognitive impairments (i.e, decreased memory) were identified. Improvement occurred in executive function, psychomotor function, and motor speed. Sackeim et al. (2001b) speculated that these cognitive improvements were attributable to decreased depression severity. Data to date have identified no substantial adverse cognitive effects. Monitoring of cognitive functioning and adverse events should be standard practice with any neuromodulation therapy. Systematic monitoring can help to detect relationships between stimulation parameter settings and adverse events, and the patient's development of tolerance.

Conclusions and future directions

VNS therapy represents a new antidepressant modality for TRD (Corcoran et al., 2006; Rush et al., 2005a). The commercial availability of VNS for treating refractory epilepsy was approved by the FDA in 1997. Eight years later, based on findings of the pilot and pivotal trials, the FDA approved VNS availability for adjunctive long-term use in chronic TRD.

Both the pilot and pivotal investigations found VNS therapy to be moderately beneficial with modest response and remission rates. No life-threatening side effects occurred, and the most troublesome effects were voice alteration and increased coughing. Most patients eventually developed tolerance to most adverse effects. VNS did not produce any identifiable neurocognitive impairment (Sackeim et al., 2001b). At two-year follow-up, 48 of 59 patients in the pilot trial were still receiving VNS (Nahas et al., 2005). Although VNS therapy has demonstrated reasonable safety and tolerability, and modest clinical benefit, questions remain unanswered about mechanism of action (Nemeroff et al., 2006; O'Keane et al., 2005), dosage (Rush et al., 2005a), predictors of response and remission (Sackeim et al., 2001a), and long-term side effects (Nahas et al., 2005).

Editor's note

Unfortunately, comorbid anxiety disorders were not accounted for in the pilot and pivotal VNS trials. They are common in mood disorders, especially when chronic, and they influence ratings of depression and quality of life. Moreover, VNS might diminish the somatic tension symptoms of anxiety disorders in a manner similar to psychotropic anticonvulsant medications, perhaps paralleling the anticonvulsant effects of VNS. Such an effect can explain some improvement shown with VNS in resistant depression.

Evaluation and treatment of anxiety disorders and their psychological and somatic
tension components should be considered along the course of treating mood disorders.
–CMS

References

American Psychiatric Association. 2000. Diagnostic and Statistical Manual of Mental Disorders, 4th edn., Text Revision. Washington, DC, American Psychiatric Association.

Ben-Menachem, E., Hamberger, A., Hedner, T., et al. 1995. Effects of vagus nerve stimulation on amino acids and other metabolites in the CSF of patients with partial seizures. Epilepsy Res 20: 221–7.

Ben-Menachem, E., Manon-Espaillat, R., Ristanovic, R., et al. 1994. Vagus nerve stimulation for treatment of partial seizures: 1. A controlled study of effect on seizures. First International Vagus Nerve Stimulation Study Group. Epilepsia 35: 616–26.

Burke, M. J. and Husain, M. M. 2006. Concomitant use of vagus nerve stimulation and electroconvulsive therapy for treatment-resistant depression. J ECT 22(3): 218–22.

Chambers, C. D., Johnson, K. A., Dick, L. M., et al. 1996. Birth outcomes in pregnant women taking fluoxetine. N Engl J Med 335(14): 1010–15.

Corcoran, C. D., Thomas, P., Phillips, J., et al. 2006. Vagus nerve stimulation in chronic treatment-resistant depression. Br J Psychiatry 189: 282–3.

Cyberonics, Inc. 2003. Physician's Manual. VNS Therapy (TM) Pulse Model 102 Generator and VNS Therapy (TM) Pulse Duo Model 102R Generator. Available at: http://www.vnstherapy.com/manuals/doc_download.asp?docid={E5D2100B A4C2-409B-B71C-E1CEA60FBD90}, accessed April 10, 2006.

Drevets, W. C. 2000. Neuroimaging studies of mood disorders. Biol Psychiatry 48: 813–29.

Fava, M. and Davidson, K. G. 1996. Definition and epidemiology of treatment-resistant depression. Psychiatr Clin North Am 19: 179–200.

George, M. S., Rush, A. J., Sackeim, H. A., and Marangell, L. B. 2003. Vagus nerve stimulation (VNS): Utility in neuropsychiatric disorders. Int J Neuropsychopharmacol 6: 73–83.

George, M. S., Rush, A. J., Marangell, L. B., et al. 2005. A one-year comparison of VNS with treatment as usual for treatment-resistant depression. Biol Psychiatry 58: 364–73.

George, M. S., Sackeim, H. A., Rush, A. J., et al. 2000. Vagus nerve stimulation: A new tool for brain research and therapy. Biol Psychiatry 47: 287–95.

George, R., Salinsky, M., Kuzniecky, R., et al. 1994. Vagus nerve stimulation for treatment of partial seizures: 3. Long-term follow-up on first 67 patients exiting a controlled study. First International Vagus Nerve Stimulation Study Group. Epilepsia 35: 637–43.

Guy, W. 1976. ECDEU assessment manual for psychopharmacology. Publication No. 76-338. Washington, DC: Superintendent of Documents, U.S. Government Printing Office, U.S. Dept. of Health, Education, and Welfare.

Hamilton, M. 1960. A rating scale for depression. J Neurol Neurosurg Psychiatry 23: 56–62.

Harden, C. L., Pulver, M. C., Ravdin, L. D., et al. 2000. A pilot study of mood in epilepsy patients treated with vagus nerve stimulation. Epilepsy Behav 1: 93–9.

Henry, T. R., Bakay, R. A., Votaw, J. R., et al. 1998. Brain blood flow alterations induced by therapeutic vagus nerve stimulation in partial epilepsy: I. Acute effects at high and low levels of stimulation. Epilepsia 39: 983–90.

Husain, M. M., McClintock, S. M., Trevino, K., et al. 2006. Vagus nerve stimulation for treatment-resistant depression. Essent Psychopharmacol 7: 91–7.

Husain, M. M., Stegman, D., and Trevino, K. 2005. Pregnancy and delivery while receiving vagus nerve stimulation for the treatment of major depression: A case report. Ann Gen Psychiatry 4: 16.

Kennedy, S. H., Evans, K. R., Kruger, S., et al. 2001. Changes in regional brain glucose metabolism measured with PET after paroxetine treatment of major depression. Am J Psychiatry 158: 899–905.

Krahl, S. E., Clark, K. B., Smith, D. C., and Browning, R. A. 1998. Locus coeruleus lesions suppress the seizure-attenuating effects of vagus nerve stimulation. Epilepsia 39: 709–14.

Marangell, L. B., Rush, A. J., George, M. S., et al. 2002. Vagus nerve stimulation (VNS) for major depressive episodes: One year outcomes. Biol Psychiatry 51: 280–7.

Mayberg, H. S., Brannan, S. K., Mahurin, R. K., et al. 1997. Cingulate function in depression: A potential predictor of treatment response. Neuroreport 8: 1057–61.

Mayberg, H. S., Brannan, S. K., Tekell, J. L., et al. 2000. Regional metabolic effects of fluoxetine in major depression: Serial changes and relationship to clinical response. Biol Psychiatry 48: 830–43.

Moses-Kolko, E. L., Bogen, D., Bregar, A., et al. 2005. Neonatal signs after late in utero exposure to serotonin reuptake inhibitors: Literature review and implications for clinical applications. JAMA 293: 2372–83.

Nahas, Z., Marangell, L. B., Husain, M. M., et al. 2005. Two-year outcome of vagus nerve stimulation (VNS) for treatment of major depressive episodes. J Clin Psychiatry 66: 1097–104.

Nemeroff, C. B., Mayberg, H. S., Krahl, S. E., et al. 2006. VNS therapy in treatment-resistant depression: Clinical evidence and putative neurobiological mechanisms. Neuropsychopharmacology 31: 1345–55.

O'Keane, V., Dinan, T. G., Scott, L., Corcoran, C. 2005. Changes in hypothalamic-pituitary-adrenal axis measures after vagus nerve stimulation therapy in chronic depression. Biol Psychiatry 58: 963–8.

Penry, J. K. and Dean, J. C. 1990. Prevention of intractable partial seizures by intermittent vagal stimulation in humans: Preliminary results. Epilepsia 31(Suppl 2): S40–S43.

Post, R. M., Denicoff, K. D., Frye, M. A., et al. 1998. A history of the use of anticonvulsants as mood stabilizers in the last two decades of the 20th century. Neuropsychobiology 38: 152–66.

Ramsay, R. E., Uthman, B. M., Augustinsson, L. E., et al. 1994. Vagus nerve stimulation for treatment of partial seizures: 2. Safety, side effects, and tolerability. First International Vagus Nerve Stimulation Study Group. Epilepsia 35: 627–36.

Rush, A. J., George, M. S., Sackeim, H. A., et al. 2000. Vagus nerve stimulation (VNS) for treatment-resistant depression: A multicenter study. Biol Psychiatry 47: 276–86.

Rush, A. J., Marangell, L. B., Sackeim, H. A., et al. 2005a. Vagus nerve stimulation for treatment-resistant depression: A randomized controlled acute phase trial. Biol Psychiatry 58: 347–54.

Rush, A. J., Sackeim, H. A., Marangell, L. B., et al. 2005b. Effects of 12 months of vagus nerve stimulation in treatment-resistant depression: A naturalistic study. Biol Psychiatry 58: 355–63.

Sackeim, H. A. 2004. Vagus nerve stimulation. In Brain stimulation in psychiatric treatment (ed., Lisanby, S. H.). Washington, DC: American Psychiatric Publishing, pp. 99–143.

Sackeim, H. A., Keilp, J. G., Rush, A. J., et al. 2001b. The effects of vagus nerve stimulation on cognitive performance in patients with treatment-resistant depression. Neuropsychiatry Neuropsychol Behav Neurol 14: 53–62.

Sackeim, H. A., Rush, A. J., George, M. S., et al. 2001a. Vagus nerve stimulation (VNS™) for treatment-resistant depression: Efficacy, side effects, and predictors of outcome. Neuropsychopharmacology 25: 713–28.

Schlaepfer, T. E. and Kosel, M. 2005. Brain stimulation in depression. In Mood disorders: Clinical management and research issues (ed., Griez, E. J. L.). Chichester, UK: Wiley, pp. 403–25.

Trivedi, M. H. 2000. Treatment-resistant depression: New therapies on the horizon. Ann Clin Psychiatry 57: 581–90.

Walker, B. R., Easton, A., and Gale, K. 1999. Regulation of limbic motor seizures by GABA and glutamate transmission in nucleus tractus solitarius. Epilepsia 40: 1051–7.

Zabara, J. 1985a. Time course of seizure control to brief, repetitive stimuli. Epilepsia 26: 518.

Zabara, J. 1985b. Peripheral control of hypersynchronous discharge in epilepsy. Electroencephelography Clin Neurophysiol 61: P26.05.

Zabara, J. 1992. Inhibition of experimental seizures in canines by repetitive vagal stimulation. Epilepsia 33: 1005–12.

Zobel, A., Joe, A., Freymann, N., et al. 2005. Changes in regional cerebral blood flow by therapeutic vagus nerve stimulation in depression: An exploratory approach. Psychiatry Res 139: 165–79.

37

Deep brain stimulation: Methods, indications, locations, and efficacy

Thomas E. Schläpfer and Bettina Heike Bewernick

Introduction

There remain a sizable number of patients who are not helped by traditional forms of pharmacological or somatic psychiatric treatment or psychotherapy. After five years of treatment, 8% to 13% of patients suffering from major depression have a poor outcome (Keller et al., 1992), and 63.2% of patients included in the Sequenced Treatment Alternatives to Relieve Depression (STAR*D) study did not achieve remission in the acute study phase (Rush et al., 2006). These patients are called "treatment resistant" and have been treated with several antidepressants (e.g., tricyclics, selective serotonin reuptake inhibitors), augmentation agents (e.g., lithium, antipsychotics), psychotherapy, and often electroconvulsive therapy (ECT). In obsessive-compulsive disorder (OCD), treatment resistance occurs in 10% to 40% (Ferrão et al., 2007; Keller and Baker, 1992). These patients have little hope of recovery, are substantially impaired, and do not enjoy a reasonable quality of life. Treatment-resistant psychiatric disorders are a significant source of worldwide disability (Murray and Lopez, 1997). For these patients, alternative treatment methods are needed. Here we review the method of deep brain stimulation (DBS), only recently applied in highly selected patients with treatment-resistant major depression or OCD.

In this review, knowledge about the neurobiology of depression and OCD and historical treatment methods are outlined. Principles of DBS and reasons for the use of DBS in psychiatry are discussed. Targets have been chosen in a hypothesis-guided approach, and first results have demonstrated that DBS can manipulate pathological neural networks in major depression and OCD. Although DBS is a unique and promising method for otherwise treatment-resistant psychiatric patients, mandatory standards are needed for patient and target selection and quality in research study protocols. This review also considers ethical aspects of DBS in psychiatric patients.

DBS method

History and principles of DBS

Electrical stimulation of the brain began in 1879, when limb movements were elicited by stimulating the motor cortex in dogs. Human studies followed in 1884 (Gildenberg, 2005). The first chronic brain stimulation was performed in the mid-20th century, when the nucleus caudatus was stimulated for eight weeks in a case of a severely depressed patient (Fins, 2003). Insights from lesioning studies, imaging studies, and animal models have contributed to the development of DBS. Chronic DBS was introduced for the treatment of movement disorders (Benabid et al., 1987). Today, this method is used clinically for the treatment of tremor associated with dystonia or Parkinson's disease and to mitigate chronic pain.

In dystonia, DBS has been applied to the internal globus pallidus and to the thalamus. Improvement rates are higher with the former, 39% to 71%. Adverse effects were primarily dysarthria, and no cognitive side effects were reported. The availability of DBS for primary generalized or segmental dystonia is approved by the U.S. Food and Drug Administration (FDA).

In Parkinson's disease, DBS of the ventral intermediate nucleus reduced tremor. Stimulation of the subthalamic nucleus produced a sustained reduction in tremor, rigidity, and akinesia with reduction in dopaminergic medication and improvements in rated quality of life. Motor side effects, speech difficulty, and induced mood elevations or depressions were reversible. DBS of the internal globus pallidus also improved tremor, rigidity, and bradykinesia but did not allow reduction in levodopa dose. Side effects such as visual phenomena are reportedly less frequent at this latter site.

The occurrence of psychiatric effects in patients receiving DBS for neurological conditions (e.g., changes in mood, hypomania, reduction of anxiety) motivated consideration that DBS might treat psychiatric disorders (Mallet et al., 2002). It also raised the possibility that the benefits of irreversible ablative neurosurgical interventions (i.e., psychosurgery) can be obtained in a focused, titratable, and apparently reversible method with DBS (see Figure 37.1).

DBS is achieved by an implanted, battery-powered neurostimulator and is usually placed subcutaneously in the chest area. The exact neurobiological mechanisms by which DBS exerts effects on brain tissue are not yet fully understood (Hardesty and Sackeim, 2007). On the neuronal level, excitatory and inhibitory processes might play a role (McIntyre et al., 2004). Most probably, DBS leads to a functional lesion of the surrounding tissue. Further mechanisms are depolarization blockade of current dependent ion channels (Beurrier et al., 2001), exhaustion of the neurotransmitter pool (Zucker and Regehr, 2002), or synaptic inhibition

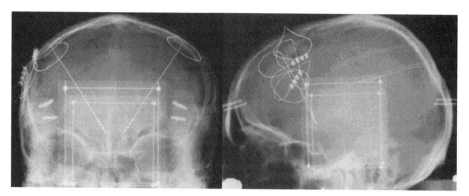

Figure 37.1   Location of the electrode leads in the postoperative control x-ray in a deep brain stimulation study for depression. Schläpfer, T. E., Cohen, M. X., Frick, C., et al. 2007. Deep brain stimulation to reward circuitry alleviates anhedonia in refractory major depression. Neuropsychopharmacology 33: 368–77.

(Dostrovsky et al., 2000). Today, it is unknown which part of the neuron (e.g., cell body, axon) is primarily modulated by DBS. Certainly, the stimulation volume is not a fixed area around the electrode, and the effect on neuronal tissue is variable. The effect of DBS on neurons depends on different factors: the physiological properties of the surrounding brain tissue, the geometric configuration of the electrode, and the distance and orientation of the neuronal elements toward the electrode (Kringelbach et al., 2007). Stimulation parameters (frequency, amplitude, pulse width, duration) clearly have an impact on the effect (Ranck, 1975). With commonly used methods, a relatively large volume of neural tissue is influenced (Kringelbach et al., 2007).

Neurophysiologic recordings during stimulation have demonstrated that the oscillatory activity between brain structures is modulated by DBS in patients with movement disorders (Kringelbach et al., 2007). Changes in neurotransmitter release (glutamate, dopamine) and brain-derived neurotrophic factor have been reported (Hilker et al., 2002; Stefani et al., 2006). Functional neuroimaging data have demonstrated that DBS changes the activity of brain areas far beyond the targeted region, and so complex neural networks are modulated (Kringelbach et al., 2007; Mayberg et al., 2005; Schnitzler and Gross, 2005; Stefurak et al., 2003). These results appear to match the long-term changes described in psychiatric patients. The reversibility of DBS effects is presumed but not proven; it is conceivable that network alterations made by DBS could eventually persist after stimulation is stopped.

In summary, short-term changes can explain the acute effects of DBS in movement disorders. In psychiatric disorders, long-term changes in symptoms have been described. These can result only from long-lasting, complex modulation of neural networks (McIntyre et al., 2004).

Safety and advantages of DBS

Side effects in DBS are related either to the operation itself (e.g., bleeding, local infections at the chest) or to the stimulation (e.g., elevation of mood, anxiety, motor slowing). The safety of the stereotactic operation technique has been markedly improved in recent years with the help of neuroimaging. The bleeding rate in DBS surgery is between 0.2% and 5% (Kühn et al., 2007). It is worth emphasizing that no side effects (such as extrapyramidal effects or weight gain) that substantially affect compliance have been reported.

DBS has many advantages over traditional therapy methods. Clinical effects can be achieved without irreversible lesioning, stereotactic operation is a minimal neurosurgical method, and electrodes can be completely removed if necessary. Brain activity can be changed in a direct, controlled manner. Furthermore, DBS offers the opportunity to continuously adjust stimulation variables for each patient to optimize therapy. The patient can turn off stimulation immediately if side effects occur. DBS is the only neurosurgical method that allows blinded studies for therapy control. It has not been found to have any effect that substantially decreases compliance or quality of life. Until extensive clinical experience and trials are obtained, it is premature to consider DBS as suitable for other than treatment-resistant patients.

Overall, DBS is a distinctive treatment method. Besides its potential use in treatment, it offers unique possibilities to gain insight into the underlying neurobiology of psychiatric disorders.

Neurobiology of depression and OCD

Characteristic symptoms of depression are sadness, lack of interest and motivation, anhedonia, disturbances in sleep and appetite, hopelessness, suicidal thoughts, psychomotor slowing, feelings of guilt, and cognitive deficits generally pertaining to attention, concentration, and problem solving. Major depression can be conceptualized by the interaction of genetic, neurobiological, environmental, and psychological factors (Belmaker and Agam, 2008). The relevance of transmitters (e.g., serotonin, noradrenaline, and dopamine; Berton and Nestler, 2006) as well as the involvement of several genes in the genesis of depression (Shelton, 2007) has been demonstrated (Berton and Nestler, 2006). However, up to today evidence of the involvement of specific genes is unclear. Life events and daily stresses clearly are examples of psychological factors that contribute to the etiology of depression (Sher, 2004).

In contrast to neurological disorders, the pathological interplay of several brain regions contributes to the development of this disease. Metabolic studies suggest that several depressive symptoms are mediated by brain regions (Yurgelun-Todd et al., 2007). A network model of depression that integrates biochemical, electro-physiological, imaging, and animal studies has been described by Mayberg (1997). According to this model, depression results from a dysregulation of limbic–cortical connections. Pathological changes in dorsal brain regions (including the dorsolat-eral prefrontal cortex, inferior parietal cortex, and striatum) are associated with cognitive symptoms (e.g., apathy, anhedonia, hopelessness, and deficits in attention and executive function). Changes in ventral areas (hypothalamic–pituitary–adrenal axis, insula, subgenual cingulate, and brainstem) contribute to the vegetative and somatic aspects of depression (e.g., sleep disturbance, appetite, endocrine dysregu-lation). This model underlines the role of the rostral cingulate cortex in regulating the network (Mayberg, 1997). The involvement of additional brain regions in depression can be considered: The hippocampus contributes to memory deficits, the nucleus accumbens is associated with anhedonia and lack of motivation, and the amygdala plays a role in the processing of aversive stimuli and avoidance (Berton and Nestler, 2006). DBS neurobiology in depression is discussed later in this chapter.

OCD is characterized by obsessions (anxiety-provoking thoughts) and compul-sions (repeated, time-consuming behaviors) (Stein, 2002). As in most psychiatric disorders, a complex interplay of genetic factors, neurotransmitter changes, and psychosocial characteristics contribute to the development of this disease. Changes in dopamine and serotonin have been reported (Stein, 2002). Dysfunctions in a network connecting the cortex and basal ganglia are thought to underlie OCD. Imaging data have demonstrated changes in orbitofrontal cortex, anterior cingu-late cortex, and caudate nucleus in OCD (Baxter, 1990). New evidence suggests that there are several different pathological patterns within these brain regions, each associated with specific symptoms. It appears that overactivation of the direct pathway of the cortico–striatal–pallidal–thalamic–cortical loop leads to intrusive thoughts and other OCD symptoms (Baxter et al., 2001).

Studies of DBS and psychiatric disorders

Problems in target selection

In DBS studies, a hypothesis-guided search for a target is necessary. In psychiatric disorders, targets have been chosen by using knowledge derived from lesion and imaging studies as well as from current understanding of the pathophysiology of the disorder. There is no single pathological structure in psychiatric illness. Several brain structures presumably play a variety of roles in the development and maintenance of symptoms. Some targets are in close anatomical or functional relationship (neural networks), and an overlap of effect is plausible. It has been shown that alteration of several targets can lead to remission. Thus, different targets can be used to manipulate the pathological network.

DBS targets in depression

The anterior limb of the internal capsule is a prominent target for DBS in depression. Historic lesion studies contributed to the hypothesis that the inactivation of larger brain areas inhibits dysfunctional connections through this region. The role of the internal capsule in depression is unclear; interest in this brain region for depression is an outgrowth of its use as a target in OCD. After one month of DBS, there was a substantial reduction in depression in a majority of patients, by Montgomery-Asberg Depression Rating scores. This outcome remained stable with some fluctuation over half a year (Malone et al., 2008).

The subgenual cingulate cortex (Brodmann area Cg25) has been stimulated with DBS (Mayberg et al., 2005). This region modulates negative mood states, is involved in the onset of sadness, and seems to be involved in the effect of some antidepressant drugs. The rostral part of the cingulate cortex plays a role in modulating the network associated with depression. Mayberg and colleagues (2005) demonstrated that, two months after surgery, five of six patients met the criterion for clinical response (decrease in baseline Hamilton Rating Scale for Depression [HRSD] score by 50%). After six months, four patients showed sustained response. Several neuropsychological functions that were impaired at baseline were significantly improved. A reduction in the pathological hyperactivity in this region has also been demonstrated using positron emission tomography in this study. During the blinded sham stimulation phase ($n = 1$), the patient's condition worsened considerably. No adverse events from stimulation were observed (Mayberg et al., 2005).

We selected the nucleus accumbens as a target for DBS because of its prominent role in the reward system. The nucleus accumbens regulates motivation for motor activity associated with the processing of emotions in the limbic system. Modulation of this structure was associated with changes in the symptoms of anhedonia and mood in three depressed patients (Schläpfer et al., 2007). The stimulation current correlated negatively with anhedonia ratings. Normalization of brain metabolism in frontostriatal networks as a result of stimulation was also observed (Schläpfer et al., 2007). No side effects were observed from DBS. Results of the nine patients in this study show acute as well as long-term antidepressant effects of DBS at this target (Bewernick et al., in preparation).

Single-case studies in OCD patients with comorbid depression have shown antidepressant effects. Bilateral stimulation of the ventral caudate nucleus in combination with the nucleus accumbens for OCD led to remission of depression

(HRSD 17-item-version, score under 7) after six months. No neuropsychological deterioration was reported (Aouizerate et al., 2004). Bilateral stimulation of the lower thalamus stem also led to remission in one depressed patient (drop in HRSD score from 42 to10). The effect remained stable for 24 months (Jiménez et al., 2005). During blind discontinuation of stimulation, the patient's condition deteriorated. Dysregulation of the connection between unspecific thalamic system and orbitofrontal cortex seems to play an important role in the development of depression (Jiménez et al., 2005).

In summary, five different targets sites are currently evaluated in scientific studies for DBS in depression therapy. Because of small sample sizes the most effective target sites have not yet been identified. Sustained antidepressant effects have been demonstrated, making DBS a desirable therapy possibility for treatment-resistant depression (see Table 37.1).

Targets in OCD

In OCD, several targets have been selected for DBS according to the underlying pathological network (see Table 37.2). Because the contribution of single brain structures to the pathology of OCD has not been elucidated, the targets have been selected from lesional and imaging studies. In most studies, the anterior limb of the internal capsule was the target for either unilateral or bilateral stimulation (Abelson et al., 2005; Anderson and Ahmed, 2003; Gabriëls et al., 2003; Nuttin et al., 1999, 2003b; Sturm et al., 2003). All studies reported promising results, ranging from response to complete remission. In terms of side effects, some studies reported symptoms of hypomania induced by stimulation. These ceased completely after reduction of stimulation intensity (Greenberg et al., 2006; Nuttin et al., 1999, 2003b).

The nucleus thalamicus-zona incerta has been studied in three patients with Parkinson's disease and comorbid OCD (Fontaine et al., 2004; Mallet et al., 2002). Both studies reported considerable amelioration of OCD symptoms.

The nucleus accumbens and nucleus caudatus were targets in one case study with comorbid depression (as mentioned earlier) (Aouizerate et al., 2004). This patient achieved remission (Aouizerate et al., 2004). Unilateral stimulation of the nucleus accumbens had good results in 14 patients with OCD (Kühn et al., 2007). Stimulation of the ventral capsule/ventral striatum led to major improvement in 50% of patients (Greenberg et al., 2006). Side effects related to stimulation were transient hypomania and increased anxiety. These effects could be counteracted by parameter change (Greenberg et al., 2006).

In summary, there are promising effects associated with several targets in OCD. As worldwide sample sizes are small, it is too early to select a single preferred target.

Table 37.1 Deep brain stimulation (DBS) studies in major depression

Reference	n	Target	Study design	Stimulation parameters	Effect	Side effects	Hypothesis
Mayberg et al., 2005	6	Anterior cingulate gyrus (Cg25)	Systematic parameter search; acute off–on–off–on trials; blinding phase; 6-mo follow-up	Monopolar stimulation; 130-Hz 60-µs voltage, increased to 9 V at each contact; mean parameters at 6 mo: 4 V, 130 Hz, 60 µs	Remission of depression in 4/6 patients; all patients reported acute effects; one patient met response criteria during first 4 mo, normalization of brain metabolism in Cg25	Dose-dependent adverse effects (lightheadedness, headache, psychomotor slowing) at high amplitudes, local skin irritations (2/6) because of which the system needed to be explanted, skin pressure, necrosis (1/6)	Inactivation of Cg25 leads to recovery based on functional neuroimaging findings
Aouizerate et al., 2004	1	Ventral nucleus caudatus (contacts 2,3); nucleus accumbens (contacts 0,1)	6-mo observation; no blinding phase		Remission of depression (HRSD score < 7); stimulation of all contacts necessary	Failure of the pulse generator battery improved visual and verbal memory	Inactivation of dysfunctional connections based on neurosurgical interventions for OCD and depression
Jiménez et al., 2005	1	Lower stem of thalamus	24-mo observation; blinding phase	2.5 V, 130 Hz, 450 µs	Remission of depression, (decrease of HRSD score from 42 to 10)	Transient decrease in learning-to-learn capabilities (WCST); improvement in verbal and nonverbal memory and abstraction tests	Dysfunctional connection between thalamic system and orbitofrontal in depression; disruption of overactivation of frontal cortex with DBS based on functional neuroimaging
Schläpfer et al., 2007	3	Nucleus accumbens	3-mo observation		Reduction of anhedonia ratings; normalization of brain metabolism in nucleus accumbens		Modulation of the nucleus accumbens, which is a central structure in the reward system, leads to improvement of anhedonia, based on clinical experience and neurobiology of reward system

HRSD, Hamilton Rating Scale for Depression; OCD, obsessive–compulsive disorder; WCST, Wisconsin Card-Sorting Test.

Table 37.2 Deep brain stimulation (DBS) studies in obsessive-compulsive disorder (OCD)

Reference	n	Target	Study design	Parameter	Effect	Side effects/problems	Hypothesis
Nuttin et al., 1999, 2003b	6	Anterior capsule	Double-blind; on–off for 3 mo (four patients), 21-mo follow-up	Different parameters, individually adjusted, up to 10.5 V, 100 Hz, 450 μs	66% of patients responded; acute effect in one patient (reduced anxiety, depression, and obsessive thoughts), worsening in stimulation-off phase	Sensation of the leads and the stimulator, fatigue, acute worsening of anxiety with some parameters, weight changes At high amplitude, cognitive and behavioral disinhibition (reversed when stimulation amplitude was decreased), short battery life (5 mo)	Relay between cortex and thalamus; based on anterior capsulotomy
Mallet et al., 2002	2	Nucleus sub-thalamicus	Clinical observations 1 mo before surgery and after 6 mo	Patient 1: 3 V, 185 Hz, 60 μs Patient 2: 3 V, 130 Hz, 90 μs	58% improvement in Patient 1; 64% improvement in Patient 2 in Y-BOCS after 2 wk		Modulates indirect OCD pathway; based on imaging studies
Anderson and Ahmed, 2003	1	Anterior limb of capsula interna	Case study; parameters set at 2 wk after implantation, reviewed at 6 wk and 3 mo	At 2 wk: 2 V, 100 Hz, 210 μs	Positive case report; decrease in Y-BOCS from 34/40 to 7/40		Relay between cortex and thalamus; based on anterior capsulotomy
Gabriëls et al., 2003	3	Anterior capsule	15- to 33-mo follow-up	High amplitude	66% of patients responded		Relay between cortex and thalamus; based on anterior capsulotomy
Sturm et al., 2003	4	Nucleus accumbens	Clinical observations, 24- to 30-mo follow-up	2 to 6.5 V	75% of patients responded		Overactivation of the direct pathway provokes OCD symptoms; based on imaging studies

Study	N	Target	Design	Stimulation parameters	Outcome	Adverse effects	Mechanism
Aouizerate et al., 2004	1	Nucleus caudatus/accumbens	Case study, 15-mo follow-up	Stimulation intensity increased 2 V, 130 Hz, 90 μs (deepest contacts used bilaterally); contacts added and voltage increased up to 4 V and 120 μs	Positive case report; remission of depressive symptoms at 6 mo; delayed remission of OCD at 12–15 mo		Modulates both direct and indirect OCD pathways; based on subcaudate tractotomy, volumetric studies, metabolic studies, imaging studies
Fontaine et al., 2004	1	Nucleus subthalamicus	Case report, 6-mo follow-up	Left electrode: 3.5 V; right electrode: 1.3 V; 185 Hz, 60 μs; chronic monopolar stimulation	Positive case report, PD motor symptoms improved, OCD symptoms disappeared, decreased anxiety		Modulates indirect OCD pathway; based on imaging studies
Abelson et al., 2005	4	Anterior capsule	2 times Double-blind for 3 weeks, open-label testing phase, 4–34 mo	5–10.5 V, 4- to 23-mo follow-up	25% of patients responded	One suicide, judged to be unrelated to stimulation	Relay between cortex and thalamus; based on anterior capsulotomy
Greenberg et al., 2006	10	Ventral capsule/striatum	Patients were blinded	Intraoperative: Different parameters; Best results: Ventral contact (0 or 1) negative, 100–130 Hz, 90–210 μs, 8–17 mA	50% of patients responded (Y-BOCS scores and level of global functioning)	Implantation: Intracerebral hemorrhage after lead insertion, a single tonic–clonic seizure, superficial surgical wound infection, all treated successfully; Stimulation: Acute anxiety mood elevation/hypomania DBS interruption: Worsening in depressed mood and OCD, short battery life (5.5–13 mo), one patient died (recurring breast cancer)	Relay between cortex and thalamus; based on anterior capsulotomy

Y-BOCS, Yale-Brown Obsessive Compulsive Scale; PD, Parkinson's Disease.

Ethical considerations and quality standards in DBS research

Introducing a new therapeutic approach requires evaluation according to high ethical standards. The high mortality, low quality of life, and social burden of inadequately treated serious psychiatric illness should favor the use of DBS for treatment-resistant patients. The potential benefit to the understanding of pathological principles in mental disorders is evident (Ford, 2007; Fuchs, 2006; Schläpfer, 2006; Synofzik, 2005, 2007).

Fundamental ethical concerns are generally applicable to all clinical interventions (e.g., pharmacotherapy, psychotherapy) including DBS in neurological disorders. Foremost, are patients able to give conformed consent? It has been demonstrated that depressed patients show no impairment in decision-making capacity related to clinical treatment research (Appelbaum et al. 1999). Another concern is how far human nature may ethically be manipulated (Fuchs, 2006). Long-term effects of DBS cannot be evaluated yet, but in comparison with pharmacotherapy, brain stimulation is a more specific and reversible intervention. No harmful effects have been reported so far. Most people would agree that trying to heal illness is a fruitful manipulation of human nature. More problematic is the danger of misuse, such as for mind control or overenhancement of normal (healthy) cognitive function ("brain doping") (Ford, 2007; Fuchs 2006). As clinical researchers in psychiatry, we aim to help patients to lead a normal life, including having normal cognitive function and personal autonomy.

More practical ethical concerns are the availability of alternative treatment methods (e.g., pharmacotherapy, ECT, psychotherapy). DBS is used only with treatment-resistant patients, who have already shown no benefit from other treatment approaches currently available. The apparent reversibility of DBS and its robust potential benefits are strong ethical arguments for considering DBS treatment for resistant psychiatric disorders (Synofzik 2005, 2007).

However, there are some notable risks with DBS (particularly intracerebral bleeding and wound infection), and its efficacy is not formally and extensively established. Accordingly, each candidate for DBS must be scrutinized, and obligatory ethical standards must be established, including inclusion and exclusion criteria. Detailed and specific criteria should inhibit researchers and clinicians from "jumping on the bandwagon."

Until the DBS treatment method is scientifically validated, obligatory standards for patient inclusion and the selection of targets are needed. In 2002, Nuttin and colleagues (2003a) advocated certain minimum requirements for using DBS in psychiatric conditions. These requirements include an ethics committee to consider the study protocol and ongoing projects. They also proposed a separate committee for reviewing patient selection. It is questionable as to whether a committee with only distant access to the individual patient should make this decision or whether an external gatekeeper (who is not involved otherwise in the study) is more suitable for this task. Despite any committee review, clinical responsibility remains with the patient's clinicians and is not shared by review committees.

According to Nuttin and colleagues (2003b), the inclusion criteria are severity, chronicity, disability, and treatment refractoriness. These criteria have to be further specified for each psychiatric disease. For example, Mink and colleagues (2006) developed criteria for Gilles de la Tourette syndrome. Our group applied the following criteria for depression (Schläpfer and Bewernick, 2006):

Inclusion criteria

- Major depression, severe, unipolar type;
- German mother tongue (in Germany);
- HRSD24 score greater than 20;
- Global Assessment of Function score less than 45;
- At least four episodes of major depression or chronic episode longer than two years;
- Five years after first episode of major depression;
- Failure to respond to adequate trials (more than five weeks at the maximum recommended or tolerated dose) of primary antidepressants from at least three different classes;
- Adequate trials (more than three weeks at the usually recommended or maximum tolerated dose) of augmentation/combination of a primary antidepressant using at least two different augmenting or combination agents (lithium, T3, stimulants, antipsychotics, anticonvulsants, buspirone, or a second primary antidepressant);
- Adequate trial of ECT (more than six bitemporal treatments) and;
- Adequate trial of individual psychotherapy (more than 20 sessions with an experienced psychotherapist);
- Ability to give written informed consent;
- No medical comorbidity; and
- Drug free or on stable drug regimen at least six weeks before study entry.

Exclusion criteria

- Current or past nonaffective psychotic disorder;
- Any current, clinically significant neurological disorder or medical illness affecting brain function, other than motor tics or Gilles de la Tourette syndrome;
- Any clinically significant abnormality on preoperative magnetic resonance imaging;
- Any surgical contraindications to undergoing DBS;
- Current or unstably remitted substance abuse (aside from nicotine);

- Pregnancy (or being of childbearing age not using effective contraception); and
- History of severe personality disorder.

In psychiatric disorders the process of diagnosis is less verifiable and observable than in neurology. There are no neurobiological markers, and psychiatrists rely on clinical impressions and the patient's subjective report. It is possible for a healthy person to pretend to suffer from several psychiatric syndromes so that even an experienced psychiatrist is unsure of genuineness. Accordingly, it is essential to corroborate the patient's life history, course of illness, and psychopathology.

Another important aspect of quality in DBS research is patient management. Clinical experience shows that it is extremely important to clarify the patient's expectations before surgery and to closely follow the patients after the operation to avoid stress, catastrophic thinking, hypomania, or suicidality, especially in the event of suboptimal acute therapy effect. In event of no response, hospitalization or other treatment options (change in medication, ECT, psychotherapy) should be offered.

As a broad variety of possible settings is available, and clinical changes generally take several weeks (rather than a few days) to develop, stimulation should be altered only after several weeks. When the stimulation settings are changed, all other therapies should be kept constant.

Each case must be documented according to high scientific and administrative expectations (standardized diagnostic tests with clinical scales, evaluation of cognitive parameters with psychological tests, reports of parameter changes, other therapies, additional neuroimaging, etc.). The quality of research procedures is a main consideration in DBS therapy: Patient selection, baseline psychiatric and neuropsychological assessment, and the operation and follow-up require a team of surgeons, psychiatrists, and neuropsychologists who have clearly developed proficiency in their fields focused towards localized brain function in psychiatric conditions. These requirements are most straightforwardly fulfilled in tertiary-care academic centers where such resources are available. Standards for target selection need to be established with clear anatomical and functional hypotheses. It is our task as neuroscientists to develop standards to ensure quality in DBS research.

Conclusions

DBS is a unique and promising method for the treatment of therapy-resistant psychiatric patients. The method consists of manipulating pathological neuronal networks in a focused and precise manner. Initial studies showed promising effects in psychiatric disorders, but the number of patients involved is too small for generalization. Still, the logic and specificity of the method represents new hope to many therapy-resistant psychiatric patients. To date, no fundamental ethical objections to its use in psychiatric disorders have appeared, but until substantial clinical data are available, mandatory standards are needed.

Editor's note

In psychosurgery (as well as antipsychotic drug treatment for mood and anxiety disorders), a substantial concern is the possible development of a pathological prefrontal syndrome. One is mesialfrontal syndrome with apathy or passivity. Another is orbitofrontal syndrome with childlike oversimplicity, loss of awareness of social complexity, and disinhibition. A third is dysexecutive syndrome with impaired problem solving and multitasking. Although some of these symptoms can be caused by the psychiatric illness itself, studies of DBS therapy should include examination for these hypofrontal syndromes as a possible result of this treatment. Presumably, different methods of DBS will vary in resulting prefrontal symptoms.

A report of 121 patients receiving DBS for Parkinson's disease noted serious adverse surgical events in 39 patients, usually infection, and mild decreases in working memory, processing speed, and recall. These were overshadowed by an average gain of 5 hours/day of good quality mobility (Weaver et al., 2009). There were no suicides but the authors noted cumulative data showing high suicide rates after DBS for Parkinson's disease; within the first year it is 13-fold and at four years it is still double the pre-surgery rate.–CMS

Weaver, F. M., Follett, K., Stern, M., et al. 2009. Bilateral deep brain stimulation vs best medical therapy for patients with advanced Parkinson disease: a randomized controlled trial. JAMA 301: 63–73.

References

Abelson, J. L., Curtis, G. C., Sagher, O., et al. 2005. Deep brain stimulation for refractory obsessive-compulsive disorder. Biol Psychiatry 57(5): 510–16.

Anderson, D. and Ahmed, A. 2003. Treatment of patients with intractable obsessive-compulsive disorder with anterior capsular stimulation. Case report. J Neurosurg 98(5): 1104–8.

Aouizerate, B., Cuny, E., Martin-Guehl, C., et al. 2004. Deep brain stimulation of the ventral caudate nucleus in the treatment of obsessive-compulsive disorder and major depression. Case report. J Neurosurg 101: 574–5.

Appelbaum, P. S., Grisso, T., Frank, E., et al. 1999. Competence of depressed patients for consent to research. Am J Psychiatry 156(9): 1380–4.

Baxter, L. R. 1990. Brain imaging as a tool in establishing a theory of brain pathology in obsessive compulsive disorder. J Clin Psychiatry 51 Suppl: 22–5; discussion 26.

Baxter, L. R., Clark, E. C., and Iqbal, M., 2001. Cortical-subcortical systems in the mediation of OCD: Modeling the brain's mediation of a classic "neurosis." In Frontal-subcortical circuits in psychiatric and neurological disorders (eds. Lichter, D. G. and Cummings, J. L.). New York: Guilford Press, pp. 207–30.

Belmaker, R. H. and Agam, G. 2008. Major depressive disorder. N Engl J Med 358(1): 55–68.

Benabid, A. L., Pollak, P., Louveau, A., et al. 1987. Combined (thalamotomy and stimulation) stereotactic surgery of the VIM thalamic nucleus for bilateral Parkinson disease. Appl Neurophysiol 50(1–6): 344–6.

Berton, O. and Nestler, E. J. 2006. New approaches to antidepressant drug discovery: Beyond monoamines. Nat Rev Neurosci 7: 137–51.

Beurrier, C., B. Bioulac, Audin, J., and Hammond, C. 2001. High-frequency stimulation produces a transient blockade of voltage-gated currents in subthalamic neurons. J Neurophysiol 85(4): 1351–6.

Dostrovsky, J. O., R. Levy, Wu, J. P., et al. 2000. Microstimulation-induced inhibition of neuronal firing in human globus pallidus. J Neurophysiol 84(1): 570–4.

Ferrão, Y. A., Diniz, J. B., Lopes, A. C., et al. 2007. Resistance and refractoriness in obsessive-compulsive disorder [in Portuguese]. Rev Bras Psiquiatr 29 Suppl 2: S66–S76.

Fins, J. J. 2003. From psychosurgery to neuromodulation and palliation: History's lessons for the ethical conduct and regulation of neuropsychiatric research. Neurosurg Clin N Am 14(2): 303–19, ix–x.

Fontaine, D., Mattei, V., Borg, M., et al. 2004. Effect of subthalamic nucleus stimulation on obsessive-compulsive disorder in a patient with Parkinson disease. Case report. J Neurosurg 100(6): 1084–6.

Ford, P. J. 2007. Neurosurgical implants: Clinical protocol considerations. Camb Q Healthc Ethics 16(3): 308–11.

Fuchs, T. 2006. Ethical issues in neuroscience. Curr Opin Psychiatry 19: 600–7.

Gabriëls, L., Cosyns, P., Nuttin, B., et al. 2003. Deep brain stimulation for treatment-refractory obsessive-compulsive disorder: Psychopathological and neuropsychological outcome in three cases. Acta Psychiatr Scand 107(4): 275–82.

Gildenberg, P. L. 2005. Evolution of neuromodulation. Stereotact Funct Neurosurg 83(2–3): 71–9.

Greenberg, B. D., Malone, D. A., Friehs, G. M., et al. 2006. Three-year outcomes in deep brain stimulation for highly resistant obsessive-compulsive disorder. Neuropsychopharmacology 31(11): 2384–93.

Hardesty, D. E. and Sackeim, H. A. 2007. Deep brain stimulation in movement and psychiatric disorders. Biol Psychiatry 61(7): 831–5.

Hilker, R., Voges, J., Thiel, A., et al. 2002. Deep brain stimulation of the subthalamic nucleus versus levodopa challenge in Parkinson's disease: Measuring the on- and off-conditions with FDG-PET. J Neural Transm 109(10): 1257–64.

Jiménez, F., Velasco, F., Salin-Pascual, R., et al. 2005. A patient with a resistant major depression disorder treated with deep brain stimulation in the inferior thalamic peduncle. J Neurosurg 57: 585–93.

Keller, M. B. and Baker, L. A. 1992. The clinical course of panic disorder and depression. J Clin Psychiatry 53 Suppl: 5–8.

Keller, M. B., Lavori, P. W., Mueller, T. I., et al. 1992. Time to recovery, chronicity, and levels of psychopathology in major depression. A 5-year prospective follow-up of 431 subjects. Arch Gen Psychiatry 49(10): 809–16.

Kringelbach, M. L., Jenkinson, N., Owen, S. L., and Aziz, T. Z. 2007. Translational principles of deep brain stimulation. Nat Rev Neurosci 8(8): 623–35.

Kühn, J., Huff, W., Lee, S.H., Lenartz, D., et al. 2007. Tiefenhirnstimulation bei psychiatrischen Erkrankungen. Fortschritte der Neurologie und Psychiatrie 75: 447–57.

Mallet, L., Mesnage, L., Houeto, J. L., et al. 2002. Compulsions, Parkinson's disease, and stimulation. Lancet 360(9342): 1302–4.

Malone, D. A., Dougherty, D. D., Rezai, A. R., et al. 2008. Deep brain stimulation of the ventral capsule/ventral striatum for treatment-resistant depression. Biological Psychiatry, in press.

Mayberg, H. S. 1997. Limbic-cortical dysregulation: A proposed model of depression. J Neuropsychiatry 9: 471–81.

Mayberg, H. S., Lozano, A. M., Voon, V., et al. 2005. Deep brain stimulation for treatment-resistant depression. Neuron 45: 651–60.

McIntyre, C. C., Savasta, M., Kerkerian-Le Goff, L., and Vitek, J. L. 2004. Uncovering the mechanism(s) of action of deep brain stimulation: Activation, inhibition, or both. Clin Neurophysiol 115(6): 1239–48.

Mink, J. W., Walkup, J., Frey, K. A., et al. 2006. Patient selection and assessment recommendations for deep brain stimulation in Tourette syndrome. Mov Disord 21(11): 1831–8.

Murray, C. J. and Lopez, A. D. 1997. Global mortality, disability, and the contribution of risk factors: Global Burden of Disease Study. Lancet 349(9063): 1436–42.

Nuttin, B., Cosyns, P., Demeulemeester, H., et al. 1999. Electrical stimulation in anterior limbs of internal capsules in patients with obsessive-compulsive disorder. Lancet 354(9189): 1526.

Nuttin, B., Gybels, J., Cosyns, P., et al. 2003a. Deep brain stimulation for psychiatric disorders. Neurosurg Clin N Am 2003; 14: xv–xvi.

Nuttin, B. J., Gabriëls, L. A., Cosyns, P. R., et al. 2003b. Long-term electrical capsular stimulation in patients with obsessive-compulsive disorder. Neurosurgery 52(6): 1263–72; discussion 1272–4.

Ranck, J. B. Jr. 1975. Which elements are excited in electrical stimulation of mammalian central nervous system: A review. Brain Res 98(3): 417–40.

Rush, A. J., Trivedi, M. H., Wisniewski, S. R., et al. 2006. Acute and longer-term outcomes in depressed outpatients requiring one or several treatment steps: A STAR*D report. Am J Psychiatry 163: 1905–17.

Schläpfer, T. and Bewernick, B. 2006. Deep brain stimulation for treatment-refractory major depression. Available at http://clinicaltrials.gov/ct2/show/NCT00122031

Schläpfer, T. E. 2006. Deep brain stimulation. Neuromodulation therapies for psychiatric disorder and their ethical implications. Akademie-Brief der Europäischen Akademie zur Erforschung von Folgen wissenschaftlich-technischer Entwicklungen 65: 1–3.

Schläpfer, T. E., Cohen, M. X., Frick, C., et al. 2007. Deep brain stimulation to reward circuitry alleviates anhedonia in refractory major depression. Neuropsychopharmacology 33: 368–77.

Schnitzler, A. and Gross, J. 2005. Normal and pathological oscillatory communication in the brain. Nat Rev Neurosci 6(4): 285–96.

Shelton, R. C. 2007. The molecular neurobiology of depression. Psychiatr Clin North Am 30(1): 1–11.

Sher, L. 2004. Daily hassles, cortisol, and the pathogenesis of depression. Med Hypotheses 62(2): 198–202.

Stefani, A., Fedele, E., Galati, S., et al. 2006. Deep brain stimulation in Parkinson's disease patients: Biochemical evidence. J Neural Transm Suppl (70): 401–8.

Stefurak, T., Mikulis, D., Mayberg, H., et al. 2003. Deep brain stimulation for Parkinson's disease dissociates mood and motor circuits: A functional MRI case study. Mov Disord 18(12): 1508–16.

Stein, D. J. 2002. Obsessive-compulsive disorder. Lancet 360(9330): 397–405.

Sturm, V., Lenartz, D., Koulousakis, A., et al. 2003. The nucleus accumbens: A target for deep brain stimulation in obsessive-compulsive- and anxiety-disorders. J Chem Neuroanat 26(4): 293–9.

Synofzik, M. 2005. Interventionen zwischen gehirn und geist: Eine ethische analyse der neuen möglichkeiten der neurowissenschaften. Fortschritte der Neurologie und Psychiatrie 73(10): 1–9.

Synofzik, M. 2007. Eingriffe in die grundlagen der persönlichkeit: Eine praxisorientierte ethische analyse von neuropharmaka und tiefhirnstimulation. Ethik in der Medizin 132: 1–4.

Yurgelun-Todd, D. A., Sava, S., and Dahlgren, M. K. 2007. Mood disorders. Neuroimaging Clin N Am 17(4): 511–21, ix.

Zucker, R. S. and Regehr, W. G. 2002. Short-term synaptic plasticity. Annu Rev Physiol 64: 355–405.

38

Transcranial direct current stimulation

Julie A. Williams and Felipe Fregni

Introduction

Brief historical facts

The use of electric current as a therapeutic tool was as early as the first century C.E., when Romans used electric currents from torpedo fish to treat a variety of ailments, including headaches and other body pains. The development of this field occurred only after the experiments of Volta and Galvani developing the first battery pile – indeed this was the first use of direct current stimulation experimentally. Significant development and systematic research in this area began in the 1950s with controlled animal studies. By the 1960s, this method of brain stimulation was also being tested in humans. Several animal studies applied direct current directly to the cortex. Researchers, including Bindman et al. (1964), and Purpura and McMurtry (1965) showed that electrical currents, much weaker than those needed to induce an action potential, induced changes in spontaneous neural activity – the hallmark of this truly neuromodulatory tool. This discovery led to human studies of the neuromodulatory effects of transcranial direct current stimulation (tDCS), with expectations of alleviating neuropsychiatric syndromes.

Few research publications using it were documented until the 1990s. The lack of study may have resulted from the absence of tools to investigate brain activity and from the mixed results of prior studies.

How it works

Transcranial direct current stimulation is a noninvasive brain stimulation technique that uses a weak continuous electric current applied through scalp electrodes to inject currents into the brain and modulate spontaneous neuronal activity in a painless manner. Whereas other noninvasive techniques, such as transcranial magnetic stimulation (TMS), may act as either a neuromodulator or a neurostimulator, tDCS is a purely neuromodulatory method. Two electrodes (anode and cathode) are placed over two different brain regions. These electrodes are connected to an electricity source that can emit currents up to 10 mA, depending on the device model.

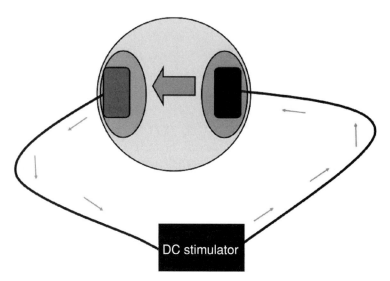

Figure 38.1   Scheme showing tDCS application – two large electrodes (cathode, right-hand electrode; anode, left-hand electrode) are placed in the scalp and connected to a source of battery. Arrows indicate the direction of the conventional positive current.

The most commonly used are in the range from 0.5 to 2 mA over a period of time ranging from seconds to minutes (Figure 38.1). Different types of electrodes can be used: The two most common are the cotton and sponge electrodes (Figure 38.2). Both of them are soaked in saline solution to increase the local conductance.

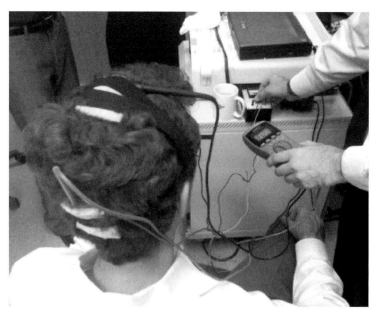

Figure 38.2   Subject receiving tDCS over the occipital cortex – the reference electrode is placed on Cz. (See Color Plate IX.)

Although frameless stereotaxic systems exist for use in conjunction with TMS, they are not used for tDCS because this technique has little focality. Currently, the method used for determining the location of the brain region to be targeted is the International 10-20 system for electrode placement, such that if the dorso-lateral prefrontal cortex (DLPFC) is the region being targeted by stimulation, F3 corresponds to this brain region.

Several electrode montages are in use, such as bipolar stimulation (with anode and cathode electrodes on the patient's scalp) and monopolar stimulation (with one electrode on the scalp and the other on the neck or shoulder). Other strategies include using three electrodes (e.g., two anodes and one cathode) but studies of these strategies are rare.

Importance as a clinical tool

Transcranial direct current stimulation offers several advantages over other techniques of noninvasive brain stimulation (specifically, rapid TMS [rTMS]) such as (a) small size of the apparatus, allowing portability; (b) possibility of increasing neuronal activity in any lesioned cortex and decreasing activity in healthy cortex (or vice versa) simultaneously because, for tDCS, two electrodes are placed (the anode apparently increases cortical activity, and the cathode decreases it); (c) longer-lasting effects than rTMS – for instance, 13 minutes of stimulation changes brain excitability for up to 90 minutes (Nitsche and Paulus, 2001); and (d) tDCS represents pure neuromodulation because it changes the membrane resting potential. Moreover, it can be controlled for by a sham method that study subjects cannot distinguish from tDCS itself.

Although the majority of recent clinical investigations show significant clinical effects associated with tDCS, it is still not known whether tDCS will be an effective clinical tool. If further studies confirm the initial results, tDCS might be useful: (a) in patients who showed no benefit from psychotropic drugs; (b) to potentiate medications; (c) in patients with intolerable adverse drug effects; or (d) as an alternative to procedures or drugs with undesirable effects (e.g., see Chapter 23).

Adverse events

Although adverse effects from tDCS have been identified, most can be avoided if the safety guidelines are followed (Iyer et al., 2005; Nitsche et al., 2003b). In addition, personnel certified for basic life support and trained in the prompt recognition of medical emergencies such as syncope or vasovagal reaction should be available.

The safety of this technique has been addressed and tested by multiple researchers, who have concluded that tDCS induces only temporary cognitive and motor effects and no severe adverse effects. More than 50 research studies on the use of tDCS involving hundreds of participants have been published. Hundreds more participants have undergone tDCS for unpublished pilot research. No undesirable or long-lasting effects have been reported, nor have any participants reportedly abandoned a study because of discomfort.

Researchers at the National Institute of Neurological Disorders and Stroke (NINDS) (Iyer et al., 2005) conducted a safety study on tDCS, investigating the safety of 20-minute sessions of 1-mA and 2-mA current stimulation with healthy controls ($n = 103$) using electroencephalography and a neuropsychological battery of tests. No adverse effects were identified. Nitsche and colleagues (2004) found no measurable structural changes in brain tissue caused by tDCS (Nitsche et al., 2004).

Additionally, studies have shown that consecutive sessions of tDCS can be used safely in patients with chronic neuropsychiatric disorders such as stroke patients (Fregni et al., 2005b; Hummel and Cohen, 2005), fibromyalgia and spinal cord injury (Fregni et al., 2006a, 2006d), and major depression (Fregni et al., 2006b). It should be noted, however, that these studies investigated a small number of participants. In these studies, only mild adverse effects (such as mild headache) have been reported. Nevertheless, these studies considered only the acute effects of tDCS, and the safety evaluation might not have been complete as the methods were noninvasive. Data from larger studies with longer follow-up evaluations are necessary for completeness.

Clinical applications

Because of its characteristics, tDCS seems to have the potential to be developed as a clinical tool and several preliminary clinical trials have been performed. We discuss in this chapter the rationale and the results of studies investigating tDCS for various neuropsychiatric disorders.

Depression

The mechanism of tDCS in alleviating depression might be related to a modulation of the activity in the DLPFC. It has been shown that tDCS changes cortical excitability by modulating synaptic transmission (long-term potentiation- and depression-like mechanisms) according to pharmacological studies (Liebetanz et al., 2002; Nitsche et al., 2003a). Therefore, it is reasonable to expect that DLPFC tDCS might induce a change in DLPFC activity, a critical area in the cortico-subcortical, mood-related neural network.

In a double-blind clinical trial, 40 medication-free patients with major depression were randomized into three groups of treatment (anodal tDCS of the left DLPFC; anodal tDCS of the occipital cortex, or sham tDCS). Anodal tDCS was applied for 10 sessions over a two-week period (Boggio et al., 2007). Both the

Hamilton Rating Scale for Depression and the Beck Depression Inventory were used to evaluate any changes in mood. A significantly larger reduction in depression scores was measured in the active group than in the two control groups. These benefits persisted for one month after the treatment.

Additional studies are needed to explore the parameters of stimulation to optimize the clinical benefits. These benefits should be studied for the treatment by itself but also in combination with cognitive behavioral therapy or antidepressant drugs. tDCS can even be used during the psychotherapy session. Larger studies and studies in varying populations are needed to confirm the results of these initial studies. Finally, studies of higher dosages of tDCS are needed, although with closer attention to safety.

Fibromyalgia

Fibromyalgia is associated with neuropsychiatric pathology. Nonrapid eye movement (non-REM) sleep is altered in patients with fibromyalgia and is associated with symptom severity. Fibromyalgia is associated with depression, and tricyclics and other antidepressants can mitigate the symptoms of both. Finally, neuroimaging studies have shown that regional cerebral blood flow in some pain-related brain areas (e.g., thalamic nuclei) in patients with fibromyalgia is different from that in healthy controls.

Only initial research has been completed using tDCS or other types of central electrical stimulation in fibromyalgia, but tDCS has been studied in chronic pain and depression. In these studies, anodal tDCS applied to either the primary motor cortex or the DLPFC was successful in alleviating symptoms. Fregni et al. (2006d) showed that anodal tDCS stimulation of the primary motor cortex in patients with fibromyalgia induces a larger and more significant lessening of pain than sham stimulation. These results are similar to those published in another tDCS study measuring the effects of tDCS on chronic pain (Fregni et al., 2006a, 2007). In a study of the effects of tDCS on sleep in fibromyalgia, the effect of anodal tDCS was specific to the site of stimulation: primary motor cortex (M1) stimulation increased sleep efficiency and decreased arousals, and this effect was associated with clinical changes in pain (Roizenblatt et al., 2007). These findings suggest that the therapeutic effects of tDCS in fibromyalgia may be via sleep modulation.

Epilepsy

Extensive studies of animals and limited work in humans have shown that epileptogenesis involves an increase in excitatory synaptic strength in a manner similar to long-term potentiation. Targeting seizure foci with cathodal tDCS may be able to reverse the hyperexcitability state of the epileptic focus, because the effects of cathodal tDCS resemble long-term depression of neuronal activity.

Noninvasive brain stimulation might help to interrupt ongoing seizure activity in epilepsia partialis continua or even in status epilepticus. Such concepts have not yet been tested.

In a study published in 2006 by Fregni et al. (2006e), cathodal direct current (DC) stimulation was used to induce a decrease in cortical excitability in patients with cortical dysplasia; it resulted in a reduction in the number of epileptiform discharges (EDs) in the electroencephalogram. Patients who received active DC polarization had a decrease in the mean number of EDs from 413.9 ± 427.1 (baseline) to 148.0 ± 168.2 (after stimulation), whereas patients who received sham DC polarization had a small decrease in EDs from 334.4 ± 619.5 to 315.0 ± 632.5. Although the data were not significant, they suggested that the effects of DC polarization on cortical excitability might last several days. None of the patients reported an increase in seizure frequency after the treatment in the active-treatment group. This analysis suggested that active cathodal DC polarization in patients with single focal abnormalities was significantly effective in seizure and epileptiform reduction compared with sham treatment in a similar group of patients. In addition, a recent animal study showed that cathodal tDCS increases the seizure threshold similarly to antiepileptic drugs (Liebetanz et al., 2006). Still, it is not clear yet if tDCS antiepileptic effects are strong enough to make clinical improvements.

Craving disorders

Craving is understood as a strong internal drive for an abusable substance, such as cocaine, alcohol, or even food. It is associated with an increase in activity in the DLPFC, and neuromodulation of DLPFC using tDCS might decrease craving. A study by Fecteau et al. (2007) showed that stimulation of the DLPFC is associated with decreased risk-taking in the Balloon Analog Risk Task, which may be itself analogous to risk-taking craving.

In reported studies on the effects of tDCS to modulate craving in food (Fregni et al., 2008b), alcohol (Boggio et al., 2008), and nicotine (Fregni et al., 2008a), respectively, active anodal stimulation of the DLPFC was associated with decreases in craving. This decrease was observed with active anodal stimulation of either the right or left DLPFC in alcohol or nicotine cravings. In food cravings, however, right anodal DLPFC stimulation led to a larger decrease in craving than left anodal DLPFC stimulation. This result could be an indication of hemispheric laterality for food craving, and it suggests that the effects of left and right stimulation may be qualitatively different.

Moreover, a significant negative correlation was observed between craving reduction and both age and number of smoking years. Accordingly, patients with longer smoking duration may be more resistant to a single session of tDCS.

The effects of tDCS may be particularly well applied to the DLPFC, as this area integrates information about internal state (craving, withdrawal), motivation, expectancy, and cues and uses this information in the regulation and planning of drug-seeking or drug-avoiding behavior. Active anodal tDCS may have prevented craving by increasing activity in the DLPFC or its connected neural networks. tDCS has not been shown to have local disruptive effects on cortical activity, although this is not entirely disproven.

Next steps for craving studies include the use of consecutive sessions of tDCS, tests for laterality of food craving, and comparisons between tDCS and medications such as topiramate to diminish alcohol cravings.

Parkinson's disease

It is possible that the effects of noninvasive brain stimulation are not limited to the directly stimulated brain region, but spread to distant cortical and subcortical structures through neuronal network connections.

As of October 2007, there were only two published reports of tDCS use in Parkinson's disease. Fregni et al. (2006c), found that anodal stimulation of the primary motor cortex (M1) was associated with a significant improvement of motor function compared to sham stimulation, cathodal stimulation of M1, and anodal stimulation of the DLPFC. These findings suggested that the observed effects were specific for tDCS polarity and site stimulation, and that the primary motor cortex may be a useful target for brain stimulation in Parkinson's patients. A nonsignificant trend to correlaton between motor function improvement and increased motor-evoked potential size suggested an increase in cortical excitability from tDCS. A further increase in cortical excitability by anodal stimulation (with higher dose or longer stimulation) might help to compensate for the underactive pallido-thalamo-cortical drive.

In another tDCS study by the same group, patients with Parkinson's disease showed a significant improvement in task accuracy, reflecting working memory, after active anodal tDCS of the left DLPFC with 2 mA. This may be useful because memory deficits usually worsen with progression of Parkinson's disease (Boggio et al., 2006). The other conditions of stimulation – sham tDCS, anodal tDCS of left DLPFC with 1 mA, or anodal tDCS of M1 – did not produce a significant task performance change, suggesting specificity of both left DLPFC site and 2-mA dose.

Memory

Transcranial direct current stimulation has been explored for enhancement of working memory. Working memory refers to the temporary storage and manipulation of the information necessary for complex tasks such as language comprehension, learning, and reasoning. Neuroimaging studies have shown that the DLPFC (Brodmann areas 9 and 46) plays a central role in working memory. There was an apparent beneficial effect of excitability-enhancing anodal DC stimulation on simple reaction times and implicit motor learning when the primary motor cortex was stimulated (Nitsche et al., 2003c). Similarly, learning of a visuo-motor coordination task was enhanced by stimulation of the primary motor area or the visual area V5 (Antal et al., 2004). These suggest that anodal tDCS may improve cognitive functions in humans.

In the study of Fregni et al. (2005a), 15 participants underwent a three-back working memory task based on letters. This task was performed during sham and anodal stimulation applied over the left DLPFC. Seven participants also performed the same task, but with cathodal stimulation of the DLPFC and anodal stimulation of M1 to test for the specificity of the effects.

In the three-back letter working memory paradigm, participants were presented with a pseudorandom set of 10 letters (A–J). Each letter was displayed on a computer monitor for 30 ms. A different letter was displayed every two seconds. Participants were asked to respond through a key press if the presented letter was the same as the letter presented three stimuli previously. Results from the study indicated that only anodal stimulation of the left prefrontal cortex increases the accuracy of the task performance when compared to sham stimulation of the same area. There was no effect by cathodal stimulation of the left DLPFC or anodal stimulation of M1.

The accuracy enhancement during active stimulation cannot be accounted for by slowed responses, as response times were not changed by stimulation. Because accuracy but not response times differed between the stimulation conditions, the results are in accordance with a critical role of the DLPFC in working memory formation rather than simply task execution because of attention enhancement.

Other evidence that anodal tDCS enhances memory comes from an elegant, recent study by Marshall et al. (2006). These investigators showed that tDCS applied (using a paradigm of oscillating potentials with a frequency of 0.75 Hz) to the prefrontal cortex during early non-REM sleep (a period of emerging slow-wave sleep) enhances the retention of declarative memories in healthy humans. Overall, tDCS shows promise in enhancing some aspects of cognition.

Anxiety disorders

There have been no reports describing tDCS in patients with anxiety disorders. tDCS might have therapeutic value in obsessive-compulsive disorder or post-traumatic stress disorder by modulating brain activity in the prefrontal cortex and indirectly affecting the neurally linked amygdala and nucleus accumbens.

Conclusions

Initial experience in clinical trials suggests the possibility that tDCS is useful in mitigating a variety of neuropsychiatric disorders. Evidence of efficacy from sham-controlled clinical trials is still insufficient to justify its widespread use, but there seems to be a great margin of safety with standard precautions. Further study is needed in comparing intermittent and constant-current tDCS (e.g., Marshall et al., 2006)and in determining the most effective settings of electrical stimulation parameters.

References

Antal, A., Nitsche, M. A., Kruse, W., et al. 2004. Direct current stimulation over V5 enhances visuomotor coordination by improving motion perception in humans. J Cogn Neurosci 16: 521–7.

Bindman, L. J., Lippold, O. C., and Redfearn, J. W. 1964. The action of brief polarizing currents on the cerebral cortex of the rat (1) during current flow and (2) in the production of long-lasting after-effects. J Physiol 172: 369–82.

Boggio, P. S., Ferrucci, R., Rigonatti, S. P., Covre, P., Nitsche, M., Pascual-Leone, A., et al. 2006. Effects of transcranial direct current stimulation on working memory in patients with Parkinson's disease. J Neurol Sci 249: 31–38.

Boggio, P. S., Rigonatti, S. P., Ribeiro, R. B., et al. 2007. A randomized, double-blind clinical trial on the efficacy of cortical direct current stimulation for the treatment of major depression. Int J Neuropsychopharmacol 11(2): 1–6.

Boggio, P. S., Sultani, N., Fecteau, S., et al. 2008. Prefrontal cortex modulation using transcranial DC stimulation reduces alcohol craving: A double-blind, sham-controlled study. Drug Alcohol Depend 92(1–3): 55–60. Epub 2007 Jul 19.

Fecteau, S., Pascual-Leone, A., Zald, D. H., et al. 2007. Activation of prefrontal cortex by transcranial direct current stimulation reduces appetite for risk during ambiguous decision making. J Neurosci 27: 6212–8.

Fregni, F., Boggio, P. S., Nitsche, M., et al. 2005a. Anodal transcranial direct current stimulation of prefrontal cortex enhances working memory. Exp Brain Res 166: 23–30.

Fregni, F., Simon, D. K., Wu, A., and Pascual-Leone, A. 2005b. Non-invasive brain stimulation for Parkinson's disease: A systematic review and meta-analysis of the literature. J Neurol Neurosurg Psychiatry 76: 1614–23.

Fregni, F., Boggio, P. S., Lima, M. C., et al. 2006a. A sham-controlled, phase II trial of transcranial direct current stimulation for the treatment of central pain in traumatic spinal cord injury. Pain 122: 197–209.

Fregni, F., Boggio, P. S., Nitsche, M. A., et al. 2006b. Cognitive effects of repeated sessions of transcranial direct current stimulation in patients with depression. Depress Anxiety 23: 482–4.

Fregni, F., Boggio, P. S., Santos, M. C., et al. 2006c. Noninvasive cortical stimulation with transcranial direct current stimulation in Parkinson's disease. Mov Disord 21: 1693–702.

Fregni, F., Gimenes, R., Valle, A. C., et al. 2006d. A randomized, sham-controlled, proof of principle study of transcranial direct current stimulation for the treatment of pain in fibromyalgia. Arthritis Rheum 54: 3988–98.

Fregni, F., Thome-Souza, S., Nitsche, M. A., et al. 2006e. A controlled clinical trial of cathodal DC polarization in patients with refractory epilepsy. Epilepsia 47: 335–42.

Fregni, F., Freedman, S., and Pascual-Leone, A. 2007. Recent advances in the treatment of chronic pain with non-invasive brain stimulation techniques. Lancet Neurol 6: 188–91.

Fregni, F., Orsati, F., Pedrosa, W., et al. (2008a). Transcranial direct current stimulation of the prefrontal cortex modulates the desire for specific foods. Appetite 51: 34–41.

Fregni, F., Liguori, P., Fecteau, S., et al. 2008b. Cortical stimulation of the prefrontal cortex with transcranial DC stimulation reduces smoking cue-provoked craving: A randomized, sham-controlled study. J Clin Psychiatry 69(1): 32–40.

Hummel, F., and Cohen, L. G. 2005. Improvement of motor function with noninvasive cortical stimulation in a patient with chronic stroke. Neurorehabil Neural Repair 19: 14–19.

Iyer, M. B., Mattu, U., Grafman, J., et al. 2005. Safety and cognitive effect of frontal DC brain polarization in healthy individuals. Neurology 64: 872–5.

Liebetanz, D., Nitsche, M. A., Tergau, F., and Paulus, W. 2002. Pharmacological approach to the mechanisms of transcranial DC-stimulation-induced after-effects of human motor cortex excitability. Brain 125: 2238–47.

Liebetanz, D., Klinker, F., Hering, D., et al. 2006. Anticonvulsant effects of transcranial direct-current stimulation (tDCS) in the rat cortical ramp model of focal epilepsy. Epilepsia 47: 1216–24.

Marshall, L., Helgadottir, H., Molle, M., and Born, J. 2006. Boosting slow oscillations during sleep potentiates memory. Nature 444: 610–13.

Nitsche, M. A. and Paulus, W. 2001. Sustained excitability elevations induced by transcranial DC motor cortex stimulation in humans. Neurology 57: 1899–1901.

Nitsche, M. A., Fricke, K., Henschke, U., et al. 2003a. Pharmacological modulation of cortical excitability shifts induced by transcranial direct current stimulation in humans. J Physiol 553: 293–301.

Nitsche, M. A., Liebetanz, D., Lang, N., et al. 2003b. Safety criteria for transcranial direct current stimulation (tDCS) in humans. Clin Neurophysiol 114: 2220–3.

Nitsche, M. A., Schauenburg, A., Lang, N., et al. 2003c. Facilitation of implicit motor learning by weak transcranial direct current stimulation of the primary motor cortex in the human. J Cogn Neurosci 15: 619–26.

Nitsche, M. A., Niehaus, L., Hoffmann, K. T., et al. 2004. MRI study of human brain exposed to weak direct current stimulation of the frontal cortex. Clin Neurophysiol 115: 2419–23.

Purpura, D. P., and McMurty, J. G. 1965. Intracellular activities and evoked potential changes during polarization of motor cortex. J Neurophysiol 28: 166–85.

Roizenblatt, S., Fregni, F., Gimenez, R., et al. 2007. Site-specific effects of transcranial direct current stimulation on sleep and pain in fibromyalgia: A randomized, sham-controlled study. Pain Pract 7(4): 297–306. Epub 2007 Nov 6.

Index

abortive seizures, 474
Abrams, Richard, 171, 173, 175
ACC. *See* American College of Cardiology
ACGME. *See* American Council on Graduate
    Medical Education
acroagonine, 176
ACT. *See* Association for Convulsive Therapy
ACTH. *See* adrenocorticotropic hormone
activity regulated cytoskeleton (Arc) genes,
    62–63
acute catatonic schizophrenia, ECT for, 131–133
    benzodiazepines v. ECT for, 132, 133
    remission rates for, 132–133
acute onset delirium, 435–436
acute schizophrenia, ECT for, 127–131
    antipsychotic drugs v., 127–128
    remission rates for, 127
    trial studies for, 128–130, 131
Aden v. Younger, 210, 219
adrenocorticotropic hormone (ACTH), 153
Advocates for Humanity, 217
AF. *See* atrial fibrillation
age of patient, ECT use and, 231
    in Asia, 260
AHA. *See* American Heart Association
All's Well That Ends Well (Shakespeare), 384
Almansi, Renato, 227
Alonso, Rafael J. Larragoiti, 281
ambulatory electroconvulsive therapy, 515–518
    ACT guidelines for, 516–517
    development of, 515–516
ambulatory insulin therapy, 25
American Academy of Child and Adolescent
    Psychiatry, 499
American College of Cardiology (ACC), 402
    CAD/post-MI guidelines under, 404
American Council on Graduate Medical
    Education (ACGME), 199–200
American Heart Association (AHA), 402
    CAD/post-MI guidelines under, 404
American Journal of Psychiatry, 212, 413
American Psychiatric Association (APA), xxi,
    208
    ECT guidelines under, in state regulations, 202

ECT Task Force under, 173, 200, 358, 516
    application guidelines under, 228
    with EEG, 468
    legislation influenced by, 214–215
    risk factor discussion guidelines of, 392
Uruguay and, guidelines for ECT use in,
    282
amnesia. *See also* memory loss
    anterograde, 493
    retrograde, 491–492
An Angel at My Table (Frame), 182–183, 193
anatomical theory, 78
    direct stimulation hypothesis in, 78
    TMS in, 78
anesthesia, for ECT, 412–425
    airway management during, 422–423
        hyperventilation and, 423
        preparation procedures for, 422–423
        with LMA, 422
    anticholinergics, 414–415
        adverse effects of, 415
        atropine, 415
        glycopyrrolate, 414–415
    atracurium, 420–421
    in *The Bell Jar,* 413
    with concomitant medications, 423–424
        anticonvulsants, 423
        for glucose control, 424
        l-dopa, 424
        lithium, 423–424
        theophylline, 424
    history of, 413–414
        with curare, 413
    induction agents, 415–418
        barbiturates, 415–416
        comparisons between, 416
        etomidate, 417
        inhalational, 418
        ketamine, 417–418
        propofol, 417
        thiopental, 416–417
        ultrashort-acting narcotics, 418
    induction, in placebo trials, 113–114
    major elements of, 413

anesthesia, for ECT (*cont.*)
    with muscle relaxants, 418–421
        cuff method, 419
        mivacurium, 420
        moderate/short-acting, 420–421
        succinylcholine, 419–420
    rationale for, 412
    rocuronium, 421
anesthetists, 323–324
    psychiatrists and, 324, 424–425
anterograde amnesia, 493
anticholinergics, 414–415
    adverse effects of, 415
    atropine, 415
    glycopyrrolate, 414–415
anticoagulation, ECT and, 406
anticonvulsant activity, from ECT, xxv
anticonvulsant medications, 423
anticonvulsant theory, 78
    seizure thresholds in, 78
antidepressant medications
    for anxiety disorders, ECT v., 348–349
    with cECT, 505–506, 507–508
    electrode placement and, 433
    for mood disorders, ECT v., 114–115, 117
        blind v. nonblind studies for, 114–116
        dosage issues in, 116
        meta-analyses failures in, 117
        new medications in, 116
        with outmoded techniques, 116
        variability in diagnoses in, 116–117
    VNS as alternative to, 549
anti-ECT movements, 212–214. *See also* Church
        of Scientology; Hubbard, Lafayette
        Ronald
    Coalition for the Abolition of Electroshock in,
        214
    Coalition to Stop Electroshock in, 214, 215
    development of, 214
    Hubbard role in, 212–213
    Insane Liberation Front in, 214
    International Coalition for the Abolition of
        Electroshock in, 214
    Mental Patients Liberation Project in, 214
    NAPA in, 214, 215
    in Russian Federation, 268
    in Scandinavia, 237
antipsychiatry opponents, ECT and, 198. *See
        also* Church of Scientology; Citizens
        Commission on Human Rights
    National Anti-Shock Action, 249
    U.S. state regulations and, influence on,
        203–204
antipsychotic drugs, xvii. *See also* hypofrontality
    for acute schizophrenia, 127–128

    for chronic schizophrenia, with ECT, 136–138
    death rates and, 371
    for depression, v. ECT, 351–352
    in DSM-IV, 363
    ECT v, xvii, 362–379
        for catatonia, 376–377
        for depression, 373–376
        hypofrontality and, 365–367
        lifespan rates and, 365
        physician behavior and, 377–379
        tardive psychosis and, 369
        therapeutic benefits with, 373–376
    for malignant catatonia, 133
    mortality rates with, 364
    for nonpsychotic indications, 363
    patient tolerance for, 372–373
        CATIE and, 372
    side effects of, 364
        aspiration pneumonia as, 371
        cancer as, 371–372
        cardiac risk factor exacerbation as,
            370–371
        hypoactivity as, 372
        hypofrontality as, 365–367
        lifespan rates as, 364–365
        mental, 364, 369–370
        neurological, 370
        NMS as, 371
        sexual dysfunction as, 372
        sudden cardiac death as, 371
        tardive dyskinesia as, 370
        tardive psychosis as, 367–369
    with SSRIs, 375–376
anxiety disorders, 342
    atypical depression and, 342
    bipolar disorder, xviii, 347
        non-ECT therapies for, 36–37
    ECT for, 343–344
        antidepressant medications v., 348–349
        patient selection for, 344
        for prevention of, 346–347
    indications for, 344–345
    OCD, 343
    PTSD, xviii, 345
    SSRIs for, 342
    tDCS for, 580
apathetic syndrome, 366
arachidonic acid cascade genes, 61–62
Arc genes. *See* activity regulated cytoskeleton
        genes
area under the curve (AUC), in prolactin release,
        156
Argentina, ECT use in, 280
Arnold, William, 192
Artaud, Antonin, 181–182

Asia, ECT as treatment throughout, 256–264.
    See also Hong Kong, ECT use in; Japan,
    ECT use in; Taiwan, ECT use in;
    Thailand, ECT use in
  age as factor for, 260
  gender as factor for, 261
  history of, 256
  indications for, 259–260
    for schizophrenia, 259–260
  professional publications about, 263–264
  rates of use for, 256–259, 263
  regulation of, 262
  technical aspects of, 261–262
    with brief-pulse devices, 262
    electrode placement and, 261, 263
    modified with muscle relaxants, 261–262
    training guidelines for, 262–263
aspiration pneumonia, 371
Association for Convulsive Therapy (ACT),
    516–517
atracurium, 420–421
atrial fibrillation (AF), 404–405
atropine, 415
atropinic agents, xxvi
atypical depression, 342–346
  anxiety disorders and, 342
AUC. *See* area under the curve, in prolactin
    release
Auditory Hallucinations Rating Scale, 530
Avrutsky, G.Y., 272

Bailine, Samuel, 175
Balloon Analog Risk Task, 578
Barber, Stephen, 181
barbiturates, 415–416
BDNF pathway, 58–61
  after chronic ECS, 58–59
  neuritin gene, 61
  Vesl/homer gene, 60–61
A Beautiful Mind, 211
Behrman, Andy, 190
Belgium, ECT in, 246–248
  rate of use, 247–248
The Bell Jar (Plath), 184–185, 188, 193,
    413
Benchmark Method, 153, 441
  for peak heart rate, 479, 481
  for stimulus dosing, 456–458
    cardiovascular reactivity in, 458
    seizure morphology in, 457–458
  technique for, 456
Bennett, Alan, 187–188, 194, 413
benzodiazepines
  for acute catatonic schizophrenia, v. ECT, 132,
    133

  ECT v., for catatonia, 376–377
  in pre-ECT protocols, xxvii
bifrontal electrode placement, 442–444
  clinical outcomes from, 443
  MMSE scores after, 443–444
Bini, Lucio, 227
Bini, Luigi, 168
bipolar depression, 530
bipolar disorders, xviii
  cECT for, 511
  mECT for, 511
  non-ECT therapies for, 36–37
bipolar mania, 531–532
bitemporal electrode placement, 438–439
  Benchmark Method and, 153, 441
  clinical application of, 438
  clinical outcomes from, 438–439
  HRSD scores after, 438
  MMSE score after, 438
  right unilateral v., 440
books and films, ECT in, 180–195, 211–212
  An Angel at My Table, 182–183, 193
  The Bell Jar, 184–185, 188, 193
  Electroboy, 190
  Family Life, 188
  Fear Strikes Out, 191–192, 193
  Frances, 188, 192
  Holiday of Darkness, 188–189
  legislation influenced by, 210–211
  Memoirs of an Amnesiac, 183
  One Flew over the Cuckoo's Nest, xviii, 172,
    188, 191, 192, 210, 321
  Out of Tune, 193
  in professional literature, 211
  psychiatrists negatively influenced by, 198
  psychiatrists' portrayals in, 210
  Shadowland, 192
  Shine, 193
  *Shock: The Healing Power of Electroconvulsive
    Therapy,* 191
  The Snake Pit, 172
  The Tender Place, 184
brain. *See also* deep brain stimulation
  DBS, 556–569
    advantages of, 559
    chronic, 557
    for depression, 561–562
    for dystonia, 557
    ethical considerations for, 566–568
    history of, 557
    neurophysiologic changes from, 558
    for OCD, 562
    patient selection for, 567–568
    principles of, 557–558
    quality standards for, 566–568

brain (*cont.*)
   safety of, 559
   surgical implantation in, 557–558
   target selection issues with, 560–561
   for treatment-resistant depression, 556
   ECT and, electrical effects of, 6
      in choroid plexus, 58
      in hippocampus, 55
   electricity effect on, overcoming inhibitions in, 82–85
   electroconvulsive therapy and, regions for, 45–46
   electrode placement and, neurobiology of, 436–438
   neuroimaging of, for ECT, 94–105
   organizational levels of, 79–82
      mental disorders and, 80–82, 89
Brazil, ECT use in, 282–283
   history of, 282–283
brief-pulse stimulus dose, 9–11
   approximation of separation in, 9
   efficiency of, 13–14
   electrode placement with, 10–11
   pulse width in, 14
   sine wave v., 12–13
   ultrabrief, 14–15
      average/range of, 15
      electrode placement with, 14–15
brief stimulus therapy (BST), 170–171
BST. *See* brief stimulus therapy
burns, ECT treatment with, 410

CAD. *See* coronary artery disease
caffeine, stimulus potentiation and, xxix
Canada, ECT use in, 198–199
cancer, from antipsychotic drugs, 371–372
capacity. *See* mental capacity
cardiovascular disorders, ECT with, 402
   anticoagulation and, 406
   CAD, 404
      ACC/AHA guidelines for, 404
      medication treatment guidelines for, 404
   CHF, 402–404
      decompensated, 403
      patient evaluation for, 403
      treatment for,
   dysrhythmias, 404–405
      AF as, 404–405
      ECG for, 405
   ECG assessment with, 405
   ICDs/pacemakers and, 405
   MI, 404
      ACC/AHA guidelines for, 404
      medication treatment guidelines for, 404
   valvular disease, 406
   vascular disease, 405–406

Cardiozol. *See* pentamethylenetetrazol, in non-ECT therapy
Castedo, Cesar, 280
catatonia
   childhood/adolescent psychoses and, 141–142
   definition of, 124
      in DSM-IV, 124
      in ICD-10, 124
   diagnostic problems with, 125
   ECT for, 124–142
      indications for, 349–350
      for malignant, 133–135
      methodological limitations of, 125–126
   lethal, 350
   malignant, ECT for, 133–135
      antipsychotic drugs v., 133
      NMS and, 133
      "shock block" method of, 134
      survival rates for, 134–135
   organic, 139–141
   pharmacological treatments for, 126
   schizophrenia and, 124
      acute, 131–133
   TMS for, 531
CATIE. *See* Clinical Antipsychotic Trials of Intervention Effectiveness
Cavett, Dick, 180, 208
CCHR. *See* Citizens Commission on Human Rights
cECT. *See* continuation electroconvulsive therapy
central nervous system (CNS), grand mal seizures and, xxiii
cerebrovascular disease, ECT with, 408
Cerletti, Ugo, 23, 168, 176, 227
Chabasinski, Ted, 214
chemical convulsants, 18–24. *See also* pentamethylenetetrazol, in non-ECT therapy
   with insulin therapy, 28–30
      application procedures for, 29
      complications from, 29–30
      indications for, 29
   "Meduna's method" and, 266
   model policy guidelines for, 292–294
      for involuntary patients, 293–294
      for voluntary patients, 292–293
   in physical therapy, 167
   PM-1090, 24
   PTZ, 19–24
      application procedure for, 19–20
      complications from, 22–23
      for depression, 21–22
      ECT replacement for, 23–24
      indications for, 20–22
      relapse rates for, 21

remission rates from, 20–21
for schizophrenia, 20–21
in Russian Federation, early use of, 266
chemical convulsive therapy, 167
CHF. *See* congestive heart failure, ECT with
childhood/adolescent psychoses, catatonia and, 141–142
children/adolescents, ECT in, 498–503
adverse events with, 502–503
tardive seizures, 502
cognitive effects of, 502–503
patient assessment for, 499–501
NICE guidelines for, 499
physical fitness as factor in, 500
treatment needs in, 499–500
rates of use for, 498–499
seizure thresholds with, 501
stimulus dosage for, 501–502
techniques for, 501–502
Chile, ECT use in, 281
choroid plexus, 58
chromatin remodeling, 58
chronic DBS, 557
chronic schizophrenia, ECT for, 136–138
antipsychotic drugs and, 136–138
definition of, 136
effect of catatonic features after, 138
Church of Scientology, 187, 208, 212, 217. *See also* Hubbard, Lafayette Ronald
CCHR and, 187, 208, 213
psychiatry and, 212
Citizens Commission on Human Rights (CCHR), 187, 208, 213
Clinical Antipsychotic Trials of Intervention Effectiveness (CATIE), 372
CME. *See* continual medical education
CNS. *See* central nervous system
Coalition for the Abolition of Electroshock, 214
Coalition to Stop Electroshock, 214, 215
Columbia University Consortium (CUC), 174
competency, 393–394
determination of, 393
legally relevant criteria for, 395–396
MacCAT-T for, 393
congestive heart failure (CHF), ECT with, 402–404
decompensated, 403
patient evaluation for, 403
treatment for,
Consortium for Research in ECT (CORE), 174
mECT study by, 520
constant-current stimulus generators, 4–5
skin burns from, 4–5
constant-current tDCS, 581
constant-voltage stimulus generators, 4
continual medical education (CME), 205

continuation electroconvulsive therapy (cECT), 505–512
for bipolar disorders, 511
for depression, 505–510, 511
with antidepressants, 505–506, 507–508
indications for, 510
with lithium, 507
praxis of, 510–511
for schizophrenia, 511
The Convulsive Therapy of Schizophrenia (Rotshtein), 266
convulsive therapy, 168
reemergence of, 175–176
CORE. *See* Consortium for Research in ECT
coronary artery disease (CAD), 404
ACC/AHA guidelines for, 404
medication treatment guidelines for, 404
corticotropin-releasing hormone (CRH), 478
cortisol hormone release, 159–160
causes of, 159
pretreatment for, 159
resting hypercortisolism and, 159
Cott, Jonathan, 190–191, 194
court-ordered treatment, 397
PADs and, 397
POA and, 397
craving disorders, 578–579
CREB pathway, 58–61
ECS and, 60
CRH. *See* corticotropin-releasing hormone
Cuba, ECT use in, 281
CUC. *See* Columbia University Consortium
cuff method, 419
curare, 23
as anesthesia, 413

DBS. *See* deep brain stimulation
deep brain stimulation (DBS), 556–569
advantages of, 559
chronic, 557
for depression, 561–562
neurobiology of, 559–560
studies for, 563
for dystonia, 557
ethical considerations for, 566–568
history of, 557
neurophysiologic changes from, 558
for OCD, 562
neurobiology of, 560
studies for, 564
patient selection for, 567–568
exclusion criteria for, 567–568
inclusion criteria for, 567
principles of, 557–558
quality standards for, 566–568
patient management in, 568

deep brain stimulation (DBS) (*cont.*)
  safety of, 559
  surgical implantation in, 557–558
  target selection issues with, 560–561
  for treatment-resistant depression, 556
deep transcranial magnetic stimulation,
  536–537
de Haviland, Olivia, 172
d'Elia, Giacomo, 237
delusions
  with melancholia, 352–353
  from TMS therapy, 536
dementia, ECT with, 407
  medication-resistant, 357–358
  medication treatments with, 407
Denmark. *See* Scandinavia, ECT as treatment
  in
depolarization, 7
depression
  antidepressant-resistant, 352–354
  atypical, 342–346
    anxiety disorders and, 342
  brain stimulation applications for, 68
  cECT for, 505–510, 511
    with antidepressants, 505–506, 507–508
    indications for, 510
    with lithium, 507
    praxis of, 510–511
  DBS for, 561–562
    studies for, 563
  diagnostic criteria for, 341
  diencephalic theory and, 77
  in DSM-IV, 341
  ECT for, 45, 109
    antipsychotic drugs v., 373–376
    antipsychotic medications v., 351–352
    for atypical, 342–346
    cECT after, 505–510, 511
    functional consequences of, 85
    neurotransmitters and, effects on, 46
    receptors and, effects on, 46
    in U.S., as treatment for, 228–229
  hippocampal volume and, 65–66
  HRSD for, 103, 345–346
    for resting hypercortisolism, 160
  indications for, 345
  MDD, 489
    VNS for, 547
  melancholia and, 347
    delusions with, 352–353
    ECT for, 347–348, 351
    psychotic, 353
  monoamine depletion and, 46
  Montgomery-Asberg Depression Rating Scale
    for, 346
  NE and, 49–51

  neurobiology of, 559–560
  NPY neuropeptide and, 53
  PTZ for, in non-ECT therapy, 21–22
  resting hypercortisolism and, 160
    HRSD scores for, 160
  serotonergic pathways and, 47–49
    serotonins in, 47–49
  STAR*D study for, 556
  stimulus dosing for, 450–454, 455–456
    fixed, 454
    formula-based, 453–454
    mECT and, 460–461
    titrated, 450–453
  suicidality and, 348
  tDCS for, 576–577
  TMS for, 528–529
    bipolar, 530
    high-frequency, 529
    low-frequency, 529
  treatment-resistant, 172–173
    DBS for, 556
    VNS for, 543
  VNS for, 546–548
    clinical outcomes for, 547
      MDD, 547
    treatment-resistant, 549
    trial studies for, 547–548
diabetes mellitus, ECT with, 410
  glucose control medications and, 424
*The Diagnostic Statistical Manual of Mental
  Disorders, 4th Edition* (DSM-IV-TR),
  124
  antipsychotic drugs in, 363
  depression diagnosis in, 341
    treatment-resistant depression in, 549
  melancholia diagnosis in, 347
Dianetics (Hubbard), 212
Dianetics, as spiritual technology, 212
  as alternative to psychiatry, 213
diencephalic theory, 77–78
  depression and, 77
diffusion tensor imaging (DTI), 94
  during interictal period, with ECT, 105
diffusion weighted imaging (DWI), 96
  during interictal period, with ECT, 105
direct stimulation hypothesis, in anatomical
  theory, 78
Disconn-ECT News, 217
disorders. *See* anxiety disorders; bipolar
  disorders; cardiovascular disorders, ECT
  with; craving disorders; major depressive
  disorder; mental disorders; mood
  disorders; movement disorders, ECT
  with; obsessive-compulsive disorder;
  panic disorder; schizoaffective disorders,
  ECT for

Donahue, Anne B., 194
dopamine hypothesis, 76. *See also* schizophrenia
dopaminergic pathways, 51
  dopamines, 51
dopamines, 51
  after ECS, 51
  HVA, 51
  hypothesis, 76
  receptors, 51
drugs, antipsychotic, xvii
"dry shock," 33
DSM-IV-TR. *See The Diagnostic Statistical*
    manual of Mental Disorders, 4th Edition
DTI. *See* diffusion tensor imaging
Dukakis, Kitty, 191, 194, 208, 212
Dukakis, Michael, 208
Duke, Patty, 208
Dutch Association for Psychiatry, 249
DWI. *See* diffusion weighted imaging
dysexecutive syndrome, 366
dysrhythmias, with ECT, 404–405
  AF as, 404–405
  ECG for, 405
dysthymic order, 530
dystonia, 557

EAAC1. *See* excitatory amino acid carrier 1
ECG. *See* electrocardiogram, with ECT
echocardiograms (ECG), with ECT
  for cardiovascular disorders,
  for dysrhythmias, 405
ECS. *See* electroconvulsive shock
ECT Accreditation Service (ECTAS), 241
ECTAS. *See* ECT Accreditation Service
ECT Handbook, 239, 241–242
EEG. *See* electroencephalography, with ECT
EFFECT, 252
electricity
  ECT and, 3–15
    on brain tissue, 6
    brief-pulse stimulus dose and, 9–11, 12–13
    conversion of energy in, 3
    dynamic impedance and, 6
    seizure generation and, 6–8
    sine wave stimulus dose and, 11, 12–13
    stimulus efficiency in, 3
    stimulus generators, 4–5
    toxic dosage range with, 5–6
  hypothesized mechanisms of action, for ECT,
      and, 82–89
    overcoming inhibitions in brain and, 82–85
  process of, 3
  properties of, 3–4
  seizure induction and, 6–8, 82
Electroboy (Behrman), 190
electrocardiogram (ECG), with ECT, 468

electroconvulsive shock (ECS), 45
  BDNF pathway and, 58–59
  CREB pathway and, 60
  dopamines after, 51
  5-HT serotonin receptors after, 47–49
  GABA pathways and, 51–52
  gene regulation after, 56
  gene transcription after, 54–55
  with MI, 404
  NE receptors, 50–51
  neurogenesis after, 64–66, 67
    regulation of, 65, 66–67
  NPY neuropeptide after, 53
  serotonins after, 47–49
  synaptic plasticity after, 64–66, 67
    neurotrophic factors for, 67
    structural changes, 65
  tachykinin neuropeptides after, 54
electroconvulsive therapy (ECT). *See also*
      anesthesia, for ECT; anti-ECT
      movements; Asia, ECT as treatment
      throughout; books and films, ECT in;
      brief-pulse stimulus dose;
      children/adolescents, ECT in;
      electroconvulsive shock;
      electroconvulsive therapy; electrodes,
      placement of; electroencephalography,
      with ECT; gene transcription, ECT
      effects on; hormones, ECT effect on;
      hypothesized mechanisms of action, for
      ECT; informed consent, for ECT;
      legislation, for ECT use; neuroimaging,
      for ECT; neuropeptides, ECT effects on;
      neurotransmitters, ECT effects on;
      nonelectrical convulsive therapies;
      physical therapies; psychiatric hospital
      programs, ECT in; psychosis, ECT for;
      seizures; sine wave stimulus dose;
      stimulus dosing, with ECT; stimulus
      generators
  for acute schizophrenia, 127–131
    antipsychotic drugs v., 127–128
    remission rates for, 127
    trial studies for, 128–130, 131
  ambulatory, 515–518
    ACT guidelines for, 516–517
    development of, 515–516
  analogous to surgery, xviii
  anesthesia for, 412–425
    airway management during, 422–423
    with anticholinergics, 414–415
    with atracurium, 420–421
    in *The Bell Jar,* 413
    with concomitant medications, 423–424
    history of, 413–414
    induction agents, 415–418

electroconvulsive therapy (ECT) (*cont.*)
  induction, in placebo trials, 113–114
  major elements of, 413
  with muscle relaxants, 418–421
  rationale for, 412
  rocuronium, 421
anterograde amnesia after, 493
antidepressants v., 114–115, 117, 348–349
  blind v. nonblind studies for, 114–116
  dosage issues in, 116
  meta-analyses failures in, 117
  new medications in, 116
  with outmoded techniques, 116
  variability in diagnoses in, 116–117
anti-ECT movements, 212–214
  development of, 214
  in Russian Federation, 268
  in Scandinavia, 237
antipsychiatry opponents and, 198
  U.S. state regulations and, influence on, 203–204
antipsychotic drugs v., xvii, 362–379
  for catatonia, 376–377
  for depression, 373–376
  hypofrontality and, 365–367
  lifespan rates and, 365
  physician behavior and, 377–379
  tardive psychosis and, 369
  therapeutic benefits with, 373–376
for anxiety disorders, 343–344
  antidepressants v., 348–349
  indications for, 344–345
  patient selection for, 344
  for prevention of, 346–347
APA Task Force on, 173, 200, 358, 516
  guidelines under, 202
in Argentina, 280
throughout Asia, 256–264
  age as factor for, 260
  gender as factor for, 261
  history of, 256
  indications for, 259–260
  professional publications about, 263–264
  rates of use for, 256–259, 263
  regulation of, 262
  technical aspects of, 261–262
  training guidelines for, 262–263
in Belgium, 246–248
benzodiazepines v., for catatonia, 376–377
in books and films, 180–195
  An Angel at My Table, 182–183, 193
  The Bell Jar, 184–185, 188, 193
  Electroboy, 190
  Family Life, 188
  Fear Strikes Out, 191–192, 193
Frances, 188, 192
Holiday of Darkness, 188–189
Memoirs of an Amnesiac, 183
One Flew over the Cuckoo's Nest, xviii, 172, 188, 191, 192, 210, 321
Out of Tune, 193
Shadowland, 192
Shine, 193
Shock: The Healing Power of Electroconvulsive Therapy, 191
The Snake Pit, 172
The Tender Place, 184
brain regions for, 45–46
in Brazil, 282–283
  history of, 282–283
with burns, 410
with CAD, 404
in Canada, as treatment therapy, 198–199
for catatonia, 124–142
  indications for, 349–350
  lethal, 350
  malignant, 133–135
  methodological limitations of, 125–126
  organic, 139–141
cECT after, 505–512
  for bipolar disorders, 511
  for depression, 505–510, 511
  for schizophrenia, 511
for cerebrovascular disease, 408
with CHF, 402–403, 404
in children/adolescents, 498–503
  adverse events with, 502–503
  cognitive effects of, 502–503
  patient assessment for, 499–501
  rates of use for, 498–499
  seizure thresholds with, 501
  stimulus dosage for, 501–502
  techniques for, 501–502
in Chile, 281
for chronic schizophrenia, 136–138
  antipsychotic drugs and, 136–138
  definition of, 136
  effect of catatonic features after, 138
clinical indications for, 341–358
  for catatonia, 349–350
  for delusions, 352–353
  for depression, 345
  for lethal catatonia, 350
  for mixed manic-depressive episodes, 350
cognitive side effects of, 485–495
  to executive functions, 493–494
  to language function, 494–495
  memory loss as, 490–493
  postictal confusion/disorientation, 486–487
in Cuba, 281

for dementia, 357–358, 407
  medication-resistant, 357–358
  medication treatments with, 407
for depression, 45, 109
  antidepressant-resistant, 352–354
  antipsychotic medications v., 351–352
  for atypical, 342–346
  brain stimulation applications for, 68
  cECT for, 505–511
  functional consequences of, 85
  neurotransmitters and, effects on, 46
  receptors and, effects on, 46
with diabetes mellitus, 410
with dysrhythmias, 404–405
with ECG, 405, 468
ECS in, 45
  BDNF pathway and, 58–59
  CREB pathway and, 60
  dopamines after, 51
  5-HT serotonin receptors after, 47–49
  GABA pathways and, 51–52
  gene regulation after, 56
  gene transcription after, 54–55
  NE receptors, 50–51
  neurogenesis after, 64–67
  NPY neuropeptide after, 53
  serotonins after, 47–49
  synaptic plasticity and, 64–67
  tachykinin neuropeptides after, 54
EEG with, 96, 468–474
  APA Task Force guidelines for, 468
  electrode placement and, 468–469
  of HR, 479
  during ictal periods, 469–472
  memory loss and, 472–473
  during postictal periods, 470–471
  seizures and, 473–474
electricity and, 3–15
  on brain tissue, 6
  brief-pulse stimulus dose and, 9–11, 12–13
  conversion of energy in, 3
  dynamic impedance and, 6
  seizures from, 6–8
  sine wave stimulus dose and, 11, 12–13
  stimulus generators, 4–5
  toxic dosage range with, 5–6
electrode placement in, 430–444
  antidepressant medication and, 433
  in Asia, 261, 263
  bifrontal, 442–444
  bitemporal, 438–439
  with brief-pulse stimulus dose, 10–11
  cognitive side effects from, 434–436
  comparison studies for, 433
  development history for, 170, 173–175

efficacy of, 434
in Europe, 252
LART technique for, 175, 441–442
neurobiology of, 436–438
pre-ECT protocol for, xxviii
right unilateral, 439–441
SSRIs and, 433
with stimulus dosing, 459–460
with ultrabrief-pulse stimulus dose, 14–15
with epilepsy, 409
in Europe, 246
  EFFECT for, 252
  electrode placement variation in, 252
  history in, 246
throughout Europe, 246
  history in, 246
evaluation after, 505–512
fractures as result of, 209
in France, 248
Friedberg opposition to, 213–214
future applications of, 176
in Germany, 248–249
history of, 167–176
  current application reduction in, 170–171
  electrode placement in, 170, 173–175
  Meduna in, 18, 168
  memory loss in, 169
  oxygenation in, 171–172
  within physical therapies, 167
  psychopharmacology in, 172
  restraint development in, 169
  Sakel in, 18, 167–168
in Hong Kong, 256
hormonal effects of, 149–161
  ACTH, 153
  comparison of changes in, 151–153
  consequences of, 150–151
  cortisol release, 159–160
  future research applications with, 160–161
  posterior pituitary, 158–159
  prolactin, 152, 153–158
  resting hypercortisolism and, 159
  as temporary, 149
in hospital programs, 201
  model policy guidelines for, 287–294, 313
  for patients from other facilities, 306–308
HR and, 477–483
  peak, 479–481
  seizure activity and, 477–479
  tachycardia duration and, 481–483
Hubbard movement against use of, 212, 213
hypothesized mechanisms of action for, 75, 76–90
  abnormal metabolism in, 85
  anatomical theory of, 78

electroconvulsive therapy (ECT) (*cont.*)
   anticonvulsant theory of, 78
   background of, 75
   development of, 79–89
   diencephalic theory of, 77–78
   functional consequences of, 85–87
   neurochemical theories of, 75–77
   neuronal network function restoration in,
      87–89
   seizure generalization theory and, 79, 89
   with ICDs/pacemakers, 405
   in India, 258
   informed consent for, xxv–xxvi, 384–398
      competency for, 393–394
      court-ordered treatment and, 397
      definitions of, 385
      discussion strategies for, 387–392
      historical development of, 385
      hospital programs policy guidelines for,
         289–292
      in Latin America, 279–280
      legislation on, for ECT use, 215
      mental capacity for, 393–394
      mental incapacity and, 393–397
      obstacles to, 392–397
      practical strategy methods for, 386–387
   in Japan, 257–258
   throughout Latin America, 276–283
      anesthesia with, 279
      applications of, 278–279
      history of use in, 276–277
      informed consent for, 279–280
      rates of, 279
      techniques for, 279
      training for, 280
   legislation for, 207–220
      APA Task Force role in, 214–215
      for banned use, 208
      in California, 214–216
      constructive lawmaking in, 218–219
      films' influence on, 210–211
      history of, 214–218
      for informed consent, 215
      litigation cases as basis for, 209–210
      in Massachusetts, 215
      proactive, 219
      state regulations and, 202–204, 233
      in Texas, 216–218
   legislative regulations against, 202–204
   for malignant catatonia, 133–135
      antipsychotic drugs v., 133
      NMS and, 133
      "shock-block" method of, 134
      survival rates for, 134–135
   malpractice concerns with, 204
   mania, 119–120

   for manic episodes, 354
   MECT and, 138–139, 518–522
      for bipolar disorders, 511
      cognitive function during, 521–522
      CORE study on, 520
      definition of, 518
      effectiveness of, 520
      electrode placement during, 522
      NICE on, 519–520
      pharmacotherapy with, 520–521
      relapse rates for, 519
      for schizoaffective disorders, 135
      with stimulus dosing, 460–461, 522
   with medical disorders, 401–410
      anticoagulation and, 406
      CAD, 404
      for cardiovascular disorders, 402
      cerebrovascular disease, 408
      CHF, 402–404
      dementia, 407
      diabetes mellitus, 410
      dysrhythmias, 404–405
      epilepsy, 409
      with ICDs/pacemakers, 405
      intracranial space-occupying lesions,
         409
      MI, 404
      neurological, 406–407
      planned management for, 401
      pretreatment assessment for, 401
      pulmonary, 410
      reevaluation during treatment in,
         401
      valvular disease, 406
      vascular disease, 405–406
   for melancholia, 347–348, 351
      with multiple medications, 348
      psychotic, 353
      SSRIs v., 347–348
   for mental disorders, 89
   in Mexico, 281–282
   with MI, 404
   for mood disorders, 109–120
      antidepressant medications v., 114–115,
         117
      mania, 119–120
      placebo trials v., 109–112, 114
      response rates for, 109, 110
      variety of treatments in, 117
   as most clinical studied procedure, 197–198
   for movement disorders, 407–408
      PD, 407–408
   muscle relaxants with, 170
   negative public impressions of, xviii, 172
      from *One Flew over the Cuckoo's Nest,* xviii,
         172

in The Netherlands, 249, 250
neurochemical effects of, 45–69
    on dopaminergic pathways, 51
    on GABA pathways, 51–52
    on gene transcription, 54–64
    on glutamergic systems, 52
    on neuropeptides, 52–54
    on neurotransmitters, 46–52
    on noradregenic pathways, 49–51
    on receptors, 46–52
    on serotonergic pathways, 47–49
neuroimaging and, 94–105
    with DTI, 94
    with DWI, 96
    with EEG, 96
    future applications for, 105–106
    during ictal period, 96–98
    during interictal period, 99–105
    with LORETA, 96
    measurement parameters for, 95–96
    with MRI, 94, 95–96
    with MRS, 94
    with PET, 94
    during postictal periods, 99–101
    purpose of, 94–95
    with SPECT, 94
    structural abnormalities under, 94
    with TCD, 96
non-ECT therapies, 17–37
    for bipolar disorder, 36–37
    chemical convulsants, 18–24
    flurothyl inhalation, 30–31
    historical background of, 17–18
    insulin therapy, after coma inducement, 18,
      24–28
    PTZ, 19–24
    theoretical implications of, 31–37
nursing guidelines for, 300–306
    inpatient transportation, 301–302
    for post-ECT duties, 305–306
    pre-ECT patient preparation, 301
    for recovery procedures, 304–305
    staff assistance during treatment, 303–304
    treatment room preparation, 302
orbitofrontal syndrome from, 367
for organic catatonia, 139–141
in Pakistan, 258
patient selection for, 341–358
    for anxiety disorders, 344
with PD, 407–408
personal accounts of, 181–184, 187, 189–191
philosophy for use of, 341–342
physical suite layout for, 314–321
    anesthetists in, 323–324
    design considerations for, 321
    for high-volume operations, 316

IV access considerations in, 317–319
    nurses in, 322–323
    outpatient considerations for, 319
    pretreatment personnel in, 322
    psychiatrists in, 323
    for recovery rooms, 320–321
    in small hospitals, 315–316
    for small-volume operations, 315–316
    surgical operating rooms and, 314
    for treatment rooms, 319–320
Plath critique of, 184–185, 211
in Portugal, 250–251
posttreatment protocol, xxix–xxx
    patient discharge considerations in,
      xxix–xxx
    patient management in, xxix
pre-ECT protocol, xxv–xxx
    atropinic agents in, xxvi
    with benzodiazepines, xxvii
    electrode placement in, xxviii
    intramuscular medication in, xxv–xxvi
    muscle relaxants in, xxvii
    narcosis agents in, xxvi–xxvii
    oral medications in,
    oxygenation during, xxvii
    physiological monitoring for, xxix
    sedation for sleep on night before, xxvi
    stimulus dose method in, xxviii
    stimulus potentiation in, xxviii–xxix
during pregnancy, 409
as prerequisite for other procedures, 357
prevention of mental illness, xvii
for prevention of threatening experiences,
    xvii–xviii
    bipolar disorders, xviii
    PTSD, xviii
psychiatrists' response to, 197–205
    in Canada, 198–199
    legislative regulations against, 202–204
    malpractice concerns, 204
    as molded by negative film portrayals,
      198
    as professional mindset, 204–205
    sociopolitical barriers to, 201–202
    training issues with, 199–200
    in treatment patterns, 198, 200–201
    in U.S., 198–199
psychological testing after, 485–490
    of general intelligence, 487–490
    with MMSE, 435, 485–486
    with SSMQ, 491
    with WAIS, 488
for psychosis, 350
    medication-resistant, 354–357
PTZ replacement by, 23–24
public perceptions of, 208

electroconvulsive therapy (ECT) (*cont.*)
  reboot theory of, xxiii–xxv
    anticonvulsant activity in, xxv
     preexisting psychiatric illness in, xxiii
    seizures' role in, xxiii
  recovery from, xxix
  in regional medical centers, guidelines for,
      308–311
    reporting requirements for, 311
  retrograde amnesia after, 491–492
  in Russian Federation, 266–273
    anti-ECT movement in, 268
    chemical convulsants and, in early use of,
        266
    contemporary applications of, 271–272
    device development in, 271
    early history of, 266–270
    "Meduna's method" and, 266
    Moscow Society of Neurologists and
        Psychiatrists in, 270
    for nonpsychiatric conditions, 272
    political influence on, 267–268
    psychiatry in, under Stalin, 267
    Soviet Scientific Society of Neurologists
        and Psychiatrists in, 268
  in Scandinavia, 236–238
    anti-ECT movement in, 237
    future applications for, 243
    history of, 236
    rates of use for, 236–237
    research tradition and, 238
    training for, 242
  for schizoaffective disorders, 135–136
    psychosis and, 355
  for schizophrenia, 124–131, 142
    acute, 127–131
    acute catatonic, 131–133
    chronic, 136–138
    continuation, 138–139
    history of, 124–125
    mECT and, 135, 138–139
    methodological limitations of, 125–126
    for schizoaffective disorders, 135–136
    for schizophreniform disorder, 126–127
  for schizophreniform disorder, 126–127
  seizures from, repeated application
      complications for, 35–36
    spontaneous v., 82–84
  "shock-block" method of, 134
  sociopolitical barriers to, 201–202
  in Spain, 251
  with spinal cord injury, 410
  stimulus dosing with, 447–463
    augmentation strategies for, 458–459
    Benchmark Method for, 456–458
    case studies of, 461–463

    cognitive side effects of, 454–455
    for depression, 450–454, 455–456
    electrode placement and, 459–460
    with mECT, 460–461, 522
    schedule for, 452
    sham studies for, 449
    units of measure for, 447–449
    waveform morphology for, 449–450
  in Taiwan, 256–257
  tardive psychosis for, 369
  in Thailand, 257
  TMS v., 36, 534–535
  training issues with, 199–200
    for nonpsychiatric physicians, 199
    during psychiatric residency, 199–200
  treatment for, xviii
  in UK, 238–242
    contemporary standards and practices for,
        241–242
    ECT Handbook in, 239, 241–242
    future applications for, 243
    under NICE, 240–241
    pre-NICE standards and practices, 238–240
    training for, 242–243
  in Uruguay, 282
  in U.S., 198–199, 209–210, 227–234
    academic medical centers as factor for, 229
    age as factor for, 231
    APA guidelines for, 228
    demographic variation in, 231–232
    for depression, 228–229
    ethnicity/race as factor in, 232
    excessive use of, 209
    future applications for, 233–234
    gender as factor in, 231–232
    inpatient v. outpatient status and, 230–231
    insurance access as factor for, 232–233
    legislation for, 207–220
    litigation over, 209–210
    overuse of, 209
    in public v. private hospitals, 230
    regional/state variation for, 229
    service sites for, 230–231
    service system variation for, 229–230
    small-area analysis for, 228–229
    socioeconomic factors for, 232–233
    state regulations over, 202–204, 233
    usage trends for, 227
    variation of, 228
  with VNS, 549–550
electrodes, placement of, 430–444
  antidepressant medication and, 433
  in Asia, in ECT treatment, 261, 263
  bifrontal, 442–444
    clinical outcomes from, 443
    MMSE scores after, 443–444

bitemporal, 438–439
  Benchmark Method and, 153, 441
  clinical application of, 438
  clinical outcomes from, 438–439
  HRSD scores after, 438
  MMSE score after, 438
  right unilateral v., 440
with brief-pulse stimulus dose, 10–11
cognitive side effects from, 434–436
  acute onset delirium as, 435–436
  gradual cumulative disorientation as, 435
  MMSE and, 435
  permanent memory loss as, 436
comparison studies for, 433
development of, in ECT history, 170, 173–175
  CUC v. CORE study in, 174
EEG and, 468–469
efficacy of, 434
  stimulus dosing as factor for, 434
in Europe, in ECT treatment, 252
LART technique, 175, 441–442
  clinical applications of, 441
  MMSE scores after, 442
during MECT, 522
neurobiology of, 436–438
  through skull bones, 437
in pre-ECT protocol, xxviii
right unilateral, 439–441
  bitemporal v., 440
  clinical application of, 439
  dosing levels for, 440–441
  rationale for, 439
SSRIs and, 433
with stimulus dosing, 459–460
in tCDS, 575
with ultrabrief-pulse stimulus dose, 14–15
electroencephalography (EEG), with ECT, 96, 468–474
  APA Task Force guidelines for, 468
  electrode placement and, 468–469
  of HR, 479
  during ictal periods, 469–472
    interpretation of, 471–472
    scalp distribution of, 471
    seizure duration during, 471
    seizure expression during, 471–472
    seizure rhythms during, 470
  memory loss and, 472–473
  during postictal periods, 470–471
  seizures and, 473–474
    abortive, 474
    missed, 473–474
    prolonged, 474

Electroshock: The Case Against (Morgan), 212
ELL2 gene, 64
emergence agitation, 150. *See also* postictal excitement
Emergency Medical Treatment and Active Labor Act (EMTALA), 287
EMTALA. *See* Emergency Medical Treatment and Active Labor Act
Endler, Norman, 188–189
England. *See* United Kingdom, ECT as treatment in
epilepsy
  ECT with, 409
  phenytoin for, 35
  schizophrenia and, 34–35
  tDCS for, 577–578
  VNS for, 543, 546
epileptic seizures, 84
epileptiform phenomena, 33
  symptoms of, 34
epinephrine, 478
ERK5 genes, 63
ethnicity, ECT use and, 232
etomidate, 417
eugenics
  psychiatrists and, 17
  schizophrenia and, 17
Europe, ECT treatment throughout, 246. *See also* Belgium; France; Germany; The Netherlands; Portugal, ECT use in; Spain, ECT use in
  EFFECT for, 252
  electrode placement variation in, 252
  history in, 246
excitatory amino acid carrier 1 (EAAC1), 52

Family Life, 188
FDA. *See* Food and Drug Administration
Fear Strikes Out, 191–192, 193
FGF-2 genes, 62
fibromyalgia, 577
films, ECT in. *See* books and films, ECT in
Fink, Max, 173, 174, 238
Finland. *See* Scandinavia, ECT as treatment in
First International Meeting on Modern Treatment of Schizophrenia, 18
5-HT serotonin receptors, 47–49
fixed-charge stimulus generators, 4
flurothyl inhalation therapy, 30–31
  application procedures for, 30
  complications from, 30–31
    from technical issues, 30–31
  historical background for, 30
  indications for, 30
  seizure onset with, 30

fMRI. *See* functional magnetic resonance
    imaging
Fontanarrosa, Orlando y, 280
Food and Drug Administration (FDA), 287
Forman, Milos, xviii, 172
Foucault, Michel, 172
fractures, from ECT, 209
Frame, Janet, 182–183, 193
France, ECT in, 248
    training issues with, 248
Frances, 188, 192
Frank, Leonard Roy, 214
Friedberg, John, 211, 212
    opposition to ECT, 213–214
Friedman, Emerick, 170
frizzled protein (Frz) genes, 64
Frz genes. *See* frizzled protein genes
functional magnetic resonance imaging (fMRI),
    96

GABA. *See* gamma-aminobutyric acid pathways
Gage, Phineas, 366
Gamito, António, 253
gamma-aminobutyric acid (GABA) pathways,
    46, 51–52
    ECS and, 51–52
    ECT and, 51–52
    in hypothesized mechanisms of action, for
        ECT, 85–86
Geddes, John, 174
gender, ECT use by, 231–232
    in Asia, 261
gene transcription, ECT effects on, 54–64. *See
        also* BDNF pathway
    arachidonic acid cascade genes, 61–62
    Arc genes, 62–63
    in BDNF/CREB pathway, 58–61
        chronic ECS and, 58–59, 60
    in choroid plexus, 58
    for chromatin remodeling, 58
    after chronic ECS, 54–55
    after ECS, 56
    ELL2 gene, 64
    ERK5/MEF2C genes, 63
    FGF-2 genes, 62
    Frz genes, 64
    in hippocampus, 55
    Kf-1 gene, 64
    Ndrg2 gene, 64
    neurochemical theories and, 76–77
    neurogenesis, 64–67
        regulation of, 65, 66–67
    NGF genes, 62
    synaptic plasticity, 64–67
        neurotrophic factors for, 64–67
        structural changes, 65

TIMP-1 and, 63
TRH and, 63
VAMP2 gene, 64
VEGF genes, 62
VGF genes, 62
Germany, ECT in, 248–249
    increased use of, 249
Glassman, Alexander, 173
glucagon, 25
glutamergic systems, 52
    EAAC1, 52
glycopyrrolate, 414–415
Goldman, Douglas, 171
Gonda, Victor, 169
gradual cumulative disorientation, 435
grand mal seizures, xxiii–xxiv
    CNS depletion in, xxiii
Grove, Andrew, 362
*Guidelines of Perioperative Cardiovascular
        Evaluation and Care for Noncardiac
        Surgery* (ACC/AHA), 402

Halstead-Reitan Neuropsychological Test
    Battery, 494
Hamilton, Max, 419
Hamilton Rating Scale for Depression (HRSD),
    103, 345–346, 489
    after bitemporal electrode placement, 438
    in placebo trials v. ECT, for mood disorders,
        110–113
Hammersley, Donald, 173
heart rate (HR), ECT and, 477–483
    peak, 479–481
        Benchmark Method for, 479, 481
        hyperventilation from, 480
    seizure activity and, 477–479
        CRH and, 478
        EEG recording of, 479
        epinephrine and, 478
        neuroanatomic rationale for, 477–478
    tachycardia duration and, 481–483
Helfgott, David, 193
Helfgott, Margaret, 193
Hemingway, Ernest, 180, 184, 185–186
    Hotchner on, 186–187
    suicide attempts of, 185–187
hippocampus, 55
    depression and, volume as factor in, 65–66
The History of Madness (Foucault), 172
Holiday of Darkness (Endler), 188–189
Holmberg, Carl Gunnar, 170, 413
homovanilic acid (HVA), 51
Hong Kong, ECT use in, 256
hormones, ECT effect on, 149–161
    ACTH, 153
    comparison of changes in, 151–153

for baseline levels, 152–153
Benchmark Method for, 153
measurement problems in, 151
medical v. psychiatric, 152
consequences of, 150–151
postictal excitement as, 150–151
during pregnancy, 151
cortisol release, 159–160
causes of, 159
pretreatment for, 159
future research applications with, 160–161
posterior pituitary, 158–159
oxytocin, 158–159
vasopressin, 158–159
prolactin, 152, 153–158
AUC and, 156
basic model for, 156–157
brain neurochemistry changes and, 154
as pituitary hormone archetype, 154–155
seizure-induced, 158
resting hypercortisolism and, 159
cognitive side effects of, 160
depression and, 160
as temporary, 149
Horowitz, Vladimir, 181, 208
hospitals. See psychiatric hospital programs,
ECT in
Hotchner, A.E., 186
on Hemingway depression, 186–187
HR. See heart rate, ECT and
HRSD. See Hamilton Rating Scale for Depression
Hubbard, Lafayette Ronald, 211, 212, 213
Church of Scientology under, 187, 208, 212
Dianetics development by, 212
Hughes, Ted, 184
HVA. See homovanilic acid
hyperventilation, 423, 480
hypoactivity, from antipsychotic drugs, 372
hypofrontality, 365–367
apathetic syndrome in, 366
behavioral/mental changes and, 366–367
dysexecutive syndrome in, 366
orbitofrontal syndrome in, 366
somnolence and, 367
hypomania, 535–536
hypothesized mechanisms of action, for ECT, 75,
76–90. See also neurochemical theories
abnormal metabolism in, 85
GABA concentrations and, 85–86
glutamate levels and, 85
imaging studies for, 85–87
anatomical theory of, 78
direct stimulation hypothesis in, 78
TMS in, 78
anticonvulsant theory of, 78
seizure thresholds in, 78

background of, 75
development of, 79–89
electrical stimulation in, 82–89
organizational levels of the brain in,
79–82
diencephalic theory of, 77–78
depression and, 77
functional consequences of, 85–87
for depression, 85
neurochemical theories of, 75–77
gene transcription in, 76–77
intracellular signaling in, 76–77
neurotransmitter theories in, 75–76
neurotrophic action in, 76–77
neuronal network function restoration in,
87–89
seizure generalization theory and, 79, 89
objections to, 79

ICD-10. See International Classification of
Diseases, 10th Revision
ICDs. See implantable cardioverter defibrillators
Iceland. See Scandinavia, ECT as treatment in
ictal periods, 95
EEG during, 469–472
interpretation of, 471–472
scalp distribution of, 471
seizure duration during, 471
seizure expression during, 471–472
seizure rhythms during, 470
neuroimaging in ECT during, 96–98
electrode placement in, 97–98
with PET, 97–98
with SPECT, 96–97
Impastato, David, 227
implantable cardioverter defibrillators (ICDs),
405
incapacity. See mental incapacity
India, ECT use in, 258
induction agents, for anesthesia, 415–418
barbiturates, 415–416
etomidate, 417
inhalational, 418
ketamine, 417–418
propofol, 417
thiopental, 416–417
ultrashort-acting narcotics, 418
informed consent, for ECT, xxv–xxvi, 384–398
competency for, 393–394
determination of, 393
legally relevant criteria for, 395–396
MacCAT-T for, 393
court-ordered treatment and, 397
PADs and, 397
POA and, 397
definitions of, 385

informed consent, for ECT (*cont.*)
  discussion strategies for, 387–392
    for adverse side effects, 391
    APA Task Force report on, 392
    for consent process, 387–389
    for ECT v. other treatments, 389–390
    for nature of illness, 389
    physician's role in, 389
    for risk factors, 391–392
    for treatment/posttreatment, 389,
      390–391
  historical development of, 385
    in legal cases, 385
    Parens Patriae doctrine and, 385
  hospital programs policy guidelines for,
    289–292
  in Latin America, 279–280
  legal applications of, 385–386
    in malpractice cases, 385
    State of California Welfare and Institutions
      Code for, 386
  legislation on, for ECT use, 215
    model for, 218
    in Texas, 216–217
  mental capacity for, 393–394
    determination of, 393
    legally relevant criteria for, 395–396
  mental incapacity and, 393–397
    National Quality Forum for, 394
  obstacles to, 392–397
    with competent patients, 392
    mental incapacity as, 393–397
  practical strategy methods for, 386–387
Inglis, James, 174, 443
Insane Liberation Front, 214
The Insulin Myth, 27
insulin therapy, after coma inducement, 18,
    24–28
  ambulatory, 25
  application procedure for, 25
  with chemical convulsants, 28–30
    application procedures for, 29
    complications from, 29–30
    indications for, 29
  complications of, 28
    fatalities as, 28
  convulsive factor in, 33–34
  "dry shock" from, 33
  epileptiform phenomena in, 33
  glucagon in, 25
  historical background of, 24–25, 167–168
  indications for, 25–27
  "moist shock" from, 33
  outcomes from, 21
  patient fear of, 31–33

  remission rates with, 26
  for schizophrenia, 26, 167
    PZT v., 26
  as symptomatic, 27
intelligence, 487–490
  WAIS for, 488
interictal periods, 95
  neuroimaging, with ECT, 99–105
    with DTI, 105
    with DWI, 105
    HRSD scores and, 103
    with MRI, 104–105
    with MRS, 104
    with PET, 102
    with SPECT, 103–104
    with TCD, 102, 103
intermittent tDCS, 581
*International Classification of Diseases, 10th
  Revision* (ICD-10), 124
International Coalition for the Abolition of
  Electroshock, 214
International Congress of Psychiatry, 26–27
intracellular signaling, 76–77
intracranial space-occupying lesions, ECT with,
  409
intramuscular medication, in pre-ECT protocol,
  xxv–xxvi

Japan, ECT use in, 257–258

Kalinowsky, Lothar, 169
Karliner, William, 170
Kesey, Ken, 172, 210
ketamine, 417–418
Kety, Seymour, 67
Kf-1 gene, 64
Kill Your Sons (Reed), 187
kindling, 7–8
Klüver-Bucy syndrome, 430
Kohloff, Roland, 208
Korsakov, S.S., 272

Lancaster, Neville, 173
LART technique. *See* left anterior right temporal
  technique
laryngeal mask airway (LMA), 422
Latin America. *See also* Argentina, ECT use in;
      Brazil, ECT use in; Chile, ECT use in;
      Cuba, ECT use in; Mexico, ECT use in
  academic research in, 278
  demographics for, 277
  ECT use throughout, 276–283
    anesthesia with, 279
    applications of, 278–279
    history of use in, 276–277

informed consent for, 279–280
rates of, 279
techniques for, 279
training for, 280
geography of, 276
mental health disorder rates in, 277–278
scarcity of resources for, 277–278
Lawson, J.S., 175
l-dopa, 424
left anterior right temporal (LART) technique, 175, 441–442
clinical applications of, 441
MMSE scores after, 442
legislation, for ECT use, 207–220
APA Task Force role in, 214–215
for banned use, 208
in California, 214–216
constructive lawmaking in, 218–219
films' influence on, 210–211
history of, 214–218
for informed consent, 215
model for, 218
in Texas, 216–217
litigation cases as basis for, 209–210
overregulation as result of, 210
in Massachusetts, 215
proactive, 219
in Texas, 216–218
for informed consent, 216–217
Texas Society of Psychiatric Physicians influence on, 216
Leicestershire trial, 118, 449
lesions. *See* intracranial space-occupying lesions, ECT with
lethal catatonia, 350. *See also* malignant catatonia, ECT for
Levant, Oscar, 183, 188, 194
Lewis, Aubrey, 22
Liberson, Wladimir, 170
Lisanby, Sarah, 174
lithium, 423–424
cECT with, for depression, 507
litigation, over ECT use, 209–210
Aden v. Younger, 210, 219
Mitchell v. Robinson, 209
overregulation as result of, 210
"therapeutic privilege" as defense in, 209
Wyatt v. Hardin, 209–210, 219
LMA. *See* laryngeal mask airway
Loach, Ken, 188
LORETA. *See* low-resolution brain electromagnetic tomography
Loudet, Osvald, 280
Lowell, Robert, 181

low-resolution brain electromagnetic tomography (LORETA), 96
during interictal period, with ECT, 103

MacCAT-T. *See* McArthur Competence Assessment Tool for Treatment
Madness and Civilization. See The History of Madness
magnetic resonance imaging (MRI), 94, 95–96
DTI, 94
fMRI, 96
during interictal period, with ECT, 104–105
magnetic resonance spectroscopy (MRS), 94
during interictal period, with ECT, 104
maintenance electroconvulsive therapy (MECT), 138–139, 518–522. *See also* continuation electroconvulsive therapy
for bipolar disorders, 511
cognitive function during, 521–522
CORE study on, 520
definition of, 518
effectiveness of, 520
electrode placement during, 522
NICE on, 519–520
pharmacotherapy with, 520–521
relapse rates for, 519
for schizoaffective disorders, 135
with stimulus dosing, 460–461, 522
major depressive disorder (MDD), 489
VNS trials for, 547
malarial-fever therapy, 167
malignant catatonia, ECT for, 133–135
antipsychotic drugs v., 133
NMS and, 133
"shock-block" method of, 134
survival rates for, 134–135
malpractice, ECT use and, 204
informed consent and, 385
psychiatric hospital programs and, 204
"therapeutic privilege" as defense against, 209
mania
ECT for, 119–120
from TMS, as side effect, 535–536
TMS for, 531–532
manic episodes, ECT for, 354
Manning, Martha, 189–190
Mayo Clinic, 317
McArthur Competence Assessment Tool for Treatment (MacCAT-T), 393
McGuire, Tobey, 190
MDD. *See* major depressive disorder
mECT. *See* maintenance electroconvulsive therapy
medical insurance, ETC use and, 232–233

medications. *See* intramuscular medication; oral
    medications
Meduna, Ladislas, 18, 168
"Meduna's method," 266
MEF2C genes, 63
melancholia, diagnosis of, 347. *See also*
    depression
    delusions with, 352–353
    ECT for, 347–348, 351
        with multiple medications, 347–348
        SSRIs v., 347–348
    psychotic, 353
Memoirs of an Amnesiac (Levant), 183
memory loss, 169. *See also* working memory
    after ECT, 490–493
        SSMQ for, 491
        subjective complaints of, 490–491
    EEG with ECT and, 472–473
    from electrode placement, 436
    from stimulus dosing, 454–455
mental capacity, 393–394
    determination of, 393
    legally relevant criteria for, 395–396
mental disorders
    ECT as treatment for, 89
    organizational levels of brain and, 80–82,
        89
        structural abnormalities in, 81–82
mental incapacity, 393–397
    National Quality Forum for, 394
Mental Patients Liberation Project, 214
"The Merry Pranksters,"
Mexico, ECT use in, 281–282
Meyer, Adolph, 18
Meyers, Jeffrey, 186
MI. *See* myocardial infarction, with ECT
Mini Mental State Examination (MMSE), 435,
    485–486
    after bifrontal electrode placement, 443–444
    after bitemporal electrode placement, 438
    after LART technique, 442
minors, ECT use for, 294–295
missed seizures, 473–474
Mitchell v. Robinson, 209
mivacurium, 420
MMSE. *See* Mini Mental State Examination
Moench, Louis, 173
"moist shock," 33
Molohov, A.I., 267
monoamine hypothesis, 76
monoamine systems
    depression from depletion of, 46
    hypothesis for, 76
Montgomery-Asberg Depression Rating Scale,
    346

mood disorders, 76. *See also* antidepressant
    medications; depression
    chemical convulsive therapy for, 167
    depression
        brain stimulation applications for, 68
        diencephalic theory and, 77
        ECT for, 45, 109–120
        hippocampal volume and, 65–66
        HRSD for, 103
        monoamine depletion and, 46
        NE and, 49–51
        NPY neuropeptide and, 53
        PTZ for, in non-ECT therapy, 21–22
        serotonergic pathways and, 47–49
    ECT for, 109–120
        antidepressant medications v., 114–115,
            117
        for mania, 119–120
        placebo trials v., 109–112, 114
        response rates for, 109, 110
        for subtypes of depression, 117–119
        variety of treatments in, 117
    mania, ECT for, 119–120
    symptoms of, 77–78
Morgan, Robert F., 212
Moscow Society of Neurologists and
    Psychiatrists, 270
movement disorders, ECT with, 407–408
    PD, 407–408
MRI. *See* magnetic resonance imaging
MRS. *See* magnetic resonance spectroscopy
Müller, Max, 18
muscle relaxants, with ECT, 170. *See also*
    succinylcholine
    with anesthesia, 418–421
        cuff method, 419
        mivacurium, 420
        moderate/short-acting, 420–421
        succinylcholine, 419–420
    in Asia, 261–262
    development of, 418–419
myocardial infarction (MI), with ECT, 404
    ACC/AHA guidelines for, 404
    medication treatment guidelines for, 404
Myth of Mental Illness (Szasz), 172

NAPA. *See* Network Against Psychiatric Assault
narcosis agents, xxvi–xxvii
Nash, John, 211
National Anti-Shock Action, 249
National Institute for Clinical Excellence
    (NICE)
    ECT guidelines under, 240–241
        for children/adolescents, 499
        on MECT, 519–520

pre-NICE standards and practices, in U.K., 238–240
National Institute of Mental Health (NIMH), 208
    ECT usage, demographics for, 227
National Institute of Neurological Disorders and Stroke (NINDS), 576
National Quality Forum, 394
NCS-1 neuropeptide, 53
NE. *See* norepinephrine receptors
Nelson, Alexander, 175, 441
nerve growth factor (NGF) genes, 62
NET. *See* norepinephrine transporter
The Netherlands
    Dutch Association for Psychiatry in, 249
    ECT in, 249–250
    National Anti-Shock Action in, 249
Network Against Coercive Psychiatry, 217
Network Against Psychiatric Assault (NAPA), 214, 215
neuritin gene, 61
neurochemical theories, 75–77
    gene transcription in, 76–77
    intracellular signaling in, 76–77
    neurotransmitter theories in, 75–76
        dopamine hypothesis in, 76
        monoamine hypothesis, 76
    neurotrophic action in, 76–77
neuroendocrine view. *See* diencephalic theory
neurogenesis, after ECS, 64–66, 67
    regulation of, 65, 66–67
neuroimaging, for ECT, 94–105
    with DTI, 94
        during interictal period, 105
    with DWI, 96
        during interictal period, 105
    with EEG, 96
    future applications for, 105–106
    during ictal period, 96–98
        electrode placement in, 97–98
        with PET, 97–98
        with SPECT, 96–97
    during interictal period, 99–105
        with DTI, 105
        with DWI, 105
        HRSD scores and, 103
        with LORETA, 103
        with MRI, 104–105
        with MRS, 104
        with PET, 102
        with TCD, 102, 103
    with LORETA, 96
        during interictal period, 103
    measurement parameters for, 95–96

with MRI, 94, 95–96
    DTI, 94
    fMRI, 96
    during interictal period, 104–105
with MRS, 94
    during interictal period, 104
with PET, 94
    during ictal period, 97–98
    during interictal period, 102
    during postictal periods, 99–101
    purpose of, 94–95
with SPECT, 94
    during ictal period, 96–97
    during interictal period, 103–104
    structural abnormalities under, 94
with TCD, 96
    during interictal period, 102, 103
neuroleptic malignant syndrome (NMS), 133
    from antipsychotic drugs, 371
neuropeptides, ECT effects on, 52–54
    in animal models, 52
    NCS-1, 53
    neuroserpin, 53
    neurotensin, 54
    NPY, 52–53
        angiogenic patterns of, 53
        after chronic ECS, 53
        depression and, 53
    tachykinins, 54
        after chronic ECS, 54
neuroserpin neuropeptide, 53
neurotensin neuropeptide, 54
neurotransmitters, ECT effects on, 46–52
    depression and, 46
    dopaminergic pathways, 51
        dopamines, 51
    GABA pathways, 46, 51–52
        ECS and, 51–52
        ECT and, 51–52
    glutamergic systems, 52
        EAAC1, 52
    noradregenic pathways, 49–51
        depression and, 49–51
        NE receptors, 49–51
    serotonergic pathways
        depression and, 47–49
        serotonins in, 47–49
neurotransmitter theories, 75–76
    dopamine hypothesis in, 76
    monoamine hypothesis, 76
neurotrophic action, 76–77
New England Journal of Medicine, 174
Newsweek, 191
NGF genes. *See* nerve growth factor genes

NICE. *See* National Institute for Clinical
    Excellence
NIMH. *See* National Institute of Mental Health
NINDS. *See* National Institute of Neurological
    Disorders and Stroke
NMS. *See* neuroleptic malignant syndrome
N-Myc downstream-regulated protein 2
    (Ndrg2) gene, 64
nonelectrical convulsive (non-ECT) therapies,
    17–37. *See also* chemical convulsants;
    insulin therapy, after coma inducement;
    pentamethylenetetrazol, in non-ECT
    therapy
  for bipolar disorders, 36–37
  chemical convulsants, 18–24
    ECT as replacement for, 23–24
    with insulin therapy, 28–30
    PM-1090, 24
    PTZ as, 19–24
  flurothyl inhalation, 30–31
    application procedures for, 30
    complications from, 30–31
    historical background for, 30
    indications for, 30
    seizure onset with, 30
  historical background of, 17–18
    Meduna role in, 18
    in mental institutions, 17
    psychiatrists as eugenicists and, 17
  insulin therapy, after coma inducement, 18,
    24–28
    ambulatory, 25
    application procedure for, 25
    with chemical convulsants, 28–30
    complications of, 28
    convulsive factor in, 33–34
    "dry shock" from, 33
    epileptiform phenomena in, 33
    glucagon in, 25
    historical background of, 24–25
    indications for, 25–27
    "moist shock" from, 33
    outcomes from, 21
    remission rates with, 26
    for schizophrenia, 26
    as symptomatic, 27
  PTZ, 19–24
    application procedure for, 19–20
    complications from, 22–23
    for depression, 21–22
    ECT replacement for, 23–24
    indications for, 20–22
    outcomes from, 21
    outcome treatments from, 21
    patient fear of, 31–33

    psychological impact from, 32–33
    relapse rates for, 21
    remission rates from, 20–21
    for schizophrenia, 20–21
  theoretical implications of, 31–37
    patient fear as, 31–33
    psychological impacts in, 32–33
nonpsychiatric physicians. *See* physicians,
    nonpsychiatric
noradregenic pathways, 49–51
  depression and, 49–51
  NE receptors, 49–51
norepinephrine (NE) receptors, 49–51
  ECS and, 50–51
  ECT effects on, 50–51
  NET and, 49
norepinephrine transporter (NET), 49
Northwick Park trial, 113, 118, 449
Norway. *See* Scandinavia, ECT as treatment in
NPY neuropeptide, 52–53
  angiogenic patterns of, 53
  after chronic ECS, 53
  depression and, 53
nursing guidelines, for ECT treatment, 300–306
  inpatient transportation, 301–302
  in physical suite, 322–323
  for post-ECT duties, 305–306
  pre-ECT patient preparation, 301
  for recovery procedures, 304–305
  in recovery room, 324–325
  staff assistance during treatment, 303–304
  treatment room preparation, 302

obsessive-compulsive disorder (OCD), 343
  DBS for, 562
    studies for, 564
  neurobiology of, 560
  tardive, 368
  TMS for, 532–533
OCD. *See* obsessive-compulsive disorder
One Flew over the Cuckoo's Nest, xviii, 172, 188,
    191, 192, 210, 321
On the Sea of Memory (Cott), 190–191
oral medications, in pre-ECT protocol, xxvi
orbitofrontal syndrome, 366
  from ECT, 367
organic catatonia, ECT for, 139–141
Ottosson, Jan-Otto, 172, 238
Out of Tune (Helfgott), 193
oxytocin, 158–159

pacemakers, 405
Pacheco e Silva, Antonio Carlos, 282
PADs. *See* psychiatric advance directives
PAHO. *See* Pan American Health Organization

Pakistan, ECT use in, 258
Pan American Health Organization (PAHO), 277
panic disorder, 533
PANSS. *See* Positive and Negative Syndrome Scale
Parens Patriae (father of his country) doctrine, 385
Parkinson's disease (PD)
 DBS for, 557
 ECT with, 407–408
 l-dopa and, 424
 tDCS for, 579
Pascal, Constance, 167
PD. *See* Parkinson's disease
peak heart rate, ECT and, 479–481
 Benchmark Method for, 479, 481
 hyperventilation from, 480
pentylenetetrazol (PTZ), in non-ECT therapy, 19–24, 168
 application procedure for, 19–20
 patient distress in, 19–20
 seizure generation from, 19
 complications from, 22–23
 fatalities from, 22
 neuropathologic, 22–23
 seizure severity as, 23
 for depression, 21–22
 ECT replacement for, 23–24
 indications for, 20–22
 illness duration and, 20
 outcomes from, 21
 patient fear of, 31–33
 psychological impact from, 32–33
 relapse rates for, 21
 remission rates from, 20–21
 for schizophrenia, 20–21
 insulin therapy v., 26
PET. *See* positron emission tomography
phenytoin, 35
physical suite layout, for ECT, 314–321
 anesthetists in, 323–324
 design considerations for, 321
 for high-volume operations, 316
 IV access considerations in, 317–319
 nurses in, 322–323
 outpatient considerations for, 319
 pretreatment personnel in, 322
 psychiatrists in, 323
 for recovery rooms, 320–321
 nurses in, 324–325
 in small hospitals, 315–316
 for small-volume operations, 315–316
 surgical operating rooms and, 314
 for treatment rooms, 319–320

physical therapies, 167. *See also* electroconvulsive therapy
 chemical convulsive, 167
 insulin, for schizophrenia, 26, 167
 malarial-fever therapy, 167
physicians, nonpsychiatric, ECT training for, 199
placebo trials
 ECT v., for mood disorders, 109–114, 111–112
 anesthesia induction and, 113–114
 HRSD scores in, 110–113
 Northwick Park trial, 113, 118, 449
 Leicestershire Trial, 118, 449
Plath, Sylvia, 184–185, 188, 211, 413
Ploticher, A.I., 268
PM-1090. *See* tetramethyl-succinamide
pneumonia. *See* aspiration pneumonia
POA. *See* power of attorney
Portugal, ECT use in, 250–251
Positive and Negative Syndrome Scale (PANSS), 530
positron emission tomography (PET), 94
 during ictal period, with ECT, 97–98
 during interictal period, with ECT, 102
 VNS under, 544
posterior pituitary hormones, after ECT, 158–159
 oxytocin, 158–159
 vasopressin, 158–159
postictal confusion/disorientation, 486–487
postictal excitement, 150–151
 prevention methods for, 150–151
postictal periods, 95
 EEG during, 470–471
 neuroimaging during, with ECT, 99–101
post-traumatic stress disorder (PTSD), xviii, 345
 TMS for, 532
power of attorney (POA), 397
prefrontal model. *See* anatomical theory
pregnancy
 ECT during, 409
 hormones production during, 151
 VNS during, 550
private hospitals, ECT use in, 230. *See also* psychiatric hospital programs, ECT in
prolactin release, from ECT, 152, 153–158
 AUC and, 156
 basic model for, 156–157
 brain neurochemistry changes and, 154
 as pituitary hormone archetype, 154–155
 seizure-induced, 158
prolonged seizures, 474
propofol, 417
psychiatric advance directives (PADs), 397

psychiatric hospital programs, ECT in, 201. *See also* nursing guidelines, for ECT treatment
  under EMTALA, 287
  under FDA, 287
  malpractice concerns with, 204
  at Mayo Clinic, 317
  model policy guidelines for, 287–294, 313
    for convulsive treatment, for involuntary patients, 293–294
    for convulsive treatment, for voluntary patients, 292–293
    departmental performance improvements under, 311–312
    development for, 287–288
    for excessive use of convulsive treatment, 296
    general, 298–299
    for informed consent, 289–292
    for inpatients from other facilities, 306–308
    for minors, 294–295
    monthly reports under, 296–297
    nursing responsibilities in, 300–306
    for outpatients, 299–300
    posttreatment audit committees in, 295–296
    quality assurance monitors under, 312–313
    for regional centers, 308–311
    scope of service under, 311
    violation penalties under, 298
  for patients from other facilities, 306–308
    for medical emergencies, 308
    posttreatment/recovery for, 307–308
    pretreatment for, 306–307
    treatment for, 307
  public v. private, 230
  in small hospitals, 315–316
  in UIHC, 317
psychiatrists, 323
  anesthetists and, 324, 424–425
  CME for, 205
  ECT and, response toward, 197–205
    legislative regulations against, 202–204
    malpractice concerns, 204
    as molded by negative film portrayals, 198
    as professional mindset, 204–205
    sociopolitical barriers to, 201–202
    training issues with, 199–200
    in treatment patterns, 198, 200–201
    in U.S., 198–199
  as eugenicists, 17
  portrayals of, in films, 210
  residency training for, 199–200
    under ACGME, 199–200
    organizational recommendations for, 200

psychiatry
  Church of Scientology and, 212
  Dianetics as alternative to, 213
  in Russian Federation, under Stalin, 267
  Psychobiology of Convulsive Therapy, 68
psychopharmacology, 172
  antipsychotic drugs, xvii
    for acute schizophrenia, 127–128
    for chronic schizophrenia, with ECT, 136–138
    for malignant catatonia, 133
psychosis, ECT for, 350
  medication-resistant, 354–357
    chronic, 356–357
    intermediate-duration, 355–356
    schizoaffective illness and, 355
    schizophrenia diagnosis v., 356–357
  tardive, 367–369
psychotic disorders. *See* catatonia; schizophrenia
psychotic melancholia, 353
PTSD. *See* post-traumatic stress disorder
PTZ. *See* pentamethylenetetrazol, in non-ECT therapy
public hospitals, ECT use in, 230. *See also* psychiatric hospital programs, ECT in

race, ECT use and, 232
Ramirez Moreno, Samuel, 281
reboot theory, of ECT, xxiii–xxv
  anticonvulsant activity in, xxv
  preexisting psychiatric illness in, xxiii
  seizures' role in, xxiii
    grand mal, xxiii–xxiv
    neurotransmitter depletion/replenishment, xxiv–xxv
receptors, effects of ECT on, 46–52
  depression and, 46
  dopamine, 51
  NE, 50–51
  serotonins, 47–49
    5-HT, 47–49
Reed, Lou, 187
regional medical centers, ECT guidelines for, 308–311
  reporting requirements for, 311
resting hypercortisolism, 159
  cognitive side effects of, 160
  depression and, 160
    HRSD scores and, 160
retrograde amnesia, 491–492
right unilateral electrode placement, 439–441
  bitemporal v., 440
  clinical application of, 439
  dosing levels for, 440–441
  rationale for, 439

rocuronium, 421
Rosenberg, Leon, 208
Rotshtein, G.A., 266
Rozhnov, V.A., 433
Rubio y Yarza, Mauricio, 281
Russian Federation, ECT use in, 266–273
  anti-ECT movement in, 268
  chemical convulsants and, in early use of,
    266
  contemporary applications of, 271–272
  device development in, 271
  early history of, 266–270
  "Meduna's method" and, 266
  Moscow Society of Neurologists and
    Psychiatrists in, 270
  for nonpsychiatric conditions, 272
  political influence on, 267–268
  psychiatry in, under Stalin, 267
  Soviet Scientific Society of Neurologists and
    Psychiatrists in, 268

Sackeim, Harold, 173, 174
Sakel, Manfred, 18, 167–168
SAPS. See Simplified Acute Physiology
    Scores
Scandinavia, ECT as treatment in,
    236–238
  anti-ECT movement in, 237
  future applications for, 243
  history of, 236
  rates of use for, 236–237
  research tradition and, 238
  training for, 242
schizoaffective disorders, ECT for, 135–136
  psychosis and, 355
schizophrenia. See also catatonia
  acute, ECT for, 127–131
    antipsychotic drugs v., 127–128
    remission rates for, 127
    trial studies for, 128–130, 131
  catatonia and, 124
    acute, 131–133
    organic, 139–141
  cECT for, 511
  chronic, ECT for, 136–138
    antipsychotic drugs and, 136–138
    definition of, 136
    effect of catatonic features after, 138
  diagnosis rates for, in Europe, 22
  ECT for, 124–131, 142
    for acute schizophrenia, 127–131
    in Asia, 259–260
    for chronic schizophrenia, 136–138
    continuation, 138–139
    history of, 124–125

mECT and, 135, 138–139
  methodological limitations of, 125–126
  for schizoaffective disorders, 135–136
  for schizophreniform disorder, 126–127
epilepsy and, 34–35
eugenics as answer to, 17
homeostatic theory of, 35
insulin therapy for, 26
  PZT v., 26
medication-resistant chronic psychosis v.,
    356–357
medication-resistant intermediate-duration
    psychosis v., 355–356
pharmacological treatments for, 126
PTZ for, in non-ECT therapy, 20–21
TMS for, 36, 530–531
  with auditory hallucinations, 530
  Auditory Hallucinations Rating Scale for,
    530
  with catatonia, 531
  with negative symptoms, 531
  PANSS for, 530
  SAPS for, 530
schizophreniform disorder, 126–127
  ECT for, 126–127
Scotland. See United Kingdom, ECT as
    treatment in
seizure generalization theory, 79, 89
  objections to, 79
seizures. See also ictal periods; interictal periods
  abortive, 474
  in anticonvulsant theory, thresholds for, 78
  Benchmark Method and, morphology of,
    457–458
  in children/adolescents, thresholds for, 501
    tardive, 502
  curare and, 23
  ECT and, repeated application complications
    for, 35–36
  electricity and, in generation of, 6–8, 82
    depolarization and, 7
    kindling and, 7–8
  epileptic v. electrically induced, 84
  epileptiform phenomena, 33
  from flurothyl inhalation therapy, 30
  forced normalization between, 35
  generalization theory for, 79
    objections to, 79
  grand mal, xxiii–xxiv
    from CNS depletion, xxiii
  HR and, 477–479
    CRH and, 478
    EEG recording of, 479
    epinephrine and, 478
    neuroanatomic rationale for, 477–478

seizures (*cont.*)
  ictal periods for, 95
    EEG during, 469–472
    neuroimaging in ECT during, 96–98
  interictal periods for, 95
    neuroimaging, with ECT, 99–105
  missed, 473–474
  neuronal network function restoration and, 87–89
  postictal periods for, 95
    neuroimaging during, with ECT, 99–101
  prolactin release from, 158
  prolonged, 474
  from PTZ, in non-ECT therapy, 19
    increased severity of, 23
    repeated application complications from, 35–36
  in reboot theory, of ECT, xxiii
    neurotransmitter depletion/replenishment, xxiv–xxv
  spontaneous, 34
    ECT-generated v., 82–84
  from TMS therapy, 535
selective serotonin reuptake inhibitors (SSRIs)
  with antipsychotic drugs, 375–376
  for anxiety disorders, 342
  ECT v., for melancholia, 347–348
  electrode placement and, 433
Sequenced Treatment Alternatives to Relieve Depression (STAR*D) study, 556
Sereysky, M.Y., 272
serotonergic pathways
  depression and, 47–49
  serotonins in, 47–49
serotonins, 47–49
  ECS and, 47–49
  5-HT, 47–49
Shadowland (Arnold), 192
Shakespeare, William, 384
Shepherd, Michael, 238
Shine, 193
"shock-block" method, of ECT, 134
Shock: The Healing Power of Electroconvulsive Therapy (Dukakis), 191, 212
shock therapies, 167. *See also* physical therapies
Shock Treatment is Not Good for Your Mind (Friedberg), 211
Simmons, Everett, 341
Simplified Acute Physiology Scores (SAPS), 530
sine wave stimulus dose, 11
  brief pulse v., 12–13
single photon emission computed tomography (SPECT), 94
  during ictal period, with ECT, 96–97
  during interictal period, with ECT, 103–104

skin burns, from constant current stimulus generators, 4–5
skull bones, electrode placement and, neurobiology of, 437
Small, Iver, 173
The Snake Pit, 172
Spain, ECT use in, 251
SPECT. *See* single photon emission computed tomography
spinal cord injury, ECT with, 410
spontaneous seizures, 34, 82–84
Squire Subjective Memory Questionnaire (SSMQ), 491
SSMQ. *See* Squire Subjective Memory Questionnaire
SSRIs. *See* selective serotonin reuptake inhibitors
STAR*D study. *See* Sequenced Treatment Alternatives to Relieve Depression study
State of California Welfare and Institutions Code, for informed consent, 386
state regulations. *See* U.S. state regulations, against ECT use
stimulus dose method, xxviii
  brief pulse, 9–11
    approximation of separation in, 9
    electrode placement with, 10–11
stimulus dosing, with ECT, 447–463
  augmentation strategies for, 458–459
  Benchmark Method for, 456–458
    cardiovascular reactivity in, 458
    seizure morphology in, 457–458
  case studies of, 461–463
  cognitive side effects of, 454–455
    memory loss as, 454–455
    from sine wave stimulus, 455
  for depression, 450–454, 455–456
    with fixed dosing, 454
    with formula-based dosing, 453–454
    mECT and, 460–461
    with titrated dosing, 450–453
  electrode placement and, 459–460
  with mECT, 460–461, 522
  schedule for, 452
  sham studies for, 449
  units of measure for, 447–449
  waveform morphology for, 449–450
stimulus generators
  constant current, 4, 4–5
    skin burns from, 4–5
  constant voltage, 4
  fixed-charge, 4
stimulus potentiation, caffeine and, xxix
Stone, Alan, 210

succinylcholine, 419–420
    metabolization of, 420
    side effects of, 419–420
suicidality, depression and, 348
surgery, ECT analogous to, xviii
Swartz, Conrad, 171, 175
Sweden. *See* Scandinavia, ECT as treatment in
synaptic plasticity, after ECS, 64–66, 67
    neurotrophic factors for, 64–67
    structural changes, 65
Szasz, Thomas, 172

tachykinin neuropeptides, 54
    after chronic ECS, 54
tachykinins neuropeptide, 54
Taiwan, ECT use in, 256–257
tardive dyskinesia, 370
tardive OCD, 368
tardive psychosis, 367–369
    ECT for, 369
tardive seizures, 502
Taylor, Michael, 175
TCD. *See* transcranial Doppler
tDCS. *See* transcranial direct current stimulation
TDMHMR. *See* Texas Department of Mental
        Health and Mental Retardation
The Tender Place (Hughes), 184
tetramethyl-succinamide (PM-1090), 24
Texas Department of Mental Health and Mental
        Retardation (TDMHMR), 217
Texas National Association of Women, 218
Texas Society of Psychiatric Physicians, 216
Thailand, ECT use in, 257
theophylline, 424
"therapeutic privilege," 209
Thesleff, Stephan, 413
Thesleff, Stephen, 170
thiopental, 416–417
Thoreau, Henry David, 393
thyrotropin-releasing hormone (TRH), 63
Tierney, Gene, 183–184
TIMP-1. *See* tissue inhibitors of
        metalloproteinases-1
tinnitus, 533–534
tissue inhibitors of metalloproteinases-1
        (TIMP-1), 63
titrated stimulus dosing, 450–453
TMS. *See* transcranial magnetic stimulation
training, for ECT, 199–200
    in Asia, 262–263
    in France, 248
    in Latin America, 280
    for nonpsychiatric physicians, 199
    during psychiatric residency, 199–200
    for psychiatrists, 199–200

in Scandinavia, 242
in UK, 242–243
transcranial direct current stimulation (tDCS),
        573–581
    advantages of, 575
    adverse effects of, 575–576
    for anxiety disorders, 580
    clinical applications for, 576–580
    clinical technique for, 573–575
    for craving disorders, 578–579
    for depression, 576–577
    electrode placement options in, 575
    for epilepsy, 577–578
    for fibromyalgia, 577
    future applications of, 581
    history of, 573
    intermittent v. constant-current, 581
    for PD, 579
    safety of, 576
    for working memory, 579–580
transcranial Doppler (TCD), 96
    during interictal period, with ECT, 102
transcranial magnetic stimulation (TMS),
        525–537, 573
    adverse effects of, 535–536
        delusions, 536
        hypomania/mania, 535–536
        seizure induction, 535
    in anatomical theory, 78
    for bipolar mania, 531–532
    contraindications to, 536
    deep, 536–537
    for depression, 528–529
        bipolar, 530
        high-frequency, 529
        low-frequency, 529
    for dysthymic order, 530
    ECT v., 36, 534–535
    neurobiological background for, 527–528
    for OCD, 532–533
    for panic disorder, 533
    for PTSD, 532
    for schizophrenia, 36, 530–531
        with auditory hallucinations, 530
        Auditory Hallucinations Rating Scale for,
            530
        with catatonia, 531
        with negative symptoms, 531
        PANSS for, 530
        SAPS for, 530
    for tinnitus, 533–534
treatment-resistant depression, 172–173
    DBS for, 556
    in DSM-IV-TR, 549
    VNS for, 543, 549

TRH. *See* thyrotropin-releasing hormone
Tye, Larry, 191, 212

UIHC. *See* University of Iowa Hospitals and
        Clinics
UK *See* United Kingdom, ECT as treatment
ultrabrief pulse stimulus dose, 14–15
    electrode placement with, 14–15
United Kingdom (UK), ECT as treatment in,
        238–242
    contemporary standards and practices for,
        ECTAS within, 241
    ECT Handbook in, 239, 241–242
    future applications for, 243
    under NICE, 240–241
    pre-NICE standards and practices, 238–240
    training for, 242–243
United States (U.S.). *See also* legislation, for ECT
        use
    ECT use in, 198–199, 209–210, 227–234
        academic medical centers as factor for, 229
        age as factor for, 231
        APA guidelines for, 228
        demographic variation in, 231–232
        for depression, 228–229
        ethnicity/race as factor in, 232
        future applications for, 233–234
        gender as factor in, 231–232
        inpatient v. outpatient status and, 230–231
        insurance access as factor for, 232–233
        litigation over, 209–210
        overuse of, 209
        in public v. private hospitals, 230
        regional/state variation for, 229
        service sites for, 230–231
        service system variation for, 229–230
        small-area analysis for, 228–229
        socioeconomic factors for, 232–233
        usage trends for, 227
        variation of, 228
    EMTALA in, 287
    legislation, for ECT use in, 207–220
        APA task force role in, 214–215
        for banned use, 208
        in California, 214–216
        constructive lawmaking in, 218–219
        films' influence on, 210–211
        history of, 214–218
        for informed consent, 215
        litigation cases as basis for, 209–210
        in Massachusetts, 215
        proactive, 219
        in Texas, 216–218
    state regulations in, against ECT use, 202–204
        in Texas, 202–203

University of Iowa Hospitals and Clinics
        (UIHC), 317
Uruguay, ECT use in, 282
    APA guidelines for, 282
U.S. state regulations, against ECT use, 202–204,
        233
    antipsychiatry groups' influence on, 203–204
    APA guidelines in, 202
    in Texas, 202–203

vagus nerve, 543
vagus nerve stimulation (VNS) therapy, 543–553
    adverse effects of, 551–552
    antidepressant medications and, as alternative
        to, 549
    application guidelines for, 549–552
        ECT with, 549–550
        parameter settings in, 550–551
        for patient safety, 551
        for patient selection, 549–550
    for depression, 546–548
        clinical outcomes for, 547
        MDD, 547
        trial studies for, 547–548
    for epilepsy, 543, 546
    future applications for, 552
    indications for, 546–549
    mechanisms of action for, 543–544
    neurochemical changes from, 544
    neurophysiological changes from, 543–544
    under PET, 544
    during pregnancy, 550
    under SPECT, 544
    surgical implant procedure for, 544–545
    Therapy Pulse Generator in, 544–546
        device parameters for, 550
        programming for, 545–546
    therapy system for, 544–546
    for treatment-resistant depression, 543, 549
valvular disease, ECT with, 406
VAMP2 gene. *See* vesicle-associated membrane
        protein gene
vascular disease, ECT with, 405–406
vasopressin, 158–159
Vedak, Chandra, 171
VEGF genes, 62
vesicle-associated membrane protein (VAMP2)
        gene, 64
Vesl/homer gene, 60–61
VGF genes, 62
VNS. *See* vagus nerve stimulation therapy
VNS Therapy Pulse Generator, 544–546
    device parameters for, 550
    programming for, 545–546
von Meduna, Ladislas, 246

von Meduna, Lazlo, 282

WAIS. *See* Weschler Adult Intelligence Scale
Wales. *See* United Kingdom, ECT as treatment
    in
Ward, Mary Jane, 172
Weiner, Richard, 173
Weschler Adult Intelligence Scale (WAIS), 488

Wilcox, Paul, 170
Wilder, Gene, 184
Witton, Kurt, 172
working memory, 579–580
World Association of Electroshock Survivors,
    217
World Psychiatric Association, 412
Wyatt v. Hardin, 209–210, 219